CLINICAL REASONING
in the HEALTH PROFESSIONS

Fourth
Edition

CLINICAL REASONING
in the HEALTH PROFESSIONS

EDITED BY

Joy Higgs, AM, PhD, MHPEd, BSc, PFHEA
Professor in Higher Education,
Charles Sturt University, Sydney, Australia

Gail M. Jensen, PhD, PT, FAPTA
Professor of Physical Therapy,
Faculty Associate, Center for Health Policy and Ethics, Dean, Graduate School,
Vice Provost for Learning and Assessment,
Creighton University, Omaha, Nebraska, USA

Stephen Loftus, PhD, MSc, BDS
Associate Professor of Medical Education, Oakland University William Beaumont
School of Medicine, Rochester, Michigan, USA

Nicole Christensen, PhD, MAppSc, BS, BA
Professor and Chair, Department of Physical Therapy, Samuel Merritt University,
Oakland, California, USA

ELSEVIER   Edinburgh London New York Oxford Philadelphia St. Louis Sydney 2019

ELSEVIER

First edition 1995
Second edition 2000
Third edition 2008
Fourth edition 2019

ISBN: 978–0-7020–6224–7

Notices

Content Strategist: Poppy Garraway, Serena Castelnovo
Content Development Specialist: Helen Leng
Project Manager: Manchu Mohan
Design: Patrick Ferguson
Illustration Manager: Teresa McBryan
Illustrator: Muthukumaran Thangaraj

your source for books, journals and multimedia in the health sciences
www.elsevierhealth.com

Working together to grow libraries in developing countries

www.elsevier.com • www.bookaid.org

The publisher's policy is to use **paper manufactured from sustainable forests**

Printed in Great Britain

Last digit is the print number: 9   8   7   6   5   4   3

CONTENTS

Section 1
UNDERSTANDING CLINICAL REASONING

Section 2
THE CHANGING CONTEXT OF CLINICAL REASONING AND PRACTICE

Section 3
COLLABORATIVE AND TRANSDISCIPLINARY REASONING

Section 4
CLINICAL REASONING AND THE PROFESSIONS

Section 5
TEACHING CLINICAL REASONING

Section 6
LEARNING CLINICAL REASONING

PREFACE

In earlier editions of this book we sought out scholars, educators and practitioners who were examining the challenges of clinical reasoning and decision making. Each edition expanded our understanding of what clinical reasoning is across the professions and how these changes in reasoning approaches are shaping both professional practice changes and how practice developments are influencing changes in clinical reasoning. The fourth edition of this book has been written to reflect these current and emerging developments in an age of digital communication and cultural and socioeconomic changes in professional practice and society. These changes include increased commodification and globalization of health services and greater expectations by consumers of their rights to share decision making about their health care. This book sets out to examine all aspects of the complex phenomenon of clinical reasoning across six areas of consideration:

1. Understanding clinical reasoning
2. The changing context of clinical reasoning and practice
3. Collaborative and transdisciplinary reasoning
4. Clinical reasoning and the professions
5. Teaching clinical reasoning
6. Learning clinical reasoning.

Key themes presented in the fourth edition are:

- Clinical reasoning as a composite of encultured capabilities
- Clinical reasoning embedded within situated practice, including the wider socioeconomic and political contexts, the practitioner's and the client's contexts and shared goals such as promoting health communities
- Clinical reasoning and practice models of knowledge-culture and practice problem spaces

- The importance of narratives, language and culture in clinical decision making
- The idea of practitioners particularly (and also clients) as perpetual learners, continually expanding their knowledge base, critically appraising their reasoning abilities and enhancing their reasoning capabilities
- Changing reasoning practices linked to increasing autonomy of practitioners working without the requirement of medical referrals
- Clinical reasoning as an increasingly team-based practice, including shared decision making with clients
- The need for sound strategies and tools to facilitate the expanding collaborations in health care across disciplines and with clients and carers
- Advanced education approaches promoting expansion and enhancement of reasoning strategies
- The importance of building good practices for learning clinical reasoning into curricula and into students' own practice development approaches
- Strengthening links between orthodox and complementary medicine reasoning practices.

CLINICAL REASONING AS THE CORE OF PROFESSIONAL PRACTICE

Professional decision making (often labelled clinical reasoning in clinical contexts) is the core competency of professional practice. In this book we focus on clinical reasoning, while recognizing that many of the practices and educational strategies discussed relate to health care in other settings such as schools. Without the capacity to make sound, client-centred clinical decisions, health practitioners cannot capably perform *professional* practice or best serve the interests of their patients, clients and communities.

In reexamining the nature of clinical reasoning in this edition, authors examined (see Chapter 1) the way professional decision making is changing in relation to changes in the world of clinical practice in this century. Chapter 2 introduces the notion of epistemic cultures and decision making in practice paradigms and presents clinical reasoning as a model of encultured decision-making practice capabilities. Section 1 also examines key aspects of clinical reasoning through the ideas of clinical problem spaces, clinical practice models and links between reasoning and practice expertise.

THE CONTEXT OF CLINICAL REASONING

Section 2 of the book provides the reader with insights into the dynamic contextual environment that is influencing evolving practices of clinical reasoning and decision making. In the fourth edition of *Clinical Reasoning in the Health Professions,* this changing context is envisioned through examination of several environmental factors such as changing demographics, high client expectations, evolving technology, increasing globalization and continued commercialization of healthcare delivery. The context of clinical reasoning is changing for all health professionals.

Health professionals are working, in many countries, with an aging population. With increased life expectancy comes the growth of noncommunicable, chronic diseases. Managing chronic health conditions brings new forms of complexity to clinical care not only from comorbidities but also from the need for the funding of health care and long-term care. Increasing ethnic and racial diversity is occurring across many countries, and with this comes the challenge for practitioners to formulate a treatment plan that fits patients' personal values and cultural customs.

Health care as a sizeable component in many countries' economies is now part of continued commercialization and privatization of healthcare delivery. Health professionals must navigate these economic influences in their clinical reasoning and decision-making process. Organizational and regulatory pressures for evidence of patient-centred care, coupled with the power of social media and patient access to health information, add another layer of complexity to health professionals' clinical reasoning processes. In addition, technology and the explosive growth of *big data* across many organizations bring an additional layer of evidence that health professionals must consider in clinical decision making.

As healthcare practice occurs in an increasingly complex, diverse and uncertain environment, how clinical reasoning is envisioned, enacted and investigated through models of practice is also evolving. Importantly, investigative methods for studying clinical reasoning also must evolve. The interdependence of clinical reasoning and clinical practice needs to remain central to both practice and research. Practitioners must engage in a critical practice model that maintains a critical view of current practices along with continual questioning of their clinical reasoning.

COLLABORATIVE AND TRANSDISCIPLINARY REASONING

Clinical decision making is rarely an isolated or independent process. Healthcare teams have been a traditional part of health care for some time, and the importance of teams is increasing. What we see today are evolutions in the idea and implementation of collaboration in practice, particularly around reasoning and decision making. This is evident in health practice models that emphasize mutual respect and collaboration, recognition of the knowledge of clients and caregivers as experts about the lives and health of clients, participation in collaborative decision making at a distance and using advanced technologies and, increasingly, transdisciplinary reasoning. Bridges are strengthening between orthodox and complementary medicine reasoning practices. The use of tools and protocols to facilitate client participation in decision making is constantly evolving.

REASONING ACROSS THE PROFESSIONS

Section 4 takes an in-depth look at clinical reasoning in different health professions. What is striking are the similarities and the differences that reflect the overlapping but different goals of the professions. For example, emergency medicine specialists, paramedics and surgical teams need to make accurate diagnoses of presenting problems and sudden changes in acute settings as promptly as possible. Accuracy and speed of diagnosis in these situations can sometimes make the difference between life and death. In contrast, other health professions are often more concerned with managing long-term relationships with patients.

Occupational therapists are usually dealing with patients for whom the diagnosis is well known. The issue for them is to work out how best to support patients over time and to co-create health enhancement or support narratives. Many disabled and elderly patients are not going to recover and can be expected to gradually deteriorate as time goes by. This means that the demands of clinical reasoning on health professionals who are managing patients with chronic conditions are quite different from those health professionals who are assessing acute conditions. Many health professions have to deal with both acute and chronic situations. Good examples are dentists and optometrists. They may spend the majority of their time working with long-term patients who will be regular visitors to the practice or clinic for years. However, health professionals must also be prepared to deal with acute emergency cases who might turn up at their practices at any time.

Other trends in clinical reasoning are apparent in the different professions. One such trend is for health professions to become more autonomous. For example, we now have physician assistants and nurse practitioners. Physiotherapists too, in a growing number of countries, are now allowed to practice as independent practitioners without referrals from a physician. The similarities in clinical reasoning across different professions reflect this. At the same time, clinical practice is becoming more interprofessional with expectations that health professionals can adapt their clinical reasoning around the activities of other health professions. This is seen most strikingly in the work of nurses, hospital pharmacists and dietitians who often need to modify their clinical reasoning according to the needs of the team. The increasing complexity of health care and the rising standards of education and training in the health professions are all reflected in the increasing complexity of clinical reasoning and how the different professions understand what this entails.

TEACHING CLINICAL REASONING

Our understanding of clinical reasoning and how we teach it continues to develop and is becoming more complex and sophisticated across all health professions. A critical challenge for educators is how we introduce newcomers to the health professions to this complexity and sophistication. Coping with the challenges of this task is the major topic of Section 5. As with the previous section there are similarities among health professions but also notable differences across the professions. The similarities reflect the commonalities that are shared in the teaching and learning processes as educators need to facilitate learning across classroom and workplace settings. The differences reflect the variations in the goals of the health professions and how they conceptualize their work with patients and clients.

For example, speech pathologists have found classification systems, such as the International Classification of Functioning, Disability and Health (ICF), to be a particularly useful framework to organize clinical reasoning and how to teach it to students. This reflects the focus of speech pathology, which is the diagnosis and remediation of specific disabilities in speech. Nursing focuses on developing students' clinical reasoning abilities through teaching and learning strategies that foster lifelong critical thinking habits. Medicine typically advocates a curriculum for clinical reasoning for undergraduate medical education that is grounded in the science of reasoning practice with knowledge acquisition and clinical skill building, as well as introduction of concepts of clinical uncertainty and diagnostic error.

A health profession may have a specific focus that distinguishes it from other professions, but we are now in a world where those health professions must collaborate as never before. Besides teaching clinical reasoning as *the way 'our' profession does it,* we now must teach our students how to modify their clinical reasoning when working in a team with other health professions and engage in shared decision making. The centrality of the situated and experiential nature of clinical reasoning is shared by all health professions. Our attempts to assess how well we teach clinical reasoning now have a long and complex history, reflecting the changes in how we define and theorize what clinical reasoning is.

LEARNING CLINICAL REASONING

This section of the book is aimed at teachers and learners who are working to facilitate, develop and better understand clinical reasoning. The focus of several chapters is on exploration of pedagogical and assessment strategies, grounded in educational theory, relevant to the teaching and learning of clinical reasoning in educational and practice-based learning contexts. Other chapters provide the reader with an understanding of research considerations and strategies for developing a better understanding of clinical reasoning and how to negotiate the integration of evidence into reasoning that leads to well-grounded clinical decisions.

Key messages of this section include the importance of integrating explicit and theoretically sound strategies that bring to the surface and make visible the aspects of clinical reasoning that exist within multiple educational contexts, knowledge areas and practice activities. This includes an overt focus on the metaskills and capabilities necessary to communicate clinical reasoning and to learn from clinical reasoning experiences. Learners have to substantiate their decisions with appropriate evidence. Those who struggle need remediation. Readers are guided through a process of developing a conceptual framework for research about clinical reasoning and the scholarship of teaching and learning of clinical reasoning.

This section contains significant updates from the previous edition, including new perspectives of ways in which today's educators can improve clinical reasoning learning and assessment outcomes by grounding their teaching and learning activities in sound educational strategies.

As well as a significant update and expansion in content, the book design has added concrete examples, cases and vignettes to bring these discussions to life for the reader. Strategically placed reflection points assist readers to extend their insights and build learning from their own practical experiences and theoretical knowledge.

As well as a key resource for practitioners, this book is a valuable resource for educators seeking to ground their teaching practices in educational theory, sound knowledge of clinical reasoning and practice-based evidence and researchers seeking to expand their research horizons. The book consolidates past knowledge and practices in the field of clinical reasoning, reflects current practices and provides insights and directions for future professional practice, learning, teaching and research of clinical reasoning.

JOY HIGGS, GAIL M. JENSEN, STEPHEN LOFTUS AND
NICOLE CHRISTENSEN

LIST OF CONTRIBUTORS

ROLA AJJAWI, BAppSc(Physio)Hons, PhD
Senior Research Fellow, Centre for Research in
Assessment and Digital Learning, Deakin
University, Geelong, Victoria, Australia

JOSE F. AROCHA, MA, PhD
Associate Professor, School of Public Health and
Health Systems, University of Waterloo, Waterloo,
Ontario, Canada

NICOLE BLAKEY, BN, Grad Dip Critical Care, MN
Senior Lecturer and National Professional Practice
Lead (Nursing), Australian Catholic University,
Brisbane, Queensland, Australia

HENNY P.A. BOSHUIZEN, PhD
Professor Emeritus Welten Institute, Open University
of the Netherlands and Visiting Professor, Faculty
of Education, Turku University, Finland

JUDITH L. BOWEN, MD
Professor and Director, Education Scholars Program,
Department of Medicine, Oregon Health and
Science University, Portland, Oregon, USA

ROSEMARY BRANDER, PhD, MSc
Assistant Professor (Adjunct), School of
Rehabilitation Therapy and Department of
Biomedical and Molecular Sciences, Queen's
University, Kingston, Ontario, Canada

CHRISTINE CHAPPARO, MA, PhD
Senior Lecturer, Discipline of Occupational Therapy,
Faculty of Health Sciences, University of Sydney,
New South Wales; Associate Professor, Southern
Cross University, Gold Coast, Queensland,
Australia

NICOLE CHRISTENSEN, PhD, MAppSc, PT
Professor and Chair, Department of Physical Therapy,
Samuel Merritt University, Oakland, California,
USA

DENISE M. CONNOR, MD
Associate Professor, Department of Medicine,
University of California, San Francisco, California,
USA

CINDY COSTANZO, PhD, RN, CNL
Senior Associate Dean, Graduate School, Department
Chair for Interdisciplinary Studies, Creighton
University, Omaha, Nebraska, USA

JENNIFER L. COX, BSc, BMedSc(Hons), PhD
Lecturer, Biomedical Science, Charles Sturt University,
Orange, New South Wales, Australia

PAT CROSKERRY, MD, PhD
Professor, Department of Emergency Medicine;
Director, Critical Thinking Program, Dalhousie
University Medical School, Halifax, Nova Scotia,
Canada

RACHEL DAVENPORT, BSc(Hons)
Clinical Education Coordinator, Speech Pathology, La
Trobe University, Melbourne, Victoria, Australia

LINDA DE COSSART, CBE, ChM, FRCS,
FAcadMed
Consultant Vascular and General Surgeon and
Director of Medical Education, Countess of
Chester Hospital; Honorary Professor, University
of Chester, Chester, UK

CLARE DELANY, PhD MHlth & Med Law, M Physio(Manip), BAppScPhysio
Associate Professor, Department of Medical Education, University of Melbourne; Clinical Ethicist, Children's Bioethics Centre, Royal Children's Hospital, Melbourne, Victoria, Australia

GURPREET DHALIWAL, MD
Professor of Medicine, University of California at San Francisco; Site Director, Internal Medicine Clerkships, San Francisco VA Medical Center, San Francisco, California, USA

JANINE MARGARITA DIZON, BSPT, MSPT, PhD
Research Fellow, International Centre for Allied Health Evidence (iCAHE), University of South Australia, Adelaide, Australia

JOY DOLL, OTD, OTR/L
Associate Professor, School of Pharmacy and Health Professions, Creighton University, Omaha, Nebraska, USA

STEVEN J. DURNING, MD, PhD, FACP
Professor and Director, Department of Medicine, Uniformed Services University, Bethesda, Maryland, USA

IAN EDWARDS, PhD, Grad Dip PT
Senior Lecturer, School of Health Sciences, University of South Australia, Adelaide, Australia

CAROLINE FAUCHER, OD, PhD, FAAO
Associate Professor, School of Optometry, Université de Montréal, Quebec, Canada

DELLA FISH, MA, MEd, PhD, PGCert
Visiting Professor, University of Chester, Education for Postgraduate Medical Practice, Chester, UK

MAUREEN HAYES FLEMING, EdD, OTR, FAOTA
Associate Professor, Department of Occupational Therapy, Tufts University-Boston School of Occupational Therapy, Medford, Massachusetts, USA

SANDRA GRACE, PhD, MSc(Res), GradCertSportsChiro, DBM, DipAcup, DC, DO, DipEd, BA
Director of Research, School of Health and Human Sciences, Southern Cross University, Lismore, New South Wales, Australia

SUSAN GRIEVE, DPT, MPT, MS, BS
Assistant Professor, Doctor of Physical Therapy, Samuel Merritt University, Oakland, California, USA

KAREN GRIMMER, PhD, MMedSc, LMusA, BPhty, Cert Health Ec
Professor Extraordinaire, Stellenbosch University, Cape Town, South Africa

JEANNETTE GUERRASIO, MD
Professor of Medicine and Director of Remediation, University of Colorado, Aurora, Colorado, USA

TERESA GWIN, EdD, FNP
MSN Family Nurse Practitioner, Samuel Merritt University, Oakland, California, USA

AMY M. HADDAD, PhD, RN
Professor, Center for Health Policy and Ethics and the Dr. C.C. and Mabel L. Criss Endowed Chair in the Health Sciences, Creighton University, Omaha, Nebraska, USA

JOY HIGGS, AM, PhD, MHPEd, BSc, PFHEA
Professor in Higher Education, Charles Sturt University, Sydney, Australia

DEBBIE HORSFALL, PhD, MA, BEd
Professor of Sociology, Western Sydney University, Sydney, New South Wales, Australia

KATHRYN N. HUGGETT, PhD
Robert Larner, MD Professor in Medical Education; Director, The Teaching Academy; Assistant Dean for Medical Education, The Robert Larner, MD College of Medicine at the University of Vermont, Burlington, Vermont, USA

GAIL M. JENSEN, PhD, PT, FAPTA
Dean, Graduate School and Vice Provost for Learning and Assessment; Professor, Department of Physical Therapy; Faculty Associate, Center for Health Policy and Ethics, Creighton University, Omaha, Nebraska, USA

ROBYN B. JOHNSON, BAppSc(Speech Pathology)
Associate Lecturer, Work Integrated Learning, Faculty of Health Sciences, University of Sydney, New South Wales, Australia

MARK JONES, CertPT, BS(Psych), Grad Dip Advan Manip Ther, MAppSc(Manip Physio)
Senior Lecturer, Program Director, Master of Advanced Clinical Physiotherapy, School of Health Sciences, University of South Australia, Adelaide, Australia

DAVID R. KAUFMAN, PhD Educational Psychology, MA Educational Psychology, BA Psychology
Associate Professor, Department of Biomedical Informatics, Arizona State University; Research Affiliate, Mayo Clinic, Scottsdale, Arizona, USA

BELINDA KENNY, PhD
Lecturer, Work Integrated Learning, University of Sydney, New South Wales, Australia

SHIVA KHATAMI, DDS, PhD, Diploma of the American Board of Orthodontics
Associate Professor, Department of Orthodontics and Dentofacial Orthopedics, Nova Southeastern University, Fort Lauderdale, Florida, USA

OLGA KOSTOPOULOU, PhD
Reader in Medical Decision Making, Department of Surgery & Cancer, Imperial College London, UK

JUAN N. LESSING, MD, FACP
Assistant Professor, University of Colorado School of Medicine; Site Director, Hospitalized Adult Care Clerkship and Subinternship, University of Colorado Hospital, Denver, Colorado, USA

TRACY LEVETT-JONES, RN, PhD, MEd & Work, BN, DipAppSc(Nursing)
Professor of Nursing Education, Discipline Lead – Nursing, University of Technology, Sydney, New South Wales, Australia

ROBIN MOORMAN LI, PharmD, BCACP, CPE
Clinical Associate Professor, University of Florida College of Pharmacy, Gainesville, Florida, USA

STEPHEN LOFTUS, PhD, MSc, BDS
Associate Professor of Medical Education, Oakland University William Beaumont School of Medicine, Rochester, Michigan, USA

BILL LORD, BHlthSc(Pre-HospCare), MEd, PhD
Associate Professor and Discipline Leader, Paramedicine, University of the Sunshine Coast, Sippy Downs, Queensland, Australia

KIRSTEN MCCAFFERY, BSc(Hons), PhD
Professorial Research Fellow, School of Public Health, Sydney Medical School; NHMRC Career Development Fellow, Deputy Director, Public Health Section, Centre for Medical Psychology and Evidence-based Decision-making (CeMPED), University of Sydney, New South Wales, Australia

MICHAEL MACENTEE, LDS(I), Dip Pros (MUSC), PhD, FCAHS
Professor Emeritus, Prosthodontics and Dental Geriatrics, University of British Columbia, Vancouver, Canada

ANNA MAIO, MD
General Internal Medicine, Department of Medicine, Creighton University, Omaha, Nebraska, USA

MARIA A. MARTIMIANAKIS, MA, MEd, PhD
Associate Professor and Director of Medical Education Scholarship, Department of Paediatrics; Scientist and Strategic Lead International, Wilson Centre, Faculty of Medicine, University of Toronto, Ontario, Canada

CHERYL MATTINGLY, PhD
Professor, Joint Appointment with the Department of
Anthropology, University of Southern California,
Dornsife College of Letters, Arts and Sciences, Los
Angeles, California, USA

W. CARY MOBLEY, BSPharmacy, PhD
Clinical Associate Professor, University of Florida
College of Pharmacy, Gainesville, Florida, USA

MARIA MYLOPOULOS, PhD
Associate Professor, Department of Paediatrics;
Scientist, The Wilson Centre, University of Toronto,
Ontario, Canada

GEOFFREY R. NORMAN, PhD
Professor Emeritus, Department of Clinical
Epidemiology and Biostatistics, McMaster
University, Hamilton, Ontario, Canada

VIMLA L. PATEL, PhD
Senior Research Scientist and Director, Centre for
Cognitive Studies in Medicine and Public Health,
The New York Academy of Medicine, New York;
Professor of Biomedical Informatics, Arizona State
University, Phoenix, Arizona, USA

NARELLE PATTON, PhD
Sub Dean Workplace Learning and Accreditation
(Faculty of Science), Charles Sturt University,
Sydney, New South Wales, Australia

JACQUELINE PICH, PhD, BNurs, BSc
Lecturer, University of Technology, Sydney, New
South Wales, Australia

JUDY RANKA, BSc(OT), MA, HlthScD
Director and Principal Occupational Therapist,
Occupational Performance Network; Honorary
Academic Affiliate, Discipline of Occupational
Therapy, University of Sydney, New South
Wales; Adjunct Research Associate, Charles Sturt
University, Albury, New South Wales, Australia

LINDA J. RESNIK, PhD, PT
Research Career Scientist, Providence VA Medical
Center; Professor, Health Services Policy and
Practice, School of Public Health, Brown
University, Providence, Rhode Island, USA

BARBARA J. RITTER, EdD, FNP
Lecturer, Sonoma State University, Rohnert Park,
California, USA

HENK G. SCHMIDT, PhD
Professor of Psychology, Institute of Psychology,
Erasmus University, Rotterdam, The Netherlands

LAMBERT W.T. SCHUWIRTH, MD, PhD
Professor of Medical Education, Director Prideaux
Centre for Research in Health Professions
Education, College of Medicine and Public
Health, Flinders University, Adelaide, Australia;
Professor for Innovative Assessment, Department
of Educational Development and Research,
Maastricht University, Maastricht, The
Netherlands; Distinguished Professor of
Medical Education, Chang Gung University,
Kwei-Shan, Taoyuan, Taiwan; Professor of
Medicine (Adjunct), Uniformed Services University
for the Health Sciences, Bethesda, Maryland,
USA

ALAN SCHWARTZ, PhD
The Michael Reese Endowed Professor of Medical
Education and Associate Head, Department
of Medical Education; Research Professor,
Department of Pediatrics, University of Illinois at
Chicago, Chicago, Illinois, USA

**MAREE DONNA SIMPSON, BPharm, BSc
(Hons), PhD, GradCert Univ Teach & Learn**
Discipline Leader Pharmacy and Health Studies,
Charles Sturt University, Orange, New South Wales,
Australia

PAUL SIMPSON, PhD, MScM, GradCert Paediatric Emergencies, GradCert Clinical Education, BHSc, BEd(PD/H/PE), AdvDip Paramedical Science
Senior Lecturer and Director of Academic Program (Paramedicine), Western Sydney University, New South Wales, Australia

MEGAN SMITH, PhD, MAppSc(Cardiopulm physio), BAppSc(Physio)
Professor and Deputy Dean, Faculty of Science, Director, Three Rivers University Department of Rural Health, Charles Sturt University, Sydney, New South Wales, Australia

CATHERINE SUTTLE, PhD
Senior Lecturer in Optometry and Visual Science, City, University of London, UK

DIANE TASKER, PhD
Partner, The Education, Practice and Employability Network, Sydney, Australia

JILL E. THISTLETHWAITE, MBBS, PhD, MMEd, FRCGP, FRACGP
Health Professions Education Consultant, Medical Adviser NPS MedicineWise, Sydney; Adjunct Professor, University of Technology, Sydney; Honorary Professor University of Queensland, Brisbane, Australia

ALIKI THOMAS, BSc, OT, MEd, PhD
Assistant Professor, School of Physical and Occupational Therapy; Research Scientist, Center for Medical Education, McGill University Centre for Interdisciplinary Research in Rehabilitation of Greater Montreal, Quebec, Canada

FRANZISKA TREDE, PhD, MHPEd, Dip Physiotherapy
Associate Professor, Institute for Interactive Media and Learning, University of Technology, Sydney, New South Wales, Australia

LYNDAL TREVENA, PhD
Professor, Primary Health Care, Sydney School of Public Health, University of Sydney, New South Wales, Australia

MERRILL TURPIN, BOccThy, Grad Dip Counsel, PhD
Senior Lecturer, School of Health and Rehabilitation, University of Queensland, Brisbane, Australia

CEES P.M. VAN DER VLEUTEN, PhD
Scientific Director, School of Health Professions Education, Maastricht University, Maastricht, The Netherlands

CELESTE VILLANUEVA, EdD, CRNA, FNAP
Assistant Academic Vice President, Director, Health Sciences Simulation Center, Samuel Merritt University, Oakland, California, USA

RUTH VO, BNutrDiet(Hons), MHSc(Edu)
Accredited Practising Dietitian (APD); PhD Candidate, Charles Sturt University, Sydney, New South Wales, Australia

JASON A. WASSERMAN, PhD
Associate Professor of Biomedical Sciences (Primary), Associate Professor of Pediatrics (Secondary), Oakland University William Beaumont School of Medicine, Rochester, Michigan, USA

MICHAEL J. WITTE, MD
Chief Medical Officer, California Primary Care Association, Sacramento, California, USA

NICOLE A. YOSKOWITZ, PhD
Postdoctoral Fellow at Behavioral Associates, New York, New York, USA

MEREDITH YOUNG, PhD
Assistant Professor, Department of Medicine; Research Scientist, Centre for Medical Education; McGill University, Montreal, Quebec, Canada

MOHAMMAD S.Y. ZUBAIRI, MD, MEd, FRCPC
Developmental Paediatrician, Holland Bloorview Kids Rehabilitation Hospital; Clinical Team Investigator, Bloorview Research Institute; Assistant Professor, Department of Paediatrics, University of Toronto, Ontario, Canada

ACKNOWLEDGEMENTS

The editor(s) would like to acknowledge and offer grateful thanks for the input of all previous editions' contributors. Their input provided an important foundation for the ideas that have been extended in this volume.

Our thanks to Ros Allum, Jennifer Pace-Feraud, and Kim Woodland for their valuable assistance in preparation of this manuscript.

Section 1   UNDERSTANDING CLINICAL REASONING

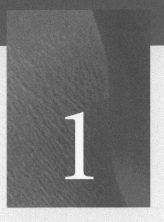

1

CLINICAL REASONING
Challenges of Interpretation and Practice in the 21st Century

JOY HIGGS ■ GAIL M. JENSEN

CHAPTER AIMS

The aim of this chapter is to introduce key themes explored in this book in relation to:

■ current understandings in the term and practice of clinical reasoning,

■ challenges faced by people engaged in decision making and

■ challenges faced by people engaged in learning and teaching clinical reasoning.

KEY WORDS

Clinical reasoning

Clinical decision making

UNDERSTANDING CLINICAL REASONING

Clinical reasoning is the core of clinical practice; it enables practitioners to make informed and responsible clinical decisions and address problems faced by their patients or clients. It involves *wise action,* meaning taking the best judged action in a specific context (Higgs, 2016); *professional action* encompassing ethical, accountable and self-regulatory decisions and conduct; and *person-centred action* that demonstrates respect for and collaboration with clients, carers and colleagues.

It has been over 20 years since the first edition of this book was produced (Higgs and Jones, 1995). While there have been changes to our editors and authors list and considerable changes to the book content, the key idea of clinical reasoning being both a simple and complex phenomenon has remained (Higgs, 2006). Simply, clinical reasoning is the thinking and decision-making processes associated with clinical practice; it is a critical capability in the health professions, central to the practice of professional autonomy that permeates clinical practice. At a complex level, clinical reasoning is a multilayered and multicomponent capability that allows practitioners to make difficult decisions in the conditions of complexity and uncertainty that often occur in health care. Such decisions require a high level of tolerance of ambiguity, reflexive understanding, practice artistry and collaboration.

There is no one model of clinical reasoning that best, or comprehensively, represents what clinical reasoning is in the contexts of different professions and different workplaces. The reason for this lies in several factors:

■ The complex nature of the phenomenon of clinical reasoning and the consequential challenges of understanding, researching, assessing and measuring it.

■ The context-dependent nature of clinical decision making in action.

■ The inherent individuality of expertise.

■ The changing conceptions of quality and error in clinical reasoning.

■ The challenge to novices in developing clinical reasoning skills and to educators in facilitating this development.

■ The changing volume and nature of the demands of factors influencing health care, its costs, its consequences and its modes of operation.

Ratcliffe and Durning (2015, p. 13) provide this overview of clinical reasoning: 'although definitions and descriptions of clinical reasoning entail the cognitive operations allowing clinicians to observe, collect and analyze information, resulting in actions that take into account a patient's specific circumstances and preferences'. They add that 'many scholars now view clinical reasoning as having both cognitive and noncognitive domains as well as being a social as opposed to an individual construct' (p. 14). These considerations are reflected in the following two definitions.

We define clinical reasoning as the cognitive and noncognitive process by which a healthcare professional consciously and unconsciously interacts with the patient and environment to collect and interpret patient data, weigh the benefits and risks of actions, and understand patient preferences to determine a working diagnostic and therapeutic management plan whose purpose is to improve a patient's well-being (Trowbridge et al., 2015, p. xvii).

Clinical reasoning (or practice decision making) is a context-dependent way of thinking and decision making in professional practice to guide practice actions. It involves the construction of narratives to make sense of the multiple factors and interests pertaining to the current reasoning task. It occurs within a set of problem spaces informed by the practitioner's unique frames of reference, workplace context and practice models, as well as by the patient's or client's contexts. It utilizes core dimensions of practice knowledge, reasoning and metacognition and draws on these capacities in others. Decision making within clinical reasoning occurs at micro, macro and meta levels and may be individually or collaboratively conducted. It involves meta skills of critical conversations, knowledge generation, practice model authenticity and reflexivity (Higgs, 2006).

The authors in this book and others across the literature often use clinical reasoning and decision making synonymously. We recognize that this interchange is common, and, alternatively, some professions and writers use the terms distinctly. Here we make the distinction that clinical reasoning is the overall process of thinking during clinical practice, while clinical decision

making could be seen to emphasize the outputs or decisions.

REFLECTION POINT 1

What is your definition of clinical reasoning? What experiences can you describe of clinical reasoning as a cognitive and noncognitive process?

CHALLENGES FACED BY PEOPLE ENGAGED IN CLINICAL DECISION MAKING

In this section, we will explore four key challenges faced by people engaged in clinical decision making:

- Dealing with a complex world
- Dealing with wicked problems in a world that looks for accountability and evidence clarity
- Addressing complex real-world problems, human tasks with consequences for life and quality of life
- Dealing with issues associated with sharing decision-making processes and outcomes

CHALLENGES OF DEALING WITH A COMPLEX WORLD

Bauman's (2000, 2005) 'liquid modernity' metaphor captures the values and desires that characterize the prosperous West today. Casting aside the attitudes that predominated in the second half of the 20th century (such as the vision that puts others first, the sense of mystery of things beyond us and recognition of the fallibility of human knowledge), liquid modernity challenges the ideals of service and moral responsibility of professions in meeting societal needs. Bauman's ideas highlight current trends, such as taking shortcuts to increase perceived efficiencies, outsourcing work and resources provision and being preoccupied with short-term goals and desires instead of long-term pursuits. This is seen in changing consumerist ideas such as replacing long-lasting products with shorter, fixed-term products and changing lifetime employment with casual jobs.

The liquid-modern age pursues instant gratification and constant movement (which goes beyond fluency and flexibility to volatility, fragmentation and short life spans of knowledge, tasks, work groups and so on).

This contrasts with the ongoing commitments of healthcare professionals to patients, to best possible care, to persistence, to resilience, to carefulness and to obligations arising from and through multiprofessional teamwork. Another problem is the changing attitude towards knowledge in the liquid-modern world, where established knowledge and know-how have an increasingly shorter shelf life. Tradition and experience seem to be no longer valued.

A key issue in clinical reasoning is the demand for practitioners to be able to explain professional matters articulately and clearly to all parties and to take proper account of their own values as well as the needs and values of all those involved or influential in patient/client care. Fish and Higgs (2008) contend that responsible members of a profession need to argue their moral position; implement their roles with proper transparency and integrity; and their clinical thinking, utilize professional judgement and practice wisdom to serve the needs of differing individuals as well as understand and work towards the common good.

A second key element of the complexity of the worlds of practice and health care today is the digital revolution, which poses both opportunities and challenges to health care, clinical reasoning and the making and communication of clinical decisions. Sennett (2005), reviewing culture and society for several decades in Britain and America, reflects on the challenges facing us all today because of the unstable, fragmentary conditions in society and work. He contends that not everyone will thrive in the face of 'hot-desking' workplaces and in 'dot.com' modelled hospital and university workplaces. O'Neill (2002) critiques today's systems of accountability that are driven by the human resources industry and are designed to provide transparent checks on the implementation of change. The critique is that constant checking on people's work progress and outcomes in support of transparency actually damages trust and does not allow change to consolidate.

Of particular interest, in relation to clinical reasoning, are the strategies and tools that have been developed with the goal of assisting decision making and communication. Studies in this area include the work of Chaudhry et al. (2006), who demonstrated improved quality and efficiency of health information technologies across four benchmark institutions. Buntin et al. (2011) provide support for the adoption of electronic health records and information technology. They found that such tools and strategies had largely positive benefits, but the 'human element' was critical to health information technology implementation. Chau and Hu (2002) examined different theories and strategies for implementing telemedicine; they reported variation in the acceptability of different telemedicine approaches, linked to differences in the essential characteristics of user, technology and context.

Osheroff et al. (2007, p. 141) examined the value of clinical decision support that provides practitioners, patients and others with 'knowledge and person-specific information, intelligently filtered or presented at appropriate times, to enhance health and health care. It encompasses a variety of tools and interventions such as computerized alerts and reminders, clinical guidelines, order sets, patient data reports and dashboards, documentation templates, diagnostic support, and clinical workflow tools'. They concluded that some healthcare institutions achieved positive benefits for knowledge users while others faced problems. The demand for reliable health information to support decisions is being driven by consumerism and moves to shift the cost of care to patients and increase client input to decision making. Koch (2006) raises the concern of the potential negative effect of home telehealth on the patient–provider relationship, particularly in relation to special user groups, such as people who are elderly or have a disability. She calls for further exploration of the use of such strategies.

REFLECTION POINT 2

How do you think we should go about linking the headspace of personal reasoning with the etherspace of technology-enabled reasoning? What experience have you had in this area? How would you advise novices about this area?

CHALLENGES IN ADDRESSING WICKED PROBLEMS AND ACCOUNTABILITY

Clinical reasoning and decision making are essentially professional problem solving – solving the problem or challenge of making decisions about diagnosis, prognosis, treatment options and preferences and so on as a way of informing healthcare actions by practitioners

TABLE 1.1
Types of Problems

Type 1 problems	are 'simple problems' that enjoy a consensus on a problem definition and solution.
Type 2 problems	are 'complex problems' that introduce conflict to the problem-solving process. While problem solvers agree on what the problem is, there is no consensus on how to solve it.
Type 3 problems	are 'wicked problems' that engender a high level of conflict among the stakeholders. The problem-solving process is not bound – it is experienced as ambiguous, fluid, complex, political and frustrating.

Based on Roberts, N., 2000. Wicked problems and network approaches to resolution. IPMR 1, 1–19.

and clients. Schön (1987) reminds us that the process of problem setting, the ability to identify the problem in the swampy lowland of practice, requires seeing the situation or context from multiple frames of reference. Roberts (2000) identifies three types of problems (Table 1.1) with different levels of complexity and solution/management solution.

Wicked problems (Roberts, 2000) have the following characteristics:

1. There is no definitive statement of the problem; indeed, there is typically broad disagreement on what 'the problem' is.
2. Without a definitive statement of the problem, the search for solutions is open ended. People who have a stake in the problem and its solution, the stakeholders, play various competing and changing roles from their perspectives including framing the problem, supporting and shaping different solutions.
3. The problem-solving process is complex because constraints, such as resources and political ramifications, are constantly changing.
4. Constraints also change because they are generated by numerous interested parties who may bring variable levels of participation to the problem solving and whose input can vary as they change their minds, fail to communicate well and change their frame of reference in addressing the problem.

The very idea of wicked problems runs contrary to the search for 'correct' answers and the unequivocal justification of clinical decisions. Consider diagnostic and treatment decisions, for instance. While in some cases a clear diagnosis is straightforward and necessary, particularly in life-threatening situations, it is often the case that comorbidities exist. The clinical condition might be rare, unfamiliar or hard to diagnose. Treatment decisions are multifactorial, facing variables like skill levels of practitioners, available funding, resourcing and client wishes. For instance, a client/patient may aspire to a health and well-being narrative that runs contrary to the 'restitution narrative' (i.e., return to normality). The latter is particularly the case for people with chronic health problems (Alder and Horsfall, 2008). Further, decision paradigms and cultures vary across different professions. Again, we see clinical reasoning and decision making as complex phenomena.

REFLECTION POINT 3

Where does evidence in support of our decisions fit with these decisions and actions? Consider the arguments put forward in Chapters 4 and 5 (expertise), Section 3 chapters (collaborative and transdisciplinary decision making) and Section 4 chapters (clinical reasoning across the professions).

CHALLENGES OF MAKING COMPLEX AND CONSEQUENTIAL DECISIONS

Orasanu and Connolly (1993) examined the real world of clinical decision making and described the characteristics of decision making in dynamic settings as follows:

- Problems are ill-structured and made ambiguous by the presence of incomplete dynamic information and multiple interacting goals.
- The decision-making environment is uncertain and may change while decisions are being made.
- Goals may be shifting, ill-defined or competing.
- Decision making occurs in the form of action–feedback loops, where actions result in effects and

generate further information that decision makers have to react to, and use, to make further decisions.

- Decisions contain elements of time pressure, personal stress and highly significant outcomes for the participants.
- Multiple players act together, with different roles.
- Organizational goals and norms influence decision making.

To work within such a practice world requires an approach to clinical reasoning that accommodates these complexities. Higgs et al. (2006) described a number of key characteristics of clinical reasoning needed to address these challenges:

- Clinical reasoning as a solo process is a complex, mostly invisible, process that is often largely automatic and therefore not readily accessible to others in practice or research.
- Clinical reasoning is linked with more visible behaviours such as recording diagnoses and treatment plans in patient histories and communicating treatment rationales in team meetings, case conferences and teaching novices.
- Clinical reasoning and practice knowledge are mutually developmental; each relies on the other, each gives meaning to the other in the achievement of practice and each is the source of generation and development of the other.
- Clinical reasoning can be implemented as a sole practitioner process or a group process.
- Clinical reasoning may be understood as both cognitive and collaborative processes; however, in either case there is a growing imperative, linked to increasing demands for evidence-based practice and public accountability, to make reasoning more explicit.
- The idea of evidence means different things in different contexts and paradigms (see Turpin and Higgs, 2017); understanding evidence is important when planning to use or require evidence-based practice.
- Core reasoning abilities, language and interactive behaviours are required for understanding and developing practice knowledge and clinical reasoning.
- It is important to understand clinical reasoning behaviours and effectiveness (including the

communication of reasoning) in relation to contextual influences, including the practice model that has been chosen or imposed.
- Clinical reasoning requires a range of capabilities including cognitive, metacognitive, emotional, reflexive and social capabilities.
- Clinical reasoning is, and for the purposes of quality assurance, should be, a reflexive process that involves practitioner(s) in critical self-reflection and ongoing development of their reasoning abilities, knowledge and communication (of reasoning) abilities.

So, what has the 21st century brought to this practice space that further challenges clinical reasoning practice? Some of the most critical factors, we believe, include:

- The technological and digital revolutions, which have increased the use of high-level technology in health care (for those who can afford it) and high-tech communication and decision-making aids in the practice of clinical decision making and its communication. Examples of these trends include robotics, telehealth, use of big data and self-doctoring.
- The further erosion of professionalism often linked to a decline in altruism and an increase in self-interest and expectations privilege by practitioners.
- An escalation in the demand by patients/clients and carers for respectful and informed participation in clinical decision making. This has been greatly effected by readily accessible information on the Internet.
- Globalization (the global spread of capitalism as an economic system) and neoliberalism (the support of a deregulated global market society) have brought increasing emphasis in health care (and therefore clinical decision making) on commodification of health care, fiscal accountability often in advance of ethical accountability, replacement of service-oriented professionals with business-oriented entrepreneurs, corporatization of professional practices, increasing litigation by consumers and more widespread adoption of systems and practices that shift the economic cost/burden of health care to the individual rather than the state.

Professionals are under increasingly more pressure on a number of fronts from higher demands for standards of professional competence and fiscal demands for increased productivity, to external regulations that require sound evidence, efficiency and accountability. These challenges also affect professional autonomy and control. Sullivan and Benner (2005, p. 79) describe this well: 'the question of how healthcare professionals can function as prudent managers in the public interest, as well as engaged autonomous professionals, takes on salience in this new environment'. Now more than ever, healthcare professionals need not only strong cognitive and analytical skills but integrity, individual self-awareness and the ability to engage in clinical reasoning that leads to wise judgement. Consider how you would respond to the situation presented in the following case study.

CHALLENGES IN SHARING DECISION-MAKING PROCESSES AND OUTCOMES

Interprofessional collaboration is being promoted by healthcare organizations, governments and regulatory groups as an important means to addressing many of the complex and wicked problems in caring for patients, improving health organization performance measures,

managing escalating costs and improving health outcomes (Frenk et al., 2010; Royeen et al., 2009). (Refer to the chapters in Section 3 of this book for further work on collaborative decision making.) Professional education accreditation requirements are moving rapidly in response to this need for interprofessional collaboration and setting standards for institutions to demonstrate that graduates are 'collaboration ready' (Prystajecky et al., 2017).

The successful care of patients and communities depends not only on the knowledge and expertise of the individual practitioner but the collective knowledge and distributed intelligence of the interprofessional team (Cooke et al., 2010; Jensen, 2011). This distributed intelligence of the team often requires a process of shared decision making as patients and the interprofessional team members work together in the decision-making process. The development of the specific health profession's clinical reasoning abilities is a central focus in professional education and often leaves little time for an intentional focus on shared decision making. Therefore it is essential that the development of clinical reasoning from novice to expert has an intentional focus on key concepts. These key concepts include the critical relationship between knowledge restructuring and clinical reasoning and level of expertise, the importance of adaptive expertise and the concept of progressive

---

CASE STUDY 1.1

Misalignment of Professional Autonomy, Accountability and Evidence

Dan, a newly licensed physical therapist, was working at a clinic where the organization had a clinical standard–to achieve at least 52 minutes and 4 billable units with each patient. He was told that this was the expectation for maintaining productivity and that as a skilled clinician he should be able to work with any patient for 52 minutes. If he couldn't, then he should not consider himself a skilled clinician. It did not take long for him to experience moral distress as he was trying to balance his ability to make clinical decisions about patient discharge and accountability for being a good steward of healthcare resources in balance with evidence-based practice guidelines and

now organizational expectations. His patient, Joan, had adhesive capsulitis of her shoulder and had reached all of her goals. Joan was well aware of everything she needed to do after therapy, was experiencing no pain, had achieved functional goals and was ready for discharge. Dan ended up keeping the patient for only 30 minutes and was confronted by the clinic manager for not maintaining productivity for that hour with that patient. Dan was following best practice clinical guidelines and believed that as a practising physical therapist, he had professional responsibility for patient-centred quality care along with being a steward of scarce healthcare resources.

problem solving, outlined in Chapters 5 and 6 on clinical reasoning expertise.

REFLECTION POINT 4

What are teaching and learning strategies that could be used to engage learners in shared decision-making processes?

How would you apply key ideas for the ongoing development of expertise in clinical reasoning and the concept of adaptive expertise in your clinical teaching?

CHALLENGES FACED BY PEOPLE ENGAGED IN LEARNING AND TEACHING CLINICAL REASONING

In this section we will explore three key challenges faced by people engaged in clinical reasoning and decision making:

- intentionally building clinical reasoning teaching and learning into pressured curricula,
- teaching and learning the often more tacit elements in clinical reasoning along with the ambiguous, complex realities and 'wickedness' of clinical reasoning and
- learning about how professionals often have to make judgements in uncertain conditions

BUILDING CLINICAL REASONING INTO CURRICULA

Health sciences curricula tend to follow a number of patterns: discipline-content driven preclinical and clinical courses, problem-based courses and practice-based curricula. These vary in the attention given to clinical problem solving, clinical reasoning and clinical decision making as part of the curricula. A key goal of this book is to emphasize the importance of overtly and experientially teaching clinical reasoning as part of any curriculum. Section 5 of the book provides multiple examples of curriculum, learning and teaching approaches adopted across the professions including:

- application of a clinical thinking pathway for surgeons that uses a formulaic approach along with humane and individualistic approaches,

- creative strategies such as deconstructing critical events and reflecting on cognitive biases as part of teaching clinical reasoning in nursing and
- understanding the centrality of context in the teaching and learning of clinical reasoning in academic and workplace environments as essential.

TEACHING AND LEARNING CLINICAL REASONING COMPLEXITIES

We have argued that clinical reasoning – once you approach it deeply and in many complex circumstances – is a challenging thing to do. Fig. 1.1 illustrates the definition of clinical reasoning by Higgs (2006). We see in this figure different types of decisions, multiple decision spaces (see Higgs and Jones, 2008), the foundational dimensions of clinical reasoning, the players in the clinical decision-making process and meta processes framing the practices of clinical reasoning and decision making. This, or any other interpretation of clinical reasoning as a complex process, highlights the challenges that even experienced practitioners, let alone novices, face when engaging in this critical component of clinical practice.

LEARNING SOMETHING THAT'S NOT SIMPLY BLACK AND WHITE

Section 6 deals with learning clinical reasoning, both from the perspective of providing learning opportunities and activities for learners, ranging from direct clinical experience, to online learning activities and self-directed learning. In each case, learners need to come to an understanding of what their job requires of them in relation to making clinical decisions, what is expected of them and what the consequences of their reasoning are for their clients, colleagues and themselves and also what strategies they can adopt as part of their lifelong learning commitment to continue to develop their reasoning abilities. Students and novice professionals often experience insecurities when they become responsible for people's lives and well-being in clinical situations. It takes time to build up the capacity to reason well in situations that are complex and to become confident in performing this core practice. Chapters 5 and 6 pursue this journey of developing confidence, capability and expertise in clinical reasoning.

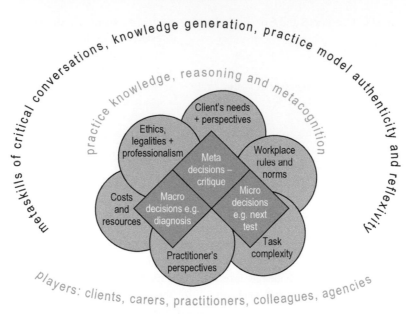

Fig. 1.1 ■ Clinical reasoning: A challenging practice. (From Higgs, J., Trede, F., Loftus, S., et al., 2006. Advancing clinical reasoning: Interpretive research perspectives grounded in professional practice. CPEA, Occasional Paper 4, Collaborations in Practice and Education Advancement. University of Sydney, Australia, with permission.)

REFLECTION POINT 5

As a novice or experienced practitioner reflect on these questions:
- What do I know about clinical reasoning? What does it mean in my practice?
- How well do I reason – not just in terms of avoiding errors and making sound decisions – but also in terms of working across different communities of practice (e.g., within my profession, across work teams, with my clients as active decision-making participants)?
- How can I improve my clinical decision making? What strategies work well for me? Who can I ask for help to further develop my clinical reasoning capability?

CHAPTER SUMMARY

In this chapter we have explored a number of arguments:

- There is no universal model of clinical reasoning that fits all settings, professions and individuals,

but we recognize this as a complex phenomenon that includes cognitive and noncognitive processes.
- Dealing with a complex world presents healthcare professionals with 'wicked problems' that require approaches to clinical reasoning that can accommodate and address these complexities.
- Increasing demands for interprofessional collaboration and client engagement bring the need for greater understanding of shared decision making.
- The challenges in teaching and learning clinical reasoning provide great opportunities for innovation, exploration and assessment of learning.

REFLECTION POINT 6

Fig. 1.1 Clinical reasoning: A challenging practice – provides an overview of many of the key concepts in this chapter that are also further detailed in the book.

What component(s) is most challenging for your learners?

What will you focus on in your teaching clinical reasoning?

REFERENCES

Alder, S., Horsfall, D., 2008. Beyond the restitution narrative: lived bodies and expert patients. In: Higgs, J., Jones, M.A., Loftus, S., et al. (Eds.), Clinical Reasoning in the Health Professions, third ed. Elsevier, Edinburgh, pp. 349–356.

Bauman, Z., 2000. Liquid Modernity. Polity Press, Cambridge.

Bauman, Z., 2005. The liquid modern challenges to education. In: Robinson, S., Katulushi, C. (Eds.), Values in Higher Education, Aureus and the University of Leeds. Leeds, UK, pp. 36–50.

Buntin, M.B., Burke, M.F., Hoaglin, M.C., et al., 2011. The benefits of health information technology: a review of the recent literature shows predominantly positive results. Health Aff. (Millwood) 30, 464–471.

Chau, P.Y.K., Hu, P.J., 2002. Investigating healthcare professionals' decisions to accept telemedicine technology: an empirical test of competing theories. Inf. Manag. 39, 297–311.

Chaudhry, B., Wang, J., Wu, S., et al., 2006. Systematic review: impact of health information technology on quality, efficiency, and costs of medical care. Ann. Intern. Med. 144, 742–752.

Cooke, M., Irby, D., O'Brien, B., 2010. Educating Physicians: A Call for Reform of Medical School and Residency. Jossey-Bass, San Francisco, CA.

Fish, D., Higgs, J., 2008. The context for clinical decision making in the 21st century. In: Higgs, J., Jones, M.A., Loftus, S., et al. (Eds.), Clinical Reasoning in the Health Professions, third ed. Elsevier, Edinburgh, pp. 19–30.

Frenk, J., Bhutta, Z., Cohen, J., et al., 2010. Health professionals for a new century: transforming education to strengthen health systems in an interdependent world. Lancet 376, 1923–1958.

Higgs, J., 2006. The complexity of clinical reasoning: exploring the dimensions of clinical reasoning expertise as a situated, lived phenomenon. Seminar presentation at the Faculty of Health Sciences, University of Sydney, Australia, 5 May.

Higgs, J., 2016. Practice wisdom and wise practice: dancing between the core and the margins of practice discourse and lived practice. In: Higgs, J., Trede, F. (Eds.), Professional Practice Discourse Marginalia. Sense, Rotterdam, The Netherlands, pp. 65–72.

Higgs, J., Jones, M.A. (Eds.), 1995. Clinical Reasoning in the Health Professions. Butterworth-Heinemann, Oxford.

Higgs, J., Jones, M.A., 2008. Clinical decision making and multiple problem spaces. In: Higgs, J., Jones, M.A., Loftus, S., et al. (Eds.), Clinical Reasoning in the Health Professions, third ed. Elsevier, Edinburgh, pp. 3–17.

Higgs, J., Trede, F., Loftus, S., et al., 2006. Advancing clinical reasoning: interpretive research perspectives grounded in professional practice, CPEA, Occasional Paper 4, Collaborations in Practice and Education Advancement, University of Sydney, Australia.

Jensen, G.M., 2011. The Forty-Second Mary McMillan Lecture: Learning: what matters most. Phys. Ther. 91, 1674–1689.

Koch, S., 2006. Home telehealth: current state and future trends. Int. J. Med. Inform. 75, 565–576.

O'Neill, O., 2002. A Question of Trust. Polity Press, Cambridge.

Orasanu, J., Connolly, T., 1993. The reinvention of decision making. In: Klein, G.A., Orasanu, J., Calderwood, R., et al. (Eds.), Decision Making in Action: Models and Methods. Ablex, Norwood, NJ, pp. 3–20.

Osheroff, J.A., Teich, J.M., Middleton, B., et al., 2007. A roadmap for national action on clinical decision support. J. Am. Med. Inform. Assoc. 14, 141–145.

Prystajecky, M., Lee, T., Abonyi, S., et al., 2017. A case study of healthcare providers' goals during interprofessional rounds. J. Interprof. Care 31, 463–469.

Ratcliffe, T.A., Durning, S.J., 2015. Theoretical concepts to consider in providing clinical reasoning instruction. In: Trowbridge, R.L., Rencic, J.J., Durning, S.J. (Eds.), Teaching Clinical Reasoning. American College of Physicians, Philadelphia, PA, pp. 13–30.

Roberts, N., 2000. Wicked problems and network approaches to resolution. IPMR 1, 1–19.

Royeen, C., Jensen, G.M., Harvan, R., 2009. Leadership in Interprofessional Health Education and Practice. Jones & Bartlett Learning, Boston, MA.

Schön, D., 1987. Educating the Reflective Practitioner. Jossey-Bass, San Francisco, CA.

Sennett, R., 2005. The Culture of the New Capitalism. Yale University Press, New Haven, CT.

Sullivan, W., Benner, P., 2005. Challenges to professionalism: work integrity and the call to renew and strengthen the social contract of the professions. Am. J. Crit. Care 14, 78–84.

Trowbridge, R.L., Rencic, J.J., Durning, S.J., 2015. Introduction/Preface. In: Trowbridge, R.L., Rencic, J.J., Durning, S.J. (Eds.), Teaching Clinical Reasoning. American College of Physicians, Philadelphia, PA, pp. xvii–xxii.

Turpin, M., Higgs, J., 2017. Clinical reasoning and evidence-based practice. In: Hoffmann, T., Bennett, S., Del Mar, C. (Eds.), Evidence-Based Practice: Across the Health Professions. Elsevier, Chatswood, pp. 364–383.

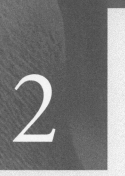

2

RE-INTERPRETING CLINICAL REASONING
A Model of Encultured Decision-Making Practice Capabilities

JOY HIGGS

CHAPTER AIMS

The aims of this chapter are to:

- re-interpret clinical reasoning as a complex practice through the lens of enculturation,
- recognize the place of social, practice and epistemic cultures in framing clinical reasoning and decision making,
- explore the connection between clinical reasoning, learning and knowing in practice,
- recognize the place of epistemic-ontological fluency as an approach to developing and practising clinical reasoning capability in professional practice and
- present a model of clinical reasoning as encultured decision-making practice capabilities.

KEY WORDS

Encultured

Epistemological practice

Fluency

Ontological practice

The complexity of clinical reasoning is inherent in the very nature of the task or challenge, faced by novice and expert alike. This challenge is to process multiple variables, contemplate the various priorities of competing healthcare needs, negotiate the interests of different participants in the decision-making process, inform all decisions and actions with advanced practice knowledge and make decisions and take actions in the accountable context of professional ethics and community expectations. By encompassing much of what it means to be a professional (autonomy, responsibility, accountability and decision making in complex situations), clinical reasoning is imbued with an inherent mystique. This mystique is most evident in the way expert practitioners make difficult decisions with seemingly effortless simplicity and justification and in the professional artistry and practice wisdom of experienced practitioners who produce, with humanity and finesse, individually tailored health management plans that address complicated health needs. To address and achieve these professional attributes, clinical reasoning is much more a lived phenomenon, an experience, a way of being and a chosen model of practising than it is simply a process. It is enacted through a set of capabilities that demonstrate current knowledge and practice expertise and the capacity to work in unknown and unpredictable situations.

RE-INTERPRETING CLINICAL REASONING

Many chapters in this book hint at or openly declare the need for re-interpretation of clinical reasoning for multiple reasons including:

- the escalation of research and scholarship on clinical reasoning, which is exploring the complexities and demands of clinical reasoning in a range of human, professional and institutional healthcare spaces;

■ the far greater current emphasis on shared decision making (among multidisciplinary teams and with clients and carers);

■ the quantum shift in the use of technology and digital communication systems to aid the reasoning, communication and collaboration involved in clinical decision making;

■ the changing local and global contexts of health care and decision making, including influences and challenges posed by and to evidence-based practice, changing expectations and capacities of healthcare consumers and healthcare economic factors (including escalating healthcare costs, the difficulty – even impossibility – of public funding of health care for all citizens and the large proportion of populations who cannot self-fund their health care);

■ the need to see clinical reasoning as knowledge use and development in practice, not the application of prior knowledge to clinical decision making and

■ the need to view clinical reasoning and decision making as collaborative, holistic practices actioned by practitioners and clients, assisted by technology as appropriate.

The re-interpretation presented in this chapter builds on the following key arguments:

■ *Encultured Practice:* Clinical reasoning is a way of thinking and decision making that is developed within the framework of various cultural arenas: the world of healthcare practice and the societal and organizational cultures that shape healthcare practices and systems, the multiple worlds and cultures of healthcare clients and professional practice cultures.

■ *Understanding Professional Practice Paradigms:* Clinical reasoning and decision making operate within communities of practice. To operate within these practice communities and their cultures requires a deep understanding of the practice paradigms underpinning them.

■ *Knowing, Being and Identity in Practice:* Deliberate choices and ownership by practitioners of their practice models and their approaches to reasoning

and collaboration are essential for advanced practice. Informed and owned practice comprises doing, knowing, being and becoming and chosen stances on practice epistemology and practice ontology.

■ *Practice-in-Action:* Practice actions, knowledge, reasoning and discourse operate symbiotically; they are essential organic aspects of practice-in-action.

■ *Pursuing Clinical Reasoning Capability:* Viewed as a capability clinical reasoning is a journey of development in self-realization, interaction and critical appraisal.

The chapter will extend this discussion and produce a revised definition of clinical reasoning and a model of modes of encultured and contextualized reasoning.

REFLECTION POINT 1

What is your understanding of clinical reasoning and decision making? Do you draw the ideas discussed earlier into your practice?

CLINICAL REASONING AS AN ENCULTURED PRACTICE

Clinical reasoning operates within practice settings and multiple cultures including socio-political and instructional cultures, client health and well-being contexts and cultures, professional practice cultures and communities of practice. These cultures are created and entered through rich social construction and interaction processes, in particular, professionalization of occupations and the professional socialization of individuals entering the profession.

Culture

Culture is the characteristics, social behaviour and customs of a particular group of people (a society, community, ethnic group). It encompasses the beliefs, language, customs and the acquired knowledge of societies, so named as a result of their ongoing interaction and patterns of expected social behaviour and organization. Culture is expressed through material forms (technologies, artefacts, tool usage, art and architecture) and nonmaterial forms (politics, mythology and science). Culture is created and transmitted through social learning in human social groups both as a means of individual enculturation and as a way of maintaining that culture through succeeding generations. Culture can also refer to the set of shared attitudes, values, conventions, goals and social practices that characterize a particular field, discipline, institution or organization.

Socio-Political and Institutional Cultures Affecting the World of Healthcare Practice

Healthcare practice and decisions occur within complex social, economic, global and political contexts. (See also Chapters 1 and 7). These contexts reflect a range of influences and trends (Fish and Higgs, 2008), including:

- Political trends:
  - political and strategic environments that are imbued with a general failure to trust and an aversion to risk
  - a world that is fragmented, complex and uncertain
- Global work context trends:
  - increased emphasis on strategies and operations that are loosely connected and short term
  - changes in work, communication and service mechanisms linked to the digital revolution, creating 'unstable, fragmentary conditions' (Sennett, 2005, p. 3) where constant checking of progress creates instability and difficulty to flourish (O'Neill, 2002)
  - rising demands for accountability for practice that is fiscally, evidentially and ethically defensible
- Communication and information trends:
  - global mass communication strategies that bring to our urgent attention the latest information and knowledge of practice, technologies, world events and dilemmas
  - escalating client access to Internet information
- Knowledge trends:
  - exponential knowledge and technological advances
  - transitory knowledge and the devaluing of history, tradition and practice cultures
- Population trends:
  - demographic changes, particularly aging populations and an increasing number of displaced persons in many areas

- changing patterns of disease and disability, changing locations for health services provision, an increased focus on chronic diseases and an increase in the need for complex disease management strategies
- Individual/lifestyle trends and expectations:
  - limited time for individuality, creativity and practice wisdom
  - increased pressures on healthcare professionals in relation to work and life balance contexts and changing roles and expectations
  - increased client expectations of quality care and participation in clinical decision making

Practice cultures are shaped by their organization's target groups, goals, structures, operational factors like hierarchies and power, economic factors, codes of conduct, legal imperatives and size of the organization. Organizations may be local, national or international, government-operated or publicly or privately funded, and they can focus on primary, secondary or tertiary health care. The ongoing debate and pressures from economic versus professionalism imperatives are a key part of institutional healthcare cultures. This debate influences expectations held by clients and colleagues of healthcare professionals but also expectations of the organization as a whole to provide competent and ethical services to clients.

Client Health and Well-Being Narratives and Horizons

In this fourth edition of the book, we have devoted a whole section to collaborative clinical reasoning and client input to decision making. This is caused by the changing behaviour and expectations of clients who have much more medical information available to them, the way society is changing (particularly in the West) in relation to the pursuit of health and well-being as a more widespread norm in the face of epidemics like obesity and diabetes, plus changes in professional practice towards greater recognition of the role clients can play in clinical decision making, as informed experts about their own life and health situations. In addition to bringing these horizons to the 'decision-making table', patients, particularly those who have chronic conditions, are bringing other perspectives and narratives to their health care that go beyond the biomedical, cure, illness or restitution narrative. People want to replace 'normal' with 'their normal', 'the professional as expert and the patient as recipient' with 'we both have knowledge to share and perspectives to consider'. And many healthcare clients want to replace 'my role is a passive, compliant patient' with 'since much of my health care is in my own time, I need to be informed so that I can take sound and chosen actions' (particularly when discharged early, learning to live with chronic disability or illness).

Professional Practice

Professional practice and health care deal with many different challenges, including wicked problems (Roberts 2000), in a context that looks for accountability and evidence, clarity addresses complex real world problems, human tasks with consequences for life and quality of life and deals with issues associated with sharing decision-making processes and outcomes. Within this arena, professions share a number of common characteristics (the expectation of ethical conduct, operation within professional codes of conduct and societal expectations of competence and professionalism) and are increasingly challenged by the complexities of the human world and the changing physical and technological worlds.

Yet each profession has its own culture, including the norms and realizations of practice, standards, language and modes of communication, tools and artefacts of practice implementation and typical locations and situations of operation. Health care comprises a collective of disciplinary and professional cultures and could be thought of as a metaculture in which key norms and ways of being and doing are manifest. For instance, across health care (professions and systems) we recognize the importance of duty of care for individuals and groups participating in health care or living in communities where health promotion seeks to affect individual and population health. The potential of healthcare interventions or restrictions to affect people's lives and well-being is a core dimension of healthcare practice and decision making at broad community and individual levels. Such potential impact demands decisions and decision-making capabilities that are commensurate with quality of life and actions of doing good.

Communities of Practice

Professions, such as the health professions, are communities of practice that occur locally, nationally and globally.

Practice communities may operate on a profession-specific or interprofessional basis within organizations. In both cases, such communities demonstrate the ability to work collaboratively as a result of shared discourse, language, goals and practices. These shared artefacts and actions constitute dimensions of culture.

The term 'communities of practice' was developed by Lave and Wenger (1991) to describe a theory of social learning that places learning 'in the context of our lived experience of participation in the world' (Wenger, 1998, p. 3). Communities of practice are dynamic and flexible as people arrive and leave and as they become more or less central to the practice of the group. Some communities of practice are formally established and managed; others are more organic and evolve, developing shared purposes based on interests or passions. Underpinning this theory are four premises: 1) that people are social beings, 2) that knowledge occurs in relation to valued enterprises, 3) that knowing results from participating and pursuing ability in these enterprises and 4) that learning produces meaningful knowledge.

Two key concepts related to communities of practice (Lave and Wenger, 1991) are the following:

- *Situated learning,* which views learning as part of an activity in the world; in that agent, activity and the world mutually constitute each other
- *Legitimate peripheral participation,* which relates to the contention that for newcomers to a practice community, learning through activity happens legitimately from the periphery towards the core of the community of practice as they progressively become full practitioners and members of the practice community, who are integral to the maturing of the field of practice.

Professionalization and Professional Socialization

Two core processes lead to the emergence of the practice of professionals within practice cultures. First, there is the socio-historical process of professionalization that transitioned their occupations into professions. These occupations defined and shaped themselves into auto-regulated, standard-setting, occupational groups with requirements of educational entry and continued membership. Second, there is the process of professional socialization. This is an acculturation process involving entry education, reflection, professional development and engagement in professional work interactions; it enables the individual's development of the expected capabilities of the profession and a sense of professional identity and responsibility (Higgs et al., 2009). Novices become members of a particular profession and a unique social group and learn to be part of the culture of that group with all its privileges, requirements and responsibilities. They learn about, and make commitments to, meeting professional and discipline-specific codes of conduct and practice. Professional socialization also refers to the way in which a profession, through its educators, practitioners and leaders, socializes or inducts new members (Higgs, 2013).

Professional socialization involves both learning through practice communities and learning to be part of communities of practice. In her research on collaboration in health care, Croker (2011) found that most healthcare professionals engage with multiple practice communities in their work (e.g., their discipline team, their local work area group such as in a specific workplace and their broader professional association). Newcomers need to learn how to relate across each of these groups and communities. A key aspect of professional socialization is the way that students develop working relationships with other practitioners and team members from a range of professions.

UNDERSTANDING PROFESSIONAL PRACTICE PARADIGMS

We can relate communities of practice and practice cultures to the notion of paradigms wherein a group of practitioners (who could be researchers in a shared research paradigm or professional/clinical practitioners in a shared practice paradigm) come together to pursue common interests and goals. By sharing cultural norms, knowledge and practices, members of the paradigm community function coherently as members of a group who walk, talk and think (reason) in shared, encultured ways. Over time, paradigms evolve their pursuits and methodologies, and their goals often become more refined and effective in relation to the interests they serve. Paradigms proliferate, and new ones emerge as interests change or evolve. This means that science (including study of the human and the physical worlds)

is not static or confined to a single strategy but responds to changing interests.

A key element of learning and working in practice paradigms is recognizing and respecting the profession's practice worldview (or practice ontology) and how that is linked to the way knowledge is determined and created within that practice world (or practice epistemology) (Higgs et al., 2004b) (Box 2.1). Being grounded in their own profession's practice, members of the profession typically work across multiple communities of practice with a range of frames of reference

---

BOX 2.1
ONTOLOGY AND EPISTEMOLOGY – DEFINITIONS

Ontology: What is? What exists? What types of entities really exist? What is reality (like)?

- 'The theory of existence, or, more narrowly, of what really exists' (Bullock and Trombley, 1999, pp. 608–609).
- A branch of metaphysics, ontology 'is the science of *being* in general, embracing such issues as the nature of existence and the categorical structure of reality' (Honderich, 1995, p. 634).
- 'Derived from the Greek word for *being*, but a 17th century coinage for the branch of metaphysics that concerns itself with what exists' (Blackburn, 1994, p. 269).
- 'Ontology comes from the Greek "ontos" meaning being and "logos" meaning logic or rationale, and means literally "the study of being" or "the study of existence"' (Everitt and Fisher, 1995, p. 9).

Epistemology: What is knowledge? What can we know? How do we know what we know? What counts as true knowledge?

- 'The philosophical theory of knowledge, which seeks to define it, distinguish its principal varieties, identify its sources, and establish its limits' (Bullock and Trombley, 1999, p. 279).
- The branch of philosophy, epistemology 'is concerned with the theory of knowledge. Traditionally, central issues in epistemology are the nature and derivation of knowledge, the scope of knowledge, and the reliability of claims to knowledge' (Flew, 1984, p. 109).
- 'The term derives from the two Greek words, "episteme" meaning knowledge and "logos" meaning logic or rationale. In modern English, epistemology means the theory of knowledge' (Everitt and Fisher, 1995, p. 1).

	TABLE 2.1		
	Practice Paradigm		
		Practice Paradigm	
	Empirico-Analytical Paradigm	*Historical-Hermeneutic/Interpretive Paradigm*	*Critical Paradigm (Critical Science)*
Practice field	Natural Sciences Biomedicine	Social Sciences Wellness-oriented health care	Critical Science Collaborative health care

Interests	Technical Cognitive:
	  Prediction
	Objective Evidence
		Practical Cognitive: Finding
		  understanding, Mediation,
		  Consensus
			Emancipatory-Cognitive:
			  Transformation
			  Emancipation

Ontology
Approach to defining
  reality
	Positivist/empiricist ontology:
	  the world is objective
	  and lawful; it exists
	  independently of the
	  knowers
		Social constructivist ontology:
		  reality is socially constructed
		Hermeneutic ontology: people
		  are being in the world of
		  social practices and historical
		  contexts
			Historical Realism: history, social
			  practice and culture shape
			  practice

Epistemology (nature
  and construction of
  knowledge)
	To positivists knowledge
	  arises from the rigorous
	  application of the scientific
	  method
		In the interpretive paradigm,
		  knowledge: comprises
		  constructions arising from the
		  minds and bodies of knowing,
		  conscious and feeling beings
		  and is generated through a
		  search for meaning.
			In the critical paradigm,
			  knowledge: is emancipatory
			  and personally developmental,
			  requires becoming aware of
			  how our thinking is socially and
			  historically constructed

Methodological tools	Controlled Observation	Understanding meaning,
		  Interpretations of texts
			Self-reflection, group critical
			  reflection

Knowledge product	Facts
	Truths
		Intersubjectively Negotiated
		  Meaning
			Critique of natural and social
			  influences
			Negotiated understanding

Evidence and expertise	Best available external evidence	Individual practice expertise	Respect for expertise of all parties

Practice	Practice is characterized as
	  objective, pure, accountable
		Practice is characterized as
		  subjective, emotional, risky
			Practice is characterized as
			  collaborative, respectful, self-
			  challenging and transformative

Based on Higgs, Trede and Rothwell, 2007, and Higgs and Trede, 2010

(profession-specific, interdisciplinary, organizational and workplace oriented).

Table 2.1 presents a categorization of three practice paradigms (the empirico-analytical, interpretive and critical paradigms) informed by Habermas' concept of interests. According to Habermas (1968/1972) our interests, while often hidden, reflect our specific viewpoints and values and are the motivational aspect of our inquiries and action. Our interests are expressed in our knowledge (which is an activity rather than a static phenomenon) and are evident in the types of questions we ask and the strategies that we apply to search for responses to these questions. Habermas differentiated three interests: technical, practical and

emancipatory interests (see Table 2.1). Habermas (1968/1972, p. 308) contended that:

> *The approach of the empirical-analytic sciences incorporates a technical cognitive interest, that of the historical-hermeneutic sciences incorporates a practical one (and emanates from a concern for understanding); and the approach of critically oriented sciences incorporates emancipatory cognitive interest.*

In Table 2.1, the three paradigms are interpreted according to the practice field, interests, ontology, epistemology, methodological tools, knowledge product, evidence and expertise and the mode of practice they epitomize. Across the health sciences, practitioners may work in areas that are typically based on the biosciences (e.g., pathology, practices that support the cure and restitution narrative), a wellness orientation (e.g., occupational therapy, narratives based on client-led ability rather than disability narratives) and collaborative health care focussed on rejection of taken-for-granted rules and practices.

Practitioners who want to work deliberately in these paradigms need to pursue practice ontologies and practice epistemologies that match their paradigms. They need to understand these practice philosophy underpinnings and make them part of their being (practice ontology), knowing (practice epistemology), doing (practice embodiment), thinking (practice reasoning) and becoming (practice development). In this way, practitioners develop and own their personal ontologies and epistemologies:

- **Personal ontologies** refers to *being* in practice and owning and embodying an ontological worldview. The ontological turn involves a shift away from technical rationality and intellectual (cognitive) capacity towards being and becoming in practice. 'This turn is primarily based on the assumption that the knowledge and skills that will be needed in future workplaces cannot be known, in advance, in detail or with any great certainty; thus, attention to "knowing the world" and "skills for doing" appears to be an unproductive focus for educating future professionals in higher education. Rather, "being in the world" – pulling disparate elements of practice together into one "assemblage of self" – needs to be at the centre of university teaching' (Markauskaite and Goodyear, 2017, p. 54).
- **Personal epistemologies:** Epistemology as a broad concept (Barton and Billett, 2017) refers to the nature and origins of knowledge and encompasses how knowledge is derived, tested and validated. Personal epistemology is about people's way of knowing and how they build their knowledge base from prior experiences and through their capacities and ongoing negotiations. Such knowledge bases evoke readiness for practice, learning and reasoning, but they can also inhibit these activities if they are narrow or unchanging.

Loftus (2009) identified the substantial influences of sociocultural factors and the personal history and socialization experiences of individual practitioners and students on the way they understood what knowledge is and how they use and name it in practice.

Further depth of information on ontological and epistemological underpinnings of different practice approaches is provided in Box 2.2.

CLINICAL REASONING AND KNOWING IN PRACTICE

Practice and knowledge are reciprocal elements; each forms part of the composite culture of professional practice. One of the responsibilities of professionals is to understand and critique the knowledge they use in practice. Professional knowledge is embedded in and arises from the context of professional practice, particularly the history of ideas and the knowledge of society (Higgs et al., 2004). The development of practice knowledge occurs within a variety of contexts including the historical era and the cultural, social and individual perspectives of practitioners, scholars and researchers engaged in the exploration of practice and practice knowledge.

Professions evolve in sociocultural, political and historical frames of reference. Traditionally, Western thought has been dominated by the Cartesian notions that reasoning and knowing are essentially activities of individuals operating in isolation. Vygotsky (1978, 1986) and Bakhtin (1986) have challenged this idea. They argued that reasoning and knowing begin as activities embedded in social interaction, and they are primarily intersubjective processes arising within cultures. We become acculturated into societies that provide us with a cognitive toolkit of knowledge and ways of using such knowledge. Professional education and training are primarily about socializing students into particular ways of knowing and thinking about the world of practice. In Vygotskian terms, professional ways of thinking and knowing are higher mental functions. Vygotsky (1978) claimed that higher mental functions, which would include clinical reasoning, are qualitatively different from lower mental functions and cannot be reduced to them. Higher mental functions need a different

---

BOX 2.2
ONTOLOGIES AND EPISTEMOLOGIES

Ontological or worldview perspectives differ across the practice paradigms (see Table 2.1).

- In the positivist/empiricist ontological tradition, the world is objective, because it is said to exist independently of the knowers, and it consists of phenomena or events that are orderly and lawful.
- In the constructivist view, knowers are seen as conscious subjects separate from a world of objects; subjects who use knowledge who have theories about their practice and who behave according to tacit rules and procedures. Multiple constructed realities are recognized to occur (i.e., different people have different perceptions of reality through their attribution of meaning to events, meaning being part of the event not separate from it) (Lincoln and Guba, 1985).
- The social constructivist view contends that reality and knowledge are socially constructed. Reality exists because we give meaning to it (Berger and Luckmann, 1985). Different cultures have different social constructions of reality. Within the interpretive tradition, the world and reality are interpreted by people in the context of historical and social practices.
- The hermeneutic view arises from the ideas of Heidegger (1962), Merleau-Ponty (1956) and Gadamer (1975). In this hermeneutic view, there is no subject/object split; people are seen as part of the world, being in it and coping with it. They are also seen as beings for whom things have significance and value, having a world of social practices and historical contexts and as being a person in time (Leonard, 1989). This view of people and the world is a relational one (Benner and Wrubel, 1989). Unlike the constructivist view of knowledge, this knowing has no mental representation and may be embodied, that is, known by the body without cognition.
- The (historical) realist is concerned with social structures and how macro- and micro-political, historical and socio-economic factors influence our lives.

Epistemological perspectives or stances within research paradigms are portrayed as follows:

- To positivists or empiricists, knowledge arises from the rigorous application of the scientific method and is measured against the criteria of objectivity, reliability and validity. In the empirico-analytical paradigm, knowledge: is discovered, i.e., universal and external truths are grasped and justified, arises from empirical processes which are reductionist, value neutral, quantifiable, objective and operationalizable; statements are valid only if publicly verifiable by sense data.
- The idealist approaches of Dilthey (1833–1911) and Weber (1864–1920) focused on interpretive understanding (Verstehen), accessing the ideas and experiences of actors, as opposed to the explanatory and predictive approach of the physical sciences (Smith, 1983). This perspective results in a focus on human behaviour as occurring within a context and the understanding or knowledge of human behaviour as requiring an understanding of this context.
- Constructivists view knowledge as 'an internal construction or an attempt to impose meaning and significance on events and ideas'. In this perspective, each person constructs a more-or-less idiosyncratic explanatory system of reality' (Candy, 1991, p. 251).
- The social constructionist approach (McCarthy, 1996) construes knowledge as a changing and relative phenomenon and examines the social and historical constructs of knowledge in terms of what knowledge is socially produced and what counts as knowledge.
- The (historical) realist is concerned with how we understand our lives in the context of socio-cultural, historical influences. Knowledge is always influenced by social interest, and it is not grasped or discovered but is acquired through critical debate. In the critical paradigm, knowledge: is emancipatory and personally developmental; requires becoming aware of how our thinking is socially and historically constructed and how this limits our actions; enables people to challenge learned restrictions, compulsions or dictates of habit; is not grasped or discovered but is acquired through critical debate; and promotes understanding about how to transform current structures, relationships and conditions that constrain development and reform (Higgs and Titchen, 1995).

---

conceptual framework, one that takes into account their cultural and historical nature.

Professional Practice Knowledge

Professional practice knowledge evolves as a consequence of the critical use and reflection on the profession's knowledge and practice by individual professionals and the profession collectively. The exploration of the *history of ideas* (see Berlin, 1979) within a practice can assist practitioners to contextualize their understanding of contemporary practice and enhance their ability to develop their knowledge and practice effectively. The discipline of the history of ideas was popularized by the American philosopher Arthur Lovejoy (1873–1962) in the 1920s (Kelley, 1990). The term 'history of ideas' encompasses approaches to study that centre on how the meaning and associations of ideas change according to history (Burke, 1988). Lovejoy (1936) argued that we understand ourselves better by understanding the ways in which we have evolved, or the manner in which we have come, over time, to hold the ideas that we do. History needs to be concerned with ideas that attain a wide diffusion and to cross barriers between different disciplines and thinking, recognizing the fact that ideas that emerge at any one time usually manifest themselves in more than one direction (Lovejoy, 1936). A history of ideas approach allows us to understand the origins of ideas and place our own ideas in perspective (Adams, 1987).

Learning, both formal and self-directed, involves understanding the way that knowledge of the discipline is created and used in practice. Epistemology and disciplinarity are related; both are concerned with knowledge and the adaptation of knowledge in particular situations of practice (Barton and Billett, 2017). Building disciplinary knowledge similarly requires this understanding and a recognition of how knowledge in the discipline and practice community is created, tested and validated.

Table 2.2 provides an overview of different ways of categorizing knowledge. This work illustrates how important knowledge is in practice and how much work over time has been spent by many scholars in recognizing different ways knowledge is created and used in practice. We need multiple forms of knowledge, including the scientific knowledge of human behaviour and body responses in health and illness, the aesthetic perception of significant human experiences, understanding of the uniqueness of the self and others and their interactions and an appreciation of morality and ethics. According to Kemmis and Smith (2008, p. 4), praxis 'is action that *is morally-committed and oriented and informed by traditions in a field*. It is the kind of action people are engaged in when they think about what their action will mean *in the world*. Praxis is what people do when they take into account all the circumstances and exigencies that confront them at a particular moment and then, taking the broadest view they can of what it is best to do, they act'.

Clinical reasoning is embedded in praxis. In the model in Table 2.2, praxis is seen as a core aspect of advanced practice because of the expertise required to engage deeply in praxis and because it epitomizes practice that embodies ethics and morality, as well as professional capabilities.

Developing Intellectual Virtues

Another way of revealing advanced and deliberately known practice is via Aristotle's (trans., 1999) three intellectual virtues or excellences of mind:

- *Epistêmê* is an intellectual virtue characterized as scientific, universal, invariable, context-independent knowledge. The concept is reflected in the terms *epistemology* and *epistemic*.
- *Téchnê* refers to craft or applied practice; it is an intellectual virtue characterized as context-dependent, pragmatic, variable, craft knowledge; it is governed by a conscious goal, and it is oriented towards practical instrumental rationality. The concept is reflected in terms such as *technique, technical and technology*.
- *Phrónêsis* refers to practical wisdom; it is an intellectual virtue characterized by values and ethics. It involves value-based deliberation and practical judgement. It is reflective, pragmatic, variable, context-dependent and action-oriented.

These ways of knowing provide a useful point of reflection on reasoning in practice – what it is and what it can be, when knowingly practiced. These virtues ask learners and practitioners to think deeply about what knowledge is, how it links to professionalism and how knowledge, reasoning and action combine in practice and to engage with these ways of knowing, doing, being and becoming in practice. (Refer to practice as doing, knowing, being and becoming in: Higgs, 1999; Higgs and Titchen, 2001.)

Epistemic Cultures

According to Nerland and Jensen (2014, in Nerland 2016, p. 137) 'professions can be regarded as distinct knowledge cultures, constituted by a set of knowledge processes and practices that define expertise in the given area and serve to distinguish professional practitioners from other actors'. To contend with the challenges related to knowledge and practice conventions faced by

TABLE 2.2
Knowledge Categorizations

Plato (400 BC) (P) Aristotle (300 BC) (A) (in Gustavsson, 2004)*	Vico (in Berlin, 1979)	Kolb (1984)	Carper (1978) Sarter (1988)	Reason and Heron (1986)	Higgs and Titchen (1995)	Bereiter (2002) Eraut (1994, 2010)
Epistémē (P) (A) Objective knowledge, represents scientific knowledge, theoretical knowledge	Deductive knowledge: things that are true either by definition or by deduction from propositions or assumptions that are themselves true purely by definition Scientific knowledge requires objectively valid, reliable and reproducible evidence. Only evidence gained by the senses, through observation, description and measurement, may be counted. Knowledge remains 'true' only for as long as it is not objectively refuted; when it fails the crucial test, it becomes obsolete, to be replaced by a superior formula/findings.		Interpretive knowledge (philosophical analysis) Empirical knowledge	Propositional knowledge: knowledge of things, gained through conversation, reading, etc.	Propositional knowledge: knowledge derived through research and/or scholarship; it is formal, explicit and exists in the public domain. It may be expressed in propositional statements that describe relationships between concepts or cause–effect relationships, thus permitting claims about generalizability. Or it may be presented in descriptive terms that allow for transferability of use.	Public knowledge (Bereiter, 2002) Theoretical/propositional knowledge (Schön, 1995)

Téchnē (A)	Experiential knowledge	Experiential knowledge:	Aesthetic	Nonpropositional	Nonpropositional/ experience-based	Collaborative knowledge building and knowledgeability:
Knowledge used in the process of producing, manufacturing and creating products	is gained by personal experience. Some crucially important human knowledge exists that is distinct from and not reducible to either scientific or deductive knowledge	concrete experience, reflective observation, abstract conceptualization, active experimentation	knowledge (artistic) pattern of knowing, derived from experience	(a) Experiential knowledge from direct encounters with persons, places/things	(a) Professional craft knowledge can be tacit and is embedded in practice; it comprises general professional knowledge gained from health professionals' practice experience and also specific knowledge about a particular client in a particular situation.	(stable, episodic, implicit, implicity, impressionistic, regulative) (Bereiter)
Phrónēsis (A)			Personal pattern of knowing self	(b) Practical knowledge gained through activity and related to skills or competencies		Professional personal knowledge and capability: codified knowledge, accumulated memories, personal understandings, self-knowledge, metaprocesses and know-how (Eraut)
Practical knowledge or wisdom used in the process of social interaction; incorporates ethical understanding of the values and norms that help people frame their ideas of a good life			Ethical (moral) pattern of knowing		(b) Personal (individual) knowledge includes the collective knowledge held by the community and culture in which the individual lives and the unique knowledge gained from the individual's life experience.	Knowing in action (Schön, 1995) Actionable knowledge (Argyris, 1999) Working knowledge (Yinger and Hendricks-Lee, 1993)

Based on Higgs, Jones and Titchen, 2008

professional communities today, argued Nerland (2016), we need a perspective that accounts for multiple and dynamic dimensions of knowledge. This would involve adopting a critically reflexive approach to the use and development of knowledge processes and development practices.

Knorr Cetina (2007) contends that different expert cultures produce knowledge in distinctly different ways, and she introduced the concept of epistemic cultures to represent the way that such expert and professional cultures generate and use their knowledge. She uses the term 'machinery of knowledge construction' to encompass sets of practices, arrangements and mechanisms bound together by necessity, affinity and historical coincidence, which, in a given area of professional expertise, make up how we know what we know (Knorr Cetina 2007, p. 363).

The notion of *epistemic culture* is a rich and deep way of understanding the worlds of practice and how the discourse of practice knowledge and knowledge-grounded practice cohabits these worlds symbiotically. Epistemic cultures comprise both knowledge as practiced and the disciplinary, expert-framed and social cultural settings in which knowledge and practices interact for the benefit of the participants in these cultures. Professional cultures are thus enacted and embodied through the group or profession and by individual practitioners. This enactment involves a critical living dialogue that occurs among practice knowledge, practice actions and practice reasoning, with each of these three existing as evolving dimensions of living practice in changing social practice arenas.

Epistemic Fluency

Beyond and within epistemic cultures, we come to the idea of *epistemic fluency* (Goodyear and Zenios, 2007). Goodyear and Ellis (2007) build on the work of Morrison and Collins (1996, p. 109), who provide Collins' key terms: *epistemic forms* to refer to 'target structures that guide inquiry' and *epistemic games* to refer to 'sets of moves, constraints, and strategies that guide the construction of knowledge around a particular epistemic form'. Epistemic forms include taxonomies, models and lists. Engaging in epistemic games in one's own disciplinary field (and others) helps build capacity to perform strategies linked to the inquiry structures of that field and others; the latter helps the learner to gain an appreciation of how others develop and use knowledge.

The concept and practice of epistemic fluency is described by Markauskaite and Goodyear (2017, p. 1) as follows: 'people who are flexible and adept with respect to different ways of knowing about the world can be said to possess epistemic fluency'. The idea of fluency, typically applied to language, the spoken word and interactive communication, is particularly useful when thinking about knowledge and clinical reasoning. First, it refers to having a command of the language, and experienced practitioners with advanced clinical reasoning capabilities need to have this ability. Technical language provides the means and tools for communicating with colleagues using the rich knowledge and shared understanding embedded in discipline-specific and generic healthcare language. It is used to record notes in patient histories, write reports to referring practitioners, record information for legal or historical records and present new ideas such as research findings for the critical appraisal of the professional and scientific communities. Interpersonal (professional) language is a means for performing the actions of practice such as taking a patient's history and seeking feedback about changes in symptoms during treatments, a way of sharing viewpoints and discussing treatment options and a tool for communicating findings, decisions, diagnoses and so on.

Linking this fluency to knowledge construction and co-construction and the derivation of knowledge from practice, we can recognize the way that clinical reasoning and decision making rely on epistemic fluency. Both reasoning and decision making involve understanding knowledge, appreciating different ways of knowing, using different sources and forms of knowledge in reasoning and placing different knowledge (including client's knowledge) as the influences and benchmarks that drive and determine decisions. We can think of epistemic fluency within clinical reasoning as a capability that is most clearly demonstrated by experienced and expert practitioners. Overall practice capability requires clinical reasoning fluency.

Developing Epistemic Fluency and Reasoning Conversation Capability

If we acknowledge that living cultures exist in health care, we recognize that culture requires communication, and decision making requires conversations. At the very least, these practice conversations involve the ascertainment of patients'/clients' needs/goals/expectations and practitioners'/professionals' expert input to decision making and treatment advice. Frequently professional practice also involves conversations and collaborative decision making among practitioners who share 'case management' responsibilities. Ideally, practice involves conversations that incorporate and respect the multiple cultures, expert and self-knowledge perspectives of the decision-making participants (including clients/patients and carers) and the perspectives and prerogatives of each player. In this way, rich collaborative clinical decision making is both encultured and conversational.

PURSUING CLINICAL REASONING CAPABILITY

Too often clinical reasoning is simply thought of as a process of thinking or a set of decisions that need to be made. Instead, clinical reasoning needs to be recognized as capability, indeed, as a set of capabilities.

Capability refers to practice-grounded ability that is demonstrable and justifiable (Stephenson, 1998); it goes beyond technical competence and encompasses agency, ingenuity and confidence in actions including decision making, problem identification and problem solving. Capability places emphasis on being able to perform well in both known and unknown contexts and the capacity to solve complex and more straightforward clinical problems. Capability is required in both task and relationship aspects of practice, in working effectively with others and confidence in the ability to navigate unfamiliar circumstances and learn from these experiences.

'Capability is a holistic concept which encompasses both current competence and future development through the application of potential. The concept is applicable across both individuals and organisations' (Cairns and Stephenson, 2009, p. 16). The three key elements of capability are ability (current competence and perceived potential), self-efficacy (confidence in capacity to perform tasks) and values (particularly the way actions in uncertain conditions are guided by values and the capacity to articulate values). 'Capability (encompasses):

- the capacity to operate in both familiar and unfamiliar circumstances
- the utilization of creativity and imagination/innovation
- being mindful about change and open to opportunities/uncertainties
- being confident about one's abilities
- being able to engage with the social values relevant to actions
- engaging with learning as a self-directed process
- operating to formulate and solve problems'. (ibid).

In the re-interpretation of clinical reasoning presented in this chapter, clinical reasoning is viewed as a set of capabilities that are cognitive, embodied, owned, collaborative and critical. Each of these words reminds us of the contexts, cultures, communities and challenges that have been presented earlier, and they epitomize the essential responsibilities of professionals to draw all of their knowledge, reasoning and technical capabilities together in practice that is of high quality in conditions of uncertainty and conditions of greater simplicity, whether these situational dimensions are caused by the inherent nature of the practice-reasoning task, setting, decision making practice or the setting.

The idea of capability is strongly supported in education and other forms of practice. Eraut (2000, p. 128), for example, identifies capability as a core element in choosing an appropriate cognitive approach in given situations. He raises the question 'What factors are likely to affect the mode of cognition employed by a particular practitioner in a particular context?' The answer, he argues, includes:

- task factors: evidence, complexity
- practitioner factors: capability and disposition
- contextual factors: time available and the crowdedness of the situation (the number of clients, activities, pieces of information and so on that are competing for the practitioner's attention.

Eraut contends (ibid) the following:

- An analytic approach is appropriate where there is 'sufficient research evidence available in which the practitioner has confidence, the problem being capable of being represented in a form which enables it to be "solved" mainly on the basis of that evidence, and the practitioner being willing

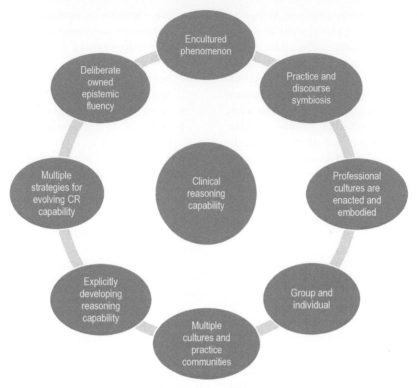

Fig. 2.1 ■ Clinical reasoning capability.

and able to do the analysis and implement the results'.

■ An intuitive approach is appropriate when 'the practitioner has considerable experience of similar situations'.

■ A deliberative approach is appropriate when the practitioner 'has both some evidence and some relevant experience, a willingness to reflect and consult and a sense of what is possible under the circumstances'.

Fig. 2.1 draws together the arguments presented earlier, in an interpretation of clinical reasoning capability built around an encultured view of clinical reasoning that is embodied and enacted in healthcare professional practice.

The evolution of clinical reasoning capability requires practitioners to pursue a deep understanding of reasoning as a complex arena of practice, to recognize the inherent contextualization of clinical reasoning, to value different approaches to reasoning suited to the reasoner's learning readiness, to develop advanced ability and fluency in the language and articulation of reasoning with diverse clinical decision-making partners and to employ learning strategies that draw each of these abilities and understandings into practice.

REFLECTION POINT 2

How do you interpret each of the dimensions and considerations of capability presented in Fig. 2.1? Do they feature in your reasoning practices?

REDEFINING CLINICAL REASONING AS A RANGE OF ENCULTURED DECISION-MAKING CAPABILITIES

In this section, I present my model and definition of clinical reasoning and decision making reconceptualized as a set of encultured decision-making capabilities. This definition and model build on my 20 years of extensive research and scholarship on clinical reasoning. This research has been challenged, filtered and re-interpreted through the process of producing the four editions of this book since 1995 and through an extensive program of research and scholarship involving a team of doctoral students, colleagues and postdoctoral fellows. Of particular interest in my research and education have been the nature of practice knowledge, multiple ways of knowing, communities of practice, the symbiosis of practice knowledge and research, philosophical views of knowledge and practice and the power of the lenses of capability and enculturation. International leaders in clinical reasoning research, scholarship and education have debated with me about the nature of clinical reasoning and how it operates in and emerges from practice. These rich debates have enriched my journey of understanding of this fascinating and vital component of professional practice.

A Revised Interpretation of Clinical Reasoning and Decision Making

Clinical reasoning is a multilayered, context-dependent way of thinking and decision making in professional practice that is embedded and enacted in healthcare professional practice through epistemic-ontological cultures.

The **purpose** of clinical reasoning is to make sound, client-centred decisions (preferably *with* clients), guide practice stances, actions and trajectories and optimize client health and well-being choices, pathways and outcomes.

Its key **dimensions** are the generation and use of practice knowledge, reasoning capabilities and metacognition.

It involves **metaskills** of reflexivity, knowledge generation through practice, ongoing learning and reasoning refinement, practice model authenticity (see Chapter 4), constructed narratives and critical, creative conversations. The construction of **narratives** helps make sense of the multiple factors and interests pertaining to the current reasoning task. The pursuit of **conversations** among colleagues, clients and carers helps construct client-optimal decisions and particularized healthcare pathways. Such 'conversations' occur when clinical reasoning is viewed as a contextualized interactive phenomenon rather than a specific process.

Practitioners interact both with the task/informational elements of decision making and with the human/collaborative elements and the interests of the various decision-making participants. These conversations involve interactions based on critical appraisal of circumstances and, where possible, critical interests in promoting emancipatory practice and the creation and implementation of particularized, person-centred healthcare programs.

It is **framed** by, and embodied in, the epistemic (knowledge) and ontological (worldview) cultures of practice communities, professionalism, ethical codes of practice, community and client expectations and the needs and perspectives of its participants.

It occurs within a range of **problem spaces** (see Chapter 3) and contexts framed by the unique frames of reference (interests, knowledge, abilities, values, experience) of the practitioners, patients/clients, carers and organizations involved.

It draws on **evidence** to support decision making that takes a range of forms and importance including clinical data, experience-based illness scripts, (qualitative and quantitative) research findings, theoretical arguments and professional experience theorizations (Higgs, 2017; 2018).

It incorporates **judgement** and decision making at micro (e.g., deciding on next steps, interpreting observed symptoms), macro (e.g., making and producing diagnoses, treatment plans) and meta (e.g., metacognitive critique of decisions in action, evaluation of proposed actions and outcome suitability and quality) levels. Judgement is both a verb (practice, process) and a noun (product and responsibility).

It may be **individually or collaboratively** conducted. Teams are often interdisciplinary and ideally involve the client (and carers). Shared reasoning and decision making values the different inputs (knowledge, interests, perspectives) that each player brings to decision making, particularly the client.

Advanced clinical reasoning involves moving beyond the acts of clinical decision making through the pursuit of epistemic and ontological **fluency** and the informed use of the language of clinical reasoning across cultures, to enhance clinical reasoning in action as an embodied, reflexive and interactive capability that is realized through clinical decision-making conversations.

A Model of Clinical Reasoning as Encultured Decision-Making Capabilities

This model (Fig. 2.2) is framed by four influence factors:

- the task facing the decision maker(s) (left side) – ranging from highly complex, challenging tasks to straightforward tasks. In the centre of this continuum lie fluctuating tasks.
- the 'scene' or context (right side) – ranging from highly fluid settings where multiple factors influence the decision-making challenge to stable, predictable situations. In the centre of this continuum lie changeable situations.
- the decision-making approach (upper continuum) – ranging from discipline-based, autonomous approaches to life-based, interdependent approaches.

- the decision makers (lower continuum) – ranging from individual and teams of professionals who lead the clinical decision making to community-based decision-making groups (including practitioners and clients).

There are five decision-making approaches with colours assigned to reflect the approach:

- **WHITE** (Novice) Decision Making – this approach matches the demands of (more) straightforward reasoning tasks in relatively stable and predictable settings. It is typical of novices who adopt a deliberate, explicit, studied approach to reasoning (e.g., hypothetico-deductive reasoning) and work individually or in professional teams; it relies on emerging disciplinary knowledge. This approach draws on *téchnê* and *epistêmê* intelligences.

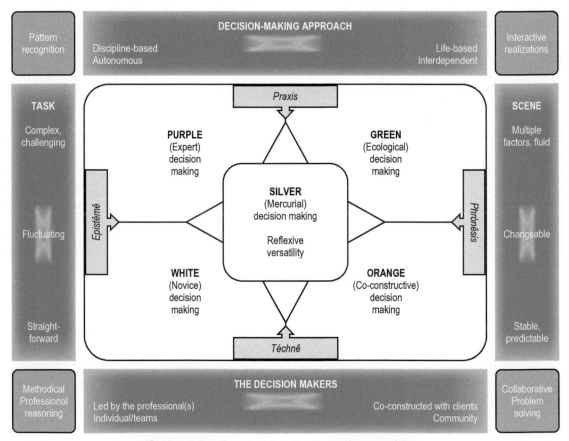

Fig. 2.2 ■ Encultured clinical decision-making capabilities.

- **PURPLE** (Expert) Decision Making – this approach matches the demands of (more) complex and challenging reasoning tasks in relatively fluid settings influenced by multiple factors. It is typical of acknowledged, expert clinical reasoners who adopt a complex reasoning approach to reasoning (e.g., pattern recognition) and the use of instantiated scripts (see Boshuizen and Schmidt, 1992) and deep rich knowledge bases. They work individually or in professional teams. This approach draws on *epistêmê* and the embedded ethicality and depth of embodied practice or *praxis*. It demands high-level fluency and rich technical, professional, critical, epistemic, ontological and interpersonal capability.
- **ORANGE** (Co-constructed) Decision Making – this approach emphasizes the demands of recent times, where clients are better informed and agentic than ever before. It can work well within the demands of (more) straightforward reasoning tasks in relatively stable and predictable settings. It may involve decision making with individual clients, groups or communities. The key element that influences this approach is co-constructed and interdependent decision making, aiming to pursue life-based rather than clinically oriented decisions. This approach draws on *téchnê* and *phrónêsis*. It requires a willingness to share expert knowledge and capabilities with clients and a commitment to valuing the perspectives and input of others.
- **GREEN** (Ecological) Decision Making – this approach matches the demands of (more) complex and challenging reasoning tasks in relatively fluid settings, influenced by multiple factors. It is typical of highly experienced but nontraditional practitioners who focus on the complexity of practice and community settings where individuals or groups of clients are looking for different narratives and solutions. The term *ecological* has been attached to this approach to highlight the interdependence of the decision-making parties and the need for mutual respect among them for their different perspectives and contributions. The processes of 'green' decision making are inherently dynamic and emergent. This approach draws on a strong ability in *phrónêsis* and the embedded ethicality and depth of embodied practice or *praxis*. It demands high-level (individual and collective)

epistemic and ontological fluency and rich critical, technical, professional, epistemic, ontological and interpersonal capability on the part of practitioners and a willingness to share expert knowledge and capabilities with clients and a commitment to valuing the perspectives and input of others to realize optimal solutions to the challenges posed. Networking of decision-making participants is a key feature of this approach to decision making.

- **SILVER** (Mercurial) Decision Making – is placed at the centre of the four continua, deliberately emphasizing that some decision-making approaches need to be highly versatile, reflexive and dynamic. This approach draws on *epistêmê, phrónêsis, téchnê and praxis* in varying ways, depending on the task, setting, practice and players. The approach is included in this model to recognize that clinical decision-making situations and players are not static, and the approaches adopted need to be knowingly responsive to these changes – or at times driving context changes. This approach demands a high level of reflexivity, versatility, fluency and rich technical, professional, critical, epistemic, ontological and interpersonal capability; a willingness to share expert knowledge and capabilities with clients; and a commitment to valuing the perspectives and input of others.

CHAPTER SUMMARY

Clinical reasoning is a sophisticated set of reflexive, encultured capabilities that are deeply contextualized in the reasoner's discipline, their ways of knowing, their owned practice model and in their work setting across multiple communities of practice. Somewhere on the journey from learning clinical reasoning as a systematic, conscious, risk-managed, novice-oriented process to the highly attuned wise practice of professional experts, practitioners should come to appreciate clinical reasoning as the most critical, integrative dimension and capability of professional practice.

REFLECTION POINT 3

What insights have you gained about clinical reasoning and decision making from this chapter? How might these insights influence your reasoning and practice?

REFERENCES

Adams, J., 1987. Historical review and appraisal of research on learning, retention, and transfer of human motor skills. Psychol. Bull. 10, 41–74.

Argyris, C., 1999. Tacit knowledge in management. In: Sternberg, R.J., Horvath, J.A. (Eds.), Tacit Knowledge in Professional Practice: Researcher and Practitioner Perspectives. Lawrence Erlbaum Associates, Mahwah, NJ, pp. 123–140.

Aristotle, 1999. Nicomachean Ethics, trans. T Irwin. Hackett Publishing, Indianapolis, IN (original work published c. 400 BC).

Bakhtin, M., 1986. Speech Genres and Other Late Essays, trans. VW McGee. University of Texas Press, Austin, TX.

Barton, G., Billett, S., 2017. Personal epistemologies and disciplinarity in the workplace: implications for international students in higher education. In: Barton, G., Hartwig, K. (Eds.), Professional Learning in the Workplace for International Students: Exploring Theory and Practice. Springer, Dordrecht, The Netherlands, pp. 98–111.

Benner, P., Wrubel, J., 1989. The Primacy of Caring: Stress and Coping in Health and Illness. Addison-Wesley, Wokingham, UK.

Bereiter, C., 2002. Education and Mind in the Knowledge Age. Lawrence Erlbaum Associates, Mahwah, NJ.

Berger, P., Luckmann, T., 1985. The Social Construction of Reality. Penguin, Harmondsworth, UK.

Berlin, I. (Ed.), 1979. Against the Current: Essays in the History of Ideas. The Hogarth Press, London, UK.

Blackburn, S., 1994. The Oxford Dictionary of Philosophy. Oxford University Press, Oxford.

Boshuizen, H.P.A., Schmidt, H.G., 1992. On the role of biomedical knowledge in clinical reasoning by experts, intermediates and novices. Cogn. Sci. 16, 153–184.

Bullock, A., Trombley, S., 1999. The New Fontana Dictionary of Modern Thought, third ed. HarperCollins, London, UK.

Burke, P., 1988. History of Ideas. In: Bullock, A., Stallybrass, O., Trombley, S. (Eds.), The Fontana Dictionary of Modern Thought, second ed. Fontana, London, UK, p. 388.

Cairns, L., Stephenson, J., 2009. Capable Workplace Learning. Sense, Rotterdam, The Netherlands.

Candy, P.C., 1991. Self-Direction for Lifelong Learning. Jossey-Bass, San Francisco, CA.

Carper, B.A., 1978. Fundamental patterns of knowing. Adv. Nurs. Sci. 1, 13–23.

Croker, A., 2011. Collaboration in Rehabilitation Teams, PhD Thesis. Charles Sturt University, Australia.

Eraut, M., 1994. Developing Professional Knowledge and Competence. Falmer Press, London, UK.

Eraut, M., 2000. Non-formal learning and tacit knowledge in professional work. Br. J. Educ. Psychol. 70, 113–136.

Eraut, M., 2010. Knowledge, working practices and learning. In: Billett, S. (Ed.), Learning Through Practice: Models, Traditions, Orientations and Approaches. Springer, Dordrecht, The Netherlands, pp. 37–58.

Everitt, N., Fisher, A., 1995. Modern Epistemology: A New Introduction. McGraw Hill, New York, NY.

Fish, D., Higgs, J., 2008. The context for clinical decision making in the twenty-first century. In: Higgs, J., Jones, M., Loftus, S., et al. (Eds.), Clinical Reasoning in the Health Professions, third ed. Elsevier, Edinburgh, pp. 19–30.

Flew, A. (Ed.), 1984. A Dictionary of Philosophy, second ed. Pan, London, UK.

Gadamer, H.G., 1975. Hermeneutics and social science. Cultural Hermeneutics 2, 307–316.

Goodyear, P., Ellis, R., 2007. The Development of Epistemic Fluency: Learning to Think for a Living. Sydney University Press, Sydney, Australia.

Goodyear, P., Zenios, M., 2007. Discussion, collaborative knowledge work and epistemic fluency. Br. J. Educ. Studies 55, 351–368.

Gustavsson, B., 2004. Revisiting the philosophical roots of practical knowledge. In: Higgs, J., Richardson, B., Abrandt Dahlgren, M. (Eds.), Developing Practice Knowledge for Health Professionals. Butterworth-Heinemann, Oxford, pp. 35–50.

Habermas, J., 1968/1972. Knowledge and human interest, trans. Shapiro. J.J. Heinemann, London, UK.

Heidegger, M., 1962. Being and Time. Harper & Row, New York, NY.

Higgs, J., 1999. Doing, knowing, being and becoming in professional practice, in Proceedings of the Master of Teaching Post Internship Conference, September, University of Sydney, Sydney, Australia.

Higgs, J., 2013. Professional socialisation including COP. In: Loftus, S., Gerzina, T., Higgs, J., et al. (Eds.), Educating Health Professionals: Becoming a University Teacher. Sense, Rotterdam, The Netherlands, pp. 83–92.

Higgs, J., 2017. Raisonnement clinique : des conversations au sein de cultures épistémiques. Pédagogie Médicale 18, 51–53.

Higgs, J., 2018. Judgment and reasoning in professional contexts. In: Lanzer, P. (Ed.), Catheter-Based Cardiovascular Interventions; Knowledge-Based Approach, second ed. Springer International, Cham, Switzerland, pp. 15–26.

Higgs, J., Andresen, L., Fish, D., 2004. Practice knowledge—its nature, sources and contexts. In: Higgs, J., Richardson, B., Abrandt Dahlgren, M. (Eds.), Developing Practice Knowledge for Health Professionals. Butterworth-Heinemann, Edinburgh, pp. 51–69.

Higgs, J., Jones, M., Titchen, A., 2008. Knowledge, reasoning and evidence for practice. In: Higgs, J., Jones, M., Loftus, S., et al. (Eds.), Clinical Reasoning in the Health Professions, third ed. Elsevier, Edinburgh, pp. 151–161.

Higgs, J., McAllister, L., Whiteford, G., 2009. The practice and praxis of professional decision making. In: Green, B. (Ed.), Understanding and Researching Professional Practice. Sense, Rotterdam, The Netherlands, pp. 101–120.

Higgs, J., Richardson, B., Abrandt Dahlgren, M. (Eds.), 2004b. Developing Practice Knowledge for Health Professionals. Butterworth-Heinemann, Oxford.

Higgs, J., Titchen, A., 1995. The nature, generation and verification of knowledge. Physiotherapy 81, 521–530.

Higgs, J., Titchen, A. (Eds.), 2001. Professional Practice in Health, Education and the Creative Arts. Blackwell Science, Oxford.

Higgs, J., Trede, F., 2010. Philosophical frameworks and research communities. In: Higgs, J., Cherry, N., Macklin, R., et al. (Eds.), Researching Practice: a Discourse on Qualitative Methodologies. Sense, Rotterdam, The Netherlands, pp. 31–36.

Higgs, J., Trede, F., Rothwell, R., 2007. Qualitative research interests and paradigms. In: Higgs, J., Titchen, A., Horsfall, D., et al. (Eds.),

Being Critical and Creative in Qualitative Research. Hampden Press, Sydney, Australia, pp. 32–42.

Honderich, T. (Ed.), 1995. The Oxford Companion to Philosophy. Oxford University Press, Oxford.

Kelley, D.R., 1990. What is happening to the history of ideas? J. Hist. Ideas 51, 3–25.

Kemmis, S., Smith, T.J., 2008. Enabling Praxis: Challenges for Education. Sense, Rotterdam, The Netherlands.

Knorr Cetina, K., 2007. Culture in global knowledge societies: knowledge cultures and epistemic cultures. Interdiscip. Sci. Rev. 32, 361–375.

Kolb, D.A., 1984. Experiential Learning: Experience as the Source of Learning and Development, vol. 1. Prentice-Hall, Englewood Cliffs, NJ.

Lave, J., Wenger, E., 1991. Situated Learning: Legitimate Peripheral Participation. Cambridge University Press, Cambridge, UK.

Leonard, V.A., 1989. A Heideggerian phenomenologic perspective on the concept of the person. Adv. Nurs. Sci. 11, 40–55.

Lincoln, Y.S., Guba, E., 1985. Naturalistic Inquiry. Sage, Newbury Park, CA.

Loftus, S., 2009. Language in Clinical Reasoning: Towards a New Understanding. VDM Verlag Dr. Müller, Saarbrücken, Germany.

Lovejoy, A.D., 1936. The Great Chain of Being: A Study of the History of an Idea. Harvard Press, Cambridge, MA.

Markauskaite, L., Goodyear, P., 2017. Epistemic Fluency and Professional Education: Innovation, Knowledgeable Action and Actionable Knowledge. Springer, Dordrecht, The Netherlands.

McCarthy, E.D., 1996. Knowledge as Culture: The New Sociology of Knowledge. Routledge & Kegan Paul, London, UK.

Merleau-Ponty, M., 1956. What Is Phenomenology? Cross Curr. 16, 59–70.

Morrison, D., Collins, A., 1996. Epistemic fluency and constructivist learning environments. In: Wilson, B. (Ed.), Constructivist Learning Environments: Case Studies in Instructional Design. Educational Technology Publications, Englewood Cliffs, NJ, pp. 107–119.

Nerland, M., 2016. Learning to master profession-specific knowledge practices: a prerequisite for the deliberate professional? In: Trede, F., McEwen, C. (Eds.), Educating the Deliberate Professional: Preparing Practitioners for Emergent Futures. Springer, Dordrecht, The Netherlands, pp. 127–139.

Nerland, M., Jensen, K., 2014. Changing cultures of knowledge and professional learning. In: Billett, S., Harteis, C., Gruber, H. (Eds.), International Handbook of Research in Professional and Practice-Based Learning. Springer, Dordrecht, The Netherlands, pp. 611–640.

ONeill, O., 2002. A Question of Trust. Polity Press, Cambridge, UK.

Reason, P., Heron, J., 1986. Research with people: the paradigm of cooperative experiential enquiry. Person-Centred Rev 1, 457–476.

Roberts, N., 2000. Wicked Problems and Network Approaches to Resolution. Int. Public Manage. Rev 1, 1–19.

Sarter, B. (Ed.), 1988. Paths to Knowledge: Innovative Research Methods for Nursing. National League for Nursing, New York, NY.

Schön, D.A., 1995. The Reflective Practitioner: How Professionals Think in Action, new ed. Ashgate, Aldershot Hants, UK.

Sennett, R., 2005. The Culture of the New Capitalism. Yale University Press, New Haven, CT.

Smith, J.K., 1983. Quantitative versus qualitative research: an attempt to clarify the issue. Educ. Res. 12, 6–13.

Stephenson, J., 1998. The concept of capability and its importance in higher education. In: Stephenson, J., Yorke, M. (Eds.), Capability and Quality in Higher Education. Kogan Page, London, UK, pp. 1–13.

Vygotsky, L.S., 1978. Mind in Society: The Development of Higher Psychological Processes. Harvard University Press, Cambridge, MA.

Vygotsky, L.S., 1986. Thought and language, trans. A Kozulin. MIT Press, Cambridge, MA (originally published 1962).

Wenger, E., 1998. Communities of Practice: Learning, Meaning, and Identity. Cambridge University Press, Cambridge, MA.

Yinger, R., Hendricks-Lee, M., 1993. Working knowledge in teaching. In: Day, C., Calderhead, J., Denicolo, P. (Eds.), Research on Teacher Thinking: Understanding Professional Development. Falmer Press, London, UK, pp. 100–123.

3

MULTIPLE SPACES OF CHOICE, ENGAGEMENT AND INFLUENCE IN CLINICAL DECISION MAKING

JOY HIGGS ▪ MARK JONES

CHAPTER AIMS

The aims of this chapter are to:

▪ recast clinical reasoning spaces from the inside out,

▪ examine reasoning strategy choices and

▪ reflect on professional development implications for the practitioner-as-reasoner.

KEY WORDS

Clinical reasoning approaches

Problem spaces

Choices

Engagement

ABBREVIATIONS/ ACRONYMS

HDR Hypothetico-deductive reasoning

INTRODUCTION

Clinical decision making involves people, information, evidence, goals and connections. Each of these elements of decision making operates in situations that could be thought of as spaces where choices, engagement and influences interact. In this chapter, we explore these elements using a model of these decision-making actions, engagement and influences in spaces viewed from the inside out.

CLINICAL REASONING SPACES FROM THE INSIDE OUT

Clinical reasoning could be interpreted as operating in spaces in which different clinical situations are considered, healthcare problem needs or issues are addressed, particular influences are experienced and unique sets of people are engaged in providing client care. Kassirer et al. (2010, p. 311) define the problem space as 'the subject's representation of the task environment that permits the consideration of different problem solutions and sets limitations on possible operations that can be applied to the problem; a sort of maze of mental activity through which individuals wander when searching for a solution to a problem'.

In Fig. 3.1, we can see a number of these clinical reasoning spaces from the inside out. At the centre are the core players, the client and the clinician, addressing the client's clinical needs/problems. Moving outwards, this core team is joined by other people who play a role in the client's care: the healthcare team, carers and other support people such as community services agencies. Many factors influence all of these core and surrounding interactions. These are discussed in Chapter 1 and across the various Section 2 chapters.

CLIENT SPACES

In this book we have elected to use the term 'client' instead of 'patient' to encompass many different roles clients/patients follow and the different approaches to care across different agencies and professions. The role

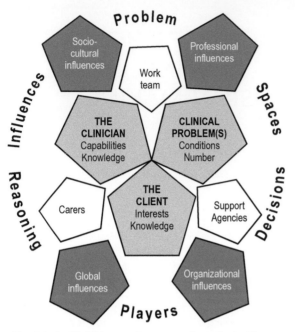

Fig. 3.1 ■ Clinical reasoning spaces from the inside out.

for the client as a consumer of health care is radically different in many respects from the dependent patient role of traditional medicine, where 'autonomy' of healthcare professionals was manifest as maximum control over clinical decision making and clinical intervention. Consumers of health care are becoming increasingly well informed about their health and about healthcare services. Self-help and holistic health care are becoming more central to health care, and the goal of achieving effective participation by consumers in their health care is widespread, requiring healthcare professionals to diminish their decision-making authority and involve their clients actively in clinical decision making when possible.

Increasingly, clients' choices, rights and responsibilities in relation to their health are changing. For some time, people have advocated client involvement in decision making about the management of their health and well-being. Payton et al. (1990), for instance, argued that this process of client participation is based on the 'recognition of the values of self-determination and the worth of the individual' (p. ix). Using understanding of their clients' rights and responsibilities, clinicians

need to develop their own approaches to involving the client in reasoning and decision making. Mutual decision making (see Section 3 chapters) requires not only a sharing of ownership of decisions but also the development of skills in negotiation and explaining to facilitate effective two-way communication. Professional autonomy becomes redefined as independence in function (within a teamwork context) combined with responsibility and accountability for one's actions (including the sharing of decision making). An important aspect of involving patients/clients in clinical decision making is determining and facilitating their appropriate level of participation and responsibility. A level of participation in clinical reasoning appropriate for the individual has been demonstrated to contribute to the client's sense of control; in this process it is important to ensure that the client's input is voluntary and the client is informed of the inherent uncertainties of clinical decision making (Coulter, 2002).

The problem space of clients plays an important role in the process of clinical reasoning because it affects framing, naming and dealing with their healthcare needs and concerns; it comprises:

■ the *personal context* of individual clients, which incorporates such factors as their unique cultural, family, work and socioeconomic frames of reference and their state of health. Each of these factors contributes to clients' beliefs, values and expectations and to their perceptions and needs in relation to their health.
■ the *unique multifaceted context of clients' healthcare needs*. This includes clients' health conditions and their unique personal, social and environmental situation. Clinical problems can be 'confusing and contradictory, characterized by imperfect, inconsistent, or even inaccurate information' (Kassirer and Kopelman, 1991, p. vii).
■ For clients who are seeking health-promotion solutions, healthcare professionals face the task of identifying and dealing with multiple personal and environmental variables to produce an optimal *client-centred solution*.
■ The nature of the *clinical practice world,* which is complex, typically with time pressures and constrained by contextual factors.

PRACTITIONER SPACES

Practitioners bring their personal and professional selves to the task of clinical decision making; these selves frame their problem space. As well as functioning within their personal frames of reference, practitioners operate within their professional frameworks (e.g., the ethical and competency standards/requirements of their profession) and within a broader context of professionalism. The term *health professional* implies a qualified healthcare provider who demonstrates professional autonomy, competence and accountability (Higgs, 1993). Professional status incorporates the responsibility to make unsupervised and accountable clinical decisions and to implement ethical, competent and person-centred practice. This requires healthcare professionals to consider the client's problem space, as described earlier, and to make decisions about the client's level of involvement. Dealing with ill-structured healthcare problems requires high-level clinical reasoning abilities, increasingly refined and elaborated medical and profession-specific knowledge (Schmidt et al., 1990) and judgement (Round, 2001). In relation to ethical issues, practitioners need the ability to deal with these matters in person-centred, professional ways. In addition, practitioners' problem spaces include their individual philosophical paradigms and approaches to practice (see Chapter 3), their clinical reasoning capability, and clinical reasoning expertise (see Chapters 4 and 5).

THE COLLABORATIVE PROBLEM SPACE OF THE TEAM

Most healthcare professionals work in collaboration with other team members, either directly or indirectly via referral. This includes work across mainstream and complementary and alternative medicine. Byrne (1999) suggested that a coordinated and integrated approach to care is particularly important in the management of chronic and complex health problems. Similarly, Grace et al. (2006) identified an increasing preference in clients with chronic health problems, particularly those dissatisfied with mainstream medicine, for practices that directly integrate complementary and alternative medicine with general practice; such models, they found, worked best for clients when both practitioners worked in collaboration. Another area in which multidisciplinary

health care has been found to be beneficial and widespread is chronic pain management (Loftus and Higgs, 2006).

The level of collaboration in clinical decision making in these settings varies considerably. Practitioners may make decisions separately and report decisions to others (e.g., via client records); they may refer clients to others to take over client care or to receive advice; they may operate as a decision-making team making decisions on behalf of their clients; or they may work with clients as members of the decision-making team. Croker and Higgs (2016) reminded us that practitioners are often members of multiple teams with different agendas and modes and roles of decision making.

REFLECTION POINT 1

Consider the changes you make to your practice and your ways of engaging with clients if you are working solo with the client or working in a team.

THE PROBLEM SPACE OF THE WORKPLACE AND THE LOCAL SYSTEM

Clinicians frequently face ill-defined problems, goals that are complex and outcomes that are difficult to predict clearly. Many aspects of the workplace influence clinical decision making, particularly levels of available human, material and economic resources. Many factors in the workplace frame our approaches to our practice of clinical reasoning. Funding pressures create 'clinical practices whose explicit demands are heavily weighted toward management and productivity rather than diagnosis and understanding' (Duffy, 1998, p. 96). Such practices are not conducive to reflecting on our understanding of practice. Further, misinterpretations of what evidence-based practice really requires (see Reilly et al., 2004) means that some clinicians do not use clinical reasoning critically and wisely to assess evidence for its applicability to individual clients (Jones et al., 2006a, 2006b).

THE KNOWLEDGE-REASONING SPACE OF CLINICAL DECISION MAKING

Three considerations are pertinent in considering this knowledge-reasoning space. First, professional judgement and decision making within the ambiguous or uncertain situations of health care are an inexact science (Kennedy, 1987). Checkland (1981) refers to 'soft systems' (like healthcare systems) as those in which goals may be unrecognizable and outcomes ambiguous; these are typically social rather than physical world focussed. In such contexts, reasoning and judgement are highly valued and essential: simple answers that neatly fit the given situation are rarely prelearnable. Second, reasoning involves the three core elements of cognition, knowledge and metacognition. Third, judgement is referential rather than absolute. It occurs within knowledge cultures and paradigms as discussed in Chapter 1. Practitioners' judgements are influenced by codes of conduct, norms, the knowledge-base of their professions and the knowledge and particular approach of the individual.

THE PROBLEM SPACE OF THE GLOBAL HEALTH CARE SYSTEM WITH ITS DISCOURSE, KNOWLEDGE AND TECHNOLOGY

Many factors of the wider healthcare environment need to be taken into consideration in clinical reasoning. Healthcare professionals need to develop a broad understanding of the environment in which they work, including knowledge of the factors influencing health (e.g., the environment, socioeconomic conditions, cultural beliefs and human behaviour). In addition, they need to understand how the information age and the technological revolutions have affected healthcare demands, provision and expectation. They need to be able to work confidently and effectively with an increasing body of scientific, technical and professional knowledge. Developing a sound individual understanding of clinical reasoning and a capacity to reason effectively will facilitate the clinician's ability to manage complex and changing information.

ERRORS

Avoiding errors in clinical reasoning requires attributes of skilled critical thinking including open-mindedness, consideration of other perspectives, awareness and critique of assumptions and more deliberate analysis as a backup of quick first-impression judgements often

based on fixed clinical patterns and habitual practice. Rather than unquestioningly accepting information, skilled critical thinking within clinical reasoning fosters a sort of healthy scepticism that appraises information for its accuracy, completeness and relevance to facilitate understanding and identification of solutions. Errors in the cognition of clinical reasoning (e.g., information perception, interpretation, analysis) can be linked to the various forms of human bias evidenced in health- and non–health-related human judgement (Hogarth, 2005; Lehrer, 2009; Schwartz and Elstein, 2008). The priming influence of prior information (e.g., diagnosis provided in a referral, imaging findings, influence of a recent publication or course) and the tendency to attend to and collect data that confirm existing hypotheses (i.e., confirmation bias) are two classic examples. These errors are commonly associated with habits of thinking and practice that themselves are a potential risk for inaccurate pattern recognition. That is, in adopting a pattern recognition approach the novice or unreflective practitioner might focus too much on looking for the presence or absence of specific patterns and overlook other potentially important information or might find it difficult to see anything outside the most familiar patterns. Patterns can become rigid, making it difficult to recognize variations or alternatives.

Within the changing face of health care and the trend towards more biopsychosocial practice that values qualitative information of the client's experience alongside quantitative biomedical measures, there is a need to look beyond the cognitive processes and cognitive errors of the clinician. Errors in psychosocial or 'narrative' focussed reasoning can be manifest as having no consideration of psychosocial factors or engaging in superficial assessment based on insufficient information.

Questionnaires relating to psychosocial status can be helpful to quantitatively score a client's status on the construct(s) assessed, but they require complementary exploration through the client interview. That is, three clients may tick the same questionnaire box but for significantly different reasons. Practitioners who wish to adopt a client-centred approach or a team approach may make errors related to inauthentic implementation of espoused models of practice, lack of valuing or inclusion of the knowledge and reasoning input of team members or clients and limitations in interpersonal communication, including cultural incompetence. Errors can also be made in the realm of ethical reasoning, for example in the application of the principles of ethics to the client's individual circumstances (see Chapter 16) and with respect to shared decision making (see Section 3 chapters) and dilemmas in dealing with the client's wishes, informed position and power, which may be in conflict with what the practitioner considers to be in the client's best interests.

Errors of reasoning can be reduced through greater understanding of clinical reasoning generally and greater understanding and critique of your own clinical reasoning. The risk for uncritical pattern recognition can be offset by strategies that minimize the assumptions frequently underpinning pattern recognition. Such error-avoidance strategies include screening to ensure information is not missed or inaccurate; qualifying clients' meanings, consideration and, if justified, testing for competing hypotheses; and openly subjecting and comparing your reasoning to others' reasoning.

REFLECTION POINT 2

Can you identify any habits of practice in your own work? What strategies could you employ to ensure any habits you may have are sufficiently justified?

CLINICAL REASONING STRATEGIES

In various chapters of this book, a number of interpretations of clinical reasoning are discussed from the perspectives of different disciplines, the history of clinical reasoning research and models of practice within which clinical reasoning occurs. In Table 3.1 we present an overview of key models, strategies and interpretations of clinical reasoning. These been divided into two groups: cognitive and interactive models.

Examining the Range of Clinical Reasoning Strategies

Many authors have written about different clinical reasoning strategies and processes. A summary of the most common ones that appear in the literature is presented in Table 3.1 based on the historical work of such researchers as Arocha et al. (1993); Barrows et al. (1978); Bordage and Lemieux (1991); Boshuizen and Schmidt (1992a, 1992b); Edwards et al. (1998); Elstein

et al. (1978); Mattingly and Fleming (1994); Neufeld et al. (1981); Patel et al. (1988); and later publications such as Coulter (2005); Lipton (2004); and Loftus (2006). Examples of scholarly reviews with critique of existing models and implications for teaching include Banning (2007); Eva (2004); Kinchin and Cabot (2010); and Norman (2005).

Factors Influencing Choices About Clinical Reasoning Strategies

Although clinical reasoning should be able to be justified in professional and public discourse, the choice of strategy cannot be prescribed beyond discipline-specific agreements regarding the breadth of scope and range of strategies appropriate. The strategies and processes described in Table 3.1 feature to some extent across most health professions represented in this book.

Hypothetico-deductive reasoning (HDR) in the health professions traditionally refers to the process of formulating hypotheses based on specific features in the client's presentation and linked to established criteria (i.e., premises) for a type of clinical judgement (e.g., diagnosis). Formal 'testing' of initial hypotheses is said to occur through the collection of additional information such that when the judgement criteria are fulfilled the healthcare professional can deduce a specific hypothesis is confirmed or at least supported. Although diagnosis is perhaps the category of clinical judgement most researched and described in the literature, other categories of judgement where profession-specific criteria exist similarly use this process, for example clinical judgements regarding the need for caution in the examination and management, the need for referral for further medical consultation and judgements regarding prognosis (see Hypothesis Category framework Chapter 23).

Pattern recognition occurs when features in the client's presentation are sufficiently familiar to the practitioner to enable recognition of a clinical pattern, and so further 'testing' through hypothetico-deductive reasoning is not essential. Pattern recognition is most commonly associated with diagnostic clinical judgements; however, pattern recognition is part of all human perception (Kahneman, 2011), and examples will be evident across all health professions' areas of practice with differences perhaps more related to the extent they are relied on. Chapter 23 provides examples of different

TABLE 3.1			
Models and Interpretations of Clinical Reasoning (CR)			
View	**Model**	**Related Terms**	**Description**
CR as Cognitive Process	Hypothetico-deductive reasoning	Procedural reasoning Diagnostic reasoning Induction-related probabilistic reasoning	The generation of hypotheses based on clinical data and knowledge and testing of these hypotheses through further inquiry. It is used by novices and in problematic situations by experts. Hypothesis generation and testing involve both inductive reasoning (moving from a set of specific observations to a generalization) to generate hypotheses and slower detailed deductive reasoning (moving from a generalization – if – to a conclusion – then – in relation to a specific case) to test hypotheses. Procedural reasoning identifying the client's functional problems and selecting procedures to manage them.
	Pattern recognition	Pattern interpretation Inductive reasoning Categorization Mental representations	Expert reasoning in nonproblematic situations resembles pattern recognition or direct automatic retrieval of information from a well-structured knowledge base. New cases are categorized, that is, similarities are recognized (signs, symptoms, treatment options, outcomes, context) in relation to previously experienced clinical cases. Through the use of inductive reasoning, pattern recognition/interpretation is a process characterized by speed and efficiency, albeit with risk for error if relied on in the absence of adequate knowledge and experience. With increasing experience, clinicians move through three kinds of mental representations, from basic mechanisms of disease to illness scripts of clinical features and semantic qualifiers to exemplars derived from experience.
	Forward reasoning; Backward reasoning Abductive reasoning	Inductive reasoning Deductive reasoning Inference to the best explanation	Forward reasoning describes inductive reasoning in which data analysis results in hypothesis generation or diagnosis, utilizing a sound knowledge base. Backward reasoning is the reinterpretation of data or the acquisition of new clarifying data invoked to test a hypothesis. Forward reasoning is more likely to occur in familiar cases with experienced clinicians and backward reasoning with inexperienced clinicians or in atypical or difficult cases. Abductive reasoning, also called inference to the best explanation, refers to theorizing, typically regarding causal mechanisms, clinicians engage in when confronted with unexpected or unfamiliar information that cannot be deduced from established or accepted prior knowledge. It is an unproven, creative explanatory hypothesis for an area of clinical judgements when clear deductions are not available.
	Knowledge reasoning integration		Clinical reasoning involves the integration of knowledge, reasoning and metacognition. Clinical reasoning requires domain-specific knowledge and an organized knowledge base. With experience, clinical reasoning and the associated knowledge drawn on may progress through stages culminating in both exemplars and memory of specific client instances.
	Intuitive reasoning	Instance scripts Inductive reasoning Heuristics Pattern matching	'Intuitive knowledge' is related to 'instance scripts' or past experience with specific cases that can be used unconsciously in inductive reasoning. Intuition may be associated with the use of advanced reasoning strategies or heuristics. Such heuristics include pattern matching and listing (or listing items relevant to the working plan).

TABLE 3.1			
Models and Interpretations of Clinical Reasoning (CR) *(Continued)*			
View	**Model**	**Related Terms**	**Description**
CR as Interactive Process	Multidisciplinary reasoning	Interprofessional reasoning Team decision making	Members of a multidisciplinary team working together to make clinical decisions for the client, about the client's condition, e.g., at case conferences, multidisciplinary clinics.
	Conditional reasoning	Predictive reasoning Projected reasoning	Used by practitioners to estimate client responses to treatment and likely outcomes of management and to help clients consider possibilities and reconstruct their lives after injury or the onset of disease.
	Narrative reasoning		Reasoning associated with understanding the client's narrative (i.e., story) with respect to his or her pain, illness and/or disability experiences incorporating the client's personal perspectives on his or her experiences.
	Interactive reasoning		Reasoning guiding the purposeful establishment and ongoing management of client-clinician rapport important to understanding the client's perspective and overall outcome.
	Collaborative reasoning	Mutual decision making	The shared decision making between client and clinician (and others) as a therapeutic alliance in the interpretation of examination findings, setting of goals and priorities and implementation and progression of treatment.
	Ethical reasoning	Pragmatic reasoning	Reasoning underpinning the recognition and resolution of moral, political and economic ethical dilemmas that impinge upon the patient's ability to make decisions concerning his or her health and upon the conduct of treatment and its desired goals.
	Teaching as reasoning		Reasoning associated with the planning, execution and evaluation of individualized and context sensitive teaching, including education for conceptual understanding (e.g., diagnosis, disability, management options), education for physical performance (e.g., rehabilitative exercises) and education for behavioural change.

types of clinical patterns described in physiotherapy practice such as diagnostic and clinical syndromes.

Narrative (or psychosocial) focussed reasoning some would argue exists as the opposite pole to diagnostic focussed reasoning with expert physiotherapists described as being able to dialectically move in their focus and reasoning between these two poles as unfolding client information requires (Edwards et al., 2004). Narrative reasoning sits in the 'Interactive Process' half of Table 3.1 as the process of coming to understand a client's narrative with respect to his or her pain, illness and/or disability experience. Incorporating the client's personal perspectives on his or her experiences is seen as a collaborative understanding reached between client and health professional rather than a biological impairment that can be reduced to objective measurement.

Selecting a Reasoning Approach

Because HDR can be applied to any reasoning that formulates and tests hypotheses, it is likely to manifest in every health profession and with all client types. As a slower analytical process, it is often associated with the novice who lacks sufficient knowledge and experience to recognize clinical patterns and hence must consider and test a broader list of hypotheses not required by the 'expert'. Experts may revert to HDR in complex or unfamiliar cases. Use of HDR will therefore depend on the experience and knowledge of the practitioner, his or her familiarity with the clinical presentation, the nature of the clinical judgements he or she is called to make (e.g., diagnostic versus narrative) and unfortunately perhaps also the time allocated per client. However, even with narrative reasoning, knowledge and experience enable identification of typical features of potentially restricting or facilitating psychosocial factors that elicit further investigation. Ultimately a hypothesis is still formed with perhaps the key difference being the validation of judgement is reached through client–practitioner consensus, not independent measurement.

Each of the other reasoning strategies categorized as interactive processes in Table 3.1 is relevant to contemporary, holistic health care across all health professions. They would occur, implicitly or explicitly, with all healthcare professionals directly involved in client assessment and management to varying extent and ability depending on their personal philosophy of practice and responsibilities they assume.

Knowledge reasoning integration relates to all reasoning strategies because all reasoning is informed by the health professions' and individuals' knowledge as shaped and organized by their ontology regarding what constitutes knowledge (fact or truth) and their combined research- and experience-based evidence. The role of intuitive reasoning in health professions' practice continues to be contentious (Banning, 2007; Hogarth, 2005; Kinchin and Cabot, 2010) featuring more strongly in Nursing and Occupational Therapy research and practice descriptions (Banning, 2007; Fleming and Mattingly, 2008) than other health professions. The issue is not so much whether intuition exists. As Herbert Simon, best known for his seminal problem-solving research with chess masters, explains, intuition is 'nothing more and nothing less than recognition' (Simon, 1992, p. 155). Accurate intuitions of experts are best explained by the effects of prolonged practice. The question is, can the tacit knowledge and intuitive reasoning skilfully used by experts, but also a bias to those who rely on first impressions without further analysis (Kahneman, 2011), be made explicit for others to learn from with safeguards in place to minimize bias?

PROFESSIONAL DEVELOPMENT OF CLINICAL REASONING CAPABILITY

In pursuit of continuing professional development in relation to clinical reasoning, we could consider expertise in reasoning to be the ultimate goal. In a review of clinical reasoning literature in medicine, Norman (2005) suggested that there may not be a single representation of clinical reasoning expertise or a single correct way to solve a problem. He noted that 'the more one studies the clinical expert, the more one marvels at the complex and multidimensional components of knowledge and skill that she or he brings to bear on the problem, and the amazing adaptability she must possess to achieve the goal of effective care' (p. 426).

Clinical reasoning and clinical practice expertise is a journey, an aspiration and a commitment to achieving the best practice that one can provide. Rather than being a point of arrival, complacency and lack of questioning by self or others, expertise requires both the capacity to recognize one's limitations and practice capabilities and the ability to pursue professional development in a spirit of self-critique. And, it is – or at least we should expect it to be – not only a self-referenced level of capability or mode of practice; it is also a search for understanding of and realization of the standards and expectations set by the community being served and the profession and service organization being represented. In Fig. 3.1, such characteristics and expectations of experts are presented.

We have added the idea of expectations to this discussion to emphasize that any human construct is sociohistorically situated. Beyond a research-driven science-based view of technical expertise, there is a need for any professional, but particularly experts, with his or her claim to superior service and performance, to address the needs of society. There is a growing expectation of client-centred humanization (including cultural competence, information sharing, collaborative decision making, virtuous practice) of expert practice that turns healthcare professional expertise into a collaborative professional relationship rather than an expert-empowered, technically superior, practitioner-centred approach. As highlighted in the research findings of Jensen et al. (2006), this client-centred approach is grounded in a strong moral commitment to beneficence or doing what is in the client's best interest. This manifests in therapists' nonjudgemental attitude and strong emphasis on client education, with expert therapists being willing to serve as client advocate or moral agent in helping them be successful.

Box 3.1 demonstrates an evolution in thinking about expertise, beginning with the classic research by Glaser and Chi (1988) of expert attributes. In 2000, we added to this view ideas of client-centredness, collaboration,

BOX 3.1

CHARACTERISTICS, EXPECTATIONS AND EMERGING ABILITIES
OF EXPERT PRACTITIONERS

a) General characteristics of experts (Glaser and Chi, 1988)
  - Experts excel mainly in their own domains.
  - Experts perceive large meaningful patterns in their domain.
  - Experts are fast: they are faster than novices at performing the skills of their domain, and they quickly solve problems with little error.
  - Experts have superior short-term and long-term memory.
  - Experts see and represent a problem in their domain at a deeper (more principled) level than novices; novices tend to represent a problem at a superficial level.
  - Experts spend a great deal of time analyzing a problem qualitatively.
  - Experts have strong self-monitoring skills.

b) Characteristics and expectations of health professional experts (Higgs and Jones, 2000)
  - Experts need to pursue shared decision making between client and clinician if 'success' is to be realized from the client's perspective.
  - Experts need to monitor and manage their cognitive processes (i.e., to use metacognition) to achieve high-quality decision-making and practice action.
  - Experts critically use propositional and experience-based up-to-date practice knowledge to inform their practice.
  - Expertise requires the informed use and recognition of patient-centred practice.
  - Expert practitioners are mentors and critical companions (see Titchen, 2000) to less experienced practitioners.
  - Experts are expected to communicate effectively with clients, colleagues and families and to justify clinical decisions articulately.
  - Experts should demonstrate cultural competence.

c) Further characteristics and expectations of expert professionals (Higgs and Jones, 2008)
  - Experts demonstrate information and communication literacy.
  - Experts value and utilize the expertise of other team members.
  - Experts own and embody their practice model.
  - Expertise goes beyond technical expertise in pursuit of emancipatory practice.
  - Expert practice is community oriented.
  - Expertise is informed by reflexive practice and research.
  - Expert decision making is informed by the health and demographic trends in the communities they serve.
  - Experts' behaviour demonstrates a strong moral commitment to beneficence through such behaviours as patient advocacy and nonjudgemental attitudes.

d) Emerging expectations of expert professionals
  - Experts retain creativity and imagination.
  - Experts appreciate the value of wisdom in practice.
  - Experts look beyond their professional backgrounds for ideas and strategies.
  - Experts look into innovative spaces for practice.
  - Experts learn to balance economics and entrepreneurship with professional practice.
  - Experts demonstrate epistemological and ontological fluency (see Chapter 2).
  - Experts survive and flourish in the face of difficult problems and situations.

metacognition, mentoring, effective communication and cultural competence (Higgs and Jones, 2000). In 2008, we added the third group of characteristics for the third edition (Higgs and Jones, 2008). The fourth section added in this edition reflects messages in this book about the evolution of context and approaches to clinical reasoning.

We propose that clinical expertise, of which clinical reasoning is a critical component, be viewed as a continuum along multiple dimensions. These dimensions include clinical outcomes, personal attributes such as professional judgement, technical clinical skills, communication and interpersonal skills (to involve the client and others in decision making and to consider the client's perspectives), a sound knowledge base, an informed and chosen practice model and philosophy of practice, as well as cognitive and metacognitive proficiency.

A related concept to expertise is professional artistry, which 'reflects both high quality of professional practice and the qualities inherent in such artistic or flexible, person-centred, highly reflexive practice' (Paterson and Higgs, 2001, p. 2). Professional artistry refers to 'practical knowledge, skilful performance or knowing as doing' (Fish, 1998, p. 87) that is developed through the acquisition of a deep and relevant knowledge base and extensive experience (Beeston and Higgs, 2001). Professional artistry reflects a uniquely individual view within a shared tradition involving a blend of practitioner qualities, practice skills and creative imagination processes (Higgs and Titchen, 2001). Paterson (2003) combined this idea with clinical reasoning to develop the concept and practice of professional practice judgement artistry (see Paterson and Higgs, 2008; Paterson et al., 2012). Similarly, 'practice wisdom' challenges our ideas of what it means to bring knowledge and wisdom, plus reasoning and judgement artistry, into the act of clinical decision making.

CHAPTER SUMMARY

In this chapter, we have portrayed clinical reasoning as a complex set of processes and interactions occurring within multiple and multidimensional problem spaces. The complexity of clinical reasoning in the health professions is evident in the scope of reasoning required to address the full range of biopsychosocial factors that can contribute to clients' health problems and experiences. Adding to this complexity, healthcare professionals have at their disposal a broad range of clinical reasoning strategies to understand their clients and their clients' health problems to assist their collaborative management. Although these reasoning processes have relevance to all areas of health professions' practice, their use varies across professions (see Section 4 of this book). Greater understanding of the spaces in which clinical reasoning occurs and of the reasoning strategies that can be used will assist healthcare professionals' understanding of their own clinical reasoning. Errors of reasoning are linked to different forms of human bias and can be reduced through greater understanding of clinical reasoning generally and greater understanding and critique of your own clinical reasoning. Professional development is an essential part of ensuring the quality of clinical reasoning and the capability of professionals performing this key practice.

REFLECTION POINT 3

What clinical reasoning strategies can you identify in your own practice? How might you improve your clinical reasoning abilities?

REFERENCES

Arocha, J.F., Patel, V.L., Patel, Y.C., 1993. Hypothesis generation and the coordination of theory and evidence in novice diagnostic reasoning. Med. Decis. Making 13, 198–211.

Banning, M., 2007. A review of clinical decision making: models and current research. J. Clin. Nurs. 17, 187–195.

Barrows, H.S., Feightner, J.W., Neufield, V.R., et al., 1978. An analysis of the clinical methods of medical students and physicians. Report to the Province of Ontario Department of Health. McMaster University, Hamilton, ONT.

Beeston, S., Higgs, J., 2001. Professional practice: artistry and connoisseurship. In: Higgs, J., Titchen, A. (Eds.), Practice Knowledge and Expertise in the Health Professions. Butterworth-Heinemann, Oxford, UK, pp. 108–117.

Bordage, G., Lemieux, M., 1991. Semantic structures and diagnostic thinking of experts and novices. Acad. Med. 66, S70–S72.

Boshuizen, H.P.A., Schmidt, H.G., 1992a. Biomedical knowledge and clinical expertise. Cogn. Sci. 16, 153–184.

Boshuizen, H.P.A., Schmidt, H.G., 1992b. On the role of biomedical knowledge in clinical reasoning by experts, intermediates and novices. Cogn. Sci. 16, 153–184.

Byrne, C., 1999. Interdisciplinary education in undergraduate health sciences. Pedagogue (Perspectives on Health Sciences Education) 3, 1–8.

Checkland, P.B., 1981. Systems Thinking: Systems Practice. John Wiley & Sons, New York, NY.

Coulter, A., 2002. The Autonomous Patient: Ending Paternalism in Medical Care. The Nuffield Trust, London, UK.

Coulter, A., 2005. Shared decision-making: the debate continues. Health Expect. 8, 95–96.

Croker, A., Higgs, J., 2016. Reinterpreting professional relationships in healthcare: the question of collaboration. In: Croker, A., Higgs, J., Trede, F. (Eds.), Collaborating in Healthcare: Reinterpreting Therapeutic Relationships. Sense, Rotterdam, The Netherlands, pp. 3–16.

Duffy, J., 1998. Stroke with dysarthria: evaluate and treat; garden variety or down the garden path. Semin. Speech Lang. 19, 93–98.

Edwards, I.C., Jones, M.A., Carr, J., et al., 1998. Clinical reasoning in three different fields of physiotherapy: a qualitative study. In: Proceedings of the Fifth International Congress of the Australian Physiotherapy Association. Melbourne, VIC, pp. 298–300.

Edwards, I., Jones, M., Carr, J., et al., 2004. Clinical reasoning strategies in physical therapy. Phys. Ther. 84, 312–315.

Elstein, A.S., Shulman, L.S., Sprafka, S.A., 1978. Medical Problem Solving: An Analysis of Clinical Reasoning. Harvard University Press, Cambridge, MA.

Eva, K.W., 2004. What every teacher needs to know about clinical reasoning. Med. Educ. 39, 98–106.

Fish, D., 1998. Appreciating Practice in the Caring Professions: Refocusing Professional Development and Practitioner Research. Butterworth-Heinemann, Oxford, UK.

Fleming, M.H., Mattingly, C., 2008. Action and narrative: two dynamics of clinical reasoning. In: Higgs, J., Jones, M., Loftus, S., et al. (Eds.), Clinical Reasoning in the Health Professions, third ed. Elsevier, Edinburgh, pp. 55–64.

Glaser, R., Chi, M.T.H., 1988. Overview. In: Chi, M.T.H., Glaser, R., Farr, M.J. (Eds.), The Nature of Expertise. Lawrence Erlbaum, Hillsdale, NJ, pp. xv–xxviii.

Grace, S., Higgs, J., Horsfall, D., 2006. Integrating mainstream and complementary and alternative medicine: investing in prevention. In: Proceedings of The University of Sydney From Cell to Society 5: Proceedings of the Health Research Conference, 9–10 November. The University of Sydney, Sydney, Australia, pp. 18–25.

Higgs, J., 1993. Physiotherapy, professionalism and self-directed learning. J. Singapore Physiother. Assoc. 14, 8–11.

Higgs, J., Jones, M., 2000. Clinical Reasoning in the Health Professions. In: Higgs, J., Jones, M. (Eds.), Clinical Reasoning in the Health Professions, second ed. Butterworth-Heinemann, Oxford, UK, pp. 3–14.

Higgs, J., Jones, M., 2008. Clinical decision making and multiple problem spaces. In: Higgs, J., Jones, M., Loftus, S., et al. (Eds.), Clinical Reasoning in the Health Professions, third ed. Elsevier, Edinburgh, pp. 3–17.

Higgs, J., Titchen, A., 2001. Towards professional artistry and creativity in practice. In: Higgs, J., Titchen, A. (Eds.), Professional Practice in Health, Education and the Creative Arts. Blackwell Science, Oxford, UK, pp. 273–290.

Hogarth, R.M., 2005. Deciding analytically or trusting your intuition? The advantages and disadvantages of analytic and intuitive thought. In: Betsch, T., Haberstroh, S. (Eds.), The Routines of Decision Making. Lawrence Erlbaum Associates, Mahwah, NJ, pp. 67–82.

Jensen, G.M., Gwyer, J., Hack, L.M., et al., 2006. Expertise in Physical Therapy Practice, second ed. Saunders-Elsevier, St. Louis, MO.

Jones, M., Grimmer, K., Edwards, I., et al., 2006a. Challenges in applying best evidence to physiotherapy. IJAHSP 4.

Jones, M., Grimmer, K., Edwards, I., et al., 2006b. Challenges in applying best evidence to physiotherapy practice: part 2—reasoning and practice challenges. IJAHSP 4.

Kahneman, D., 2011. Thinking, Fast and Slow. Allen Lane, London, UK.

Kassirer, J.P., Kopelman, R.I., 1991. Learning Clinical Reasoning. Williams & Wilkins, Baltimore, MD.

Kassirer, J., Wong, J., Kopelman, R., 2010. Learning Clinical Reasoning. Wolters Kluwer, Lippincott Williams & Wilkins, Philadelphia, PA.

Kennedy, M., 1987. Inexact sciences: professional education and the development of expertise. Rev. Res. Educ. 14, 133–168.

Kinchin, I.M., Cabot, L.B., 2010. Reconsidering the dimensions of expertise: from linear stages towards dual processing. London Rev. Educ. 8, 153–166.

Lehrer, J., 2009. How We Decide. Houghton Mifflin Harcourt, Boston, MA.

Lipton, P., 2004. Inference to the Best Explanation, second ed. Routledge, London, UK.

Loftus, S., 2006. Language in Clinical Reasoning: Learning and Using the Language of Collective Clinical Decision Making. Doctoral thesis. University of Sydney, Sydney, NSW. Available from: http://ses.library.usyd.edu.au/handle/2123/1165. viewed 20 February 2017.

Loftus, S., Higgs, J., 2006. Clinical decision-making in multidisciplinary clinics. In: Flor, H., Kalso, E., Dostrovsky, J.O. (Eds.), Proceedings of the 11th World Congress on Pain: International Association for the Study of Pain. IASP Press, Seattle, WA, pp. 755–760.

Mattingly, C., Fleming, M.H., 1994. Clinical Reasoning: Forms of Inquiry in a Therapeutic Practice. FA Davis, Philadelphia, PA.

Neufeld, V.R., Norman, G.R., Barrows, H.S., et al., 1981. Clinical problem-solving by medical students: a longitudinal and cross-sectional analysis. Med. Educ. 15, 315–322.

Norman, G., 2005. Research in clinical reasoning: past history and current trends. Med. Educ. 39, 418–427.

Patel, V.L., Evans, D.A., Groen, G.J., 1988. Biomedical knowledge and clinical reasoning. In: Evans, D.A., Patel, V.L. (Eds.), Cognitive Science in Medicine: Biomedical Modeling. MIT Press, Cambridge, MA, pp. 49–108.

Paterson, M.L., 2003. Professional Practice Judgement Artistry in Occupational Therapy, Doctoral Thesis. University of Sydney, Sydney, NSW.

Paterson, M., Higgs, J., 2001. Professional Practice Judgement Artistry. CPEA Occasional Paper 3. The Centre for Professional Education Advancement. University of Sydney, Sydney, NSW.

Paterson, M., Higgs, J., 2008. Professional practice judgement artistry. In: Higgs, J., Jones, M., Loftus, S., et al. (Eds.), Clinical Reasoning in the Health Professions, third ed. Elsevier, Edinburgh, pp. 181–189.

Paterson, M., Higgs, J., Donnelly, C., 2012. Artistry and expertise. In: Robertson, L. (Ed.), Clinical Reasoning in Occupational Therapy: Controversies in Practice. Wiley-Blackwell, Oxford, UK, pp. 93–106.

Payton, O.D., Nelson, C.E., Ozer, M.N., 1990. Patient Participation in Program Planning: A Manual for Therapists. FA Davis, Philadelphia, PA.

Reilly, S., Douglas, J., Oates, J., 2004. Evidence-Based Practice in Speech Pathology. Whurr, London, UK.

Round, A.P., 2001. Introduction to clinical reasoning. J. Eval. Clin. Pract. 7, 109–117.

Schmidt, H.G., Norman, G.R., Boshuizen, H.P.A., 1990. A cognitive perspective on medical expertise: theory and implications. Acad. Med. 65, 611–621.

Schwartz, A., Elstein, A.S., 2008. Clinical reasoning in medicine. In: Higgs, J., Jones, M., Loftus, S., et al. (Eds.), Clinical Reasoning in the Health Professions, third ed. Elsevier, Edinburgh, pp. 223–234.

Simon, H., 1992. What is an 'explanation' of behavior? Psychol. Sci. 3, 150–161.

Titchen, A., 2000. Professional Craft Knowledge in Patient Centred Nursing and the Facilitation of its Development. Ashdale Press, Oxford, UK.

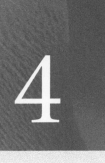

4

CLINICAL REASONING AND MODELS OF PRACTICE

JOY HIGGS ■ FRANZISKA TREDE

CHAPTER AIMS

The aims of this chapter are to:

- reflect on factors influencing practice approaches in general and clinical reasoning in particular,
- critically present different models for practice,
- support a Critical Social Science Model as a basis for practice and
- encourage practitioners to critically develop their own practice models.

KEY WORDS

Practice models
Clinical reasoning
Critical social science

INTRODUCTION

Healthcare practice operates in increasingly more complex, diverse and uncertain environments. Patients and clients of health care are better informed, technology is advancing, and healthcare practice is constantly changing. It is important in this context to adopt an informed and critical stance to practice. Being aware of the interests that drive and frame practice and practice models and understanding the way these models influence practice actions and clinical reasoning are necessary aspects for practitioners to be responsible and critically competent in demanding work environments. In this chapter, we examine different practice models and propose advantages in relevant contexts of adopting a critical practice model. The importance of critique in today's challenging and dynamic healthcare environments is linked to practitioners reclaiming their human agency and critical reflection capacity in practice models that underpin practice reasoning, action and reflexive review.

RECOGNIZING OUR PRACTICE CONTEXT AND INFLUENCES

Neither clinical reasoning nor professional practice, as a whole, occurs in a vacuum. We can think of acts of health care, client–practitioner(s) interactions and the progress of clients towards well-being as occurring in layered contexts of practice. These layers include (from the inside out) the immediate situation and needs of clients, the particular goals and interests of the practitioners working with clients to facilitate their well-being, the roles and inputs of clients' families and carers, the influences and inputs of the local healthcare setting, the wider influences of the communities of professional practice that set standards and norms of practice and the wider systems of institutional, healthcare system requirements and resources and the national and global healthcare arenas. All of these influences affect the nature of healthcare choices made by and centred on clients as part of collaborative clinical decision making and their health outcomes. In this chapter, we explore the place of models of practice created and enacted by practitioners, professions and healthcare teams as

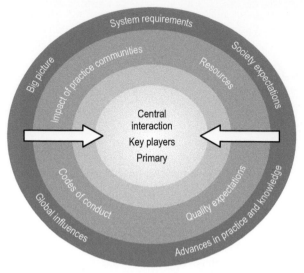

Fig. 4.1 ■ Influences (local and global) in healthcare interactions.

they work across these layered contexts of practice (Fig. 4.1).

REFLECTION POINT 1

We invite you to think about the outer circle of Fig. 4.1 and take seriously our opening statement that *Neither clinical reasoning nor professional practice, as a whole, occurs in a vacuum.* What are the world's biggest health problems and recent policies of the World Health Organization that national healthcare systems and healthcare professions are engaging with? Can you list a few of the global agendas? We often lose the connection between the global, national and local picture, and it is seductive to reduce health models to the biomedical level. Starting to think about the big picture first influences practice models and clinical reasoning processes at the micro level. What connections exist between how these global influences, society expectations, advances in technology and research knowledge influence your central interaction with patients and colleagues?

Understanding and Valuing Interests and Priorities

Clinical reasoning is a challenging undertaking. It is influenced by a complex interplay between different interests and priorities that can range from wanting to

assert professional authority and control over healthcare situations, to wanting to negotiate common ground with clients and create meaning, to striving to learn, transform and change oneself and one's clients. This discussion is framed by Habermas' (1972) theory of cognitive interests, in which he argued that ideas shape our interests and actions. Here we explore the link between interests and the actions of clinical reasoning and clinical practice. Interests can be thought of as the motivation for wanting to think and act in certain ways. Such motivation can be internally driven by values, attitudes and desires, such as a humanistic perspective, valuing of rationality or wanting to be patient-centred. Interests can also be shaped by external interests, such as pressures to adhere to the dominant healthcare practice model, system imperatives such as economic rationalism, society and peer expectations of professional behaviour and trends and discourse in health care.

Healthcare professionals are accountable and accept responsibility for their decisions and actions. What values, assumptions and reasons underpin and guide their thinking and decisions? Often such interests are subconscious and have been acquired through the pervasive and often osmotic process of professional socialization (Eraut, 1994) rather than being consciously learned and adopted through critical self-appraisal and informed choice of a desired model of practice. Once practitioners are aware of their interests and understand what motivates these interests, they are in a better position to make critically conscious choices as to how they seek to frame their clinical reasoning and consequent actions.

The Social and Historical Construction of Practice Approaches

Professional practice is socially and historically constructed (Higgs, 2016, p. 191): "it comprises individual and shared activities and expectations across a community of practice; it is manifest in language, discourses and traditions; its conduct is linked to morality and ethical conduct; its standards and implementation are regulated and evaluated by individual practitioners as well as the practice community, external authorities and society; it is manifest in a range of levels of expertise development; and beyond all of this, practice is embodied through practical consciousness". Deliberate professionals need this understanding of practice as they knowingly create their practice models and take ownership of their clinical reasoning, decision making and, ultimately, the outcomes of their practice actions.

The Shaping of Practice Models: The Place of Ideology

We tend to interpret and justify our clinical reasoning processes with theoretical knowledge and research findings without acknowledging the interests and assumptions that inform our practice. Practice is justified with theories, guidelines and professional training. The ideology behind these theories and training remains hidden. To bring the assumptions out of hiding and question our way of reasoning enhances our practice awareness and provides us with real choices about practicing optimally in each given clinical context.

It would be simplistic and limiting for a profession to define its practice purely on the basis of technical knowledge and skills (Schön, 1987). This would reduce practice to the aspects that can be measured with empirico-analytical evidence only. What we observe and what we do must be interpreted to make sense for us and to be communicated to others. Measurements and numbers on their own are meaningless. As professions develop and mature, they become more involved with questions of expertise development and knowledge growth. Higgs et al. (1999) claimed that a mature profession is one that enters into dialogue about its practices, is self-reflective and proactively transforms with global changes.

Professional ideology and interests, whether consciously or unconsciously enacted, inform practice models and professional practice (Newman, 1994). Professional ideology is made up of the values, assumptions and prejudgements that guide our thinking (Therborn, 1999). The type of practice we aspire to enact, the type of knowledge and evidence we value and utilize in practice, the way we justify our way of practicing and our clinical reasoning are all informed by interests that guide our curiosity in the first place.

Workplace Influences

Trede's (2006) research on clinical practice approaches identified the importance and effect of external context factors on the preferred or existing practice model of the practitioners and the workplace. She found that the level of acceptability of the technical biomedical model was high in situations where the environment was 'hi-tech', and healthcare delivery relied on advanced technology and in acute care or emergency situations where patients were very ill or required critical care. In such arenas, there was an unchallenged focus on pathological diagnoses and biomedical intervention approaches, with the expectation of patient compliance. In less acute and less technology-dependent healthcare settings, participants in Trede's research considered that there was greater opportunity for patient-centred care that involved patient participation in clinical decision making. The notion of emancipatory practice was foreign to most of the participants, and in early discussions they considered that in their workplace situations, with high workloads, time pressures, medical model frameworks, traditional approaches to professional hierarchies and an emphasis on evidence-based practice and cost efficiency, that moves to treat patients on an equal footing in terms of clinical decision making were not particularly feasible, expected or needed.

Working Across and Within Different Practice Communities

Work by Croker (2011) into collaboration between healthcare professionals and in teams identified the importance of understanding how different communities of practice influence workplace expectations of how professionals work and of how they work together. Her research explored the ways practitioners often work across multiple practice communities including their direct work teams, their disciplines and their workplaces. Not only do they need to respond to the norms, expectations and practices of each community, but they may well be faced with challenges associated to each of these communities having different, and possibly contradictory, practice models. A practitioner could work in both a patient-centred palliative care unit and a protocol-driven cardiac surgery biomedical-model ward yet desire to be a client collaborator who helps clients conduct their own wellness narratives, in rejection of the restitution narrative (Alder, 2003).

In her research into practice models, Trede (2006) identified that practitioners unknowingly adopted their practice models. Much of their practice was unreflective and taken for granted. Most of these practitioners, as physiotherapists, identified a preference for the biomedical practice model, as the hegemonic system and educational model of the participants' workplaces and professional socialization. Most of these research participants claimed to be patient-centred but generally reverted therapist-centred approaches based on technical interests. For a minority, the practice model preferred by the practitioner was so incompatible with the workplace model that the practitioner chose to leave that workplace.

Being Deliberate: Making Choices About Our Practice Models

Another key influence on our chosen practice model is how we consciously position and act in the world. As Arendt (1996) reminds us, practice or action is no neutral activity, and if we do not understand the wider influences on us and choose how to position ourselves, reason and be in practice, then others will choose it for us. Trede and McEwen (2016a, p. 7) introduced the term deliberate professional to 'define ways of developing moral, thoughtful, purposeful and agentic stances that enable practitioners to counterbalance one-dimensional and instrumental practices'. Deliberate professionals are people who are informed by moral consideration of self and others; they have the capacity and drive to promote positive changes through their professional practice. 'The deliberate professional is aware of complex and ever-changing relational dimensions in practice that shape the way practitioners think, talk and relate to self, others and the wider context around them; behave thoughtfully and courageously; resist unreflected conformity and notions of neutrality, repair and change conditions; and not disavow accepted practices, but rather acknowledge, appreciate, critique and change aspects of practices that need improving' (Trede & McEwen 2016b, p. 22). Because, by definition, our practices are pursued deliberately, knowingly and informedly, practitioners need to realize and enact their practices within a coherent and deliberately owned practice model (Higgs, 2016).

REFLECTION POINT 2

When we consider the global, national and local interests on how practice should be done, it could be assumed that practice models and clinical reasoning processes are predetermined and prescribed. Could you argue that your way of practicing and reasoning is informed by the ideas of the deliberate professional as outlined earlier?

MODELS OF PRACTICE

Clinical reasoning occurs within models of practice. These models can be tacit (understood and largely unquestioned), controversial (known and debated), hegemonic (dominant and widely supported) and chosen (knowingly adopted). Practice models occur at different levels: they identify the broad strategy (such as the biomedical model) that operates at the level of a system, organization or workplace; they frame the interactions of team members (such as patient-centred care); and they give meaning and direction to the actions of individual practitioners (such as an evidence-based or humanistic orientation). In each case, they reflect or challenge the interests (benefits and motivations) of the people working within the systems in which these models operate.

Models of practice are abstract ideas of what practice should look like if it followed a given framework. These frameworks comprise a variety of interests, criteria, norms, practice principles and strategies and behavioural expectations that inform clinical reasoning and practice. Models can be thought of as mental maps that assist practitioners to understand their practice. They serve to structure and to fine-tune practitioners' clinical reasoning. Whether they are learned, chosen or unconsciously acquired through professional socialization, practice models generate the principles that guide practice and create the standards practitioners strive towards and the behavioural expectations that determine performance.

Professional practice models can be categorized in a number of ways. One such categorization is based on the theory of knowledge and human interest (Habermas, 1972). According to this theory, there are three types of interest: technical, practical and critical, each of which generates a certain type of knowledge. Each interest directs the types of question that can be asked in practice, in turn dictating the type of knowledge that is generated and used in practice and the way we practice. These interests not only shape the professional practice we enact and determine which modes of practice we see as valuable, but they also influence the identity we adopt as professionals, how we see the role of patients, how we believe clinical decisions should be made and how we justify and argue our professional roles and actions. Table 4.1 presents the illness, wellness and capacity practice models and their inherent interests, based on the three Habermasian interests. We argue that practice and reasoning require critical thinking that is based on critical interests; critical thinking based on technical and practical interests is important but incomplete in meeting the challenging demands of current practice.

Table 4.1 illustrates how interests shape practice models, knowledge and clinical reasoning in practice. Some aspects are of particular relevance in this discussion of clinical reasoning.

■ The focus and definition of health selected influence healthcare goals pursued. When healthcare focuses on illness and biomedical pathology, the goal of care is limited to reducing deficit or merely helping patients cope with current situations.

When health is seen as a potential, the focus of reasoning and health care is on building capacity. A capacity practice model transcends the dualism of the illness and wellness models.

■ The relative power of the clinician and patient varies significantly across different practice models and is reflected in clinical reasoning strategies. For instance, in an emancipatory model collaboration, inclusiveness and reciprocal facilitation of responsibility are embedded in clinical decision making.

■ The type(s) of knowledge that practitioners value is grounded in their professional socialization. Practice knowledge is inclusive of dominant scientific (empirico-analytical) and psychosociocultural (ethnographic, phenomenological) constructs of knowledge.

TABLE 4.1
Three Frameworks for Professional Practice Models in Health

Practice Model	Illness Model	Wellness Model	Capacity Model
Kind of interest	Technical	Practical	Emancipatory
Approach	Clinician-centred	Patient-centred	Patient-empowered
Philosophical paradigm	Empirico-analytical	Interpretive	Critical
Health definition	Reductionist	Holistic	Holistic
Focus of health	Technical	Practical	Political
Clinician has power	Clinician has power	Clinician may share some power	Equal power sharing
Patient power	Disempowered	Empowered	Empowered in a way that can be sustained
Practice knowledge	Propositional-technical	Propositional-technical and experiential	Propositional-technical, experiential and political
Stance towards status quo	Taking things for granted, accepting, reinforcing	Being aware of taken-for-granted things	Challenging status quo and changing frameworks
Role of patient	Passive, obedient, not asked to think for self	Interactive, participative but obedient, encouraged to think a bit for self	Interactive, participative, contributing, self-determining, learn to think for self
Role of clinician	Teacher/provider	Listener	Facilitator
Context of decision making	Out of context	Psychocultural context (definitely not political)	Historical-political context
Clinician as helper	Helping to survive	Helping to cope	Helping to liberate
Clinicians helping patients	To comply	To cope	To liberate
Clinician self-awareness	Unreflective	Reflective with the aim to empower	Reflective with the aim to transform

- The relative roles of practitioners and patients are significantly influenced by practice approaches, whether chosen or unconsciously adopted. Biomedical practice models speak of providers and recipients of practice. In an emancipatory/capacity model, patients and practitioners engage in dialogues and learn from each other, both accepting the roles of listening and negotiating.
- The level of critique and reflexivity that practitioners bring to their practice is grounded in practice and reasoning approaches. Critical self-awareness of professional or personal interests is the key to consciously choosing a practice model.

Traditionally in orthodox Western medicine, most practitioners acquire a biomedical science or medical practice model during their education and practice acculturation. This acquisition frequently occurs with limited critique or questioning of this model. Such practitioners are commonly unaware of their practice model because it represents the unquestioned norm, and they are consequently unaware of how this model influences the way they reason. They reason within their adopted practice model without challenging the values and interests their practice model may entail. The key features of this model and reasoning are an emphasis on cure and the restitution of health, the role of the practitioner as professional authority in the decision-making process, and the patient being regarded as 'the one without expertise'. At times practitioners even disregard the patient's knowledge of self and his or her ability to participate in health care apart from being compliant and seeking cures. Reasoning in this model is largely performed by the expert/practitioner and is hypothetico-deductive in nature following the hypothesis generation and testing strategy of the hegemonic scientific model.

REFLECTION POINT 3

The illness, wellness and capacity models outlined earlier are theoretical constructs that do not exist in their purity in practice realities. However, what do you think are the benefits of this framework of conceptualizing professional practice models in health? How could you work with this framework in your teaching or clinical practice?

REASONING IN A CRITICAL SOCIAL SCIENCE MODEL FOR PRACTICE

To consider how a practitioner's chosen and enacted model of practice influences his or her clinical reasoning, we now turn to an in-depth interpretation of a particular model – the Critical Social Science (CSS) Model – as researched by Trede (2006). The primary goal of the research (see Trede, 2006; Trede and Higgs, 2003) was to understand how a CSS perspective, with its inherent emancipatory interests, might influence and transform healthcare practice. The development of the CSS model for practice resulted from four cycles of critical transformative dialogues based on critique and reflexivity and the pursuit of change that led to liberation. The dialogues involved two-way conversations with self and others (including other participants, patients, colleagues) using critical reasoning. The first dialogue described the status quo of the CSS and health-related literature and developed a conceptual approximation of a CSS model for healthcare practice. The second dialogue involved critique and interpretation of the related physiotherapy literature followed by a critical dialogue with the first group of physiotherapist participants to critique the status quo of physiotherapy practice. In the third dialogue, a group of practitioners trialled a CSS approach using action-learning strategies. The fourth dialogue, with another physiotherapy participant group, envisioned a CSS approach to practice.

In discussion of the status quo of practice, a few participants in Trede's study, either through dissatisfaction with their model or prompted by further education, consciously chose to adopt an alternative model based in humanistic philosophy or, less frequently, a CSS perspective. The more conscious the choice of practice model and the more this model differed from hegemonic practices, the more likely it was that the practitioners adopted a heightened level of awareness into their reasoning and behaviour. Instead of reasoning against scientific knowledge, evidence, established practice guidelines or learned behaviour expectations set by their professions, workplaces or society at large, these practitioners sought to critically construct their own set of practice standards and ways of being in the world of practice, and they monitored their behaviour against these standards. These participants, without theoretical understanding of CSS theory, had created a critical practice model.

A critical practice model starts with the assumptions that practice is complex, outcomes are uncertain and perceptions and interpretations of patient presentations are diverse. This means that a patient with an arthritic knee is not simply 'an arthritic knee' – an *object* of treatment. Instead, practitioners need to consider patients wholistically; this includes age, gender, attitude towards pain and physical activity and expectations of practitioners and themselves. Gaining a critical perspective means becoming aware of the interests that collide in practice and questioning these interests.

Critical social science is distinguished from the natural and social sciences in that it focuses on critique that leads to change and emancipation (Fay, 1987). Critique is raising awareness about interests that have arisen in the sociocultural historical worlds that influence clinical reasoning and practice approaches. From a CSS perspective, critical thinking means being able to take a sceptical stance towards self, culture, norms, practices and institutions and policy and regulations. Critical thinking questions the very roots of discipline-accepted knowledge and how it informs clinical reasoning (Brookfield, 2012; Trede and McEwen, 2015). During clinical reasoning, this scepticism is both a conscious and a metaprocess; the practitioner would explicitly challenge data, decisions and treatment alternatives and bring a heightened awareness of his or her own thinking and actions into the moments of practice, not just to posttreatment reflections.

CSS starts from the assumption that the influences listed earlier are human-made and therefore can be changed. Before these aspects of practice and reasoning are accepted and adopted, they should be challenged and checked for their intentions and assumptions. CSS separates truth from ideology, reason from power and emancipation from oppression. The agenda of CSS is to critique, engage in dialogue and transform the status quo at an individual and a collective level, working towards transformation through professional development and maturity to become a self-aware and articulate professional who works with patients, policy and institutions that respect diversity and support social justice. The focus is on transforming unnecessarily constraining policies and oppressive practices that restrict workforce development and patient empowerment.

REFLECTION POINT 4

The CSS model may appear to advocate thinking against the grain at all costs because it has critique and scepticism about current ways of thinking and practicing at its core. The purpose of a CSS perspective is not criticism and identifying deficits but rather to inclusively understand current practices with their economic, political and cultural influences to identify the way forward to strengthen what is already working well and to change what needs to be improved. What are the economic, political and cultural influences that need to be improved in your clinical environment?

During Trede's (2006) research, some of the participants trialled and experienced what it was like to transform their practice into (or towards) a critical practice model. This dialogue cycle included a preimplementation workshop, an action-learning phase and a critical appraisal workshop. Participants were informed about the findings from the first phase of the research investigating the status quo of physiotherapy practice models. They were educated about the dimensions of critique, power and emancipation of CSS, and they were invited to critically discuss our critique of current practices. The findings from this phase indicated that the practitioners had varied levels of readiness (cognitive, emotional and pragmatic) to engage in practice reflection and change and different perceptions of the value of CSS as a basis for practice. Different levels of engagement with CSS were identified. Some of the participants were happy to help with the research but persisted with their more traditional biomedical model approaches. Others practiced a patient-centred model closely related to the emerging CSS model.

The CSS Model

The CSS model (Trede, 2006) for practice has two core dimensions.

An Emancipatory Dimension

The emancipatory dimension entails recognition that to adopt a CSS or emancipatory model in a world of practice where such practice is a minority view requires a journey of critical transformative dialogues of emancipation for the practitioner. The research identified five modes of engagement with CSS as a practice model. These were labelled:

1. *The Uninformed* — those who had not heard of CSS
2. *The Unconvinced* — those who trialled CSS but did not change their current practice, which remained in the biomedical model
3. *The Contemplators* — those who trialled CSS and thought that some aspects of CSS were convincing but encountered too many perceived barriers to transform their practice substantially
4. *The Transformers* — those who were convinced of CSS and were transforming aspects of their practice

5. *The Champions* — those who were convinced of the value of CSS and embodied CSS in their practice

Across these five levels, the participants progressively engaged more deeply in transforming their practice towards a CSS approach, learning more about CSS, came to value these principles and practices more deeply, and journeyed further away from their traditional practice knowledge base and practices. Table 4.2 details the interests, practices and characteristics of each of these modes. Of particular relevance here are the changing patterns of interaction, power use and reasoning approaches, ranging from therapist-centred and therapist-empowered decision making for patients to

TABLE 4.2

Practice Dimension	The Uninformed	The Unconvinced	The Contemplators	The Transformers	The Champions
Definition	Those who have not heard of CSS	Those who have trialled CSS but do not change their current practice	Those who have explored CSS in their practice and have chosen to adopt some aspects of CSS in their practice	Those who are convinced of critical practice and are transforming their practice to this model	Those who are convinced of the value of critical practice and advocate it
Practice model	Typically the biomedical model	Typically the biomedical model	Mixed biomedical and critical model	Approximating a critical practice model	Critical model
Interests	Technical/practical	Technical/practical	Practical/technical/ emancipatory	Emancipatory (plus technical/ practical)	Predominantly emancipatory
Self-appraisal	Mastering technical application	Mastering technical application	Mastering technical application and acknowledging patients' interests	Acknowledging own assumptions and unreflected ideology	Seeking critical self-understanding, reflexive
Mode of critique	Critiquing practice from an empirico-analytical, technical perspective	Critiquing practice from an empirico-analytical, technical perspective	Critiquing practice from practical perspectives working within systems that are taken for granted or at least assumed unchangeable	Critiquing practice by starting with self-critique and awareness of system challenges	Being open, sincere, curious; avoiding making generalizations and unreflected judgements; paying attention to detail (rethinking practice dimensions through relational thinking)
Approach to reasoning	Linear, cause and effect, minimal contextual consideration	Linear, cause and effect, minimal contextual consideration	Appreciate critical reasoning without adopting it	Adopting critical reasoning in aspects of practice	Critical, dialogical reasoning

TABLE 4.2 *(Continued)*				
Practice Dimension	**The Uninformed**	**The Unconvinced**	**The Contemplators**	**The Transformers**	**The Champions**
Approach to knowledge	Propositional-technical	Propositional-technical	Propositional-technical and experiential	Propositional-technical, experiential and critical	Propositional-technical, experiential and critical
Patient relationships	Therapist is the expert and dominates	Therapist is the expert and dominates	Therapist is the expert but acknowledges patient experience	Democratizing patient-therapist relationship	Dialogical, reciprocal relationship where expertise of therapist and patient is acknowledged
Power/authority	Owned by physiotherapist's propositional knowledge	Owned by physiotherapist's propositional knowledge	Owned by propositional knowledge and some nonpropositional knowledge	Shift from propositional to critical knowledge. System propositional knowledge dominant	Shared as critical knowledge
Context interpretation	Within biomedical domain	Within biomedical domain	Within biopsychosocial domain	Within cultural and biopsychosocial domain	Within critical cultural biopsychosocial domain
Professional identity and role	Technical and telling patients what they need	Technical and telling patients what they need	Technical, practical and empathic, guiding patients	Moving to a facilitating role of emancipatory learning in self. Asking patients what they need	Moving to a role of facilitating emancipatory learning in self and patients and chosen and self-owned identity
Goals	Achievement of positive technical, biomedical outcomes	Achievement of positive technical, biomedical outcomes	Achievement of functional and practical outcomes	Achievement of negotiated outcomes	Emancipation of self, others and the system for enhancement of patient outcomes in a critical framework

Five Prototypical Engagements With CSS (Trede, 2006).

patient-centred and mutually empowered decision-making dialogues with patients.

REFLECTION POINT 5

The prototypical categorization of how professionals engage with the CSS model is intended to help readers identify themselves where they fit and where they might possibly want to position themselves on the table. It can be used as a discussion starter in teams to clarify purposes of clinical reasoning processes.

A Critical, Lived Dimension

In advocating consideration and adoption of a CSS practice model, we recognize that critical practice has variable relevance and potential across the range of practice contexts and that other models (as discussed earlier) may be preferable or more feasible in certain contexts. Critical physiotherapy practice is the practice model of choice in situations of emancipatory need, predilection and support. The ultimate value of critical practice is its capacity to enhance the quality of life of its protagonists through critical appraisal, particularization, empowerment and constructive collaboration in shared vision and actions.

CSS practice is an accessible and acceptable choice when four situations coincide: a) when there is a perceived need for patients and physiotherapists to collaborate in clinical decision making and to liberate practice; b) when it is the preferred practice model of a practitioner (or group) who is a champion of critical practice; c) when other team members are supportive of this approach and keen to embody authentic critical practice; and d) where management and organizational systems support rather than restrict critical approaches. These four situations create a facilitative and supportive environment for embedding a critical practice perspective in the existing discourse. Critical practice would then be the practice model of choice because marginalized voices of patients and practitioners are heard and acted upon in a system-based environment that is sensitive, supportive and responsive to critique and emancipation.

Practitioners bring their assumptions, values and prejudgements and professional experiences to the clinical situation. Practitioners with a critical perspective are aware of the interests that collide in practice, and they question these interests. Practicing in a CSS model involves engaging in critical transformative dialogues that enable practitioners to make practice model choices and living CSS in the every day.

Practicing and reasoning within a CSS model require practitioners to:

- challenge models of practice, practice cultures and taken-for-granted practice interests,
- choose CSS as the overall practice framework for decision making and action,
- be accountable to self and to those influenced by their professional practice,
- analyze what practice knowledge is valuable and situationally applicable,
- critically and responsibly exercise choice about courses of action,
- negotiate a practice approach with patients/clients,
- engage patients (and carers) in transformative dialogue,
- plan a team CSS approach,
- imagine alternatives,

- be willing to question their sense of self, their professional identity and their chosen model of practice,
- critically appraise their reasoning and practice on a big-picture level (is my practice model relevant and meaningful?) and within the moments of reasoning and practice and
- adopt a critical pedagogy approach to teaching and learning. Such an approach involves and enhances learners' capacity to question existing assumptions and current practices.

The relevance of CSS for healthcare professional practice is that such a practice model:

- builds the capacity of practitioners for critical self-reflection as a tool for practice development,
- democratizes professional relations and ensures inclusive, appropriate and ethical practice that empowers patients,
- raises awareness of interests and values that inform clinical reasoning,
- redefines professional identity within a constantly changing world to empower practitioners and liberate them from restrictive hegemonic practice rules and
- encourages rethinking of the boundaries and inclusions of the practice context.

A critical practice model is challenging because practitioners must constantly question their clinical reasoning and maintain a critical stance to current practices. This critical stance to self and others can only be sustained within a supportive environment that facilitates such emancipatory learning. Adopting a CSS perspective requires advanced clinical reasoning skills that allow critical reflection about self, patients and the wider practice context and open, yet sceptical, professional relationships with patients.

CHAPTER SUMMARY

In this chapter we have presented:

- practice models and their importance,
- the interdependence between reasoning and practice in the context of models of practice and
- the implication of a critical social science practice model for practice and reasoning.

REFLECTION POINT 6

In current times of rapid and relentless change, the CSS model can shape clinical reasoning processes to help students and practitioners steer through uncertainty and complexity. There is an urgent need to educate deliberate professionals with critical-thinking skills that opens up new possibilities of practicing. Where in your teaching do you explicitly discuss different professional models of health? How do you cultivate critical-thinking approaches that encourage students to think for self and imagine how to practice otherwise? How could you assess students' capabilities to engage with the CSS model and become deliberate professionals?

REFERENCES

Alder, S., 2003. Beyond the restitution narrative. PhD thesis. University of Western Sydney, Sydney, Australia, viewed 1 June 2017. Available from: http://handle.uws.edu.au:8081/1959.7/22873.

Arendt, H., 1996. Ich will verstehen: Selbstauskünfte zu leben und werk. Ursula Ludz. München: Piper.

Brookfield, S., 2012. Teaching for Critical Thinking: Tools and Techniques to Help Students Question Their Assumptions. Jossey-Bass, San Francisco, CA.

Croker, A., 2011. Collaboration in Rehabilitation Teams. PhD thesis. Charles Sturt University, Australia.

Eraut, M., 1994. Developing Professional Knowledge and Competence. The Falmer Press, London, UK.

Fay, B., 1987. Critical Social Science. Cornell University Press, Ithaca.

Habermas, J., 1972. Knowledge and human interest. trans. JJ Shapiro. Heinemann, London, UK.

Higgs, J., 2016. Deliberately owning my practice model: realising my professional practice. In: Trede, F., McEwen, C. (Eds.), Educating the Deliberate Professional: Preparing Practitioners for Emergent Futures. Springer, Dordrecht, The Netherlands, pp. 189–203.

Higgs, J., Hunt, A., Higgs, C., et al., 1999. Physiotherapy education in the changing international healthcare and educational contexts. Adv. Physiother. 1, 17–26.

Newman, M., 1994. Defining the Enemy: Adult Education in Social Action. Stewart Victor Publishing, Sydney, Australia.

Schön, D.A., 1987. Educating the Reflective Practitioner. Jossey-Bass, San Francisco, CA.

Therborn, G., 1999. The ideology of power and the power of ideology. Verso, London, UK.

Trede, F., Higgs, J., 2003. Re-framing the clinician's role in collaborative clinical decision making: re-thinking practice knowledge and the notion of clinician–patient relationships. Learning in Health and Social Care 2, 66–73.

Trede, F., McEwen, C., 2015. Critical thinking for future practice. In: Davies, M., Barnett, R. (Eds.), Palgrave Handbook of Critical Thinking in Higher Education. Palgrave Publishers, New York, NY, pp. 457–475.

Trede, F., McEwen, C., 2016a. Scoping the deliberate professional. In: Trede, F., McEwen, C. (Eds.), Educating the Deliberate Professional: Preparing Practitioners for Emergent Futures. Springer, Dordrecht, The Netherlands, pp. 3–14.

Trede, F., McEwen, C., 2016b. Carving out the territory for educating the deliberate professional. In: Trede, F., McEwen, C. (Eds.), Educating the Deliberate Professional: Preparing Practitioners For Emergent Futures. Springer, Dordrecht, The Netherlands, pp. 15–28.

Trede, F.V., 2006. A critical practice for physiotherapy. PhD thesis. University of Sydney, Sydney, Australia.

5

THE DEVELOPMENT OF CLINICAL REASONING EXPERTISE

HENNY P.A. BOSHUIZEN ■ HENK G. SCHMIDT

CHAPTER AIMS

The aims of this chapter are to:

■ examine the development of clinical reasoning expertise, particularly in medicine,

■ answer the question of whether clinical reasoning can be taught to medical students and

■ present approaches to clinical reasoning skills training building on the stage theory.

KEY WORDS

Clinical expertise

Stage theory

Knowledge structures

INTRODUCTION

The main objective of medical schools is to turn relative novices into knowledgeable and skilled professionals who are able to solve clinical problems and are aware of the reach of their knowledge and skills and what goes beyond their capacities. In this chapter, we seek to answer the question of whether clinical reasoning can be taught to medical students. We start by describing the development from novice in medicine to expert, providing a theoretical cognitive psychological framework. Several approaches to clinical reasoning skills training are then described, and the implications of this theory are considered for the way medical education can improve students' clinical reasoning.

A THEORY OF THE DEVELOPMENT OF MEDICAL EXPERTISE

For a long time, it has been thought that the human mind can be trained in logical thinking, problem solving or creativity and that these skills could transfer to all domains of daily and professional life. For this purpose, children are encouraged to play chess or to learn Latin in school. Polya's (1957) problem-solving training program also cherishes this general idea about the human mind. In the same vein, it was thought that experts in an arbitrary domain had trained their minds and had developed general problem-solving and thinking skills. This opinion has, however, been superseded, because research outcomes have shown that experts in a specific domain have not developed problem-solving skills that can be applied across domains. Instead, domain knowledge and the associated skills to use this knowledge in problem solving develop simultaneously and interdependently.

In medicine, research has shown that clinical reasoning is not a separate skill acquired independently of medical knowledge and other diagnostic skills. Instead, research suggests a stage theory of the development of medical expertise, in which knowledge acquisition and clinical reasoning go hand in hand (Boshuizen and Schmidt, 1992; Schmidt and Boshuizen, 1992; Schmidt et al., 1992; Schmidt et al., 1990). This theory of medical diagnosis is essentially a theory of the acquisition and development of knowledge structures upon which a student or a physician operates when diagnosing a case. Dramatic changes in problem solving or clinical

	TABLE 5.1
	Lines of Reasoning by a Fourth-Year Medical Student
Case Item (Number and Text)	**Think-Aloud Protocol**
31. (History) Defecation: paler and more malodorous stools according to the patient	... not so much undermines that idea ... er . their frequency . and their pattern compared with colour and the like . their smell er ... yes ... no problems with defecation, that means in any case no constipation, which you wouldn't expect with an obstruction of the biliary tract ... well yes
32. (History) Last bowel movement was yesterday	...
32. (History) Temperature: 37°C at 6 P.M.	so no temperature
33. (Physical examination) Pulse rate: regular, 72/min.	... er . yes ... the past two ... together . means that there's er no inflammation ... and that would eliminate an er ... an er . cholecystitis ... and would rather mean an ... er ... obstruction of the biliary tract ... caused by a stone, for instance ... or, what may be the case too, by a carcinoma, but I wouldn't ... although, it might be possible, lost 5 kilograms in weight ...

Note. Protocol fragment obtained from a fourth-year medical student working on a pancreatitis case showing detailed reasoning steps. See Boshuizen and Schmidt (1992) for a detailed description of the experiment.

reasoning are the result of structural changes in knowledge, whereas knowledge structure and quality are affected by the quality of the reasoning process that operates on the knowledge base. Clinical reasoning leaves its traces in the knowledge structure directly by strengthening or weakening links between concepts and indirectly as a result of concurrent or post hoc evaluation thereof and the knowledge actions of the learner that may follow from that.[i]

During the first stage of expertise development, medical students acquire large amounts of knowledge about the biomedical basic sciences. They acquire concepts that are linked together in a semantic, knowledge network. Gradually, more concepts are added and refined, and more and better connections are made. Knowledge accretion and validation are the students' main concerns in this period of their study. This process takes much more time than teachers might expect. In particular, the integration and integrated use of knowledge from different domains (e.g., the clinical sciences, biochemistry, pathophysiology, and micro-anatomy) is not self-evident (Boshuizen and van de Wiel, 1998; Groothuis et al., 1998). During this stage, the clinical reasoning process is characterized by lines of reasoning consisting of chains of small steps

commonly based on detailed biomedical concepts. An example of detailed reasoning is given in Table 5.1. It has been taken from a longer protocol in which a fourth-year medical student is dealing with a case of pancreatitis. His initial hypothesis set contained gall-bladder and pancreas disease. Apparently, this student is entertaining the hypothesis of biliary tract obstruction. First, he reasons whether the new finding about the patient's stools affects this hypothesis and decides that this is not the case. Next, three items later, he combines the information acquired and concludes that there is no inflammation (causing this obstruction) [step 1], hence, no cholecystitis [step 2], hence the biliary tract must be obstructed by something else, a stone for instance [step 3] or a carcinoma [step 4], which might be the case because the patient has lost weight [step 5].

By the end of the first stage of knowledge acquisition, students have a knowledge network that allows them to make direct lines of reasoning between different concepts within that network. The more often these direct lines are activated, the more these concepts cluster together, and students become able to make direct links between the first and last concept in such a line of reasoning, skipping intermediate concepts. We have labelled this process 'knowledge encapsulation', a term that refers to the clustering aspect of the process and can account for the automatization involved (e.g., Boshuizen and Schmidt, 1992; Schmidt and Boshuizen,

[i]We use the term 'learner' to emphasize the learning process taking place. Being a learner is independent of level of expertise reached.

1993). Many of these concept clusters have (semi-) clinical names, such as *microembolism, aortic insufficiency, forward failure,* or *extrahepatic icterus,* providing a powerful reasoning tool. Encapsulation of biomedical knowledge results in the next stage of development of clinical reasoning skills, in which biomedical knowledge has been integrated into clinical knowledge. At this stage, students' clinical reasoning processes no longer involve many biomedical concepts. Students tend to make direct links between patient findings and clinical concepts that have the status of hypotheses or diagnoses in their reasoning process. However, if needed, this encapsulated biomedical knowledge can be unfolded again, for instance when dealing with a very complicated problem. van de Wiel et al. (2000) showed that experts' clinical knowledge structures subsumed biomedical knowledge. Rikers et al. (2005) demonstrated that in expert clinical reasoning, biomedical knowledge is also activated, operating in a sort of stand-by mode.

At the same time, a transition takes place from a network type of knowledge organization to a structure referred to as 'illness scripts'. Illness scripts have three components. The first component refers to enabling conditions of disease: the conditions or constraints under which a disease occurs. These are the personal, social, medical, hereditary, and environmental factors that affect health in a positive or negative way or affect the course of a specific disease. The second component is the fault: the pathophysiological process that is taking place in

a specific disease, represented in encapsulated form. The third component consists of the consequences of the fault: the signs and symptoms of a specific disease (also see Feltovich and Barrows [1984], who introduced this theoretical notion). Contrary to (advanced) novice knowledge networks, illness scripts are activated as a whole. After an illness script has been activated, no active, small-step search within that script is required; the other elements of the script are activated immediately and automatically, which results in a major cognitive advantage. While solving a problem, a physician activates one or a few illness scripts. The illness script elements (enabling conditions and consequences) are then matched to the information provided by the patient. Illness scripts not only incorporate matching information from the patient, but they also generate expectations about other signs and symptoms the patient might have. Activated illness scripts thus provide a list of phenomena to seek in history taking and in physical examination. In the course of this verification process, expected values are substituted by real findings, instantiating and further activating the script. Illness scripts that fail in this respect will become de-activated. The instantiated script yields a diagnosis or a differential diagnosis when a few competing scripts remain active. An example of script activation by an experienced physician, dealing with the same clinical case as the student in Table 5.1, is given in Table 5.2. The information about the patient's medical past and psycho-social circumstances

TABLE 5.2	
Illness Script Activation by a Family Physician	
Case Item (Number and Text)	**Think-Aloud Protocol**
8. Complaint: Continuous pain in the upper part of the abdomen, radiating to the back	... well, when I am visiting someone who is suffering an acute ... continuous – since when? – pain in his upper abdomen, radiating to the back, who had pancreatitis a year before ... of whom I don't know for sure if he still drinks or not after that course of Refusal, but of whom I do know that he still has mental problems, so still receives a disability benefit, then I think that the first thing to cross my mind will be: well, what about that pancreas, ... how's his liver ... and also that – considering his age – eh it is not very likely that there will be other things wrong in his abdomen ... eh ... of a malign thing er nature ... of course eh if he's taking huge amounts of alcohol there's always the additional possibility of a stomach eh problem, a stomach perforation ... excessive drinking can also cause eh serious cardiomyopathy, which eh may cause heart defects mm I can't er judge the word 'continuous' very well yet in this context

Note. Protocol fragment obtained from an experienced family physician working on a pancreatitis case. Earlier, he had received information about enabling conditions such as mental problems and alcohol abuse. See Boshuizen and Schmidt (1992).

(summarized in the protocol), combined with the presenting complaint, activated a few competing illness scripts: pancreatic disease, liver disease and abdominal malignancy (which he considers implausible because of the patient's age), and stomach perforation. In addition, he thought of cardiomyopathy as an effect of excessive drinking. In the course of the think-aloud protocol, he seemed to monitor the level of instantiation of every illness script. Except for gallbladder disease, no new scripts were activated.

So far, we have seen that expert and novice knowledge structures differ in many respects. As a consequence, their clinical reasoning differs as well. Medical experts, who have large numbers of ready-made illness scripts that organize many enabling conditions and consequences associated with a specific disease, will activate one or more of these illness scripts when dealing with a case. Activation will be triggered by information concerning enabling conditions and/or consequences. Expert hypothesis activation and testing can be seen as an epiphenomenon of illness script activation and instantiation. These are generally automatic and 'unconscious' processes. As long as new information matches an active illness script, no active reasoning is required. Only in cases of severe mismatch or conflict between activated scripts does the expert engage in active clinical reasoning. During this process either illness-script-based expectations are adjusted based on specific features of the patient or the expert reverts to pure biomedical reasoning, drawing on de-encapsulated biomedical knowledge. Our old-time favourite example of deliberate script adjustment is given by Lesgold et al. (1988), who described expert radiologists' interpretations of an enlarged heart shadow on an x-ray screen. These experts took into consideration the marked scoliosis of the patient's thoracic spine, which affected the position of his heart relative to the slide. Hence, they concluded that the heart was not actually enlarged.

Students, on the other hand, can rely only on knowledge networks, which are less rich and less easily activated than experts' illness scripts. They require more information before a specific hypothesis will be generated. Semantic networks must be reasoned through step by step. This is a time-consuming process and often requires active monitoring. Hence, contrary to illness scripts, the knowledge structures that students activate do not automatically generate a list of signs and symptoms that are expected. Active searching through their networks is needed to generate such a list that might verify or falsify their hypotheses. In general, students' clinical reasoning is less orderly, less goal-oriented and more time consuming, and it is based on less plausible hypotheses resulting in less accurate diagnoses than those of experts.

The differences described thus far were all investigated in the context of solving cases that did not require further data collection. This rather artificial task has the advantage that participants can devote all their time and attention to the cognitive processing of the information given. However, authentic clinical reasoning takes place during the action of data gathering and evaluation. Recently we investigated clinical reasoning of pathologists. Similar to radiologists, their material is mostly visual: pathological slides that are inspected under a microscope. Information must be extracted by inspecting the slides at several levels of magnification. Verbal data, combined with eye movement data, suggested that students described their 'findings' in rather perceptual terms such as form and colour and searched for cues they could interpret in pathological terms without being able to come to a satisfactory conclusion. Experts and intermediates (residents) differed in the number of specific pathologies mentioned (intermediates mentioned more) and in the way they checked alternative scripts: experts actively searched for alternatives of their diagnosis at the end of the inspection, while intermediates appeared to have more scripts open already in the beginning (Jaarsma et al., 2014).

A study by Wagenaar (2008) has shown that third-year students have great difficulty combining data collection and clinical reasoning. They are very dependent on the information the client volunteers and seem unable to reason in action. Instead, they try to collect as much information as possible, and only after they have completed the interview do they review the information collected to formulate a diagnosis. Experts, on the other hand, think on their feet, adapting their data collection to the level of verification or falsification of their hypotheses and to the time available. Table 5.3 summarizes these differences between novices, intermediates, and experts. The picture that emerges here is that novices and intermediates are handicapped in two ways: their knowledge is insufficient, and it requires extra cognitive capacity when solving problems. Both

TABLE 5.3

Knowledge Restructuring, Clinical Reasoning and Levels of Expertise

Expertise Level	Knowledge Representation	Knowledge Acquisition and (Re)-Structuring	Clinical Reasoning	Control Required in Clinical Reasoning	Demand on Cognitive Capacity	Clinical Reasoning in Action
Novice	Networks	Knowledge accretion and validation	Long chains of detailed reasoning steps through preencapsulated networks	Active monitoring of each reasoning step	High	Difficulty to combine data collection and evaluation and clinical reasoning
Intermediate	Network	Encapsulation	Reasoning through encapsulated network	Active monitoring of each reasoning step	Medium	...
Expert	Illness scripts	Illness script formation	Illness script activation and instantiation	Monitoring of the level of script instantiation	Low	Adjust data collection to time available and to verification/ falsification level of hypotheses

aspects negatively influence clinical problem solving; they also hinder learning.

TEACHING CLINICAL REASONING

Until this moment we have avoided definition of the concepts of clinical reasoning and clinical reasoning skills, first giving attention to the knowledge structures upon which these reasoning processes operate. Nor have we explicitly addressed the question of whether clinical reasoning can be taught. Yet there is huge pressure on the profession to improve the quality of diagnosis and treatment, which is apparent from the numerous publications on medical error and patient safety (e.g., Brennan et al., 1991) and evidence-based medicine (Sackett et al., 1996). Generally, clinical reasoning equals the thinking process occurring when dealing with a clinical case. Most researchers who investigate teaching clinical reasoning differentiate between different phases in the clinical reasoning process (e.g., Bowen, 2006): beginning with hypothesis generation, inquiry strategy, data analysis, problem synthesis or diagnosis and finally ending with diagnostic and treatment decision making.

REFLECTION POINT 1

- The quality of a clinical reasoning process depends on the quality of the knowledge it operates on; case, knowledge and regulation together determine the quality of the result.
- Knowledge networks are transformed into illness scripts as a consequence of dealing with real or simulated patients.
- Encapsulating concepts integrate biomedical and clinical knowledge; to play their role in the communication with colleagues, they need to have a shared meaning.
- Illness scripts are powerful cognitive structures that allow automatic processing; their validity deserves continuous attention.

Clinical reasoning, its form and quality, is thus affected by the features of the case and the validity and structure of the knowledge base. Typical cases activate one illness script, plus maybe some alternatives you should always be aware of, not because of their plausibility but because of their severity (Custers et al., 1996). Atypical cases may activate several scripts that have to be sorted out by checking the script elements that are part of one but not of other scripts (Mamede et al., 2007) or that have to be further reasoned through by means of basic science knowledge (see the Lesgold et al., 1988, example described earlier). Invalid knowledge jeopardizes the validity of the whole process. Apart from these two factors, a third factor plays a role in the quality of the reasoning process. This factor is the 'regulation of the decision-making process' itself, which may vary between automatic and deliberate analytic processing.

Decision making as a general human information processing activity has a couple of features that can make it prone to biased reasoning and others that can protect against that. For instance, the speedy activation of one illness script may lead to confirmation bias (the tendency to confirm a diagnosis or to fill the open slots in an illness script instead of searching for information that might contradict that) or to premature closure (the tendency to accept a diagnosis before other relevant options have been excluded). Also priming of one illness script (e.g., as a result of recent exposure to a similar case or a presentation in the media) leads to easier activation of the same script at the cost of others, which in turn may lead to premature closing. In the medical literature, these biases have been frequently described as a cause of medical error (Croskerry, 2003). The way these three factors interact works out differently on the way from novice to expert.

More recently, researchers have investigated whether information processing in 'careful mode' helps overcome such biases. In turned out that for residents this was indeed the case but not for students (Mamede et al., 2010) and for complex cases only (Mamede et al., 2008). In a later study, Mamede et al. (2012) found that fourth-year students performed worse when stimulated to process cases very carefully than in unreflective or in 'light' mode; however, after 1 week, careful processing led to better diagnostic scores compared with their own previous performance and with the other groups. Other studies (e.g., Schmidt et al., 2014) directed the participants' attention to their conclusions afterward and so could override bias. Some of the manipulations studied had a positive effect on later case processing. A similar phenomenon was found by Grohnert (2017) in a very different domain, i.e., auditing. Grohnert found that having made a certain kind of mistake before and *not*

seeing a certain task as pure routine was beneficial for later performance.[ii]

The interventions in these studies all related to regulation of the process. The positive results related to the effects on present and future problem solving. Our conclusion from these studies is that thoughtful case processing by students as well as reflection on performance improves the quality of their knowledge structure. Discussions on the process of clinical reasoning and its fallibilities may furthermore provide students with the vocabulary and metaknowledge that can help them reflect on their performance (Kassirer, 2010).

After this analysis, we return to the question how clinical reasoning expertise can be stimulated, and whether clinical reasoning skills can be taught and trained as such, or other educational measures will be needed to improve students' clinical reasoning. It might be evident that our theory and previous experiences with direct training programs suggest direct training of the different phases of clinical reasoning does not provide a general solution and that other measures are needed, as far as the reasoning component of the diagnostic process is concerned. What is more important, our theory suggests that to improve clinical reasoning, education must focus on the development of adequate knowledge structures. Similar conclusions permeate recent publications such as Bowen (2006) and Lubarsky et al. (2015). Hence, teaching, training, coaching, modelling, or supervising should adapt to the actual knowledge organization of the student. During the first stage in which knowledge accretion and validation take place, students should be given ample opportunity to test the knowledge they have acquired for its consistency and connectedness, to correct concepts and their connections and to fill the gaps they have detected. Students will do many of these things by themselves if they are provided with stimuli for thinking and with appropriate feedback. This stuff for thinking does not necessarily have to consist of patient problems. One could also think of short descriptions of physiological phenomena (e.g., jet lag) that have to be explained. Self-explanations (e.g., Chamberland et al., 2013) and mind-mapping (Daley

---

[ii]Grohnert (2017) also found that having made a mistake and being provided with a checklist led to increased confidence but not to better performance.

et al., 2016) are powerful learning instruments for students to explore and validate their knowledge.

During the next stage of knowledge encapsulation, students should deal with more elaborate patient problems. As students go through the process of diagnosing a patient and afterwards explaining the diagnosis to a peer or supervisor, biomedical knowledge will become encapsulated into higher-level concepts. For instance, diagnosing a patient with acute bacterial endocarditis will first require detailed reasoning about infection, fever reaction, temperature regulation, circulation, hemodynamics and so on. Later on, a similar case will be explained in terms of bacterial infection, sepsis, microembolisms and aortic insufficiency (Boshuizen, 1989). These problems are not necessarily presented by real patients in real settings. Paper cases and simulated patients will serve the same goal, sometimes even better. Especially during the earlier stage of knowledge encapsulation, when students have to do a great deal of reasoning, it might be more helpful to work with paper cases that present all relevant information. Reasoning through their knowledge networks to build a coherent explanation of the information available, students need not be concerned whether the information on which they work is complete and valid. Later in this stage, when knowledge has been restructured into a more tightly connected format, greater uncertainty can be allowed.

Finally, the stage of illness script acquisition requires experience with real patients in real settings. Research by Custers et al. (1996) suggests that at this stage, practical experience with typical patients (i.e., patients whose disease manifestations resemble the textbooks) should be preferred over experiences with atypical patients. With increasing knowledge, a confrontation with sets of related cases is helpful to learn about the possible manifestations of diseases, while well-chosen combination of cases with similar signs and symptoms but different underlying diseases is essential to improve the knowledge structure (Huwendiek et al., 2013). There are no empirical data that can help to answer the question of whether illness script formation requires active dealing with the patient or whether observing a doctor–patient contact could serve the same goal. On the other hand, because encapsulation and script formation go hand in hand, especially earlier on in this stage, it is probable that 'hands on' experience is to be preferred. Having to reason about the patient would result in

further knowledge encapsulation, while direct interaction with the patient provides the opportunity for perceptual learning, adding 'reality' to the symbolic concepts learned from textbooks. During this phase, students might initially be overwhelmed by the information available in reality. They can easily overlook information when they do not know its relevance. This will especially affect their perception of enabling conditions. Therefore it might be helpful to draw the student's attention to the enabling conditions operating in specific patients, to make sure that their illness scripts are completed with this kind of information. Boshuizen et al. (1992) emphasize that in this stage of training a mix of practical experience and theoretical education is needed. They found that during clinical rotations students tend to shift towards the application of clinical knowledge, although it is not yet fully integrated in their knowledge base. A combination of the two ways of learning can help students to build a robust and flexible knowledge base.

Thus we see that working on problems and diagnosing and explaining patient cases, applying biomedical knowledge and providing feedback on students' thinking might help them to form a knowledge system that enables efficient and accurate clinical reasoning that does not require all control capacity available (monitoring of reasoning on encapsulated concepts in a network requires less control than monitoring of reasoning on preencapsulated, detailed concepts; see Table 5.3). However, in practice, clinical reasoning must be performed in a context of real patients. In the end, students should be able to collect information through history taking, physical examination, and laboratory tests, guided by their clinical reasoning process, and to find a (preliminary) diagnosis in the time available.

Again there are indications that students have problems with collecting information in real settings (Wagenaar, 2008). A well-organized knowledge base is a first requirement, along with well-trained social, perceptual and psychomotor skills.[iii]

Hence, students must learn to do their clinical reasoning and to perform these skills in a coordinated

---

[iii]These skills have a knowledge component, which makes it quite difficult to train them in isolation, separate from knowledge acquisition.

way. This again necessitates training and practice on whole training tasks that stimulate the integration of knowledge and skill into a further integrated knowledge base (Patrick, 1992). The same discussion as occurred earlier in this chapter concerning the possibility of separating knowledge acquisition and the acquisition of clinical reasoning can be repeated regarding the question of whether a well-organized knowledge base and well-trained social, perceptual, and psychomotor skills could be acquired independently. Van Merriënboer et al. (2003) have shown that good planning and design of the learning process, such that integration and automatization are fostered, are very important. A good combination of learning environments like part-task practice timely presentation of information, whole-task practice and elaboration and understanding, adjusted to the student's mastery and knowledge and the cognitive demand of the task, might be the key to success. As we have seen, working with cases plays an essential role, integrated in an educational program, based on an insight into the different obstacles that students experience at successive stages of development towards expertise. Refer to Fig. 5.1 illustrating the relationship between case, knowledge and regulation in expert clinical reasoning.

CHAPTER SUMMARY

In this chapter we have presented:

- a stage theory of development of medical expertise,
- differences in expert and novice knowledge structures,
- case examples to review the points above and
- implications for teaching clinical reasoning.

REFLECTION POINT 2

Consider how these points relate to your practice:
- Case processing in 'careful mode' does not necessarily lead to better outcomes.
- Post hoc reflection on errors in clinical reasoning improves the knowledge structure and future clinical reasoning.
- Teaching with cases requires a well-designed set of cases with similar features (but dissimilar Fault) and dissimilar features (but similar Fault); this improves the richness of illness scripts as well as the network they are part of.
- Teaching with cases should be adapted to the level of expertise development of the students' semantic networks, encapsulation or illness scripts.

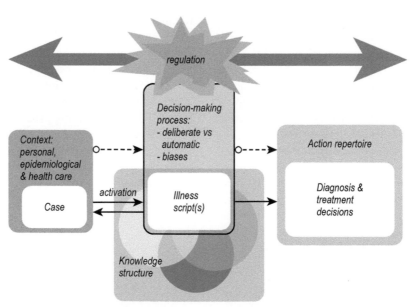

Fig. 5.1 ■ The relationship between case, knowledge and regulation in expert clinical reasoning. The underlying knowledge structure can be further activated when no acceptable solution is found.

REFERENCES

Boshuizen, H.P.A., 1989. De ontwikkeling van medische expertise: een cognitief-psychologische benadering (The Development of Medical Expertise: A Cognitive-Psychological Approach). Doctoral thesis. University of Limburg, Maastricht, The Netherlands.

Boshuizen, H.P.A., Hobus, P.M., Custers, E.J., et al., 1992. Cognitive effects of practical experience. In: Evans, D.A., Patel, V.L. (Eds.), Advanced Models of Cognition for Medical Training and Practice. Springer Verlag, New York, NY, pp. 337–348.

Boshuizen, H.P.A., Schmidt, H.G., 1992. On the role of biomedical knowledge in clinical reasoning by experts, intermediates and novices. Cogn. Sci. 16, 153–184.

Boshuizen, H.P.A., van de Wiel, M.W.J., 1998. Multiple representations in medicine: how students struggle with it. In: van Someren, M.W., Reimann, P., Boshuizen, H.P.A., et al. (Eds.), Learning with Multiple Representations. Elsevier, Amsterdam, The Netherlands, pp. 237–262.

Bowen, J.L., 2006. Educational strategies to promote clinical diagnostic reasoning. N. Engl. J. Med. 23, 2217–2225.

Brennan, T.A., Leape, L., Laird, N.M., et al., 1991. Incidence of adverse events and negligence in hospitalized patients: results of the Harvard Medical Practice Study I. N. Engl. J. Med. 324, 370–376.

Chamberland, M., Mamede, S., St-Onge, C., et al., 2013. Students' self-explanations while solving unfamiliar cases: the role of biomedical knowledge. Med. Educ. 47, 1109–1116.

Croskerry, P., 2003. The importance of cognitive errors in diagnosis and strategies to minimize them. Acad. Med. 78, 775–780.

Custers, E.J., Boshuizen, H.P., Schmidt, H.G., 1996. The influence of medical expertise, case typicality and illness script component on case processing and disease probability estimates. Mem. Cognit. 24, 384–399.

Daley, B.J., Durning, S.J., Torre, D.M., 2016. Using concept maps to create meaningful learning in medical education, MedEdPublish, vol. 5. Available from: <https://doi.org/10.15694/mep.2016.000019>.

Feltovich, P.J., Barrows, H.S., 1984. Issues of generality in medical problem solving. In: Schmidt, H.G., De Volder, M.L. (Eds.), Tutorials in Problem-Based Learning: A New Direction in Teaching the Health Professions. Van Gorcum, Assen, The Netherlands, pp. 128–142.

Grohnert, T., 2017. Judge | Fail | Learn. Enabling auditors to make high-quality judgments by designing effective learning environments. Doctoral thesis. Maastricht University, Maastricht, The Netherlands.

Groothuis, S., Boshuizen, H.P.A., Talmon, J.L., 1998. Analysis of the conceptual difficulties of the endocrinology domain and an empirical analysis of student and expert understanding of that domain. Teach. Learn. Med. 10, 207–216.

Huwendiek, S., Duncker, C., Reichert, F., et al., 2013. Learner preferences regarding integrating, sequencing and aligning virtual patients with other activities in the undergraduate medical curriculum: a focus group study. Med. Teach. 35, 920–929.

Jaarsma, T., Jarodzka, H., Nap, M., et al., 2014. Expertise under the microscope: processing histopathological slides. Med. Educ. 48, 292–300.

Kassirer, J.P., 2010. Teaching clinical reasoning: case-based and coached. Acad. Med. 85, 1118–1124.

Lesgold, A.M., Rubinson, H., Feltovich, P.J., et al., 1988. Expertise in a complex skill: diagnosing X-ray pictures. In: Chi, M.T.H., Glaser, R., Farr, M.J. (Eds.), The Nature of Expertise. Lawrence Erlbaum, Hillsdale, NJ, pp. 311–342.

Lubarsky, S., Dory, V., Audétat, M., et al., 2015. Using script theory to cultivate illness script formation and clinical reasoning in health professions education. Can. Med. Educ. J. 6, 61–70.

Mamede, S., Schmidt, H.G., Penaforte, J.C., 2008. Effects of reflective practice on the accuracy of medical diagnoses. Med. Educ. 42, 468–475.

Mamede, S., Schmidt, H.G., Rikers, R.M., et al., 2010. Conscious thought beats deliberation without attention in diagnostic decision-making: at least when you are an expert. Psychol. Res. 74, 586–592.

Mamede, S., Schmidt, H.G., Rikers, R.M., et al., 2007. Breaking down automaticity: case ambiguity and the shift to reflective approaches in clinical reasoning. Med. Educ. 41, 1185–1192.

Mamede, S., van Gog, T., Moura, A.S., et al., 2012. Reflection as a strategy to foster medical students' acquisition of diagnostic competence. Med. Educ. 46, 464–472.

Patrick, J., 1992. Training: Theory and Practice. Academic Press, London, UK.

Polya, G., 1957. How to Solve It. Doubleday, Garden City, NY.

Rikers, R.M., Schmidt, H.G., Moulaert, V., 2005. Biomedical knowledge: encapsulated or two worlds apart? Appl. Cogn. Psychol. 19, 223–231.

Sackett, D.L., Rosenberg, W.M., Gray, J.M., et al., 1996. Evidence based medicine: what it is and what it isn't. Br. Med. J. 312, 71–72.

Schmidt, H.G., Boshuizen, H.P.A., 1992. Encapsulation of biomedical knowledge. In: Evans, A.E., Patel, V.L. (Eds.), Advanced Models of Cognition for Medical Training and Practice. Springer Verlag, New York, NY, pp. 265–282.

Schmidt, H.G., Boshuizen, H.P.A., 1993. On acquiring expertise in medicine. Educ. Psychol. Rev. 5, 205–221.

Schmidt, H.G., Boshuizen, H.P.A., Norman, G.R., 1992. Reflections on the nature of expertise in medicine. In: Keravnou, E. (Ed.), Deep Models for Medical Knowledge Engineering. Elsevier, Amsterdam, The Netherlands, pp. 231–248.

Schmidt, H.G., Mamede, S., van den Berge, K., et al., 2014. Exposure to media information about a disease can cause doctors to misdiagnose similar-looking clinical cases. Acad. Med. 89, 285–291.

Schmidt, H.G., Norman, G.R., Boshuizen, H.P.A., 1990. A cognitive perspective on medical expertise: theory and implications. Acad. Med. 65, 611–621.

van de Wiel, M.W.J., Boshuizen, H.P.A., Schmidt, H.G., 2000. Knowledge restructuring in expertise development: evidence from pathophysiological representations of clinical cases by students and physicians. Eur. J. Cogn. Psychol. 12, 323–355.

Van Merriënboer, J.J.G., Kirschner, P.A., Kester, L., 2003. Taking the load off the learner's mind: instructional design for complex learning. Educ. Psychol. 38, 5–13.

Wagenaar, A., 2008. What and how students learn from experience. Doctoral thesis. Maastricht University, Maastricht, The Netherlands.

6

EXPERTISE AND CLINICAL REASONING

GAIL M. JENSEN ▪ LINDA J. RESNIK ▪ AMY M. HADDAD

CHAPTER AIMS

The aims of this chapter are to:

- describe why expertise is essential but not sufficient for providing excellent health care,
- discuss the critical importance of the integrative bridge across the concepts of expertise and clinical reasoning,
- illustrate the concept of adaptive expertise and provide considerations for teaching and learning strategies and
- propose considerations for novice development of habits of mind.

KEY WORDS

Expertise

Clinical reasoning

Adaptive expertise

Novice development

INTRODUCTION

Our challenge in professional education is how to prepare learners who can engage in analytical thinking, skilful practice and wise judgements, often in uncertain conditions. As Schön (1987) argued, we are preparing professionals to practice in that *swampy lowland of practice.* In all professions, there are individuals who perform exceptionally well and who are held in high regard by their colleagues and their patients – in other words, experts. A core assumption in our chapter is that we must not separate expert knowledge from expert

activity including the development of clinical reasoning and deliberate action. This is an interactive relationship in which knowledge development, analysis and action each influence the other (Woods and Mylopoulos, 2015).

There is continued focus on the argument that expertise is much more of a process or continuum of development than a static state resulting from a cluster of attributes such as knowledge and problem-solving skills or high-level performance (Bereiter and Scardamalia, 1993; Cooke et al., 2010). The process of moving towards expertise is not based merely on years of experience, but there is something central about the continued development of the learner. Ideally, an enhanced understanding of what distinguishes novices from experts should facilitate learning strategies for more effective professional education. We know that experience alone does not lead to more expertise, but it is the reflection on that experience that is critical for the learner (Boshuizen et al., 2004).

We begin this chapter with a 'deconstruction of the interrelated concepts of expertise and clinical reasoning' through a brief, analytical overview of key domains of theory and research. Next we argue that the integration of context is inherent in clinical reasoning and an essential element in adaptive expertise. From this review, we generate a working list of attributes that we believe need to be considered when talking about clinical reasoning and decision making. In the final section of the chapter, we engage in a discussion of strategies for facilitating learning and novice development in clinical reasoning that focuses on developing essential habits of mind. The goal of understanding expertise and clinical reasoning is, first, to promote effective reasoning in practice and, second, the translation of understanding about good reasoning into more effective teaching and student learning and ultimately the delivery of the highest-quality care.

DECONSTRUCTING THE INTERRELATED CONCEPTS OF EXPERTISE AND CLINICAL REASONING

Expertise as Mental Processing and Problem Solving

Expertise is a complex, multidimensional concept that has captured the interest of researchers for over 50 years (Ericsson, 2009; Rikers and Paas, 2005). The early work in this area came from cognitive psychology and accepted a tradition of basic information-processing capabilities of humans. Initial work in expertise concentrated on mental processing or, more simply, the conceptualization of problem solving. In deGroot's (1966) well-known work with chess players, he began to look at differences among chess players with varying levels of expertise. He found that chess masters were able to recognize and reproduce chess patterns more quickly and accurately than novice players. Subsequent studies in areas such as chess (Chase and Simon, 1973) and physics (Chi et al., 1981) revealed that expertise depended not only on the method of problem solving but also on the expert's detailed knowledge in a specific area, ability to memorize and ability to make inferences.

One of the most fundamental differences between experts and novices is that experts will bring more and better organized knowledge to bear on a problem. In medicine, the ability to determine the proper patient diagnosis was discovered to be highly dependent on the physician's knowledge in a particular clinical specialty area, called *case specificity* (Rikers and Paas, 2005; Schwartz and Elstein, 2008). Case specificity implies that a successful reasoning strategy in one situation may not apply in a second case, because the practitioner may not know enough about the area of the patient's problem. Identification of case specificity focused attention on the role of knowledge in expertise. Both clinician experience and the features of the case are factors that affect the problem-solving strategy that is used. Experts appear to have not only methods of problem solving but also

the ability to combine these methods with knowledge and an understanding of how the knowledge necessary to solve the problem should be organized (Boshuizen et al., 2004; Brandsford et al., 2000; Chi et al., 1988). Experts can make connections or inferences from the data by recognizing the pattern and links between clinical findings and a highly structured knowledge base. This explains why experts tend to ask fewer more relevant questions and perform examinations more quickly and accurately than novices. Novices and intermediate subjects tend to use hypothetico-deductive processes that involve setting up hypotheses and gathering clinical data to prove or disprove them (Schwartz and Elstein, 2008). Thus less experienced clinicians tend to ask patients more questions (and in the same order) than do experts, regardless of their relevance to the case (Rivett and Higgs, 1995).

Expertise as Skill Acquisition

Moulton et al. (2007) argue that there has been far too much focus on diagnostic performance and the role of experience. For health professions in which diagnosis is not the predominant decision point, there has been perhaps no more influential work in expertise than that by Patricia Benner in nursing (Benner, 1984; Benner et al., 1996, 1999, 2010). In her original work, Benner applied a model of skill acquisition developed by Hubert Dreyfus, a philosopher, and Stuart Dreyfus, a mathematician and system analyst (Dreyfus and Dreyfus, 1980). The Dreyfus' work came out of a reaction to the cognitive psychology tradition that intelligent practice is not just the application of knowledge and rules for instrumental decision making. A central premise in this work is that human understanding is a skill akin to knowing how to find one's way about the world, rather than knowing a lot of facts and rules for relating them.

The Dreyfus' conception of expertise is much more focused on the context of actual practice. Several critical elements emerged from the Dreyfus and Dreyfus model (1980, 1996): 1) expertise is more about 'knowing how' (procedural knowledge, knowing how to do things) rather than knowing what (declarative knowledge, knowing information and facts), 2) expert knowledge is embedded in the action of the expert rather than propositional knowledge, 3) experience is a critical factor in the development of expertise, 4) much of expert performance is automatic and nonreflective (but when

TABLE 6.1
Aligning Teaching Strategies With Key Concepts From the Dreyfus and Dreyfus (1980, 1996) Model of Skill Acquisition

Stage	Key Concepts	Teaching Strategies
Novice	Factual, rule driven, relies on others Cannot see whole situation	Point out meaningful diagnostic information Eliminate irrelevant information and highlight discriminating evidence Encourage learners to work with multiple hypotheses
Advanced beginner	Objective facts Begins to use intuition in concrete situations Uses both analytic reasoning and pattern recognition	Build what the learner knows, and work from common ground to uncommon ground Facilitate learners' ability to verbalize thinking and differentiation of diagnoses and treatments
Competent	Can devise new rules based on the situation Sees the big picture Better use of pattern recognition with common problems	Balance supervision with autonomy in decision making Expose learners to breadth and depth of cases Identify learners' developmental stage as may not be in the competent category across all areas
Proficient	Is comfortable with evolving situations Intuitive behaviours replace reasoned responses Can tolerate uncertainty	Expose learners to a balance of cases, not all complex Learners have to know when to trust intuition and when to slow down and be more analytical Facilitate learners' ability to self-regulate and know when they do not know
Expert	Can align thought, feeling, and action into intuitive problem recognition Where intuition is not developed, reasoning is applied	Keep experts challenged with complex cases Apprentice expert to a master who models the skills of a true reflective practitioner
Master	Demonstrates practical wisdom Sees the big picture Reflects in, on and for action Demonstrates moral agency	Master clinician is self-motivated and engages in lifelong learning Challenged by complex cases and habitually engaged in learning more

Source: Adapted from Benner, 1984; Carraccio, Benson, Nixon & Drestine, 2008

a situation is novel, experts engage in deliberation before action) and 5) intuition of experts or the knowing how to do things is both experiential and tacit.

The principles of the Dreyfus and Dreyfus Model of Skill Development (Table 6.1) remain a useful framework to look at learner skill development and continue to be used across the health professions (Carraccio et al., 2008).

Key Elements in Expertise and Adaptive Expertise

Although there has been prolonged debate and controversy in expertise research on the acquisition of expert characteristics, there continues to be strong agreement on the characteristics of experts (Box 6.1) (Ericsson, 2009).

BOX 6.1
CHARACTERISTICS OF EXPERTS

- Experts mainly excel in their domain of expertise.
- Experts are faster than novices in performing skills.
- Experts can solve problems more quickly and with little error.
- Experts have superior short-term and long-term memory.
- Experts can see the problem in their domain at a deeper more principled level than novices, who have a more superficial representation of the problem.
- Experts spend more time trying to understand the problem, and experts have strong self-monitoring skills.

Encouraging Adaptive Learning

You have an experienced student, with an exceptional academic record, completing her last clinical rotation in your clinic. The student demonstrates generally good judgement and always seems to be the first to respond with routine cases. Here are some things that you can do to facilitate bringing out the adaptive learner. Try focusing your questions on reflection by framing the case as follows: "Most cases are more complex than they initially appear. If they seem too simple, ask 'What am I missing?' 'What else could be going on?'" Challenge the student about how a routine approach to this case will not work – so now what? Have the student share the assumptions she has made about the patient. Collaborate with the student in reconstructing how you both can think about this case differently.

Although these characteristics of experts maintain consistency, educators are deeply interested in the development of the learner. How does expertise develop? What does expert practice look like? Education researchers have taken their understandings of expert processes and applied these to learners and learning. This has resulted in a distinction between routine expertise and adaptive expertise.

The argument is that routine experts possess mastery of knowledge in their domain and can apply that knowledge effectively and efficiently to well-known problems, but they are challenged by novel problems. A key premise in adaptive expertise is the experts' ability to break away from the routines and be adaptable as they practice in what is called the 'optimal adaptability corridor' (Mylopoulos and Woods, 2009; Cutrer et al., 2016). There is a need to balance the efficiency of routine expertise with the ability to innovate and engage in progressive problem solving. A major criticism of professional education is that we overemphasize the efficiency dimension of learning and practice. We place major emphasis on certainty and right answers and little focus on how the learner can manage uncertainty (Irby et al., 2010; Shulman, 2004).

How do we facilitate the development of expert-like learners who can engage in progressive problem solving and are on a path towards the development of adaptive expertise? Adaptive expertise requires: 1) an openness to reflecting on practice, 2) metacognitive reasoning skills to recognize that a routine approach to the problem will not work, 3) critical thinking to challenge current assumptions and beliefs and 4) the ability to reconstruct the problem space (Cutrer et al., 2016).

The major components of a master adaptive learner process (Cutrer et al., 2016) include the following activities:

- *Planning:* Identify a gap between what is and what should or could be; select an opportunity for learning; search for resources for learning.
- *Learning:* Engage in learning; critically appraise different sources for learning; move beyond traditional learning strategies such as rereading or highlighting to more effective strategies such as spaced repetitions, elaboration and concept integration.
- *Assessing:* Try out what is learned; engage in informed self-assessment that uses external feedback.
- *Adjusting:* Incorporate what is learned into daily routines; reexamine new learning, and consider opportunities and barriers needed to adjust practice; determine individual versus system implementation.

In summary, we know that experts are knowledgeable because they have extensive, accessible, well-organized knowledge and that they continue to build their practical knowledge base through a repertoire of examples, images, illness scripts and understanding that has been learned through experience (Boshuizen et al., 2004). We also see elements of the critical importance of adaptive learning as experts learn from experience by using reflective inquiry or metacognitive strategies to think about what they are doing, what worked and what did not work (Cutrer et al., 2016). Creating a learning environment that supports learners' development of creative exploration and adaptive expertise is also critical for the health professions.

EXPERTISE AND CLINICAL REASONING IN EVERYDAY PRACTICE

Qualitative research methods have been central tools in investigative, grounded theory work done in several applied professions such as nursing (Benner, 1984; Benner et al., 1996, 1999, 2010), teaching (Berliner, 1986; Sternberg and Horvath, 1995; Tsui, 2003), occupational therapy (Fleming and Mattingly, 2000; Mattingly and Fleming, 1994; Robertson et al., 2015) and physical therapy (Black et al., 2010; Edwards et al., 2004; Jensen et al., 2000, 2007; Resnik and Jensen, 2003; Shaw and DeForge, 2012). These are all professions in which human interactions and care are central aspects of practice. In these studies, we find that clinical reasoning has to include both an analytical and a narrative approach as the focus of care extends beyond the identification of a diagnosis. The clinical reasoning process is iterative and ongoing. Knowing a patient, understanding his or her story, fitting the patient's story with clinical knowledge and collaborating with the patient to problem-solve are the kinds of integral components of clinical reasoning that emerge from these studies.

In analysis of nursing practice, Benner found that much of expert performance in nursing emphasizes individual perceptions and decision-making abilities rather than just the performance of the skill. Benner et al. used observations and narrative accounts of actual clinical examples as primary tools for understanding the everyday clinical and caring knowledge and practical reasoning that were used in nursing practice. Clinical skills were identified as an overall approach to professional action that includes both perception and decision making, not just what we would think of as technical skill or technique (Benner, 1984; Benner et al., 1996, 1999, 2010). It is the integration of the knowledge with skilled know-how (i.e., knowing how to perform a skill in its real setting), along with ethical comportment, that was foundational to expertise in practice. Ethical comportment, simply stated, is the ability to engage in

ethical reflection to discern moral dilemmas. This is more fully described in the last section of the chapter on habits of mind.

In physical therapy, Jensen et al. developed a grounded theory of expert practice in physical therapy (Jensen et al., 2000, 2007). This model of expertise in physical therapy is a combination of multidimensional knowledge, clinical reasoning skills, skilled movement and virtue. All four of these dimensions (knowledge, reasoning, movement and virtues) contribute to the therapist's philosophy of practice. For novices, each of these core dimensions of expertise may exist, but they do not appear to be as well integrated. As novices continue to develop, each of the dimensions may become stronger, yet they may not be well integrated for proficient practice. When the expert therapist has fully integrated these dimensions of expertise, this in turn leads to an explicit philosophy of practice (Fig. 6.1) (Jensen et al., 2007).

Subsequent work by Resnik and Jensen (2003) corroborated the presence of a patient-centred approach to care in collaborative clinical reasoning and promotion of patient empowerment. At the foundation of the patient-centred approach, this research identified an ethic of caring and a respect for individuality, a passion for clinical care and a desire to continually learn and improve. The primary goals of empowering patients, increasing self-efficacy beliefs and involving patients in the care process are facilitated by patient–therapist collaborative problem solving and enhanced through attentive listening, trust building and observation. The patient-centred approach is exemplified by the therapist's emphasis on patient education and by strong beliefs about the power of education. This approach alters the therapeutic relationship and enhances patients' abilities to make autonomous choices. Resnik and Jensen (2003) reported that these efforts not only promoted patient empowerment and self-efficacy but also resulted in greater continuity of services, more skilful care and more individualized plans of care and ultimately better outcomes.

Although experts in that study possessed a broad, multidimensional knowledge base, Resnik and Jensen (2003) discovered that (many) years of clinical experience and specialty certification did not appear to be mandatory in achieving expertise. This seemed to challenge a basic assertion of the Dreyfus model – that

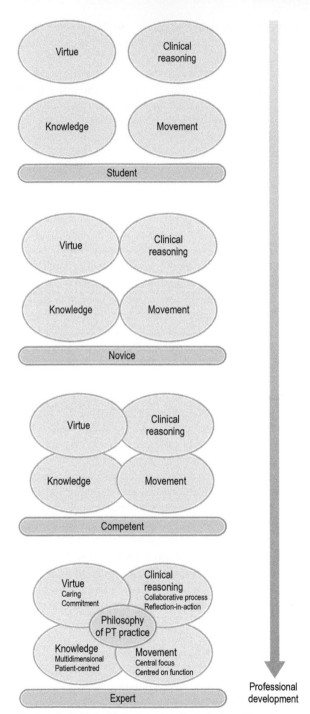

Fig. 6.1 ■ Model of expertise in physical therapy. (From Jensen, G.M., Gwyer, J., Hack, L.M., Shepard, K.F., 2007. Expertise in Physical Therapy Practice, second ed. Saunders-Elsevier, St. Louis, MO, with permission.)

(ongoing) experience is a critical factor in development of expertise. In Resnik and Jensen's (2003) study, this was not observed, and, in fact, some therapists classified as experts were relatively new physical therapists or perhaps expert-like novices (see also Resnik and Hart, 2003). In these instances, the researchers theorized, knowledge acquisition was facilitated by work and life experience before attending physical therapy school, by being in a work environment that offered access to pooled collegial knowledge and by practitioners' values and virtues of inquisitiveness and humility, which drove their use of reflection.

In-depth ethnographic work by Edwards et al. (2004) on expert physical therapists' clinical reasoning strategies has further revealed an interplay of different reasoning strategies in every task of clinical practice (e.g. interactive reasoning, diagnostic reasoning, narrative reasoning, ethical reasoning, reasoning about teaching). Rather than contrasting the cognitively based rational models of reasoning and interactive models of reasoning, Edwards et al. (2004) proposed a dialectic model of clinical reasoning that moves between the cognitive and decision-making processes required to diagnose and manage patients' physical disabilities and the narrative or communicative reasoning and action required to understand and engage patients and carers. Critical reflection is required with either process.

In their classic ethnographic study of clinical reasoning in occupational therapy, Mattingly and Fleming (1994) originally proposed three types of reasoning in their 'theory of the three-track' mind:

1. *Procedural reasoning* (similar to hypothetical-propositional reasoning but in the case of occupational therapy the focus is on identifying the patient's functional problem and selecting procedures to reduce the effects of the problem)
2. *Interactive reasoning* (Active interaction and collaboration with the patient are used to understand the patient's perspective)
3. *Conditional reasoning* (based on social and cultural processes of understanding and is used to help the patient in the difficult process of reconstructing a life that is now changed by injury or disease)

A fourth form of reasoning, narrative reasoning (Fleming and Mattingly, 2000; Mattingly and Fleming, 1994), was subsequently identified.

4. *Narrative reasoning* is used to describe the story-telling aspect of patient cases. Often therapists use narrative thinking and telling of a kind of 'short story' in coming to understand or make sense of the human experience.

REFLECTION POINT 1

What do these examples of investigative work centred on everyday practice tell us about clinical reasoning and expertise?

Across these studies, we see striking similarities that emerge from understanding the contextual factors that are essential in the clinical reasoning process (Box 6.2). Specifically, the integration of knowledge and context is critical for understanding and facilitating expertise. It is the human or relationship side of practice that emerges as a central component of clinical reasoning and, we would argue, part of progressive problem solving that is part of adaptive expertise.

CLINICAL REASONING AND NOVICE DEVELOPMENT: DEVELOPING HABITS OF MIND

If understanding and integrating context are so critical in the clinical reasoning process and in models of

---

BOX 6.2
CONSIDERING SIMILARITIES ACROSS REASONING STUDIES

- Hypothetico-deductive reasoning is used for specific procedural issues.
- The patient is a respected and central aspect of the work.
- Collaboration with the patient is a critical strategy in clinical reasoning and decision making.
- Metacognitive skill (reflection) is an integral aspect of patient care.
- Narrative is a critical tool for understanding the clinical situation including patient, carers and the clinical knowledge that is part of the story.
- Moral agency and deliberate actions are essential elements of what it means to be 'good' at one's work (it is difficult to separate clinical and ethical reasoning).

---

adaptive expertise, then finding ways to facilitate habits of mind is essential. The university setting does well in training the analytic 'habits of mind', but it does far less in developing practical skills and capacity for professional judgement (Colby and Sullivan, 2008). Although expert practitioners bring scientific evidence, analysis and problem-solving skills to the clinical situation, they also bring the skills of practical reasoning as they listen to patients and reflect on and make meaning of what they hear. It is this narrative understanding and practical reasoning that are informed by scientific knowledge but guided by concern for human well-being that are central to expertise. The challenge for professional education is finding the balance between the dominant analytic model of thinking with narrative thinking that can result in skilful practice and wise judgement. How do we go about developing habits of mind in our students? We argue that the relationship between patient and practitioner is a critical element of skilful ethical comportment and is *foundational* in expert work. Therefore focus on the patient and practitioner relationship is an essential foundation for novice development.

The choice of the metaphor of *foundation* is important in that it emphasizes the supportive nature of ethical comportment. A foundation allows something, in this case expert work, to stand on a solid base. If something is lacking in a foundation, or is shakily built, then it will not be strong enough to withstand the stresses encountered in clinical practice. Skilful ethical comportment draws on at least three basic approaches to ethics: principled reasoning, virtue and a care orientation. A solid moral foundation includes all these approaches because an expert needs to understand moral norms and theories and to be adept at using such tools to examine moral problems and practices. However, 'theories and principles are only starting points and general guides for the development of norms of appropriate conduct' (Beauchamp and Childress, 2001, p. 2). An expert must also possess the virtues or character to do the right thing. If a clinician knows the correct moral action but lacks the courage or compassion to act, then the knowledge is of little significance. Lastly, a solid foundation in ethics includes the ability to discern what is worth caring about in healthcare practice. A care orientation considers what values should be pursued, nurtured or sustained and, conversely, what should be

Consider a review of a 'routine' clinical activity such as an interdisciplinary patient care meeting from an unusual perspective to raise awareness of unseen factors that can have a direct effect on the healthcare professional and patient interaction. Ask students to make a list of all kinds of power and authority of those involved in the discussion, i.e., degrees/education level, expertise, gender, seniority, title, control of resources and so on). In light of the list, as part of an individual reflection or small-group discussion, ask students to examine how people are addressed and how they speak to each other in the care meeting. What does this tell you about hierarchies of power within the team and the institution?

disvalued. Approaches that include only abstract principles or duties often lead to conclusions that minimize the particulars of individual circumstances that are considered morally relevant to care orientation.

Within the realm of expert practice, the emotions of compassion, sympathy and empathy have a central place in our understanding of humane and ethical treatment of patients. Beyond these basic expressions of care, patients expect a range of emotional responsiveness from healthcare professionals that is appropriate to context. For example, in an emergency situation, most patients would prefer quick and competent action to save their lives rather than heartfelt empathy. However, it is clear that in certain cases, the emotional tone matters deeply. It is the life work of healthcare professionals to recognize those situations and adapt their emotional response to the particular needs of the patient at that time.

The processes of self-reflection, reflecting together between novice and expert at the moment of a clinical encounter, or small-group discussion on the identification and understanding of emotions are steps in strengthening novices' capacity to hold on to and name their emotional experiences. Rather than novices being told what they should feel or should have felt (such as empathy and compassion) when interacting with patients or others, opportunities should be provided to let novices interact with simulated patients or real patients in clinically complex situations and then reflect on their experiences in their own words.

Although emotions are sometimes seen as a somewhat fragile platform upon which to build such heavy obligations as moral duty or care, by attending to emotions we can see that they highlight certain aspects of a situation, serve as a mode of communication, lead to deeper self-knowledge and provide insight into motivation. Grounding and naming emotions in specific examples from novices' and experts' experiences in clinical practice begins to create a framework that legitimizes this component of the self in one's professional role. Novices can then examine, question and develop their skills in emotional sensitivity; this is an important part of ethical comportment and caring for others.

It is essential that novices have multiple opportunities to act on ethical judgements in a safe environment and reflect not only on the reasons for a particular action or set of actions but also on the thinking and responses that led up to the action. Novices need to hear experts 'think out loud' after a particularly difficult exchange with a patient or colleague so that the process of arriving at a sound decision becomes more transparent. The habit of reflecting on what is going on ethically in a situation, what should be done about it and the meaning for the broader professional and public community *can and must* be fostered throughout professional education.

CHAPTER SUMMARY

- Expertise is not a static state, a list of specific attributes or something that is obtained through years of experience but a continuum of development and a dynamic process in which critical reflection and deliberate action are central components.
- Adaptive expertise requires 1) an openness to reflecting on practice, 2) metacognitive reasoning skills to recognize that a routine approach to the

problem will not work, 3) critical thinking to challenge current assumptions and beliefs and 4) the ability to reconstruct the problem space.

- Clinical reasoning is a complex process in which critical analysis and reflection take place in the context of the action and interaction with the patient.

- Experts demonstrate their patient-centred focus through a consistent commitment to knowing the patient, intense listening that leads to a rich understanding of the patient's perspective and character to do the right thing.

- The challenge in professional education is to teach the complex ensemble of analytic thinking, skilful practice and wise judgement that is required in the health professions. This skilful ethical comportment based on principled reasoning, virtue and a care orientation is the foundation of expertise.

REFLECTION POINT 2

How does this discussion fit in with your previous ideas on expertise? What are the implications for your practice and teaching or learning?

REFERENCES

Beauchamp, T., Childress, J., 2001. Principles of Biomedical Ethics, fifth ed. Oxford University Press, Oxford, UK.

Benner, P., 1984. From Novice to Expert: Excellence and Power in Clinical Nursing Practice. Addison-Wesley, Menlo Park, CA.

Benner, P., Hooper-Kyriakidis, P., Stannard, D., 1999. Clinical Wisdom and Interventions in Critical Care. WB Saunders, Philadelphia, PA.

Benner, P., Sutphen, M., Leonard, V., et al., 2010. Educating Nurses: A Call for Radical Transformation. Jossey-Bass, San Francisco, CA.

Benner, P., Tanner, C.A., Chesla, C.A., 1996. Expertise in Nursing Practice. Springer Press, New York, NY.

Bereiter, C., Scardamalia, M., 1993. Surpassing Ourselves: An Inquiry into the Nature and Implications of Expertise. Open Court Press, Chicago, IL.

Berliner, D., 1986. In pursuit of the expert pedagogue. Educ Res 15, 5–13.

Black, L., Jensen, G.M., Mostrom, E., et al., 2010. The first year of practice: an investigation of the professional learning and development of promising young novice physical therapists. Phys. Ther. 90, 1758–1773.

Boshuizen, H., Bromme, R., Gruber, H., 2004. Professional Learning: Gaps and Transitions on the Way From Novice to Expert. Kluwer Academic, Norwell, MA.

Brandsford, J., Brown, A., Cocking, R., 2000. How People Learn: Brain, Mind, Experience and School. National Academy Press, Washington, DC.

Carraccio, C., Benson, B., Nixon, J., et al., 2008. From the educational bench to the clinical bedside: translating the Dreyfus Developmental model to the learning of clinical skills. Acad. Med. 83, 761–767.

Chase, W., Simon, H.A., 1973. Perception in chess. Cogn Psychol 4, 55–81.

Chi, M.T., Feltovich, P.J., Glaser, R., 1981. Categorization and representation of physics problems by experts and novices. Cogn Sci (Hauppauge) 5, 121–152.

Chi, M.T., Glaser, R., Farr, M., 1988. The Nature of Expertise. Lawrence Erlbaum, Hillsdale, NJ.

Colby, A., Sullivan, W., 2008. Formation of professionalism and purpose: perspectives from the preparation for the professions program. University of St Thomas Law Journal 5, 404–426.

Cooke, M., Irby, D., O'Brien, B., 2010. Educating Physicians. Jossey-Bass, San Francisco, CA.

Cutrer, W.B., Miller, B., Pusic, M., et al., 2016. Fostering the development of master adaptive learners: a conceptual model to guide skill acquisition in medical education. Acad. Med. 92, 70–75.

deGroot, A., 1966. Perception and memory versus thought. In: Kleinmuntz, B. (Ed.), Problem Solving Research, Methods, and Theory. Wiley Press, New York, NY, pp. 19–50.

Dreyfus, H.L., Dreyfus, S.L., 1980. A five stage model of the mental activities involved in directed skill acquisition. Unpublished report supported by the Air Force of Scientific Research (AFSC), USAF (Contract F49620-79-C-0063), University of California, Berkeley, CA.

Dreyfus, H.L., Dreyfus, S.E., 1996. The relationship of theory and practice in the acquisition of skill. In: Benner, P., Tanner, C.A.Chesla, C.A. (Eds.), Expertise in Nursing Practice. Springer Press, New York, NY, pp. 29–48.

Edwards, I., Jones, M., Carr, J., et al., 2004. Clinical reasoning strategies in physical therapy. Phys. Ther. 84, 312–335.

Ericsson, K. (Ed.), 2009. Development of Professional Expertise. Cambridge University Press, New York, NY.

Fleming, M.H., Mattingly, C., 2000. Action and narrative: two dynamics of clinical reasoning. In: Higgs, J., Jones, M. (Eds.), Clinical Reasoning in the Health Professions, second ed. Butterworth-Heinemann, Oxford, UK, pp. 54–61.

Irby, D., Cooke, M., O'Brien, B., 2010. Calls for reform of medical education by the Carnegie Foundation for the Advancement of Teaching: 1910–2010. Acad. Med. 85, 220–227.

Jensen, G.M., Gwyer, J., Hack, L.M., et al., 2007. Expertise in Physical Therapy Practice, second ed. Saunders-Elsevier, St. Louis, MO.

Jensen, G.M., Gwyer, J., Shepard, K.F., et al., 2000. Expert practice in physical therapy. Phys. Ther. 80, 28–43.

Mattingly, C., Fleming, M.H., 1994. Clinical Reasoning: Forms of Inquiry in a Therapeutic Practice. FA Davis, Philadelphia, PA.

Moulton, C., Regehr, G., Mylopoulos, M., et al., 2007. Slowing down when you should: a new model of expert judgment. Acad. Med. 82, S109–S116.

Mylopoulos, M., Woods, N., 2009. Having our cake and eating it too: seeking the best of both worlds in expertise research. Med. Educ. 43, 406–413.

Resnik, L., Hart, D., 2003. Using clinical outcomes to identify expert physical therapists. Phys. Ther. 83, 990–1002.

Resnik, L., Jensen, G.M., 2003. Using clinical outcomes to explore the theory of expert practice in physical therapy. Phys. Ther. 83, 1090–1106.

Rikers, R., Paas, F., 2005. Recent advances in expertise research. Appl. Cogn. Psychol. 19, 145–149.

Rivett, D., Higgs, J., 1995. Experience and expertise in clinical reasoning. New Zealand J Physiother 23, 16–21.

Robertson, D., Warrender, F., Barnard, S., 2015. The critical occupational therapy practitioner: How to define expertise? Aust Occup Ther J 62, 68–71.

Schön, D., 1987. Educating the Reflective Practitioner. Jossey-Bass, San Francisco, CA.

Schwartz, A., Elstein, A.S., 2008. Clinical reasoning in medicine. In: Higgs, J., Jones, M., Loftus, S., et al. (Eds.), Clinical Reasoning in the Health Professions, third ed. Elsevier, Boston, MA, pp. 223–234.

Shaw, J., DeForge, R., 2012. Physiotherapy as bricolage: theorizing expert practice. Physiother. Theory Pract. 28, 420–427.

Shulman, L., 2004. The Wisdom of Practice. Jossey-Bass, San Francisco, CA.

Sternberg, R.J., Horvath, J.A., 1995. A prototype view of expert teaching. Educ Res 24, 9–17.

Tsui, A., 2003. Understanding Expertise in Teaching. Cambridge University Press, New York, NY.

Woods, N., Mylopoulos, M., 2015. On clinical reasoning research and applications: redefining expertise. Med. Educ. 49, 542–544.

Section 2

THE CHANGING CONTEXT OF CLINICAL REASONING AND PRACTICE

THE CONTEXT OF CLINICAL REASONING ACROSS THE HEALTH PROFESSIONS IN THE 21ST CENTURY

MOHAMMAD S.Y. ZUBAIRI ▪ MARIA MYLOPOULOS ▪ MARIA A. MARTIMIANAKIS

CHAPTER AIMS

The aims of this chapter are to:

- discuss the effect of neoliberal policies and globalization on education and practice in the health professions,
- identify how a changing context influences identity, evidence and knowledge politics and
- introduce critical reflexivity as a mechanism to think beyond the clinical encounter.

KEY WORDS

Globalization

Neoliberalism

Context

Identity

Reflexivity

ABBREVIATIONS/ ACRONYMS

EBM Evidence-based medicine

IEHP Internationally educated healthcare professional

INTRODUCTION

This section of the book deals with the changing context of clinical practice and clinical reasoning. In this chapter, we use a case exemplar to set the broad scene for the chapters that follow by exploring several key movements and trends emerging from contemporary neoliberal policies and globalization more broadly. We further explore the effect of these trends on knowledge and reasoning, practice models and expectations of health professions education. Subsequent chapters will address other influences, including the effect of the information evolutions, and changes in clients' expectations and input to decision making.

REFLECTION POINT 1

In Case Study 7.1, there is an evident difference (in terms of racial background but also in English language proficiency) between the parents and the paediatrician that can be assumed to affect their interaction. What about situations in which differences between patient/families and carers are not evident? Is the verbatim message subject to influences by any sociocultural interpretation that may take place in the conversations between patient and interpreter?

The discourse of neoliberalism, consisting of socio-economic policies and practices that reify and value free markets, is often linked to globalization and the amplification of the movement of services, ideas and people across borders (Spring, 2008). This variably leads to diversification and standardization across many domains including health and education. With the increased mobility of people, numerous healthcare professionals are now studying and/or practicing beyond

A junior resident who completed her medical school in Ethiopia is working with a Canadian-trained paediatrician, who identifies as a White Anglo-Saxon male and wants to discuss a case he has encountered. He tells the resident about a 4-year-old boy who just started school and whose family is originally from Bangladesh. They migrated to Canada almost 2 years ago amid the 2008 economic crisis. The boy's father is an engineer and mother stays at home, and his primary language exposure in the household up until the start of school was Bengali. The boy has slowly picked up some single words in English, but the teachers are concerned about language delay even as he interacts with other Bengali-speaking children in the classroom. Parents speak enough English for the paediatrician to communicate with them, but he finds that the typical strategies he might use (i.e., humour

or talking about popular culture) don't work either with the parents or the child. As a result, developing rapport has been difficult. He has worked with visibly and linguistically Bangladeshi families before and tells the resident that he is trying to approach the case the same way as with others.

The paediatrician goes on to tell the resident that he struggles with explaining particular developmental diagnoses, such as autism or global developmental delay, when a language barrier is present and when cultural differences are perceived. Although this family speaks English, he wonders about the use of an interpreter particularly when time comes to give feedback to the family. He tells the resident 'If I have an interpreter, at least I know the verbatim message is getting across, and I am being culturally sensitive'.

the physical borders of their individual nation states. These trends have spurred the sharing of curricula and educational practices, with the goal of attaining greater standardization in the training of healthcare professionals and the delivery of health services (Timmermans and Almeling, 2009). In recent years, for example, there has been a proliferation of interprofessional, patient-centred and person-centred care models across the world calling for stronger collaborative and bidirectional interactions with patients (Haddara and Lingard, 2013; Pluut, 2016).

Through such movement of people, practices and ideas, there is now an increased recognition of the internationally educated healthcare professional or IEHP. The resultant challenges IEHPs face and/or create as they try to integrate into work contexts different from the ones in which they trained requires further attention (Paul et al., 2017). This is highlighted in the initial interactions between the resident trainee in Case Study 7.1 and the paediatrician.

Although discourses of globalization perpetuate the notion that the training of healthcare professionals and the object of medical practice can be standardized (Schwarz and Wojtczak, 2002; Timmermans and Epstein, 2010), the realities of being an IEHP make visible the

knowledge politics underpinning contemporary healthcare educational practices. For instance, IEHPs experience exhaustive licensure requirements in contrast to those who have trained locally. Such requirements more often than not end up leaving them outside the workforce (Paul et al., 2017; Yen et al., 2016). The perceived differences in how IEHPs orient to the delivery of care often evoke client safety concerns. Thus IEHPs who do make it into the workforce often experience discrimination and stigma.

Relatedly, the phenomenon of medical tourism, spurred by ideas of standardization of healthcare delivery, along with broader immigration and refugee trends, affects patient demographics across the world. As a result, healthcare professionals are frequently exposed to patients and colleagues with cultures, values, histories and beliefs related to health and illness that are different from their own (McKimm and McLean, 2011; Perfetto and Dholakia, 2010; Seeleman et al., 2009; World Health Organization, 2010). Healthcare professional educators are starting to report the challenges of applying curricula, pedagogies and educational tools across different healthcare contexts (Ho et al., 2011, 2012), drawing attention to how these differences affect how we operationalize 'competence' as a construct, particularly in relation to clinical reasoning (Hodges and Lingard, 2012).

SHIFTING CONTEXTS AND IDENTITIES

Although the tensions discussed earlier are amplified by growing resource constraints and efficiency mandates, globalization has conceptually and materially blurred our understanding of what constitutes context, learning and expertise. This has implications for how we think about clinical reasoning. Whether homogeneity or heterogeneity is the outcome, the interconnected movement of ideas and people across borders challenges contemporary healthcare professional educators to be attentive to knowledge flow and politics. Specifically, the types of knowledge that come to be valued and/or emerge as dominant in clinical contexts affect how healthcare professionals conduct their work and how patients and their families experience health care (Bleakley et al., 2008; Hodges et al., 2009; Martimianakis and Hafferty, 2013). As one example, the physician can play several different roles in the globalized context (Box 7.1). In our case, the paediatrician, to some extent, exemplifies the 'culturally versed global physician' drawing from an understanding of his specific context.

BOX 7.1
DISCOURSES OF THE
GLOBAL PHYSICIAN

UNIVERSAL GLOBAL PHYSICIAN

This global physician is someone who can be trained anywhere in the world using a set of universally applicable standards of competency.

CULTURALLY VERSED GLOBAL PHYSICIAN

This global physician is someone who has acquired culturally specific knowledge and training through exposure and experience. This knowledge can be applied in culturally specific contexts (locally or internationally).

GLOBAL PHYSICIAN ADVOCATE

This global physician is a socially minded individual trained to understand the economic, cultural and political determinants of health. Global physicians promote global health and use their positions of authority to advocate for marginalized populations.

Derived from Martimianakis and Hafferty, 2013, p. 32.

Contemporary educators face tensions and challenges associated with reconciling competing mandates of standardization and diversification. These challenges provide researchers with a unique opportunity to clarify and critique emergent definitions of clinical reasoning. Specifically, quality control on the one hand and attunement to patient and learner needs on the other bring into focus competencies that may be at odds with one another (Gregg and Saha, 2006; Koehn and Swick, 2006).

As a result, there is a rethinking of how people, including healthcare professionals, are disciplined into their profession and within a particular work context. This has implications for the positions we take in relation to clinical reasoning and expert development. Although multidirectional healthcare professional interactions and patient-centred approaches to care are by no means universal, and may often be limited to Western contexts, clinical reasoning is generally agreed to be a core standard component of practice in the health professions. The proliferation of Western models of care has affected notions of what make a 'good' healthcare professional and how clinical reasoning is executed. Trainees in the health professions around the world are routinely first taught a standard mix of basic science and clinical approaches through combinations of didactic lectures and small-group learning. They then have the opportunity to interact with patients they see as part of their education. Finally, they may become members of teams. This sequence in and of itself is quite standardized and has been implemented in medical schools, for example, around the world (Waterval et al., 2015).

The adoption of similar approaches to clinical practice has not resulted in sameness in how health is experienced and health care is provided. The complexity of what healthcare professionals engage with may be influenced by structures, processes and belief systems that did not evolve or emerge from the same context as their training. This is further complicated by interprofessional models of care, which call for knowledge sharing and team problem solving. We cannot assume that everyone has been socialized into health care in the same way. Given that clinical reasoning informs a large component of a practitioner's identity, it is extremely important to consider how such an identity engages with the identities of other team members,

CASE STUDY 7.2

The paediatrician, introduced in Case Study 7.1, tells the resident that there are very clear guidelines in establishing a diagnosis of autism or global developmental delay, and although there may be some cultural differences in how such diagnoses may be understood, 'a diagnosis is a diagnosis is a diagnosis, and there are standardized ways to come to that diagnosis, such as intelligence testing, or using tools such as the autism diagnostic observation schedule, better known as the ADOS'. The resident, aware that she had limited training in developmental disorders in Ethiopia, has read up on autism ahead of her current placement. She quickly points out that in some cultures people do not look people directly in the eye, yet diagnostic criteria for autism include absent or reduced eye contact.

The paediatrician reminds the resident that 'they've come to me as the doctor, so although there is some room for negotiation, I need to make sure I get the diagnosis right (implying there can only be one right diagnosis) to support the child best'. The resident wonders what is meant by 'negotiation' in the clinical setting and is confused how to think about cultural variance in diagnostic criteria.

The paediatrician goes on to tell the resident that he makes an extra effort to ensure that families who are new to Canada 'who don't speak much English' or 'who don't quite know the system yet' get connected with culturally appropriate resources. He wants to be able to meet with the child's extended family (if available) but often does not have the time and even has less time to connect with agencies directly, including those that provide therapy and the school. He gives a diagnosis and plans to see the family back in 4 to 6 months. The resident walks away asking herself 'does that mean that culture and race only affect communication in health encounters?'

---

administrators and patients (Frost and Reghr, 2013; Rummens, 2003). When the identities of the latter are different from one's own or change as a result of globalization and exposure to other health contexts, we should expect a corresponding change in how clinical reasoning occurs in day-to-day practice.

Clinical reasoning in the globalized workforce then can be conceptualized as an ongoing negotiation of the discrepancies in knowledge, attitudes and practices stemming from cultural differences in what constitutes 'good care', as more likely than not there are marked differences between where healthcare professionals are currently located and where they originally trained (Hodges et al., 2009). It is not unreasonable, then, to speculate that healthcare professionals find themselves challenged by such discrepancies in their daily practice, as in the example of our case, and they may over time resort to choosing one way to practice (most likely the dominant way in the context of their current work) as a way to adhere to notions of quality and standardization. Clinical care guidelines are facilitative mechanisms for such standard setting, where standardization of process becomes a proxy for quality care. However, what happens when clinical care guidelines call for attention to culture and differences? How is clinical reasoning affected by growing demands to attend to sociocultural differences?

REFLECTION POINT 2

When do race and culture factor into encounters with patients? How would one distinguish whether the challenges experienced by the white physician are related to cultural differences?

CLINICAL REASONING: VALUING EVIDENCE

In contrast to traditional dominant models of expertise, clinical reasoning is more frequently being defined as the 'creative and open-ended exploration of a (clinical) problem that aims to develop an understanding of a situation … (and where) a diagnosis can be a valuable aid to reasoning, but it does not define the entirety of the reasoning process … converging (only) on an answer that is either right or wrong' (Ilgen et al., 2016, p. 436).

(See Mylopoulos and Woods, 2017, for further discussion on adaptive expertise.) This is closely related to case formulation, which may involve making a diagnosis as the paediatrician, in our case, prioritizes. However, his understanding and/or explanation of the patient's presentation only superficially address context and the perspectives available to him (including those of the parents and resident trainee from Ethiopia).

In this regard, clinical reasoning, as a process of exploring problems emerging from and being influenced by globalization, becomes greater than the individual practitioner, team or organization. Although clinical reasoning could be described as application of specific algorithms and thinking very categorically about patients and their diseases (Norman, 2005), as our case highlights, globalization is challenging such a categorical and algorithmic approach. As one example, related to the developmental difficulties that children may face, it is important to consider that some diagnostic categories such as those of attention deficit hyperactivity disorder or autism may not have the same uptake as diagnoses in particular parts of the world.

This has implications for both how patients from such parts of the world interact with healthcare professionals in contexts where such categories do matter. Simultaneously, how clinical reasoning may be taught to trainees in countries where such categories do not matter also needs to be addressed. Curricular strategies, diagnostic criteria and treatment algorithms developed in one context may not apply in other contexts or vice versa (Bleakely et al., 2008). Such differences are increasingly seen as important in the provision of patient-centred care models. A good example of this might be guidelines related to management of diabetes, and similarly some guidelines around end-of-life care may pose unique challenges in places where death and dying are very much governed by religious and cultural norms. In our case, a difference in eye contact is invoked by the resident highlighting the situated nature of knowledge.

Expertise in a traditional sense, therefore, is very much a product of utilizing expert knowledge. In many contexts, clinical experts are predominantly situated within the biomedical model. Lawlor (2010, p. 169) challenges this notion of expertise by asking 'What if expertise were considered to be more multiply located or distributed? Perhaps even more radically, what if the

expertise of parents or children and adults with [specific disease] were foregrounded or privileged over other sources of knowledge … Strengthening reflections on the nature of expertise and domains of local knowledge will generate more deliberate attempts to examine multiple perspectives on understandings and events in which expertise is enacted'.

Drawing from the medical education literature, on the one hand, healthcare professionals hold all power of knowing, and on the other, knowing is strategically co-constructed and distributed between the practitioner and patient (Kawamura et al., 2014). With the latter, it becomes very relevant to identify, incorporate and consider all elements, including those that are nonhuman, symbolic and discursive, at multiple levels, including the individual, organization, community and beyond (Zubairi et al., 2016). Such a reframing of expertise, to which clinical reasoning is fundamental, challenges both our definitions of the reified 'single expert' and what it means to make meaning of complex situations. In an evidence-based world, it allows us to expand what we value as evidence in our clinical reasoning (Mylopoulos et al., 2017).

Specifically, the emergence and continual proliferation of EBM have created challenges in identifying and addressing context-specific pockets of cultural, religious and social knowledge pertinent in the delivery of patient-centred care. Some of our own work has demonstrated how objective diagnostic formulations and treatment recommendations are determined at the expense of broader sociopolitical considerations that are patient-specific, including race, class and gender (Zubairi et al., 2016). As a result, 'good' healthcare professionals in today's context may be the ones who are best at practicing EBM, but using said scientific evidence runs the risk for perpetuating inequities when sociocultural knowledge related to the patient is ignored. At the same time, there are frequent 'intercultural exchanges where hybridity has become significant in health care encounters, because this is where the culture of medicine collides with patients' ways of knowing and being' (Nielsen et al., 2015, p. 2).

Such varying contextual factors may challenge the practitioner to think differently about a case and influence his or her decision to take into account (or not) such elements as culture or socioeconomic differences, religion and sexual orientation. More specifically, this can challenge a healthcare professional's comfort with more standardized biomedical approaches that he or she would have learnt through education and an emphasis towards a specific diagnosis. There is evidence to suggest that although some practitioners draw more and more strictly on EBM, there are others who still rely on experience and context (Peters et al., 2016).

CRITICAL REFLEXIVITY AND 'NEGOTIATION'

It has been suggested that educating healthcare professionals to be able to orient themselves to different forms of knowledge requires the practice of critical reflexivity (Ng et al., 2015). Certainly, now more than ever before, in light of global events and shifting ideologies, critical reflection allows healthcare professionals to think about their practice in deeper ways, evaluating their own beliefs, values and context within the social and systemic boundaries of their clinical practice. There is potential for practitioners to identify how they are exercising or activating the power that rests within their work (Frambach and Martimianakis, 2017). The new dominant voice has become that of the patient, and it continues to collide with the historical dominance of the healthcare professional. In the context of person- or patient-centred care, there is thus the potential of greater awareness of the hierarchies of knowledge and a relative flattening of such hierarchies. Different contexts around the world have differential attitudes to hierarchy and power among practitioners and different attitudes around avoiding uncertainty in the practice of clinical reasoning (Findyartini et al., 2016).

Although there may be multiple social negotiations taking place between providers and patients who come to an encounter with different ideologies and knowledge, in the absence of an awareness of the power differentials, there may be perpetuation of inequities through hidden and differential expressions of racism and colonial practices (Bleakley et al., 2008). The spaces for negotiations and co-construction of knowledge are those 'grey' spaces where the pendulum continues to swing between how practitioners define their own roles in clinical encounters and how their engagement with patients is defined.

It is in these spaces where neoliberal constructs designed to be taught and/or measured, such as 'cultural competency', run the risk for 'othering' the patients (Betancourt, 2006; Pon, 2009; Wear, 2003) while separating clinical reasoning from important contextual factors. Such constructs are intended to standardize how care is delivered and to develop efficiencies in the health system. However, in the process, culture can become reduced in clinical encounters to a limited number of situations, for example when 1) it is visible from the perspective of the practitioner, 2) evidence and guidelines isolate culture as a variable, perpetuating race-based stereotypes, and 3) physicians use their power to treat culture as secondary to diagnostic considerations (Zubairi et al., 2016). These very spaces, therefore, permit a reconceptualization of the clinical encounter, necessitating reflection on the intended purpose of the interactions between healthcare professionals and patients/family members.

CHAPTER SUMMARY

The 21st century has brought with it emerging and evolving trends that directly and indirectly influence clinical reasoning in health care. These trends will be explored further in the chapters that follow.

In this chapter we have outlined:

- how neoliberal policies and globalization intersect with one another to influence clinical reasoning in current models of practice and education in health care,
- how shifting contexts influence identities and affect the types of knowledge that are valued and made dominant and
- how practitioners can begin to reflect on the challenges and opportunities that emerge as a result of multiple trends in health care.

REFLECTION POINT 3

Is the healthcare professional, for example, the expert (and keeper of knowledge) or a resource to the client/family? Additionally, the differences that emerge between a professional and patient and the family/carer can become points of tension or conflict that can be used as starting points for ongoing reflection.

REFERENCES

Betancourt, J.R., 2006. Eliminating racial and ethnic disparities in health care: what is the role of academic medicine? Acad. Med. 81, 788–792.

Bleakley, A., Brice, J., Bligh, J., 2008. Thinking the post-colonial in medical education. Med. Educ. 42, 266–270.

Findyartini, A., Hawthorne, L., McColl, G., et al., 2016. How clinical reasoning is taught and learned: cultural perspectives from the University of Melbourne and Universitas Indonesia. BMC Med. Educ. 16, 185.

Frambach, J.M., Martimianakis, M.A., 2017. The discomfort of an educator's critical conscience: the case of problem-based learning and other global industries in medical education. Perspect. Med. Educ. 6, 1–4.

Frost, H.D., Regehr, G., 2013. 'I AM a doctor': negotiating the discourses of standardization and diversity in professional identity construction. Acad. Med. 88, 1570–1577.

Gregg, J., Saha, S., 2006. Losing culture on the way to competence: the use and misuse of culture in medical education. Acad. Med. 81, 542–547.

Haddara, W., Lingard, L., 2013. Are we all on the same page? A discourse analysis of interprofessional collaboration. Acad. Med. 88, 1509–1515.

Ho, M.J., Lin, C.W., Chiu, Y.T., et al., 2012. A cross-cultural study of students' approaches to professional dilemmas: sticks or ripples. Med. Educ. 46, 245–256.

Ho, M.J., Yu, K.H., Hirsh, D., et al., 2011. Does one size fit all? Building a framework for medical professionalism. Acad. Med. 86, 1407–1414.

Hodges, B.D., Lingard, L. (Eds.), 2012. The Question of Competence. Cornell University Press, Ithaca, NY.

Hodges, B.D., Maniate, J.M., Martimianakis, M.A.T., et al., 2009. Cracks and crevices: globalization discourse and medical education. Med. Teach. 31, 910–917.

Ilgen, J.S., Eva, K.W., Regehr, G., 2016. What's in a label? Is diagnosis the start or the end of clinical reasoning? J. Gen. Intern. Med. 31, 435–437.

Kawamura, A.A., Orsino, A., Mylopoulos, M., 2014. Integrating competencies: exploring complex problem solving through case formulation in developmental pediatrics. Acad. Med. 89, 1–5.

Koehn, P.H., Swick, H.M., 2006. Medical education for a changing world: moving beyond cultural competence into transnational competence. Acad. Med. 81, 548–556.

Lawlor, M.C., 2010. Autism and anthropology? Ethos 38, 167–171.

Martimianakis, M.A., Hafferty, F.W., 2013. The world as the new local clinic: a critical analysis of three discourses of global medical competency. Soc. Sci. Med. 87, 31–38.

McKimm, J., McLean, M., 2011. Developing a global health practitioner: time to act? Med. Teach. 33, 626–631.

Mylopoulos, M., Borschel, D., O'Brien, T., et al., 2017. Exploring integration in action: competencies as building blocks of expertise. Acad. Med. 92, 1794–1799.

Mylopoulos, M., Woods, N.N., 2017. When I say ... adaptive expertise. Med. Educ. 51, 685–686.

Ng, S.L., Kinsella, E.A., Friesen, F., et al., 2015. Reclaiming a theoretical orientation to reflection in medical education research: a critical narrative review. Med. Educ. 49, 461–475.

Nielsen, L.S., Angus, J.E., Howell, D., et al., 2015. Patient-centered care or cultural competence: negotiating palliative care at home for Chinese Canadian immigrants. Am. J. Hosp. Palliat. Care 32, 372–379.

Norman, G., 2005. Research in clinical reasoning: past history and current trends. Med. Educ. 39, 418–427.

Paul, R., Athina, M., Martimianakis, T., et al., 2017. Internationally educated health professionals in Canada: navigating three policy subsystems along the pathway to practice. Acad. Med. 92, 635–640.

Perfetto, R., Dholakia, N., 2010. Exploring the cultural contradictions of medical tourism. Consumption Markets & Culture 13, 399–417.

Peters, A., Vanstone, M., Monteiro, S., et al., 2016. Examining the influence of context and professional culture on clinical reasoning through rhetorical-narrative analysis. Qual. Health Res. 27, 866–876.

Pluut, B., 2016. Differences that matter: developing critical insights into discourses of patient-centeredness. Med. Health Care Philos. 19, 501–515.

Pon, G., 2009. Cultural competency as new racism: an ontology of forgetting. J. Progress Hum. Serv. 20, 59–71.

Rummens, J.A., 2003. Conceptualising identity and diversity: overlaps, intersections, and processes. Can. Ethn. Stud. 35, 10–25.

Schwarz, M.R., Wojtczak, A., 2002. Global minimum essential requirements: a road towards competence-oriented medical education. Med. Teach. 24, 125–129.

Seeleman, C., Suurmond, J., Stronks, K., 2009. Cultural competence: a conceptual framework for teaching and learning. Med. Educ. 43, 229–237.

Spring, J., 2008. Research on globalization and education. Rev. Educ. Res. 78, 330–363.

Timmermans, S., Almeling, R., 2009. Objectification, standardization, and commodification in health care: a conceptual readjustment. Soc. Sci. Med. 69, 21–27.

Timmermans, S., Epstein, S., 2010. A world of standards but not a standard world: toward a sociology of standards and standardization. Ann. Rev. Sociol. 36, 69–89.

Waterval, D.G.J., Frambach, J.M., Driessen, E.W., et al., 2015. Copy but not paste: a literature review of crossborder curriculum partnerships. J. Stud. Int. Educ. 19, 65–85.

Wear, D., 2003. Insurgent multiculturalism: rethinking how and why we teach culture in medical education. Acad. Med. 78, 549–554.

World Health Organization, 2010. How Health Systems Can Address Health Inequities Linked to Migration and Ethnicity. WHO Regional Office for Europe, Copenhagen.

Yen, W., Hodwitz, K., Thakkar, N., et al., 2016. The influence of globalization on medical regulation: a descriptive analysis of international medical graduates registered through alternative licensure routes in Ontario. Can. Med. Educ. J. 7, 19–30.

Zubairi, M., Kawamura, A., Mylopoulos, M., et al., 2016. The cultural encounter in developmental paediatrics. Unpublished MRP. Ontario Institute for Studies in Education, University of Toronto, Canada.

8

CHANGING DEMOGRAPHIC AND CULTURAL DIMENSIONS OF POPULATIONS
Implications for Health Care and Decision Making

JASON A. WASSERMAN ■ STEPHEN LOFTUS

CHAPTER AIMS

The aims of this chapter are to:

■ articulate how shifts in the composition and character of populations promote greater complexity in diagnosis and treatment,

■ elaborate how greater complexity in the diagnostic and treatment processes challenges traditional forms of clinical reasoning,

■ use the examples of aging and increasing race/ethnic diversity to underscore the ways that demographic shifts confound traditional clinical reasoning and

■ consider the characteristics that need to attend clinical reasoning to navigate these new complexities, including the incorporation of reflexive logics and the recognition of intersubjective processes.

KEY WORDS

Demographic

Aging

Culture

Diversity

Complexity

Reflexivity

INTRODUCTION

Clinical reasoning is not practiced in a vacuum but rather takes place against any number of different social contexts. One of these concerns the composition and characteristics of populations of patients and the sometimes dramatic shifts these populations can undergo. Even though a healthcare professional usually is dealing at any given time only with one patient, it is often forgotten just how much the demographics of patient populations shape clinical reasoning. In this chapter, we draw attention to the importance of understanding demographics and their profound influences on clinical reasoning.

Social changes, including shifts in the composition and character of populations, affect clinical reasoning through a variety of mechanisms. Ways of thinking about health are themselves nested in culturally dependent beliefs, attitudes and ways of knowing. This is true not just of the patient population but also of the healthcare professionals who provide health care. A simple example is the traditional belief that both infants and older persons did not feel as much pain as the rest of the population. This myth likely emerged because these age groups could not express pain easily, yet it took root in ways that dramatically affected clinical reasoning. For example, those who believed this myth were unlikely to take the need for pain management sufficiently into consideration for these patients.

Such examples underscore that clinical reasoning is not simply something the healthcare professional does alone. Instead, clinical reasoning occurs within a dialogical relationship between healthcare professional and patient (at the individual level), nested in as a social structural relationship between health care and society. In this way, the clinical relationship is bidirectional, sometimes called intersubjective. The scientific basis of health care is, clearly, highly influential. At the same time, social norms and the particular tendencies of social groups place demands on health care that affect how it is practiced. For example, different beliefs and values about contraception and abortion may profoundly affect the clinical reasoning surrounding fertility and family planning. The controversies in this example are not dependent on scientific facts but on the values of those involved and, moreover, the comingling of their perspectives as they interact in a clinical dialogue. Health care and clinical reasoning, therefore, are not value-free activities. The personal and professional values of the healthcare provider and the values of his or her client play important roles. Moreover, the values that patients and providers have are partly individual but are also shaped by the wider society and especially the social groups with which they identify. Our focus in this chapter concerns how many of these wider social groups recently have experienced dramatic change.

We now live in an increasingly globalized world that can affect clinical reasoning and healthcare decision making. The coming together of diverse populations with varied beliefs about the body, disease, expectations of health and normative practices places demands on the exercise of clinical reasoning. Everywhere, we encounter greater social complexity than in the past, and, like other areas of social life, clinical reasoning must shift accordingly. In what follows, we first briefly describe key social changes that affect clinical practice, particularly through introduction of new complexities. We also underscore the challenges of adapting how healthcare professionals think about disease and their roles in the diagnosis and treatment process with diversifying populations. We conclude with some theorizing about the future direction of these trends.

CHANGING POPULATIONS

Providing a comprehensive description of demographic shifts in populations in various countries around the world is beyond the scope of this chapter. Instead we focus on a few key demographic shifts that highlight how increased complexity in disease epidemiology dramatically affects clinical reasoning (something elaborated later). Among many important demographic shifts, we find that a particularly instructive examination concerns how the changing age structure and the cultural diversification that attend globalization and mass migration are significantly disruptive to traditional forms of clinical reasoning.

Industrialized countries around the world have, for over a century or more, witnessed marked increases in the life expectancy of their populations. Despite recent data suggesting a small decline in the United States from 78.9 years in 2014 to 78.8 years in 2015 (Xu et al., 2016), long-standing trends towards greater longevity represent greater complexity for health care and society at large.

Although we often think of aging as something experienced by individuals, aggregate increased longevity can be thought of as the aging of society. As people live longer, the average age of a population increases, meaning that older people make up a greater percentage of the population. This is particularly important because social systems, including health care, often tier social support in a way that assumes healthy, working persons will care for both the young and old. At its simplest, this means that primary caregivers within family units are likely to be caring for more older family members than they did in the past. At the societal level, social service programs are funded by contributions from those in the workforce to support those who are not. As populations age, the foundations of this system of support will be more heavily stressed, a phenomenon that is already occurring in developed countries around the world and projected to increase dramatically into the future.

Data from the European Commission in the European Union (EU) show striking degrees of population aging (EU, 2015). Between 2005 and 2015, the percentage of the EU population 65 years of age and older increased 2.3% (EuroStat, 2016). Projections find the life expectancy for men increasing from 77.6 years in 2013 to a projection of 84 years by 2060. Similarly, women in the EU lived an average of 83.1 years in 2013 but are projected to live an average of 89.1 years by 2060. Importantly, this means that the relative proportion of workers will decline by nearly 10% in light of dramatic increases in the population older than 65 years of age. In fact, individuals 65 to 79 years of age made up 13.3% of the EU population in 2013 but are projected to make up 16.6% by 2060. More striking still, individuals older than 80 years of age made up only 5.1% of the population in 2013 but are projected to make up 11.8% of the population by 2060. This is associated with significant costs, with the percentage of GDP represented by health care increasing from 6.9% to 7.8% and long-term care from 1.6% to 2.7%. Although these may seem like comparatively small increases, the problem represented by an aging population is exacerbated by the declining number of workers relative to pensioners, which was 4 : 1 in 2013 but is projected to be 2 : 1 in 2060. That is, far fewer workers will support these costlier populations.

Trends from Australia and the United States parallel those of the EU. The percentage of Australians 65 years of age and older is expected to increase from 13% to 25% by 2042, representing an additional 4 million individuals in that age group (Commonwealth of Australia, 2004). Although in 2002 there were over five workers for every person older than 65 years of age in Australia, just as in the EU, by 2042, this number will decline to 2.5. In the United States, the percentage of the population 65 years of age and older increased from about 8% in 1950 to about 14% in 2013 (Martin et al., 2015). As mirrored in other Western nations, the US birth rate in the two decades after the Second World War was significantly elevated compared with the preceding decades and those that followed. Members of this 'baby boomer' cohort currently are aging into retirement, representing a population 'bubble' that will have to be supported by a relatively small number of people in the workforce.

One clinical challenge in aging societies concerns the complexity of geriatric health. Older persons frequently have several chronic health conditions, each with its own treatment that carries potential for adverse interactions. Aging populations pose challenges for healthcare professionals on an individual level but also at the societal level where questions about funding, capitation and rationing emerge. However, aging is not the only demographic challenge to health care and clinical reasoning.

Increasing race/ethnic diversity also presents new forms of complexity that challenge clinical care. This occurs not only as a result of shifting internal demographics of different nations but also because of the interlinked nature of a global society. Although there are many different often value-laden definitions of globalization, here we are primarily concerned with it as the increasingly dynamic and rapid flow of

populations and their characteristics (e.g., values, beliefs and customs) across national borders. New technologies, along with increasingly interwoven economic systems, have promoted greater laxity in national boundaries and a corresponding increase in cultural diversity within countries that, historically, were culturally homogenous by comparison. For example, 20 EU countries experienced increases in the percent of foreign-born population between 2009 and 2015; 13 of those saw increases of more than 10% in that period. Australia also witnessed a marked increase in net overseas migration (Australian Bureau of Statistics, 2016). In the United States, increasing race/ethnic diversity is being driven by increases in the populations of minority groups and migration patterns, particularly of immigrating Hispanic populations. Pol and Thomas (2013, p. 87) write that 'Current figures reveal an America that is becoming less "white", while African American, Asian American, and American Indian/Alaskan Native populations are becoming proportionately larger'.

The increasing diversity of race/ethnic groups in most developed countries holds significance for clinical reasoning that must match symptoms presented by a patient to a diagnosis and then formulate a treatment plan that not only fits within the patient's values but also that patients often must carry out themselves and with their families. Each stage of this process can be significantly affected by the cultural and social norms of the patient.

CHANGING POPULATIONS AND CLINICAL REASONING

The foundations of clinical reasoning in the Western world are grounded in modernist forms of rationality tracing back to Cartesian thought. This means that ideas such as the logic of cause and effect are largely taken for granted. It is also often assumed that the body is a biological machine, where disease is a problem to be solved. Moreover, there is an implicit assumption that the 'disease problem' can *always* be solved if we have sufficient scientific data and the technological capacity to intervene. In this model, healthcare professionals are also assumed to be technicians who can act on the body and solve those problems (Scott, 2013). However, the demographic changes we are currently witnessing challenge this worldview. One reason for this concerns the growing incidence of chronic diseases. Acute conditions may fit well in a model that conceptualizes disease as a biophysical problem. But with chronic conditions, often the problems are never solved but instead managed over long periods of time. Well-known examples involve chronic pain and diabetes. Over time, the management often has to be adjusted and may become more complex. Individuals with diabetes can slowly deteriorate over the years, even with the best management. Patients with chronic pain can acquire other health problems that may complicate palliative care. In this situation, patients need to have significant input into the clinical reasoning required and not just provide information as part of the history-taking process. Even the many well-intentioned attempts at patient-centred care often utilize strategies of relationship building largely for the purpose of getting better diagnostic information from patients. However, traditional forms of paternalism in the clinical relationship, where physician expertise and decision making go relatively unquestioned and often utilize relatively little input from the patient beyond the eliciting of diagnostically necessary somatic information, are more fundamentally undermined in an era of both epidemiological and demographic complexity. We next take a closer look at this issue of complexity and how it manifests in both aging and increasingly diverse populations.

Epidemiological Complexity, Aging and Clinical Reasoning

In the later decades of the 20th century, developed nations experienced an epidemiological shift in which chronic illnesses surpassed acute illnesses as the most significant mortality threats (Hinote and Wasserman, 2016; Omran, 1971). As a class of ailments, acute conditions can be successfully treated using a relatively simple causal profile. For example, the traditional model of disease can be understood in terms of an agent (microbe or virus) infecting a host (a person or, more specifically, an organ, tissue, blood, etc.). The miracles of modern medicine developed around disrupting the causal pathways within that paradigm, either by eliminating the pathogen from the host (antisepsis) or by steeling the host against the pathogen to prevent infection (vaccination). As notions of public health took a more significant role throughout the 20th century, the role of environment was incrementally added to create the 'epidemiological triad', but it remained conceptualized in a relatively limited way, focusing primarily on the contexts of contagion (Dubos, 1965). Importantly, this model becomes insufficient for complex chronic diseases (at least without significant reformulation of what is traditionally meant by 'environment').

Chronic diseases represent a paradigm shift in complexity in at least two ways. The first is ontological; that is, chronic illnesses are paradigmatically different *kinds* of diseases compared with acute illnesses. Chronic diseases are different kinds of entities, and therefore, the clinical reasoning required needs to be different. Although infectious diseases typically involve agents that are foreign to and distinct from the human body, most chronic illnesses involve not the presence of something foreign but elevated or depleted levels of things endemic to the human body (e.g., cholesterol or blood sugar that is too high). The targets of treatment for chronic illnesses are therefore less discrete and are natural and necessary to the body itself. Secondly, chronic illnesses emerge not from acute moments of contagion but frequently from thousands of decisions across a person's life course, each nested within different social contexts (e.g., culture, class, community, neighbourhood). Well-known examples of such decisions include smoking, alcohol use, lack of exercise and diets high in fat and sugar. These decisions are not always freely made. For example, low-income families may not have access to affordable or fresh food, and a poor diet may be the only realistic option. Thus values, beliefs, purchasing power, proximity to healthy or unhealthy opportunities and other social factors are fundamental causes of disease that can no longer be excised from our thinking about it (Link and Phelan, 1995). Put another way, rather than intervening in a single causal pathway (i.e., between agent and host), the multifactorial nature of chronic illness necessitates drawing together understandings of physiology and biochemistry on the one hand and sociological and psychological insights on the other. Insofar as traditional forms of clinical reasoning were able to disregard much of that information, clinical reasoning now needs to be just as multifactorial and wide ranging as the causes of disease in the contemporary epidemiological landscape.

As populations age, the proportion of chronic illnesses increases. In one US study, for example, nearly 86% of adults 65 years of age and older had at least one chronic condition, over 60% had two or more, and about one-third had three or more (Ward et al., 2014). The successes of modern health care have presented new complexities that cannot be met with an old logic, and the demand on health care now concerns its attentiveness to a larger case narrative inclusive of social and psychological features of a patient's illness experience.

The increasing focus on patient-centred care over the last several decades might be read as an implicit recognition of the salience of this growing complexity, but a fully delineated corresponding form of clinical reasoning has yet to take root in any widespread way. Still, efforts at elaborating and promoting narrative medicine (Charon et al., 2017; Loftus and Greenhalgh, 2010) and the generation of schemas for inductive logics inclusive of the humanistic aspects of disease today (Wasserman, 2014) suggest that attending to new forms of illness complexity and their attendant social and humanistic elements is entirely possible. Patient narratives can be read for insights into aspects of illness complexity. These include, for example, patient values or the challenges posed by contexts in which they get sick, experience illness and carry out treatment, such as their families and neighbourhoods. Utilizing such information, not just to make the patient feel more 'accompanied' by the physician but rather by fully integrating it into the diagnostic and treatment processes, will be a key task for clinical practice over the coming years and decades. However, the nature of disease in aging populations and growing diversity suggest doing so is necessary.

In the chronic illness era, seeking a single biomedical diagnosis on the basis of pathophysiological signs and symptoms alone is frequently no longer sufficient. For some years now, there have been calls to replace the biomedical model of clinical reasoning with a biopsychosocial model that takes social and psychological factors into account (Engel, 1977). However, even the biopsychosocial model has been critiqued as not going far enough. Morris (1998) has called for a biocultural model of health care that puts more emphasis on sociocultural factors. We would argue that this biocultural model can be part of a more relationship-centred approach to clinical reasoning that allows insights about the nature of disease and the direction of treatment to be genuinely co-created by physician and patient, but this requires the healthcare professional to abandon some assumptions about definitions of disease and his or her role as a paternalistic practitioner. Only from a basis of greater epistemological freedom—where clinicians are free to rethink traditional assumptions of clinical science to better collaborate with their patients' ways of thinking—can healthcare professionals and patients co-create an understanding of illness truly grounded in patients' experiences and values and develop a treatment plan best fit to each patient's life. This is especially true among aging populations where value-driven decisions related to cost and quality of life may call for a fundamental reconsideration of a traditionally unquestioned drive to treat all 'problems' (see Case Study 8.1).

REFLECTION POINT 1

For Case Study 8.1, articulate the various ways that this case entails different aspects of complexity (in terms of how the patient became ill, the providers that must treat her illnesses, the contexts in which

---

CASE STUDY 8.1

Mattie is an 83-year-old woman with a history of chronic obstructive pulmonary disease (COPD) and diabetes. Because of her diabetes, she has a very difficult time healing when she is scraped or cut and has been prone to infection of even minor skin contusions. She has discussed her end-of-life wishes with her primary care physician and signed a do-not-resuscitate order. On a routine visit to her pulmonologist, she notes that she's begun having palpitations in her heart. She's referred to a cardiologist, who recommends a catheter ablasion, which involves the insertion of catheter wires into the groin or neck that are sent down to the heart and which intentionally destroy the tissue causing the palpitations. The cardiologist tells Mattie and her son Mitch that the procedure is noninvasive. Mitch insists that she needs to consent to the procedure, but Mattie is hesitant. She consults with her primary care provider (PCP).

she faces those illnesses and treatments, the personal values she might bring to the experience, how her age might affect her treatment goals and/or those of her providers, and so on). What challenges does each of these complexities pose for clinical reasoning?

The increasingly complex pluralistic world in which practitioners meet patients today would seem to include new more reflexive forms of clinical reasoning. By 'reflexive', we mean forms of clinical reasoning that are more dialogical and intersubjective. Reflexivity in clinical reasoning gives permission to go beyond thinking only with simplistic cause-and-effect mechanisms, for example, by recognizing that cause and effect can be linked together in multifaceted ways in complex relationships that persist over time. This is the reality of chronic disease where complex long-term relationships need to be maintained and developed over months or years (Tasker et al., 2017). For example, in Case Study 8.1, a reflexive reconsideration of what is the best course of treatment calls us to ask whether we ought to treat the problem at all, interrogating the underlying values and goals of treatment. Building on this idea, it could even be argued that we need a form of clinical reasoning that thinks about the nature of clinical reasoning itself at the outset of each patient encounter, rather than carrying a universalized clinical logic into each encounter.

Reflexive thinking brings social and psychological features of a patient's life into consideration but also considers other important issues. The increasing complexity of health care that comes with an aging population stresses health systems such that values-based decisions become more important, which can affect clinical reasoning. Health care resources are finite, and consideration of who gets them and who does not stretches the boundaries of the single case narrative to include the larger social context. In the early 1970s, there was both a cultural upswing in individualism and rapid scientific advances that promoted new capacities for extending life. For example, once medical science *could* keep someone alive on a ventilator and/or feeding tube, new questions emerged about whether it *should* do so and under what conditions. Similarly, as the complex illnesses of aging populations present resource challenges at the clinical, institutional and national levels,

decisions about what to treat, when to treat and how to treat inevitably must account not only for the values of the patient but also the institution and the broader society in which they are made. Put another way, modernist clinical reasoning traditionally was underpinned by an assumption that if an intervention could be performed, it should be performed. Today, that assumption and others must be interrogated with a new more complex form of reflexive clinical reasoning.

Cultural Complexity, Race/Ethnic Diversification and Clinical Reasoning

The traditional paradigm of clinical reasoning—a Cartesian process of diagnosis using a differential logic applied to pathophysiological symptoms (Scott, 2013)—tends not to encourage reflexivity, particularly in regard to value-laden assumptions of health care. Perhaps most generally, there is an implicit assumption that disease *should* be treated (as underscored in Case Study 8.1). However, the success of modern medicine and the tacit crises that emerge from these successes have underscored the value-laden nature of clinical science. Increasingly, in the era of chronic illness and long-term care, science may supply the information and the technology needed to intervene, but sometimes it is inappropriate to do so. With respect to these issues, our clinical reasoning needs to make use of perspectives from disciplines such as philosophy, anthropology, sociology and psychology. Shifting race/ethnic demographics further complicate such values questions because cultural experiences shape the value orientations of different groups in ways that might not align with the traditional practices of modern health care. A moving account of how different value systems can collide in health care is the tragic story of a child with epilepsy from Southeast Asia being raised in an immigrant family in the United States (Fadiman, 2012).

This situation is complicated by the mass movement of people between countries as immigrants and refugees. At the time of writing, millions of refugees are seeking asylum, the largest number since the Second World War. Healthcare professionals may have to cope with both enculturated ways of thinking about health and the body and what seem like exotic physiological conditions they may have not previously encountered (see Case Study 8.2).

CASE STUDY 8.2

An Australian medical student (George) in his final year was doing an elective study in the emergency department of a hospital in a major American city with a large immigrant population from many parts of the world. The demographic mixture brought a number of challenges that stretched his clinical reasoning ability.

'I had a gentleman that I saw in the emergency department in the US who came in with seizures and lots of neuro signs. So I went through the history, and he's a young guy – would've been about 18 and so I was thinking epilepsy, brain tumour. Ran through everything quite well, obviously ordered a CT scan and it came back cysticercosis … now I would never have thought of that diagnosis in a million years. I'd never heard of it, but I was able to work through the process and do the appropriate investigations' (Loftus, 2009, p. 142).

Cysticercosis is an infection by *Taenia solium*, the pork tapeworm, acquired by eating raw or undercooked pork containing the larval form of the worm. The larvae can migrate to the brain and cause epilepsy. George's patient was an immigrant from Mexico where he had presumably contracted the disease.

George also described a patient with koro.

'He [the patient] was standing in the doorway of the room, clutching himself. The registrar thought he had to go to the toilet. So he indicated the toilet, and he [the patient] said "No, no", and he's pointing and indicating, and we have no idea what's going on, absolutely no idea, and eventually got a Laotian interpreter and from there it became quite obvious. He said "It's going to crawl back up inside me and I'm gonna die". No matter what clinical reasoning skills that I had there I don't think I would've been prepared for it' (Loftus, 2009, p. 148).

Koro is described in South East Asia, although cases have been reported in Africa. It is the morbid fear that one's genitals are retracting into one's body and will bring about a rapid death when they do so. Sufferers have been known to go to extreme lengths to prevent what they see as their imminent demise, such as impaling the offending member or cutting it off. George's patient was, apparently, seriously considering these options. Koro should not be confused with kuru. Kuru is a neurodegenerative disorder, a form of Creutzfeldt-Jakob disease, and caused by infection by a prion. It was described in parts of Papua New Guinea in regions where cannibalism was practiced. It was contracted by eating the brains of one's close relatives as part of a funerary practice.

REFLECTION POINT 2

For Case Study 8.2, articulate the various ways that this case entails different aspects of complexity (in terms of how the patients became ill, the providers that must treat these illnesses, the cultural values that both patient and provider bring to the encounter, the contexts in which the patient faces those illnesses and treatments, the cultural lens through which each patient might view and experience illness, the personal and cultural values each might bring to the experience and so on). What challenges does each of those complexities pose for clinical reasoning?

Cultural diversity forces reconsideration of commonly held ethical practices, and thus of clinical decisions, in a number of ways. First, Western orientations towards ethics, generally, and medical decision making, in particular, focus squarely, and often exclusively, on the individual patient. Take, for example, the notion of truth-telling, which has, since the 1970s, been a staple of ethical practice in most Western societies. It is taken for granted that patients must be autonomous and fully informed to exercise that autonomy. However, in other countries, including many Eastern and Middle Eastern cultures (e.g., China and Japan), the orientation towards collectivities making decisions, especially in terms of the family, undercuts the individualism of Western ethics (Zahedi, 2011). As healthcare professionals treat patients from increasingly diverse backgrounds, they may need to be more reflexive about the assumptions built into their communication and their ethical decision making.

Whether to disclose an illness, who serves as the primary communicator and decision maker (the patient or a family member), the terms used in the discussion – all of these affect how the relationship between the patient and the healthcare professional proceeds. These sociocultural considerations are relatively new challenges in the process of clinical reasoning, and they become even more pressing as the race/ethnic and cultural composition of various societies becomes more diverse.

Other kinds of complexity regarding values decisions may take on greater import as race/ethnic and cultural diversity increases. The diagnoses and prognoses made by healthcare professionals are, at least ideally, based on scientific evidence and a scientific logic. But other orientations may reject altogether the validity of the scientific perspective or define core understandings of things like hope and futility in radically different ways. For example, cultural or religious orientations towards life may reject definitions of futility based on neurological activity, favouring the idea that the soul resides in the body as long as the heart is still beating. If this is the case, then questions about discontinuing life support must contend not only with questions about physiological futility but also broader notions about the meaning of life. It may no longer be sufficient, at least from a functional perspective, to anchor clinical reasoning solely around pathophysiological data and evidence-based science to the exclusion of the social and religious values that patients and their families bring to bear. Deciding what is medically futile can be fraught with complexity on pathophysiological grounds alone, but considering different orientations towards the meaning of life makes it all the more complex. There are yet other challenges facing clinical reasoning in this changing world.

CLINICAL REASONING IN A POSTINDUSTRIAL WORLD

In the preceding section, we discussed the challenges to clinical reasoning faced at the nexus of science and values in a globalizing world. But there are other challenges posed besides growing social, cultural and religious pluralism. There is a general push towards a warmer and more engaged patient-centred care that can conflict with the cold, calculating objectivity of modern science. In recent decades, different strategies designed to 'meet the patient where he or she is' have become popular, but there has been little thought given to how clinical reasoning fits this approach. This is particularly true where clinical reasoning is traditionally seen as a rather deductive process involving the straightforward computation of medical facts. It can be argued that demographic shifts and their attendant complexities now require healthcare professionals to function as scientists in what might be called a posttruth environment. That is, healthcare professionals must not only attend to the medical evidence in a classic process of diagnosis and prognosis, but at the same time they must weave all this together with a socially sensitive and individualized understanding of who the patient is and how he or she sees the world. This more complex view of clinical reasoning is not new; it has simply been ignored. The pioneers of evidence-based medicine recognized this when they stated that good decision making required the integration of not only the best available evidence and the expertise of the professional but also the views, values and desires of the patient (Sackett et al., 1996). Many health professions have paid attention only to gathering the best available evidence and have ignored the other two components. This is probably because of the grounding of the health professions in the biomedical sciences. Healthcare professionals are comfortable discussing and working with the best scientific evidence, but many are poorly equipped to talk about personal expertise and the values of patients. However, the medical humanities and social sciences do have vocabularies that can enable healthcare professionals to engage these neglected components of clinical reasoning. The huge demographic and social changes we now face mean that clinical reasoning will require social science and humanities discourses to adequately perform not only the social and emotional aspects of patient care but also its diagnostic and treatment functions. This clearly provides a warrant for more significant inclusion of the social science and humanities, something we are beginning to witness in evolving medical, nursing and allied health curricula, and on gateway examinations into these programs (e.g., the MCAT in the United States).

Clinical reasoning will have to become more reflexive. It will no longer be sufficient to apply the modernist form of deductive logic to medical problems. The case studies in this chapter underscore how the challenge to our clinical reasoning is growing. In this environment of complexity, clinical reasoning becomes a negotiation, not just about what to do, where the healthcare professional tries to get the patient closest to what is in his or her own 'best interest', but where there are no longer *a priori* criteria for determining what that best interest might be. Instead, healthcare professionals in a postindustrial world must not only think about the relationship of symptoms to diagnosis but must also reflect on their own thinking about these things. This will require an unprecedented form of openness about the nature of health care, its goals and our roles as healthcare professionals (e.g., curing versus helping people die; helping the patient versus keeping the family whole).

CONCLUSION

In this chapter, we have chosen to focus on two demographic shifts common to most Western nations that underscore the core problem of changing demographics vis-à-vis clinical reasoning. The aging of the population and increasing cultural diversity represent growing complexity at both the medical and sociological levels. Modern clinical reasoning emerged to match a set of observable pathophysiological factors to an underlying disease process, but it is poorly equipped to manage the complexity of multiple morbidities and pluralistic value systems. Reshaping it to match the challenges of postindustrial complexity will represent an enormous change in how healthcare professionals think.

CHAPTER SUMMARY

In this chapter, we have outlined:

- how shifts in the composition and character of populations amplify the complexity of disease and its treatment, which in turn affects clinical reasoning,
- how the aging of populations brings about new complexities with respect to comorbid disease processes that are difficult to navigate within clinical medicine, which has high degrees of specialization,
- how mass migration and resulting cultural diversity challenge not only may present clinicians with unfamiliar diseases but also bring the relevance

of values and beliefs in the diagnosis and treatment processes into sharp relief and
- how the new terrain of disease complexity that results from demographic shifts calls for new more reflexive and intersubjective forms of clinical reasoning.

REFLECTION POINT 3

Why are chronic diseases such a challenge for clinical reasoning? Consider not only how traditional forms of clinical reasoning are mismatched to the complexity of contemporary disease but also how the increased specialization of clinical medicine confounds treatments of comorbid diseases and so on.

Consider how other demographic shifts might affect clinical reasoning (e.g., the feminization of medicine, rising social inequality in some countries).

REFERENCES

Australian Bureau of Statistics, 2016. Australia Today. http://www.abs.gov.au/ausstats/abs@.nsf/mf/2024.0.

Charon, R., DasGupta, S., Hermann, N., et al., 2017. The Principles and Practice of Narrative Medicine. Oxford University Press, New York, NY.

Commonwealth of Australia, 2004. Australia's demographic challenges. Viewed 10 February 2017. Available from: <http://demographics.treasury.gov.au/content/discussion.asp>.

Dubos, R., 1965. Man Adapting. Yale University Press, New Haven, CT.

Engel, G., 1977. The need for a new medical model: a challenge for biomedicine. Science 196, 129–136.

European Union (EU), 2015. The 2015 aging report: projected demographic changes in the European Union. Viewed 6 February 2017. Available from: <http://ec.europa.eu/economy_finance/graphs/2015-05-12_ageing_report_en.htm>.

EuroStat, 2016. Population age structure by major age groups: 2005 and 2015 (% of the total population). Viewed 6 February 2017. Available from: <http://ec.europa.eu/eurostat/statistics-explained/index.php/File:Population_age_structure_by_major_age_groups,_2005_and_2015_(%25_of_the_total_population)_YB16.png>.

Fadiman, A., 2012. The Spirit Catches You and You Fall Down: A Hmong Child, Her American Doctors, and the Collision of Two Cultures. Farrar, Strauss and Giroux, New York, NY.

Hinote, B., Wasserman, J., 2016. Social and Behavioral Science for Health Professionals. Rowman & Littlefield, Lanham, MD.

Link, B., Phelan, J., 1995. Social conditions as fundamental causes of disease. J. Health Soc. Behav. 35 (extra issue), 80–94.

Loftus, S., 2009. Language in Clinical Reasoning: Towards a New Understanding. VDM Verlag, Saarbrücken, Germany.

Loftus, S., Greenhalgh, T., 2010. Towards a narrative mode of practice. In: Higgs, J., Fish, D., Goulter, I., et al. (Eds.), Education for Future Practice. Sense Publishers, Rotterdam, The Netherlands, pp. 85–94.

Martin, J.A., Hamilton, B.E., Osterman, M.J.K., et al., 2015. Births: final data for 2013. National Vital Statistics Reports, 64. National Center for Health Statistics, Hyattsville, MD, viewed 28 March 2017. Available from: <http://www.cdc.gov/nchs/data/nvsr/nvsr64/nvsr64_01.pdf>.

Morris, D., 1998. Illness and Culture in the Postmodern Age. University of California Press, Berkeley, CA.

Omran, A.R., 1971. The epidemiologic transition: a theory of the epidemiology of population change. Milbank Mem. Fund. Q. 49, 509–538.

Pol, L., Thomas, R., 2013. The Demography of Health and Healthcare, third ed. Springer, Dordrecht, The Netherlands.

Sackett, D., Richardson, S., Rosenberg, W., et al. (Eds.), 1996. Evidence-Based Medicine: How to Practice and Teach EBM. Churchill Livingstone, New York, NY.

Scott, J., 2013. Complexities in the consultation. In: Strumberg, J., Martin, C. (Eds.), Handbook of Systems and Complexity in Health. Springer, New York, NY, pp. 257–278.

Tasker, D., Higgs, J., Loftus, S. (Eds.), 2017. Community-Based Healthcare: The Search for Mindful Dialogues. Sense, Rotterdam, The Netherlands.

Ward, B., Schiller, J., Goodman, R., 2014. Multiple chronic conditions among US adults: a 2012 update. Prev. Chronic Dis. 11, 130389. Available from:: http://dx.doi.org/10.5888/pcd11.130389.

Wasserman, J., 2014. On art and science: an epistemic framework for integrating social science and clinical medicine. J. Med. Philos. 39, 279–303.

Xu, J., Murphy, S., Kochanek, K., et al., 2016. Mortality in the United States: 2015, NCHS data brief no. 267. Centers for Disease Control and Prevention, Atlanta, GA.

Zahedi, F., 2011. The challenge of truth telling across cultures: a case study. J. Med. Ethics Hist. Med 4, 11.

9

CLINICAL THINKING, CLIENT EXPECTATIONS AND PATIENT-CENTRED CARE

DELLA FISH ■ LINDA DE COSSART

CHAPTER AIMS

The key aims of this chapter are to:

■ provide an overview of the current context of client expectations and patient-centred care that is raising new questions and responses about healthcare practitioners' expertise (HCPs),

■ demonstrate the significance of clinical thinking as the HCP's central expertise and the consequent need for this to be better understood both among HCP and also by patients who now have greater medical knowledge but still inevitably lack the professional's expert judgement and

■ identify the critical importance of the nature of the HCP professionalism focused on uncovering its transformative potential.

KEY WORDS

Professionalism

Transformative professionalism

Clinical thinking

Professional judgement

Healthcare practitioner

Patient-centred care

ABBREVIATIONS / ACRONYMS

NHS National Health Service (United Kingdom)

GMC General Medical Council (United Kingdom)

HCP Healthcare professional

INTRODUCTION

This chapter contextualizes current concepts of client expectations and patient-centred care and considers their implications for practitioners. It then looks at the complexity of the HCP's expertise in clinical thinking, which goes beyond the factual knowledge laypeople can pick up from the Internet and illustrates how all HCPs and patients need to respect and understand this expertise. Finally we propose and explore four competing visions of professionalism held among both patients and practitioners, which shape how they can meet each other and offer critique and debate about a fifth 'transformative' view of professionalism. We believe that this transformative view of professionalism offers a new dynamic for change in patient-centred care.

CURRENT CONCEPTIONS OF CLIENT EXPECTATIONS AND PATIENT-CENTRED CARE

The aim to make the patient the key driver of his or her own healthcare plans and to be involved in the decision making has challenged thinking in the Western world professionally, fiscally and organizationally over the past 40 years (Health Foundation, 2014; National Health Service, 2015). Our thinking supports strongly the importance of the patient's best interests being at the centre of any healthcare interaction. If person-centred care is to develop further, as is likely given current organizational thinking, it will demand a change of mind-set, particularly of HCPs but also of society. There is a critical need for HCPs and patients to be involved in prevention and active care. Developing such a new mind-set and way of seeing professionalism (both in practitioner and in patients) needs to be achieved through education and learning rather than training. We argue that this focus on education is vital because this is about conduct (what we do as driven by who we are, what we believe and how we think). This is not about training (behaviour learnt by rote or through newly required and assessed competencies or protocols) (Fish, 2012). In ensuring the care of the whole patient by the whole practitioner, the importance of the education of a professional's heart and head cannot be overestimated.

The spectrum of health provision is wide ranging, from prevention at one extreme to the care of the emergency patient at the other, with a wide range of support and therapeutic possibilities in between. Each domain of care (like nursing or physiotherapy) often sees itself in isolation to others and has its own language, and this brings its own dynamics and dilemmas. The fiscal divisions driven by the consumerist approach to health care in the UK's NHS over the past 30 years have exhausted imaginative thinking by diverting energy into maintaining budgets rather than seeing things anew and from a different perspective. Fire-fighting to maintain resources has become the norm.

The concept of the patient as a guest (Berwick, 2009) is an attractive one and fits the model of 'Medical Home' being explored in the United States. The simile falls short, however, in the operating room when the surgeon inflicts harm on her patient as part of a therapeutic process. However, common to both scenarios are principles and themes that place the patient's well-being at the centre of the transaction and which should be honoured and respected.

Little et al. (2001) identified three key areas that patients want from patient-centred care: communication, partnership and health promotion. The concept of partnership was avoided by Berwick, we think in an attempt to emphasize the importance and vulnerability of the patient. Partnership, as we see it, is a must between two (and maybe more) human beings, respecting that all bring their unique knowledge and expertise. Distortedly, however, examples of 'patient-centred' being 'what the patient wants' (rather than needs) have crept into the surgical arena, where young surgeons, unchecked, list patients for elective procedures 'because they [the patients] want it'. The case of an 89-year-old man turning up on the day case list for a hernia repair comes to mind. The patient had an uncomplicated direct inguinal hernia that had been present, unchanged, for 30 years. The clinical thinking processes, which we see as incorporating both clinical reasoning and deliberation to come to a clinical decision (a professional judgement), are here open for critique, particularly with respect to the role of the surgeon and whether to operate or not to operate. Not to operate takes more thought and courage than just to do something. The great challenges to HCPs are not just 'to do more stuff' but more profoundly how we think about our roles as professionals within the healthcare specialty in which we work and how these collaborate with and support the other elements so necessary to successful therapeutic intervention.

All of these ideas come against the backdrop of three key facts.

1. *The exponential growth of knowledge and understanding* about disease and its treatment and the resources are now freely available to all patients on the Internet.
2. *The presentation and use of this information are a matter of interpretation* and exist against the backdrop that it: is always incomplete; evolves during collaborative relationship with colleagues and patients; works *with* not *on* patients; involves professional judgement that opens professionals (and their patients) up to taking risks and thus to risk being wrong; is characterized by mystery at its heart; is based more upon uncertainty than upon total expertise; involves a spiritual dimension; opens professionals up to moral answerability; involves theorizing about practice during practice; is about creating new understanding during practice and espouses moral and ethical approaches to practice, demanding from practitioners an endless critical examination of their beliefs (de Cossart, 2005).
3. *The burgeoning number of systems and processes of regulation and governance* in the NHS in the UK and more generally in the Western world assume that being a HCP is a masterable practice and that pathways of care and outcomes can be predicted and controlled by regulation, thus, by these means making the care of patients safer.

HOW HEALTHCARE PROFESSIONALS THINK: THE CENTRAL EXPERTISE OF HCPS NEEDS TO BE BETTER UNDERSTOOD BY PATIENTS

In health care, expertise coalesces into many distinct professional groups, each with its own traditions, ways of seeing the world and ways of educating new members into the fold. Friedson (2005) and Judge Jackson (quoted in Hilborne, 2015) challenged the perceived power that this expertise gives professionals. Further, in the care of an individual patient, each professional offers unique clinical thinking and experience when working as part of a cohesive team. The problem often is that, in our experience, these invisible thinking processes that lie at the heart of their expertise (see later in the chapter and also Chapter 36) are rarely made explicit by practitioners. Thus they cannot defend their decision making in crucial cases, nor can they provide evidence that they reflect on such processes on a regular basis and so develop their thinking and decision making. Attending to explicating this process can hugely enhance the quality of care for the patient and, additionally, the quality of care for each member of the team. In well-functioning teams, respect and understanding of each other's roles and responsibilities and thinking processes are at the heart of quality care of a patient. When the team works collaboratively, understanding the processes of clinical thinking as we have defined it, we believe it is a force for good and is inspirational (see also Montgomery, 2006).

Over the past 40 years, the bureaucracy developed as part of each professional group establishing its individual expertise and power has been considerable. Many differing words exist to describe functions and roles across different healthcare professions, and little attempt has been made to create common ground. Our research and practice with not only doctors but also a wide range of HCPs on 'how doctors think' (see de Cossart and Fish, 2005; Fish and de Cossart, 2007; Thomé, 2012) have led us to identify some common ground on this element of understanding clinical thinking, because the processes, although dependent on specific expertise, are not unique to physicians and surgeons (Brigley and Jasper, 2008).

An invisible complex set of decisions and tacit professional judgements underpins the fluent everyday practice of senior professionals. Their smooth and apparently unthinking performance, as observed by others, leaves unexplained the complex mental 'workings out' that shape their actions. In fact, without an intentional exploration of what underpins these actions, these matters may also remain tacit even to the practitioner (Fish and de Cossart, 2013). If these actions are to be understood and developed further, there must be a means of making them explicit and exploring them, because the quality of professional judgements made by HCPs are at the heart of safe patient care.

Our use of 'The Clinical Thinking Pathway' (de Cossart and Fish, 2005; Fish and de Cossart, 2007) developed for physicians and surgeons and with other HCPs has led us to understand that professional judgements made about the care of each individual patient are case-specific and driven strongly by six key things related to the case:

- the specific context of that case,
- the kind of person the professional brings to that case (their personal identity, values, beliefs, spiritual focus and character traits),
- the kind of professional the HCP brings to that particular case (we all respond differently in differing contexts),
- the range of knowledge the professional draws on within that case,
- the therapeutic relationship developed with that patient and
- how the professional sees the wider context of her or his role in that case.

The following expands briefly on each of these.

1. The importance of the context of a case or event will involve the HCP's interpretations, with events being seen through different professional lenses. This is highly sensitive in all cases, and the failure to realize it often leads to misunderstanding and conflict.
2. The kind of person the professional brings to the case/event is founded on his or her personal values and beliefs, assumptions, feelings and attitudes, previous experience, expectations and insights and imagination.
3. The HCP's view of his or her own professionalism is a major driving influence, and we discuss this further in the next section.

4. Knowledge is often assumed to be largely empirical knowledge, facts that are irrefutable and procedural knowledge of what to do in specific circumstances. However, this is very simplistic, and we have identified fourteen forms of knowledge that need to be taken into account when exploring professional judgements. This includes self-knowledge, practice-based knowledge, intuitive knowledge, knowledge arising from improvisation and knowledge gained through practice rather than theory (de Cossart and Fish, 2005; Fish and de Cossart, 2007, 2013). Further, of course, there is a great deal of difference between knowing and understanding! This would suggest that more thought needs to be given to what professionals mean by knowledge as they discuss and explore cases.

5. How the HCP sees his or her relationship with the patient is highly sensitive and is specific to his or her professional group. For example: the doctor and the nurse may, on a superficial level, see their roles differently, but with deeper mutual understanding they will see they are much closer together than it first appears. How each professional relates to the wider perspective of the case, not only within his or her own institution but also in the wider global context, is highly influential in his or her decision making.

In our publications, we regularly use the term 'clinical thinking' as an overall term for the whole process from meeting the individual patient to coming to a professional judgement about his or her care. This is, of course a cycle that may happen many times during the care of the patient, because many key decisions about patient care can occur during treatment. The whole clinical thinking pathway of these processes will usually lie at the basis of all patient care but will be used with emphasis on differing points of the pathway by differing professionals at differing stages in the patient's care. Experienced professionals may run more quickly than the less experienced through the first section of the pathway as described later. Further, it is not a protocol but a guideline.

We see clinical thinking as divided into two main sections. The first we call 'clinical reasoning' because it is more objective than the second process. Clinical reasoning, as we express it, starts – from first meeting the patient – with data collection and interpretation leading to a differential diagnosis and the forming of a general clinical solution or solutions (the right thing/s to do in general). The second process, or second half of the pathway, we call 'deliberative thinking', which is focused on finding a way forward for that particular patient that is tailored to his or her unique context and unique ethical, spiritual and physical needs.

Although both of these main processes (clinical reasoning, which is more formulaic and uses applied science, and deliberation, which attends to the humane needs of the specific patient) are essential and mutually dependent and carried out across professional groups' thinking, the deliberative process is usually (but not exclusively) the domain of the more experienced practitioner. It requires a greater depth of development. Both need to be accounted for as part of good professional practice (de Cossart and Fish, 2005; de Cossart et al., 2012; Fish and de Cossart, 2013). We have expanded this further in Chapter 36 of this book.

We have observed clinical teams, in a safe and supportive environment use our *Clinical Thinking Model* to reflect on their own responsibilities in practice. Group reflection (following an event) using our model was both revealing about professional judgement and their interpretation of the event. It helped to increase understanding about formulaic decision making and deliberative decision making. This area is not only ripe for further research but would also benefit by sharing the principles of this thinking in real practice with patients, who are at the centre of the clinical thinking but have no access to the tacit thinking processes going on in the minds of the professional/s who look after them.

THE IMPORTANCE OF THE NATURE OF THE HCP'S PROFESSIONALISM: UNCOVERING ITS TRANSFORMATIVE POTENTIAL

If client expectations and patient-centred care are to become increasing realities and successful components of health care, then the patient and clinical practitioner will need to see each other's thinking more clearly. They will need to understand themselves and each other better and create a much closer and more respectful partnership in which their equally significant but differing individual expertise can be drawn together, appreciated and used to create more effective care. This is not an institutional and managerial matter but inevitably an individual 'bottom-up' one, in which change will be brought about when each person enacts the change he or she wants to see happen.

This not only means the practitioner must know more about himself or herself as a person and a professional but now urgently requires practitioners to build a more up-to-date conception of professionalism. Unfortunately, professionalism has recently been much maligned and distorted by many writers and is distant from the grounding concept of professions as a 'profession of faith' (Palmer, 2007).

Next, we therefore review some recent conceptions of professionalism and propose the groundwork for a new and transformative version of professionalism that might better sustain practitioners in the complex demands of their work and be seen by patients as more seriously authentic.

Four Current Ways of Seeing Professionalism

In this section, we characterize and explore four broad versions or categories of professionalism that we currently see in education and health care and described by the work of many recent writers (Berwick, 2009; Blond et al., 2015; Canter, 2016; Freidson, 2005; The Jubilee Centre for Character and Virtues, 2016; Palmer, 2007). These four versions run across a spectrum from three negative views about professionalism, none of which, we contend, would promote and support a genuinely closer working together of practitioner and patient. Only one view (the fourth) contains elements that are conducive to seeing the patient as a human being in a more focused way, and therefore treatment of him or her as a person evolves from a foundation of respect and trust. Our four categories are as follows.

1. 'Professionalism discounted' is what we have come to call the moral vacuum left within the radical consumerist view of education and health care when professionalism is sidelined (Berwick, 2009; Blond et al., 2015; Palmer, 2007).
2. 'Managerially compliant professionalism' is our term for the attempt to cling on to professionalism

by turning it into a managerial poodle (Canter, 2016).
3. 'Self-seeking professionalism' is our term for the distortion of professionalism as nothing but 'a self-serving protectionist racket', a metaphor possibly started by George Bernard Shaw (1934) with his idea that the professions are a conspiracy against the laity (Blond et al., 2015).
4. 'Classically shaped professionalism', which we use to refer to professionalism based on values, virtues, character development and practice wisdom (Jubilee Centre for Characters and Virtues, 2016). This version has an Aristotelian basis and a language derived from pre-Christian times, where qualities later called spiritual values are labelled and discussed as 'classical virtues'. The term 'virtues' is convenient in a multicultural society as avoiding any reference to specific religious belief.

We present our interpretation of these categories of professionalism containing different ways of seeing the 'world in which workers work' as a sharply focused polemic to prompt discussion and debate about what kinds of professionalism would be conducive to health care that was more patient-centred.

In our analysis of these four categories (Table 9.1), we have looked, for each category, at its shaping tradition, its main driving force, what it ignores or de-emphasizes, its literal or surface focus, its tacit agenda, its view of the patient, how it relates to clinical thinking and what sustains its character and succours its practitioners. Reading each column downwards reveals an overall view of each particular kind of professionalism. Thus seeing health care in consumerist terms renders care as a product, the processes of health care as conveyer belts and the patients as receivers of a satisfactory delivery. This requires streamlining practitioners' thinking into templates and pathways, leaving little place for human interaction let alone human relationship, and is kept in place as a system by extrinsic drivers and rewards. This is a world in which practitioners' compliance is required and only fiscal interests keep them going. The managerially compliant version (category 2) is much the same as this, whereas category 3, self-seeking professionalism, is seen as a system set up by professionals who are their own agents, but who in the current world

TABLE 9.1

A Range of Interpretations of Professionalism: for Critique and Debate

Key Characteristics	1 Professionalism Discounted	2 Managerially Compliant Professionalism	3 Self-Seeking Professionalism	4 Classically Shaped Professionalism	5 Transformative Professionalism
Shaping tradition	Industrial work	Management theory	Exclusiveness of professionalism	Aristotle	A recognition of the spiritual elements of who and what we are and thus building on the roots of Aristotle
Driving force	Radical consumerism in which all transactions between HCP and patient are shaped by seeing health care as a product to be delivered with utmost efficiency	Organizational management Focusing on fulfilling the demands of what it sees as the realities of the world of work and where the individual is a cog in the machine	Deficit and defensive view of professionals' status/power (focused on maintaining power and status at all stages in the professional career as the first priority)	Character education and professional wisdom/virtues (focused on bringing the best of themselves as human beings to the service of the patient, but subject to being derailed by the difficult realities of the world in which they work).	Reconciling and coping with the reality of the world of work through commitment to nonphysical values that arise from a source that transcends everyday concrete physical experience
De-emphasizes	All individual sense of service Values, virtues, individual as a talent	Individual	The positive and individual character, values and virtues of the practitioner	That which needs to succour this when times are rough	The single importance of the human values of this world
Literal focus	HCP is employee Patient is consumer Health care is a product	Being professional within the demands of the management without critique	Fighting to maintain status and importance	Professionals are good people who seek the good of the patient but relying essentially on their own inner strength	Professionals recognizing that their inner strength comes from sources beyond own self and own character

Tacit agenda	Supports government power to shape workforce	Yields all agency to management	To maintain exclusivity as power over the laity	Virtue, values and character of HCP will assure best practice (but only while human energy lasts)	Each practitioner has to 'be' what he or she seeks to develop by drawing on strength beyond self
View of patient	End consumer	Consumer with power who needs to be satisfied	Person who deserves best clinical treatment as practitioner deems best	One who deserves the best care and who can contribute to that care	Sees the patient as human and humane with physical and spiritual needs best met in a trusted partnership
How it relates to clinical thinking	Expedient and fiscally satisfactory outcomes usually addressed through pathways and protocols that override deliberative thinking	Conceives clinical thinking as 'serving' what the patient wants irrespective of his or her needs!	Practitioner thinks within the bounds of his or her expertise and leaves patient in background not engaging him or her in any deliberations	Practitioner seeks best and most wise practice for each patient	Practitioner seeks to share his or her thinking with the patient so that each understands more and better of each other
What sustains and succours its practitioners	Monetary rewards and status plus laws, rules and protocols keep it in place. No direct succour beyond recognition of compliance	Avoiding threat of losing job; seeking managers' approval and rewards sustain it. No direct succour; requires detachment from their professional beliefs and critique	Recognition of status sustains this, and self-worth and wider approval as a practitioner using critique to justify actions succour it	Recognition of integrity wisdom and expertise sustains this. Self-worth and wider approval as a person and practitioner using critical reflective practice to improve their practice succour it	Recognition of virtues and where they come from and a belief in ability to contribute to change for the good of patients. Succoured by self-awareness and the recognition of strength from human and spiritual dimensions nurtured by critical reflective practice

are increasingly seen as both self-seeking and under siege. Clearly, in all of these three categories the role of the patient within his or her health care is sidelined. In the first category, as consumers, they judge the outcome and must be satisfied. This is not conducive to working in tandem.

Only the fourth category offers a positive view of what professionals can offer their patients in working together, but even then, this is not working in tandem with the patient. Thus it is not surprising that even category 4 (classically shaped professionalism) is now being castigated as 'nostalgic' and outdated (Canter, 2016). Further, we have seen that even it fails to enable practitioners to flourish in the current realities of having simultaneously to serve various masters and to compromise their own values in relation to those of the organization they work in. Although the aims and intentions of the classically shaped version are still topical and laudable and unselfishly seek 'the good' of all, crucially the basic concept offers no succour, outside strength or support to its proponents when the going gets rough. We believe that this category needs further development.

Transformative Professionalism

In considering the four categories discussed earlier, we came to the conclusion that what is lacking is the spiritual dimension of human identity and its transformative power. This resonates with Pellegrino (1999) and much of the work of Parker Palmer (e.g., his 1993 publication). This we contend is what enables practitioners, drawing on their inner strengths, to meet both their irritatingly difficult daily bureaucratic demands and also their patients, with a humanity augmented by 'agape' (a love that is without self-seeking and works from a detachment that is correctly referred to as 'disinterested', meaning 'without seeking selfish gain'). It seems to us that the spiritual aspects of the human and the professional that make up the practitioner were lost (or left implicit) when the classically shaped version was reclarified in Aristotelian terms in the first decade of this century (Carr, 2003, 2004). Even at that time, something of the spiritual was still implicit in the way most people lived, but more recently our multicultural society seems to have demanded a sensitivity that requires no direct reference to such matters that are now left entirely tacit. We see an emergence of renewed

sensitivity appearing now in the UK. Examples are found in Wattis and Curran (2016) and also the General Medical Council's 'Good Medical Practice' (2013), which make clear the importance of spirituality, although here the focus is seen only in terms of caring for patients rather than as important for the development of professional practitioners themselves.

We offer, in the final column of Table 9.1, a view of professionalism and the world of professional work as building on the classical version through a commitment to nonphysical values that arise from a source that transcends everyday concrete physical experience and that we believe can be transforming of the professions and of the relationships between patient and practitioner.

The writing of Richard Brock (2015) and Wattis and Curran (2016) supports our deliberate use of the term 'spiritual'. It captures a set of values that work independently of the physical world and can be seen as independent of religion (although for us personally it has a Christian basis). Such values have their origins in love and humility; selflessness and self-awareness; and appreciation of beauty and wonder. The classical version attributes these values to Aristotelian thought, but they have since been transformed through the work of Christian writers like Augustine into spiritual values!

Brock makes the point that some might argue that the source that originates and sustains them is 'located beyond our everyday concrete physical experience' and 'might be seen as being the innate human potential for good, while most might see the source as the ultimate ground of existence, the absolute, the sacred, the divine — or simply God'. But this is not dependent on any one time period or religion. Indeed, probably, as Aldous Huxley argued (see Brock, 2015): 'spirituality transcends time and religion and outlasts them both'.

Spirituality, as Brock (2015, p. 10) says, is:

a process of personal transformation through which a person seeks to integrate both the values of the world and the non-physical values that arise from a transcending source into their life. To balance the material alongside the spiritual and vice versa is to harmonise the two and make them one – much like a pair of binoculars …

This is not a recipe for scrambling to the hermit's hut with nothing but sacred thoughts for company. Properly conceived, spirituality is about reconciling the difficult physical world of reality in which we still have to live and work with the one in which transcendent values can be honoured. Although difficult to put into language at one level, there are plenty of phrases in worldwide poetic and philosophical literature that describe this metaphorically.

As our working definition, we follow Wattis and Curran (2016, p. 500) who say:

Spirituality can be broadly understood as what gives meaning and purpose to life, a sense of connectedness and a source of hope. It at least includes the possibility of transcendence in the sense of moving beyond physical needs and realities.

Where that paper is about attending to the spiritual needs of patients, we are more concerned here with the needs of professionals themselves and their personal reservoirs of energy and hope that sustain them in the spirit of public service during the many difficult times found within daily practice and in seeking to meet the patient halfway. We see this not as 'being trained in resilience', where the means to rise above and beyond difficulties as a professional comes from a newly learnt 'skill' added to our repertoire but as stemming from the kind of person we seek to be and become and the inner source that feeds our being. This is what many argue is the means to cope with the world by bringing together 'the things of Time with the Timeless' (that is: confront the temporary material or physical matters of this world with enduring values from beyond it) so that the physical is transformed. As Plato wrote, 'the human soul sits on a horizon between Eternity and Time and is nourished by both' (Brock, 2015, p. 7).

Equipped with this explanation and now reading across the table, clear distinctions of key characteristics are visible between each professional category. Further, the bottom row of the table particularly shows an interesting continuum from the need in category 1 for extrinsic motivation and legal requirements to keep the professional in place through to category 5, where what is needed to keep the system working well is the practitioners' own character, drive and abilities, supported by self-awareness and the recognition of strength from

human and spiritual dimensions nurtured by critical reflective practice (Fish and de Cossart, 2013). Such a practitioner can then meet the patient on human and humane terms, with physical and spiritual needs attended to in a trusted partnership. The key to all this is who you are not what training you have had in new strategies to conform to the newest move in patient care.

This concept of transformational professionalism links with work we have already done (helped by Campbell, 1984), on the person and professional being an influential dimension within the clinical thinking processes (de Cossart and Fish, 2005; Fish and de Cossart, 2007, 2013). The concept goes beyond our earlier work, in that we are now beginning to try to explore the importance in the life of a professional of agape, of disinterest and of detachment. This is about seeing the world we work in as only a part of life as a whole. We fully recognize that this is aspirational rather than totally achievable, but at least that will enable professionals to aspire to the best and to be succoured when their journey becomes temporarily almost too wearying to be continued.

Our experience over the past 2 years of exploring some of these ideas with 75 senior medical practitioners as part of a teaching program has convinced us that there is a considerable need for this element of professional practice to be explored. The positive energy released in our learners' response to the matter has inspired and energized us to pursue this further. We invite you to explore the significance of all this for yourself by reading and critiquing Table 9.1 and responding to Reflection Point 1.

CHAPTER SUMMARY

In this chapter we have addressed the following:

- The current dilemma for all HCPs in battling with more worthwhile partnership with patients is that many of the things that they hold dear as being a good professional and humane carer will be lost if they do not take time to consider and share the unmeasurable but highly significant elements of their practice.
- We explored the concept of the HCP's clinical thinking, expertise and ability to engage in patient-centred care.

- We argued that HCPs have had a predominant focus on traditional conceptions of professionalism and that there has been little attention to the spiritual qualities in their practice.
- We proposed our Clinical Thinking Pathway and the idea of 'Transformative professionalism' as resources to be a means of exploring and developing the spiritual elements of professionalism and of sustaining and energizing the professional in providing whole patient-centred care.

REFLECTION POINT 1

1. Read through Table 9.1, and reflect on how this might help you to express your professional identity more authentically and to confront the personal demands of providing patient-centred care.
2. We suggest that 'The key to all this is who you are, not what training you have had in new strategies to conform to the newest move in patient care'. Critique this statement.
3. How would you prepare to teach these ideas to those preparing for or engaged in patient-centred care?
4. What resources might you need to help you teach this in real practice, and how does what we offer here resonate with what follows in this book?

REFERENCES

Berwick, D.M., 2009. 'Patient-centred' should mean: confessions of an extremist. Health Aff. (Millwood) 28, w555–w565.

Blond, P., Antonacopoulou, E., Pabst, A., 2015. In professions we trust: fostering virtuous practitioners in teaching, law and medicine. ResPublica, London, UK. Viewed 20 January 2016. Available from http://www.respublica.org.uk/wp-content/uploads/2015/02/In-Professions-We-Trust.pdf.

Brigley, S., Jasper, M., 2008. An evaluation of: a multi-disciplinary approach to surgical education and training: report for the Department of Surgery, Countess of Chester Hospital NHS Foundation Trust, Chester, UK.

Brock, R., 2015. Four Quartets: TS Eliot and Spirituality. Patrician Press, Manningtree, Essex.

Campbell, A., 1984. Moderated Love: A Theology of Professional Care. SPCK, London, UK.

Canter, R., 2016. The new professionalism. Bulletin 10–13.

Carr, D., 2003. Making Sense of Education: An Introduction to the Philosophy and Theory of Education and Teaching. Routledge Falmer, London, UK.

Carr, D., 2004. Rival conceptions of practice in education and teaching. In: Dunne, J., Hogan, P. (Eds.), Education and Practice: Upholding the Integrity of Teaching and Learning. Blackwell Publishing, Oxford, UK.

de Cossart, L., 2005. A question of professionalism: leading forward the surgical team. Ann. R. Coll. Surg. Engl. 87, 238–241.

de Cossart, L., Fish, D., 2005. Cultivating a Thinking Surgeon: New Perspectives on Clinical Teaching, Learning and Assessment. TFM Press, Shrewsbury, UK.

de Cossart, L., Fish, D., Hillman, K., 2012. Clinical reflection: a vital means of supporting the development of wisdom in doctors. Curr. Opin. Crit. Care 18, 712–717.

Fish, D., 2012. Refocusing Postgraduate Medical Education: From the Technical to the Moral Mode of Practice. Aneumi Publications, Cranham, Gloucestershire.

Fish, D., de Cossart, L., 2007. Developing the Wise Doctor. Royal Society of Medicine Press, London, UK.

Fish, D., de Cossart, L., 2013. Reflection for Medical Appraisal: Exploring and Developing Your Clinical Expertise and Professional Identity. Aneumi Publications, Cranham, Gloucestershire.

Friedson, E., 2005. Professionalism: The Third Way. Polity Press, Oxford, UK.

General Medical Council, 2013. Good medical practice. Viewed 17 May 2016. Available from http://www.gmc-uk.org/guidance/good_medical_practice/apply_knowledge.asp.

Health Foundation, 2014. Patient centred care made simple: the health foundation inspiring improvement. Viewed 13 January 2017. Available from http://www.health.org.uk/sites/health/files/PersonCentredCareMadeSimple.pdf.

Hilborne, N., 2015. Jackson: 'professional negligence' could disappear as attitudes to professionals change. Legal Futures (online). Viewed 7 October 2016. Available from http://www.legalfutures.co.uk/latest-news/jackson-professional-negligence-could-disappear-as-attitudes-change.

The Jubilee Centre for Character and Virtues, 2016. The Jubilee Centre for Character and Virtues statement on character, virtue and practical wisdom in the professions. University of Birmingham, UK. Viewed 15 October 2016. Available from http://www.jubileecentre.ac.uk/userfiles/jubileecentre/pdf/Statement_Character_Virtue_Practical_Wisdom_Professional_Practice.pdf.

Little, P., Everitt, H., Williamson, I., et al., 2001. Preferences of patients for patient centred approach to consultation in primary care: observational study. BMJ 322, 1–7.

Montgomery, K., 2006. How Doctors Think: Clinical Judgement and the Practice of Medicine. Oxford University Press, Oxford, UK.

National Health Service (NHS), 2015. The NHS Constitution: The NHS belongs to us all. Department of Health, London, UK. Viewed 13 January 2017. Available from https://www.gov.uk/government/uploads/system/uploads/attachment_data/file/480482/NHS_Constitution_WEB.pdf.

Palmer, P.J., 1993. To Know as We Are Known: Education as a Spiritual Journey. HarperCollins, San Francisco, CA.

Palmer, P.J., 2007. A new professional: the aims of education revisited. Change: The Magazine of Higher Learning 39, 6–13.

Pellegrino, E.D., 1999. The commodification of medical and health care: the moral consequences of a paradigm shift from a professional to a market ethic. J. Med. Philos. 24, 243–266.

Royal College of Nursing, 2012. Spirituality in nursing care: a pocket guide. Viewed 23 January 2017. Available from https://www.rcn.org.uk/professional-development/publications/pub-003887.

Shaw, G.B., 1934. The Doctor's Dilemma. Odhams Press Ltd, Watford, UK.

Thomé, R., 2012. Educational Practice Development: An Evaluation (an exploration of the impact on participants and their shared organisation of a Postgraduate Certificate in Education for Postgraduate Medical Practice 2010–2011). Aneumi Publications, Cranham, UK.

Wattis, J., Curran, S., 2016. The importance of spirituality in caring for patients. Br. J. Hosp. Med. 77, 500–501.

10

NEXT-GENERATION CLINICAL PRACTICE GUIDELINES

KAREN GRIMMER ■ STEPHEN LOFTUS ■ JANINE MARGARITA DIZON

CHAPTER AIMS

The aims of this chapter are to:

- Reflect on the past decade of activity in clinical practice guidelines (CPGs) and
- Consider the ways in which the next generation of CPGs will integrate with clinical decision making.

KEY WORDS

Clinical reasoning

Clinical practice guidelines

Evidence-based practice

Evidence implementation

ABBREVIATIONS/ ACRONYMS

ACA Adopt, Contextualise, Adapt approach

CPGs Clinical practice guidelines

DALYs Disability-Adjusted Life Years

EBP Evidence-based practice

EIP Evidence-informed practice

G-I-N Guidelines International Network

HIC High-income countries

iCAHE International Centre for Allied Health Evidence

IOM Institute of Medicine

LMIC Lower- to middle-income countries

NICE National Institute for Health and Care Excellence

PROMS Patient Reported Outcome Measures

QALYs Quality-Adjusted Life Years

SAGE South African Guidelines Excellence

SIGN Scottish Intercollegiate Guideline Network

WHO World Health Organization

INTRODUCTION

Clinical practice guidelines (CPGs) have long been considered an important element of good quality health practice (Field and Lohr, 1990). Since the last edition of this book, CPG activity internationally has escalated. New terms, new methods and more in-depth understanding have emerged regarding how research evidence can better inform clinical practice. As a consequence, much new work is presented in this chapter. This progress has been underpinned by activities of Guidelines International Network (G-I-N),[i] a vibrant international group of CPG enthusiasts who collaborate to develop better ways of CPG writing, presentation, implementation and evaluation, with the aim of fostering safe and effective patient care around the world.

FRAMEWORKS OF CLINICAL PRACTICE GUIDELINES APPLICATION

Since 2000, the Sackett et al. (2000) evidence-based practice (EBP) model has been used to promote the

---

[i]Guidelines International Network (G-I-N): http://www.g-i-n.net/home

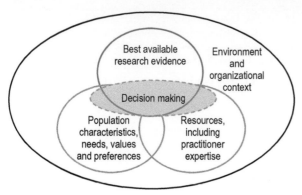

Fig. 10.1 ■ The evidence-informed practice model. (From Satterfield, J.M., Spring, B., Brownson, R.C., Mullen, E.J., Newhouse, R.P., Walker, B.B., Whitlock, E.P., 2009. Toward a transdisciplinary model of evidence-based practice. Milbank Q. 87, 368–390, with permission.)

balance of research evidence, clinical judgement and patient choices within local contexts to ensure the correct decisions are made for individual patients. In 2009 Satterfield et al. proposed the notion of evidence-informed practice (EIP) (Fig. 10.1). This model recognizes the inherent uncertainties in current best research evidence, clinical judgement and patient responses to, and understanding of, the evidence, within local contexts. This model may better align with allied health practice because of variability and uncertainties in the research evidence, patient choice and values and clinician reasoning, training and judgement.

REFLECTION POINT 1

CPGs need to be written in a manner that helps clinicians to integrate best evidence, their own clinical judgement, the desires and values of the patient within local contexts. Do you use CPGs regularly in your practice as a 'one-stop-shop' for evidence? Have the CPGs you are familiar with been written this way? How did the way they were written affect your ability to use them in your clinical reasoning?

CURRENT STATE OF PLAY IN CLINICAL PRACTICE GUIDELINES

The evolution of CPGs is exemplified by changing definitions over time. The Institute of Medicine (IOM) described CPGs in 1990 as 'systematically developed statements to assist practitioner and patient decisions about appropriate health care for specific clinical circumstances' (Field and Lohr, 1990, p. 38). This definition was updated in 2011 to emphasize the need for rigorous methodology: 'Clinical guidelines are statements that include recommendations intended to optimize patient care that are informed by a systematic review of evidence and an assessment of the benefits and harms of alternative care options' (Graham et al., 2011, p. 1). CPG research has rapidly evolved since then, with a current definition: 'Guidelines are considered a convenient way of packaging evidence and presenting recommendations to healthcare decision makers' (Treweek et al., 2013, p. 2).

Over the past decade, respected CPG developers' organizations have been established, such as the National Institute for Health and Care Excellence (NICE)[ii] and the Scottish Intercollegiate Guideline Network (SIGN).[iii] These and other international CPG writing groups have produced so many CPGs on so many topics that it would be difficult not to find some CPG for a clinical question, somewhere. There are also regularly updated repositories of CPGs such as NICE, SIGN, the International Centre for Allied Health Evidence (iCAHE) (University of South Australia[iv]) and the United States of America Guidelines Clearing House.[v] Professional associations also often host discipline-specific CPGs, but these may only be available to members. Identifying useful CPGs may require lateral thinking. For example, recommendations on how best to treat chronic low back pain may be found in a condition-specific CPG, or they may be found in a CPG about chronic pain or musculoskeletal disorders.

REFLECTION POINT 2

Well-developed CPGs can be readily found in a number of freely available Internet sites. Which guideline repositories do you use to find CPGs relevant to your area of practice?

[ii]National Institute for Health and Care Excellence (NICE): www .nice.org.uk/
[iii]Scottish Intercollegiate Guideline Network (SIGN): www.sign.ac.uk
[iv]University of South Australia: www.unisa.edu.au/cahe
[v]U.S. Department of Health and Human Services, Agency for Healthcare Research and Quality. National Guideline Clearinghouse: https://www.guideline.gov/

CRITICAL ELEMENTS OF USING CLINICAL PRACTICE GUIDELINES

Before implementing the recommendations reported in any CPG, end-users should first question its quality. Thus end-users should be comfortable in critically assessing a CPG and in making informed judgements about its usefulness to their clinical contexts. The recently published standards for CPG writing are considered industry best practice (Schünemann et al., 2014).

A good quality CPG should be easy to read and navigate. It should be written by credible methodologists, working with clinical experts. CPGs must have a clearly defined purpose and must target group and end-users. A good quality CPG should have a comprehensive Methods section that outlines a comprehensive process by which the relevant evidence was identified, collated, critically appraised to detect bias and transparently summarized into recommendations. A good CPG may also provide implementation strategies, and many quality improvement initiatives are often now linked with implementation and evaluation of CPGs. Kredo et al. (2016) provide a useful explanation of the current situation in CPG activities. Table 10.1 provides examples of tools to assist CPG writers.

With so much freely available information on CPGs methods, one could expect that the concerns raised by Shaneyfelt et al. (1999) about the quality of CPGs would have been addressed by now. However, a review in 2015 of the methodological quality of 16 current primary care CPGs developed by professional associations in South Africa, government agencies and academic institutions highlighted variability in CPG quality and construction (Grimmer et al., 2016a; Machingaidze et al., 2017). This highlights the need to educate CPG writers around the world about CPG quality elements and how to address them.

REFLECTION POINT 3

It is essential to determine the quality of the CPGs that you use, particularly in terms of how well they have been constructed and the recommendations reported. Do you assess the quality of the CPGs that you use? What are the most important aspects of CPG quality to you?

NEXT-GENERATION CLINICAL PRACTICE GUIDELINES

The South African Guidelines Excellence (SAGE) project team from South Africa reports innovative approaches to CPG writing, presented in a manner relevant to primary care in developing countries (Grimmer et al., 2016b; Machingaidze et al., 2015). The Project SAGE team proposed a three-tier CPG model, with Tier 1 being the evidence base, Tier 2 being 'expert' input to the evidence base to ensure its applicability and

TABLE 10.1		
Selected Advice to Support Clinical Practice Guideline Writing and Implementation		
Term	Explanation	References
Critically appraising CPG quality	iCAHE tool: A 14-item binary tool developed for clinicians, managers and policy-makers to assess the methodological quality of a CPG.	Grimmer et al. (2014); Dizon et al. (2016)
	Grades of Recommendation, Assessment, Development and Evaluation (GRADE): A detailed decision-making approach that establishes risk for bias and how this translates to clinical decision making	Schünemann et al. (2014)
Communicating findings	Developing and Evaluating Communication Strategies to Support Informed Decisions and Practice Based on Evidence project (http://www.decide-collaboration.eu) (DECIDE) GuideLine Implementability Appraisal (GLIA) (BridgeWhiz)	Treweek et al. (2013) Shiffman et al. (2005)
Fitting CPG recommendations to local contexts	ADAPTE Adopt, Contextualize, Adapt (ACA) approach	The ADAPTE Collaboration (2009); Dizon et al. (2016)

CPG, clinical practice guideline; iCAHE, International Centre for Allied Health Evidence.

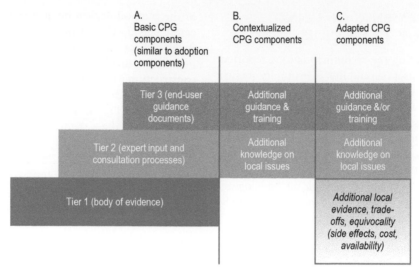

Fig. 10.2 ■ The clinical practice guideline tier approach.

generalizability to local circumstances and Tier 3 being CPG 'products' for end-users. There may be more than one Tier 3 product from a CPG depending on end-user needs (e.g., treatment protocols, patient decision-making tools, short-form recommendations, information sheets). See the first column in Fig. 10.2.

Kumar et al. (2010) spoke about the confusion around CPG terminology and the SAGE tiered approach attempts to demystify and standardize this. Project SAGE highlighted lower- to middle-income countries (LMICs). The high-income countries' (HICs) CPGs generally have extensively researched Tier 1 material, written with appropriate Tier 2 input from relevant end-users but with little focus on Tier 3 material. This might be a set of recommendations published in an academic journal or made available on a phone 'app' for clinical end-users. Conversely, in LMICs there seems to be a greater interest in Tier 3 products (how to do it) than in the evidence base (Machingaidze et al., 2015). When there is limited money for CPG writing, as often occurs in developing countries, the Project SAGE model offers an efficient and transparent approach to constructing and presenting CPGs. The Project SAGE three-tier CPG model could increase CPG construction efficiency.

REFLECTION POINT 4

Terminology around CPG writing varies, and there is no standard agreement about what constitutes a 'full'

CPG and what constitutes components of a CPG (such as a protocol). What terminology do you use when you discuss 'guidance' from CPGs?

IMPLEMENTATION

It is widely recognized that simply producing a CPG will not ensure that its recommendations are adopted by end-users. Many theories have been developed in the past decade to improve CPG implementation, and there is consistent evidence of the effectiveness of different implementation approaches. For instance, disseminating CPGs in paper copy has little effect, didactic presentations had moderate effect and there is stronger evidence for the effectiveness of peer-leaders, audit and feedback and self-reflection (Grol et al., 2013). However, there continues to be uncertainty as to how to address local barriers and clinician behaviours to sustainably improve practice.

One continuing concern is the fear expressed by many clinicians that CPG use will undermine their clinical decision-making autonomy. This can be expressed as disbelief in the nature or strength of the research evidence, or skepticism of the independence of the CPG writing group, or dismissal of CPGs as not relevant to their patient population. In response to this, work has been undertaken in the past few years to address barriers to successful implementation so that end-users can be provided with a CPG that already addresses important implementation barriers (Grimmer et al., 2016b). This work is described by Dizon et al. (2016), who proposed the Adopt, Contextualise, Adapt (ACA) approach to CPG implementation.

Clinical Practice Guideline Adoption

To adopt a CPG is straightforward across settings with similar environments and similar patient types. For instance, a CPG for the management of hypertension in 2016 in the UK (National Institute for Health and Care Excellence [NICE], 2016) could be simply adopted in similar countries, such as Australia. The adoption process does not require change to any CPG tier (Tier 1 evidence base, Tier 2 clinical expert input or Tier 3 product).

Clinical Practice Guideline Contextualization

To adopt an existing CPG into a very different setting (say from an HIC to LMIC) may require additional effort, as the CPG evidence may need additional contextualization to make the recommendations relevant and implementable. This means that the CPG Tier 1 could be adopted (no change), but additional information may be required at Tiers 2 and 3 to ensure that the CPG recommendations reflect local contexts and end-user needs. For example, one recommendation from NICE clinical guideline 68 for stroke (2008, updated March 2017) is that an appropriately trained healthcare professional should assess the swallowing ability of people suffering an acute stroke before being given anything by mouth. In most HIC settings, a speech pathologist, dietician or doctor would perform the swallowing test. However, in many LMICs where there may be few available trained specialist healthcare providers to perform this test, other healthcare professionals (such as nurses) could be trained. See the contextualization approach in the second column in Fig. 10.2.

CPG contextualization makes use of Tier 1 – evidence base (unchanged). However Tiers 2 and 3 are layered with additional information to ensure that the recommendation can be implemented in local context situations. Experts (end-users, target audience) are required to discuss how the CPG and the recommendations will work in the local context and to provide Tier 2 modification. Successful implementation of the recommendation in local contexts may require locally specific Tier 3

products, such as protocols, algorithms, training documents or checklists. CPG contextualization is an efficient implementation approach that bridges the gap between the parent CPG and its local application, without 'recreating the wheel'. This approach addresses often insurmountable LMIC challenges of limited time, CPG writing expertise and/or resources.

Clinical Practice Guideline Adaptation

To adapt means *to change something to suit different conditions or a different purpose.* This is where the Dizon ACA model (Dizon et al., 2016) adds subtleties to the ADAPTE model (Amer et al., 2015). Adaptation should occur where an adopted CPG cannot be implemented in its current form in a local environment. A recommended treatment may not be affordable, culturally acceptable, stored safely as is required for drugs or even readily obtained. Thus alternative, locally affordable, available and/or culturally acceptable treatments may be substituted for the recommended care to provide appropriate effective local treatment. Thus an additional evidence base may need to be developed that summarizes additional literature sources about alternative treatment methods. By considering and including local evidence, the CPG recommendation may thus change. For example, the NICE CPG (2015) for diabetes type I recommends rapid-acting insulin analogues be injected before meals. Where there is poor refrigeration, the use of injected insulin may not be a viable local option, and an alternative form of insulin may be required (for instance in tablet form). Adaptation will generally mean a difference between the parent CPG recommendations and locally relevant/acceptable recommendations. This may include different treatments with different forms of administration, where there are considered tradeoffs between treatment effects, side effects, costs, acceptability and shelf-life. In the Project SAGE three-tier CPG model, adaptation entails integration of an additional layer of evidence to Tier 1, which provides the basis for the substitute treatment recommendations. This may then require changes in Tiers 2 and 3. See column 3 in Fig. 10.2.

REFLECTION POINT 5

Ensuring that CPG recommendations can be implemented efficiently in the local environment is a critical part of evidence-based practice uptake and

---

CASE STUDY 10.1

Next-Generation Clinical Practice Guidelines

Ann was quite excited about the chance to work with an non-government organization in a developing country where she hoped she would be able to make a real difference in people's lives. She soon found that the health problems she was seeing were often different from those she was used to at home. This was because problems that were often quickly dealt with in an industrialized country were left untreated for much longer in a place with few resources, poor transport and a great shortage of accessible health care. Ann turned to available clinical practice guidelines for help and was pleased to find several that seemed relevant but was disappointed to find that most were oriented towards the industrialized societies she had left behind and didn't seem useful when deciding what to do with the patients she was seeing

now. However, she did have some access to the Internet and found that a group was trying to adapt some of the guidelines for settings just like hers. She was reassured when she discovered that the group was not only using the rigorous SAGE model but was focussing on the Tier 3 level and looking for low-cost and effective ways that the local population would be able to implement. Ann volunteered to become a contributor to the team and as someone 'on the ground' felt that she could make a real difference by testing out some of the proposals and giving feedback as the work developed. She knew that involvement by people like her, who knew just what the local problems were, would give credibility to the adapted guidelines that would eventually be produced and shared.

CPG implementation. What factors in your own local contexts might affect the implementation of recommendations from CPGs relevant to your field?

CONSUMER ENGAGEMENT

The term 'consumers' refers to CPG end-users. Identifying and addressing the needs of all end-users are essential elements of CPG writing quality (Eccles et al., 2012). Consumers include patients, healthcare professionals, managers, policy-makers and funders. Engaging consumer representatives during the CPG writing process is essential to ensure that the CPG is written in such a way that it resonates with all who use it (Grimmer et al., 2016b). Public consultation for a draft CPG is also a way of ensuring consumer engagement with the CPG before implementation.

REFLECTION POINT 6

CPGs must be written with consideration of patient needs and preferences. How these are built into the CPGs whilst they are being constructed should be transparent and valid (i.e., the information should come from the patients not from healthcare

providers who purport to know what patients need). Have you considered how relevant the recommendations in the CPGs are to your patients? Do you use recommendations in the CPGs as a form of communication of the evidence with your patients?

CLINICAL PRACTICE GUIDELINES, CLINICAL REASONING AND PATIENT OUTCOMES

CPGs are intended to promote better clinical reasoning and health outcomes. Local applicability and relevance are the factors that have the strongest influence on compliance (Eccles et al., 2005). Thus CPGs are more likely to be implemented if produced by locally credible CPG writers and if they do not require significant change in usual activities (Grol et al., 2013). This can be counterproductive if the international best evidence in a CPG is rejected as not being applicable locally and no alternative care approaches are substituted. This is where the value of the ACA model becomes obvious (Dizon et al., 2016). CPG-based care considered within the Satterfield et al. (2009) model of evidence-informed practice provides a framework for decision making by clinicians and enhances the value of clinician–patient interactions and decision-making processes. There is continuing debate about whether CPGs really do improve patient outcomes and decrease costs. These concerns are particularly relevant when CPG recommendations contradict current clinical practice or when significant change in practice behaviours is required to implement guidelines in a sustainable manner (Grol et al., 2013).

To measure change that could be attributed to CPG implementation (be it adopted, contextualized or adapted CPGs), strategies must be developed to monitor pre- and post-implementation practices. Audits are usually used to provide this information. Audits use checklists of items that are related to CPG implementation. Accurate and comprehensive record keeping in clinical practice is essential for clinical audits or reviews. In addition to patient details, information such as diagnosis and clinical reasoning prompts, potential risk factors, the recommendations in the CPG, requisite interventions and relevant outcome measures should be recorded on patient notes at regular points in the episode of care. Examples of audit planning and protocols include Gonzalez-Suarez et al. (2015).

There are now many standard outcome measures available to evaluate aspects of the effectiveness of management for most health conditions. Thus it is a matter for end-users to identify useful outcome measures and implement them on a regular basis throughout treatment. Health outcome measures should be applied at least twice across an episode of care to demonstrate change in health status (such as on first and last contact with the patient). This would be the minimum number of measures required to demonstrate change. Outcome measures need to reflect issues that are important to clinicians, patients, funders, managers, policy-makers and referrer. In some circumstances, they may reflect issues that are important to the family (or carer) and/ or to the employer. The most appropriate outcome measured to use to demonstrate the effectiveness of a CPG remains undetermined. Patient Reported Outcome Measures (PROMS) are currently being discussed as a way forward. These assist *patients to provide direct feedback to clinicians about their health experiences.* There are a multitude of published patient health outcome measures that have been developed for research and

clinical uses for many conditions and patient types. The iCAHE website provides a manual of freely available patient outcome measures.[vi] With the recent emergence of health economic evaluations of CPG effectiveness, the availability of quality-of-life measures is increasingly important. Quality-of-life measures are reported as QALYs (Quality-Adjusted Life Years) or DALYs (Disability-Adjusted Life Years) (World Health Organization, 2015). As allied health effectiveness is generally considered in terms of reduced morbidity rather than reduced mortality, evidence of improved quality of life is essential. Allied health clinicians could assist health economic evaluations of CPG effectiveness by routinely measuring patient quality of life.

REFLECTION POINT 7

Good quality recent CPGs provide an invaluable summary source of evidence for clinicians. Recommendations from CPGs could form the 'research' element of how you implement EBP in your practice. Do you use CPGs regularly in your practice as a 'one-stop-shop' for evidence? How do you interpret this evidence into your clinical reasoning, and how do you share this evidence with your patients?

THE FUTURE

There is a trend to computerize CPGs, particularly Tier 3 recommendations. Although this is not commonplace at present, its use is increasing, especially with recent advances in artificial intelligence. Attempts to use CPGs as interactive decision support systems have been attempted for decades, but with improvements in computer power and the widespread uptake of digital health records, we may now be reaching a tipping point where such support systems can become an everyday reality (Musen et al., 2014). The early systems, which were rule based, made use of so-called 'inference engines', and could be queried and made to show the procedures by which they made their conclusions. There was hope that such systems could be used to help teach newcomers how to be more rigorous in their clinical thinking by

---

[vi]International Centre for Allied Health Evidence (iCAHE): http://www.unisa.edu.au/Research/Sansom-Institute-for-Health-Research/Research/Allied-Health-Evidence/Resources/OC/

showing them the ways in which the underlying rules had been used to reach a conclusion. Modern systems, however, tend to be based on machine learning and work in ways that the human brain can never hope to emulate. Machine learning requires that the systems be exposed to millions of data records (so-called 'Big Data') and look for patterns, sometimes with sophisticated statistical techniques, to query that data. Therefore these systems cannot be used to show humans how they should reason. However, the promise is that these systems will be able to quickly advise clinicians of what they should be paying attention to in a particular case and how to proceed and thus support clinical reasoning. The more adaptable systems should be able to customize their recommendations to local circumstances as they gradually acquire more data and 'learn' about the local settings in which they are used. CPGs will be an important data source for developing such systems. The more rigorously a CPG is developed then the more rigorously a computerized decision support system will be able to support the decisions of clinicians in different circumstances.

REFLECTION POINT 8

Computerized decision support systems are a next logical step in the future use of CPGs. The development of increasing computer power, machine learning and the availability of 'Big Data' sets mean we may now be at a tipping point where these systems may become an everyday reality. What are some implications of this for you in your practice?

CHAPTER SUMMARY

- High-quality CPGs should be based on the best-available most recent evidence.
- They should be constructed using transparent processes that evaluate the volume and quality of available evidence, frame the recommendations in local contexts and support sound clinical reasoning.
- Healthcare professionals should therefore consider using high-quality, locally relevant CPGs to underpin their practice, as these guidelines can be applied to develop individual care plans for patients.
- In a world where 'evidence-based practice' is a common catchphrase, high-quality CPGs provide

health practitioners with a persuasive, cost-efficient and effective mechanism with which to evaluate and improve practice.
- CPGs are likely to play a key role in the computerized decision support systems of the future.

REFLECTION POINT 9

CPGs have seen rapid change and development in recent years. There are many more of them available. They are now more sophisticated, more rigorous, more adaptable to local settings and more user-friendly than ever. Critical use of CPGs can underpin clinical reasoning that can be justified as evidence-based and in the best interests of individual patients. How have/can CPGs positively influence your own decision making in practice?

REFERENCES

The ADAPTE Collaboration, 2009. The ADAPTE process: resource toolkit for guideline adaptation: version 2.0. Viewed 19 May 2017. Available from: http://www.g-i-n.net/document-store/working-groups-documents/adaptation/adapte-resource-toolkit-guideline-adaptation-2-0.pdf.

Amer, Y.S., Elzalabany, M.M., Omar, T.I., et al., 2015. The 'Adapted ADAPTE': an approach to improve utilization of the ADAPTE guideline adaptation resource toolkit in the Alexandria Center for Evidence-Based Clinical Practice Guidelines. J. Eval. Clin. Pract. 21, 1095–1106.

Dizon, J.M.R., Machingaidze, S.G., Grimmer, K.A., 2016. To adopt, adapt or contextualise? That is the question. BMC Res. Notes 9, 442.

Eccles, M.P., Grimshaw, J.M., Shekelle, P., et al., 2012. Developing clinical practice guidelines: target audiences, identifying topics for guidelines, guideline group composition and functioning and conflicts of interest. Implement. Sci. 7, 60.

Eccles, M., Grimshaw, J., Walker, A., et al., 2005. Changing the behaviour of healthcare professionals: the use of theory in promoting the uptake of research findings. J. Clin. Epidemiol. 58, 107–112.

Field, M.J., Lohr, K.N., 1990. Clinical Practice Guidelines: Directions for a New Program. National Academies Press, Institute of Medicine, Washington, DC.

Gonzalez-Suarez, C.B., Dizon, J.N.R., Grimmer, K.A., et al., 2015. Protocol for the audit of current Filipino practice in stroke in-patient rehabilitation. J. Multidiscip. Healthc. 8, 127–138.

Graham, R., Mancher, M., Wolman, D.M., et al. (Eds.), 2011. Clinical Practice Guidelines We Can Trust. National Academies Press, Institute of Medicine, Committee on Standards for Developing Trustworthy Clinical Practice Guidelines, Washington, DC.

Grimmer, K., Dizon, J.M., Milanese, S., et al., 2014. Efficient clinical evaluation of guideline quality: development and testing of a new tool. BMC Med. Res. Methodol. 14, 1–10.

Grimmer, K., Dizon, J.M., Louw, A.Q., et al., 2016a. South African Guidelines Excellence (SAGE): efficient, effective and unbiased clinical practice guideline teams. S. Afr. Med. J. 106, 440–441.

Grimmer, K., Machingaidze, S., Kredo, T., et al., 2016b. South African clinical practice guidelines quality measured with complex and rapid appraisal instruments. BMC. Res. Notes 9, 244.

Grol, R., Wensing, M., Eccles, M., et al., 2013. Improving Patient Care: The Implementation of Change in Health Care, second ed. BMJ Books, Wiley-Blackwell, Hoboken, NJ.

Kredo, T., Bernhardson, S., Young, T., et al., 2016. Guide to clinical practice guidelines: the current state of play. Int. J. Qual. Health Care 28, 122–128.

Kumar, S., Young, Y., Magtoto-Lizarando, L., 2010. What's in a name? Current case of nomenclature confusion. In: Grimmer-Somers, K., Worley, A. (Eds.), Practical Tips in Clinical Guideline Development: An Allied Health Primer. UST Publishing House, Manila, Philippines.

Machingaidze, S., Kredo, T., Young, T., et al., 2015. South African Guidelines Excellence (SAGE): clinical practice guidelines—quality and credibility. S. Afr. Med. J. Editorial Series. 105, 743–745.

Machingaidze, S., Zani, B., Abrams, A., et al., 2017. Quality and reporting standards of South African primary care clinical practice guidelines. J. Clin. Epidemiol. 83, 31–36.

Musen, M., Middleton, B., Greenes, R.A., 2014. Clinical decision-support systems. In: Shortliffe, E., Cimino, J.J. (Eds.), Biomedical Informatics: Computer Applications in Health Care and Biomedicine, fourth ed. Springer, New York, NY, pp. 643–674.

National Institute for Health and Care Excellence (NICE), 2015. Type I diabetes in adults: diagnosis and management. Viewed 19 May 2017. Available from: https://www.nice.org.uk/guidance/NG17.

National Institute for Health and Care Excellence (NICE), 2016. Hypertension in adults: diagnosis and management. Viewed 19 May 2017. Available from: https://www.nice.org.uk/guidance/cg127.

National Institute for Health and Care Excellence (NICE), 2017. Stroke and transient ischaemic attack in over 16s: diagnosis and initial management. Viewed 19 May 2017. Available from: https://www.nice.org.uk/guidance/cg68.

Sackett, D.L., Straus, S.E., Richardson, W.S., et al., 2000. Evidence-Based Medicine: How to Practice and Teach EBM, second ed. Churchill Livingstone, Edinburgh.

Satterfield, J.M., Spring, B., Brownson, R.C., et al., 2009. Toward a transdisciplinary model of evidence-based practice. Milbank Q. 87, 368–390.

Schünemann, H.J., Wiercioch, W., Etxeandia, I., et al., 2014. Guidelines 2.0: systematic development of a comprehensive checklist for a successful guideline enterprise. CMAJ 186, E123–E142.

Shaneyfelt, T.M., Mayo-Smith, M.F., Rothwangl, J., 1999. Are guidelines following guidelines? The methodological quality of clinical practice guidelines in the peer-reviewed medical literature. JAMA 281, 1900–1905.

Shiffman, R.N., Dixon, J., Brandt, C., et al., 2005. The GuideLine Implementability Appraisal (GLIA): development of an instrument to identify obstacles to guideline implementation. BMC Med. Inform. Decis. Mak. 5, 23.

Treweek, S., Oxman, A.D., Alderson, P., et al., 2013. Developing and evaluating communication strategies to support informed decisions and practice based on evidence (DECIDE): protocol and preliminary results. Implement. Sci. 8, 1–12.

World Health Organization (WHO), 2015. The global burden of disease concept. Viewed 19 May 2017. Available from: http://www.who.int/quantifying_ehimpacts/publications/en/9241546204chap3.pdf.

11

ACTION AND NARRATIVE
Two Dynamics of Clinical Reasoning

CHERYL MATTINGLY ▪ MAUREEN HAYES FLEMING

CHAPTER AIMS

The aims of this chapter are to:

- look beyond hypothetical deductive reasoning to understand clinical reasoning as action and narrative,

- focus on ways of understanding clients as people who are making meaning of their illness or injury in the context of their lives,

- present findings from ethnographic research that illustrates clinical reasoning as action and narrative and

- invite readers to reflect on their reasoning in the light of the arguments and case study presented.

KEY WORDS

Two streams of reasoning

Active judgement

Narrative

INTRODUCTION

Research in clinical reasoning emerged from the medical problem-solving tradition, which emphasized the hypothetical deductive method. Recently many theorists have argued that this strictly cognitive view is too narrow to encompass the myriad ways in which healthcare professionals devise solutions for clients' needs. We have found that the desire to conduct effective treatment, especially in the rehabilitation professions, directs the clinician to understand the client as a person who makes meaning of the illness or injury in the context of a life. By emphasizing the social dimension of clinical reasoning, we are highlighting a quality of expert judgement, which is by nature improvisational, flexible and highly attuned to the specifics of the person, the condition and the context.

In this chapter, we discuss two streams of reasoning, active judgement and narrative. Working out narrative possibilities and making active judgements are two dynamic processes that intertwine while the clinician carries out the best treatment with and for the individual patient. We further submit that through making and reflecting on these active judgements and narrative possibilities, clinicians develop their own stock of tacit knowledge and enhance their expertise. We draw upon ethnographic research projects we have conducted over the past decade, primarily (but by no means exclusively) among occupational therapists. This chapter is not a report of findings. We refer to these studies in a general way to illustrate and support a conceptualization of clinical reasoning and expertise grounded in the complexities and nuances of everyday practice in the world of rehabilitation.

ACTION AND JUDGEMENT

Action is the essence of clinical practice. In occupational, physical and speech therapy, the patient must act. Without the patient's participation, there is no therapy. One common view of action is that action takes place after one has carefully thought about the problem and its possible resolution. The assumption is that one thinks

119

carefully about the problem, decides what the central issue is, determines the best solution and takes action. This sequence may often be the case, but not always. Some philosophers, particularly phenomenologists, claim that thought and action occur in a rapid dynamic relation to one another, not in a fixed sequence. The word 'judgement' is often used to express this dynamic relationship. Buchler (1955), following on the work of John Dewey, C.S. Pierce and others, pointed out that action not only expresses the results of a judgement, it can be a judgement itself. Buchler (1955, p. 11) commented 'every action is itself a judgement'.

Schön (1983) submitted that reflective practitioners act first and judge the results afterward. Architecture students develop their expertise by looking at an area of land and sketching out versions of the structure they envision for that space. This action (sketching) is a way of seeing and a way of thinking. It is an act of both imagination and production, in which an image becomes visible and can be judged. The imagined building comes briefly to life in the form of a drawing. The structure is 'built' in imagination, action and judgement long before the backhoe arrives. Between the imaginative eye and the artful hand, the practitioner negotiates the route between the creative image and the concrete restrictions of the size, slope and orientation of the site, using a dynamic process of active judgement.

Healthcare practitioners also use imagination and action to make professional judgements about clients' problems and potential solutions. The patient is a 'site' where the best structure must be not constructed but reconstructed. Healthcare practitioners work with persons in crisis, with whom action must be taken immediately. Many judgements are made before, during and after action. In professional work, action and judgement merge. The practitioner often has the advantage of having the patient – the person – as a partner or at least informant in the endeavour. Usually the patient trusts the clinician and is willing to respond to requests for action. The actions that the patient executes give the practitioner a great deal of information. Conversely, the clinician might take action on or with the patient, which provides another source of information. The clinician and patient become involved in a coordinated set of actions and interactions that many observers have characterized as a therapeutic dance.

Many professional judgements are based on observations and interpretations of patients' actions. Clinicians want to see if and how a patient can perform an action. The practitioner judges the quality of a motion to make clinical judgements regarding the current level of strength or range of motion and to estimate the possible functional gains the patient may make during treatment. By judging today's action, the clinician can gauge the potential for future functional performance. The patient is often asked to perform specific motions or sets of movements and with frequent numbers of repetitions. Isolated motions, such as elbow flexion or thumb–finger prehension, are requested. Every day the therapist asks for more repetitions, more weight, more concentration and so on.

Therapists remind patients that they couldn't do this last week or yesterday and point out what they can do today and where they could be tomorrow or next week. The story of progress towards reconstruction is played out in increasingly better and more functional actions. Therapists want the patient's movements to match the image in the therapist's mind – to meet the perceived potential. Eventually the motions are combined into actions or sets of motions with a motive such as shoulder rotation, elbow extension, wrist stabilization, finger extension and flexion to reach for an object. Later these and other motions and actions are combined so that desired functional activities, such as eating, may be performed. In a sense, it is not the professional who is the therapist but rather the patient and his or her ability to invest in meaningful action. Through this investment, the patient rebuilds the body and reconstructs a sense of self as a person who can function in the world, an actor.

Practitioners take many actions while treating their patients. They also gain information from their interpretations of the sensations they receive from the patient, and they learn from their own actions. The therapist tests muscle tone, adjusts the position of finger and thumb in a tenodesis grasp or balances a child in her lap while he works with a toy. In the interest of improving patients' potential for future action, experts evaluate patients' actions, guide their own actions, make interpretations simultaneously, make rapid judgements and change actions smoothly and rapidly. Action is both a concrete event and a reasoning strategy that mediates the flow of therapy from image to result. Simultaneously, clinicians learn if and how their own actions work as effective treatment strategies. In this way, a wealth of personal/professional expertise is developed.

TACIT KNOWLEDGE AND PROFESSIONAL JUDGEMENT

When we conducted our first study (Mattingly and Fleming, 1994) we were confident that we would discover that therapists had a great deal of professional knowledge and skill and had a great stock of tacit knowledge. We did not anticipate the degree to which they were unaware of the amount of knowledge they had. Polanyi (1966, p. 4) coined the term 'tacit knowledge' and described it as the stock of professional knowledge that experts possess that is not processed in a focussed cognitive manner but rather lies at a not quite conscious level, where it is accessible through acting, judging or performing. This level of awareness is what Polanyi called 'the tacit dimension'. It is a type of knowledge that is acquired through experience. Polanyi called it tacit knowledge because experts were able to act on it but could not always verbalize exactly what they were doing or why. He expressed this concisely with the words, 'we know more than we can tell'.

In daily practice, the clinician encounters a new situation, takes action, perhaps several variations of a set of actions, and reflects on them to evaluate whether the action 'worked'. Was it effective in solving a problem with this particular patient who in some ways was subtly different from the last patient of the same age, gender and diagnosis? Through this action and reflection, the therapist builds a stock of tacit knowledge that becomes increasingly nuanced with further experience. Tacit knowledge has some advantages and disadvantages. It contributes to efficiency. The expert can do what is required, quickly and smoothly in much less time than it takes to explain. Because tacit knowledge is developed in action, it remains accessible to immediately guide action.

Clinicians often literally act before they think. This is not mindless action; it is an automaticity of expertise that does not have to be processed through the lengthier channels of formal cognition. However, the inability to explain all that one knows can cause others to question the credibility of the professional's knowledge. Occupational therapists in our study had a particular problem with this credibility issue because they had a wealth of practical tacit knowledge and confidence in their clinical skills but did not have a rich language to explain or describe their practice, as do physicians and some other practitioners in the clinical environment. Giving language to some aspects of their practice (Mattingly et al., 1997) gave the therapists a clearer perspective on their practice and a vehicle to examine and advance it.

Tacit knowledge works in the immediate situation resulting from its development in the past. It can also work to help a clinician formulate an image of the potential future situation, both as an image and a guide to plan treatment. Following is an example of a clinician whose tacit knowledge was copious and who could also articulate that knowledge given very little prompting.

NARRATIVE REASONING

One might assume that narrative reasoning is related strictly to telling and interpreting stories. However, it has come to be associated with a much broader human capacity. It constitutes a form of meaning making that is pervasive in human activity (Bruner, 1986, 1990, 1996; Carr, 1986; MacIntyre, 1981; Nussbaum, 1990; Ricœur, 1984). In recent years, narrative thinking has been recognized as important in clinical judgement (Frankenberg, 1993; Good, 1994; Hunt, 1994; Hunter, 1991; Mattingly, 1991, 1998a, 1998b, 2004, 2007, 2010; Mattingly and Fleming, 1994). Narrative reasoning is necessary to interpret the actions of others and to respond appropriately to the social context. Bruner (1986, 1996) referred to such reasoning as a capacity to 'read other minds', that is, to make accurate inferences about the motives and intentions of others based on their observable behaviour and the social situation in which they act (Mattingly, 2008). When we try to make sense of what another person is up to, we ask, in effect, what story is that person living out? Narrative thinking, as the anthropologist Michael Carrithers (1992, pp. 77–78) observed, 'allows people to comprehend a complex flow of action and to act appropriately within it … narrative thinking is the very process we use to understand the social life around us'.

When occupational therapists reason narratively, clinical problems and treatment activities are organized in their minds as an unfolding drama (Mattingly, 1998b, 2010). A cast of characters emerges. Motives are inferred

CASE STUDY 11.1

Narrative Reasoning

A Norwegian therapist we know read a transcript of an American therapist's report on her work with a man with a crush injury to his hand. The report was basically a long list of abbreviations about DIP (Distal joint), PIP (Proximal Interphalangeal joint) and other joints and various soft-tissue injuries. This therapist looked up from the notes and sighed. We asked, 'What is the matter?' and she said, 'I can just see it all now. This man is going to get very depressed, lose his job, probably become an alcoholic and his wife will divorce him. He will probably have bad contractures, more surgery, be committed to therapy for a while and cycle back and forth between depression and attempts to get his life and therapy back on track'. We looked at her in astonishment. That was exactly what happened to him. 'How did you know?' we asked. She said, 'I've seen it all before. I have been a hand therapist for several years. As soon as I read the description of his injuries, his hand just lit up in my mind. I could just see it. Then his life just rolled along in my mind as well. I knew just how it was going to be. This is a very difficult injury and very devastating to the person'. This experienced therapist knew similar people in the past and was able to envision this person's situation. The strong imagistic quality, to say nothing of the accuracy, of her comments demonstrates more than simple memory. Her capacity to suddenly see this patient in her mind's eye is part of her expertise. The image is a vivid and powerful portrayal of the person's future life. This therapist's ability to create vivid images of a patient's life, to take a minimal description of a hand injury and envision a host of life consequences, including how they might affect the emotions and motives of the patient, also reveals well-developed skills in narrative reasoning.

---

or examined. Narrative reasoning is needed when clinicians want to understand concrete events that cannot be comprehended without relating an inner world of desire and motive to an outer world of observable actions and states of affairs. Narrative reasoning concerns the relationship among motives, actions and consequences as they play out in some specific situation (Bruner, 1986; Dray, 1954; Ricœur, 1980, 1984).

REFLECTION POINT 1

Have you had this experience of your mind 'lighting up' about a client's potential clinical and life pathway? Did your prediction come about? What did you learn from this experience?

However, attention to the specifics of context is not sufficient to distinguish narrative reasoning from other modes of clinical thinking. As Hunter (1991, p. 28) noted, 'The individual case is the touchstone of knowledge in medicine'. The hallmark of narrative reasoning is that it utilizes specifics of a very special sort: it involves a search for the precise motives that led to certain key actions and for how those critical actions produced some further set of consequences. Although narrative reasoning is

evidently a generic human capacity, it is prone to tremendous misjudgement. As we all know, it is quite easy to misinterpret the motives and intentions of others, especially if they are strangers and come from unfamiliar social or cultural backgrounds. In some cases, and for some practices, interpretive errors are not especially important. One can make a splint, for example, without needing to have tremendous skill in interpreting the meaning of splint wearing for one's client. But one cannot make a good decision about when to give a client a splint or figure out how to get that client to wear it without developing a capacity to assess the beliefs, values and concerns of the client.

There are practical reasons why expert rehabilitation professionals, in particular, hone their narrative reasoning skills. The most obvious reason is that effective treatment depends on highly motivated patients. As occupational therapists often say, in therapy, patients are not 'done to' but are asked to 'do for themselves'. This 'active healing' process means that patients cannot passively yield their bodies to the expert to receive a cure; rather they need to become highly committed participants in the rehabilitation process.

This presents a special challenge to the professional: How do I foster a high level of commitment in my patients? This task calls upon narrative reasoning as the practitioner tries to design a treatment approach that will appeal to a particular patient. Occupational therapists refer to this as 'individualizing treatment'. Narrative reasoning figures centrally in those health professions, such as rehabilitation therapies, where efficacious practice requires developing a strong collaboration with clients. When motives matter, narrative reasoning is inevitable, and poor skills in such reasoning will mean that therapy is likely to fail.

PROSPECTIVE STORIES: THERAPY AND LIFE STORIES

In occupational therapy at least, narrative reasoning is not merely directed at the problem of obtaining the cooperation of a patient during a particular clinical encounter. The therapist's ability to employ narrative reasoning sensitively is essential to another clinical task, helping patients link their past (often a time before illness or disability) to their present and to a future worth pursuing. When therapists ask themselves, 'Who is this patient?' they are asking a fundamentally narrative question. They are wondering what might motivate this particular patient in treatment and, beyond that, which treatment activities and goals would be most appealing and useful, given the life this person will likely be living once therapy is completed. Therapists routinely struggle to develop images of their patients as individuals with unique needs and commitments, with singular life stories. 'Curing' is rare in the world of rehabilitation, and, in any case, it is not possible to transport a patient back in time to younger and healthier years. Instead, occupational therapists work to connect with patients to judge which treatment goals are most fitting and which treatment activities make most sense given the patient's conceptions of what is important in life.

Collaboration with patients is so central, it is probably more accurate to speak of the co-construction of treatment goals and activities. In fact, recognizing how complex and important a co-constructive process was, and how crucial it was to developing effective treatment goals, has led one of the authors (Mattingly) to carry out several longitudinal studies that have focussed on patient and especially family caregiver perspectives. This research has precipitated a deepening recognition of how powerful narrative is not only for the reasoning of clinicians but for patients and family members as well. Notably, it plays a crucial role in the fashioning and refashioning of hope over time (Mattingly, 2010, 2014).

The power of narrative is an ongoing, largely tacit, reasoning process that guides action and becomes most evident in clinical situations when things break down – when it is difficult for the practitioner to make narrative sense of the clinical encounter or the patient. When practitioners confront patients who are incomprehensible in some significant way, the whole direction of treatment may falter. The tacit narrative reasoning that practitioners carry into clinical encounters is likely to turn into explicit storytelling as they try to discern what is going on and 'what story they are in' with a particular client. For instance, a patient may insist that he wants to return to his job, show up to all his clinical appointments faithfully and comply with all the tasks set before him during his therapy hour but never manage to 'get around' to doing the exercises he is supposed to be carrying out at home.

Without these home exercises, the therapist may explain several times, treatment will not be successful. He will not be able to use his hand. He will not be able to return to work. And yet, nothing helps. Things continue just as before. Perhaps he has been lying or deceiving himself. Perhaps he doesn't want his job back after all. But if he were merely noncompliant and uninterested in returning to work, why does he show up to every appointment so faithfully, even arriving early? Why does he try so hard during therapy time? Such mysteries are common. Therapists become increasingly unclear about how to proceed in their treatment interventions, even when 'the good' (outcome) for a patient (say, maximal return of hand function) remains fixed in an abstract sense.

Narrative reasoning is a guide to a therapist's future actions because it provides images of a possible future for the client. When reasoning narratively, practitioners are trying to assess how to act in particular clinical situations, taking into consideration the motives and desires of themselves, their clients and other relevant actors. The ongoing construction of a narrative framework provides clinicians with historical contexts in which certain actions emerge as the inevitable next steps leading to the most promising future.

Although the question of what the good future is for any particular patient may never be explicitly asked, the process of treatment itself is very often a process of exploring and negotiating a vision of the future good. When clinicians assess how they can help patients reshape their situation for the better, this assessment is often informed by a 'prospective story,' an imagined future life story for the individual. Thus clinicians contemplate how to situate their therapeutic interventions (a kind of 'therapeutic present') in light of a patient's past and some hoped-for vision of what will follow in the future when the patient is discharged.

Narrative reasoning is directed to the future in the sense that it involves judgements about how to act to 'further the plot' in desirable directions and to subvert, as far as possible, undesirable ones. Although our traditional concept is that stories recount past events, stories in the clinical world are often directed to future possibilities. How are such 'prospective stories' communicated to patients or negotiated with them? Generally, it is not by telling the stories in detail. Rather, the stories are sketched through subtle hints or cues or enacted in clinical dramas that prefigure life after therapy.

The prospective story is offered, like the architect's sketch, as a possibility, something to be looked at, viewed from different angles, something to make a judgement about. When therapists offer short stories to their patients about what their life will be like 'in a few weeks' or 'when the halo comes off' or when 'you are home with the kids', they are offering images and possibilities of a meaningful future. Therapists hope that a commitment to these narrative images, images that point towards a future life story, will carry the patients through the long, tedious, often painful routines of treatment.

ACTIVE JUDGEMENTS, TACIT KNOWLEDGE AND NARRATIVE IMAGES: A CASE STORY

The interplay of actions, judgements, tacit knowledge and narrative image making is dauntingly intricate to describe in the abstract but becomes easily visible when examining concrete instances of practice. The following case story, written by an experienced occupational therapist, illustrates how image, action and narrative come together in expert therapeutic practice.

REFLECTION POINT 2

Would you have handled Ann's situation like Maureen? Would your workplace have allowed the flexibility that Maureen achieved to support Ann's transition? What might you have done differently?

ACTION, JUDGEMENT, NARRATIVE AND EXPERTISE IN ANN'S STORY

In the story, an experienced clinician (Maureen) orchestrated a therapy program for a somewhat unusual patient. Maureen began her story with a typical medical case history approach, but it quickly became evident that the patient's particular life situation shaped Maureen's judgements about how to design treatment. It mattered, for instance, that one of the primary consequences of Ann's stroke was that Ann is fearful about her ability to care for her newborn baby. Maureen also immediately took into account key elements that would be at play in Ann's 'future story'. Maureen noted the particular situation to which Ann would be returning as a mother unable to afford child care, with no family to turn to except her husband, who worked all day. Maureen judged what actions Ann would need to relearn and selected and invented therapeutic activities based on her perception of the social context and personal goals of Ann and her husband. Maureen was sensitive to the husband's insight about the need for Ann's transformation from patient to wife and mother. She situated her treatment goals within the notion of transformation. Her treatment approach developed as a powerful 'short story' that assisted in Ann's transformation from fearful patient to confident mother, able to handle even the difficult task of carrying her baby in her arms. Maureen made continual judgements about how to shift treatment from safer and easier tasks to those more closely approximating Ann's 'real-world' life situation.

In creating this unique treatment story, Maureen relied on her accumulated tacit knowledge culled from years of experience. She drew upon a typical treatment sequence, from building individual motions, to actions, to coordinated functional skills. She clearly had a great deal of tacit knowledge regarding how to help patients build their ADL skills. Although this occupational therapist was able to draw upon a wealth of tacit

CASE STUDY 11.2

The Story of Ann[1]

Ann was a 26-year-old woman who had given birth and subsequently had a stroke. She was admitted to a rehabilitation hospital with right hemiparesis. When I first met Ann, she was very depressed about being separated from her new baby, and her main fear was that she would not be able to adequately care for the baby on her own. Adding to this fear was the knowledge that her insurance would not cover any in-home services. Her husband was her only family, he worked construction every day and they lived in a trailer park. To go home with the baby, she would need to be very independent.

The initial therapy sessions were centred around tone normalization, with an emphasis on mat activities, along with traditional ADL (activities of daily living) training in the mornings. Ann's husband visited daily and usually brought the baby with him. At first, this was extremely frustrating to Ann because she could not hold the baby unless she was sitting down with pillows supporting her right arm. She continued to voice anxiety around the issue of going home and being able to care for the baby. Her husband was also very worried about how this transformation would take place – from Ann as a patient to Ann as wife and mother. I spent a lot of time talking to both Ann and her husband about the necessity of normalizing the tone and improving the movement of the upper extremity as a sort of foundation to the more complex functional skills Ann was so anxious to relearn.

Eventually it was time to spend the majority of the treatment time on functional skills. The two areas we focussed on were homemaking and child care. The homemaking sessions were fairly routine and traditional in nature. However, it proved to be a bit more difficult to simulate some of the child-care activities.

Our first obstacle was to find something that would be like a baby. We settled on borrowing a 'resusc-a-baby' from the nursing education department. We used this 'baby' for the beginning skills such as feeding and diaper changing. Ann had progressed to a point where she had slight weakness and incoordination in the right arm, and she was walking with a straight cane. The next step was to tackle walking with the baby. We of course practiced with a baby carrier. We also had to prepare for the event of carrying the baby without the 'carrier'. I wrapped weights about the 'baby' to equal the weight of the now 3-month-old infant at home. Ann walked down the hall carrying the 'baby', and I would follow behind jostling the 'baby' to simulate squirming (we became the talk of the hospital with our daily walks!). Ann was becoming more and more comfortable and confident with these activities, so it was time to make arrangements to have the real baby spend his days in the rehabilitation with his mother.

This was not as easy as it might seem. The administration of the hospital was not used to such requests. But with the right cajoling in the right places this was eventually approved. The real baby now replaced 'resusc-a-baby' on our daily walks and in the clinic. Although these successes were comforting to Ann and her husband, the fact remained that we were still in a very protective environment. The big question was yet unanswered: Would these skills hold up under the stresses of everyday life – alone – in a trailer for 8 hours daily?

Never being one to hold to tradition, I decided to go to administration another time with one more request. I wanted to do a full day 'home visit' with Ann and her baby. This too was approved, and 1 week before Ann's scheduled discharge, she and I set out for a rigorous day at the home front. Once there, all did not go smoothly; Ann fell once and practically dropped the baby. She was very anxious and stressed, but we managed to get through the day. We talked and problem solved every little real or perceived difficulty. Both Ann and the baby survived the fall and the 'almost' dropping. When we got back to the hospital, Ann, her husband, the social worker and I sat down and realistically discussed and decided what kind of outside help was a necessity and what Ann could really accomplish in a day. Ann's husband adjusted his schedule, a teenage neighbour was brought in for 2 to 3 hours a day and Ann was able to do the majority of the care for her baby.

[1]by Maureen Freda, MA, OTR.

knowledge, in many ways she faced a singular situation that required her to make judgements specifically tailored to Ann's needs.

The symbolic plays a powerful role in this treatment. Maureen saw the need for a substitute or symbolic baby, not just a pretend baby in the form of a pillow. She borrowed a model from another clinical department, and this seemed to do the trick. Maureen moved on with Ann from sedentary baby care activities to the more challenging, complex and risky activity of walking with the baby. She rose to this challenge by developing novel therapeutic activities, such as adding weights and simulating the baby's squirming. These increasingly active qualities of the resusc-a-baby were proxy for the real baby, who then entered the picture as a more viable image. The more realistic the 'baby's' actions became, the more Ann became prepared to make the transition from patient to mother. Maureen judged when it is time for the real baby to make an appearance on the rehabilitation floor. Maureen's confidence in her judgements prepared her to make and win the case with administration for the baby to participate in his mother's therapy. The therapy worked. It was clear to everyone that this move beyond conventional practice reaped benefits far greater than would have been obtained had Maureen stuck to conventional exercise and routine ADL activities.

Finally, the therapist determined that it was time to take what they had learned and see how they worked in the real-life situation of Ann's home. Here we see that Maureen's perceptions of her own judgement and her tacit knowledge differed. She was thoroughly confident that the home visit was the right thing to do. However, she was somewhat less confident regarding the potential success that Ann would have in some of the specific activities of baby care. Ann and Maureen now had enough trust in each other and in the plan to believe that this practice session was well worth any potential risks. Although she didn't say so, we can infer that Maureen was constantly attentive to the small details of the activities that she asked Ann to carry out in the home and set up subtle safety features, including her heightened attention and undoubted physical closeness to mother and child.

This confluence of image and action is typical of experienced therapists who are able to see opportunities in the midst of action to gradually or dramatically change

their treatment plan in response to particular details of a patient's skills and needs. Notably, this capacity for flexible plan development is central because, as Ann illustrates, a patient's needs and concerns often change over the course of therapy. Maureen, through her sensitivity to this patient and her personal and social context, was able to both speed up and individualize treatment to maximize her ability to act and return Ann to her desired social roles.

We have described this treatment process as the creation of a 'short story' within the larger life story of the patient, Ann (and, of course, the life stories of her husband and baby as well). Notably, this is a short story that not only connects to Ann's past, as a young woman who has recently given birth, but also to a future, that is, to events and experiences that have not yet taken place. With the careful guiding of treatment activities, the therapist was able to steer Ann towards her hoped-for future, the one where she could independently care for her child, and steer her away from a very undesirable future, one in which she remained depressed and fearful of her capacities to take on such care.

The power of any therapeutic short story is its capacity to help patients and their families realize some future story that deeply matters to them. The therapist cannot simply impose this desired future upon Ann, even if it is a future Ann dearly wants. She must look for signals that Ann is ready to move towards it. This requires the therapist's continual judgement about what constitutes the 'just right challenge' (Csikszentmihalyi, 1975) for Ann at any moment in therapy. Such judgements involve assessing Ann's physical capabilities but also require narrative reasoning, assessing the state of Ann's inner world of emotions, desires and beliefs, as they are expressed in her outward actions and words.

Narrative reasoning is also utilized when Maureen helped to create symbolically potent images for Ann, helping her to envision what life will be like with her baby. Maureen created dramatic situations in which Ann could test her abilities and face her fears. This dramatic play allowed Ann to face one of her worst nightmares, as she nearly dropped her child upon returning home for a trial run with Maureen. Notably, these experiences helped Maureen to talk with Ann, her husband and a social worker to make a more realistic plan about how Ann might care for her child upon discharge, including changes in the husband's work schedule and bringing in a neighbourhood babysitter to help out.

CHAPTER SUMMARY

We have found that clinical reasoning is not just one cognitive process and is not limited to the task of making decisions about concrete biological problems. We claim that to be truly therapeutic, clinicians must understand their patients and the ways in which they make meaning in lives that are changed by illness or injury. Two of the ways practitioners perceive patient's perceptions of their past and future lives and orchestrate treatment programs to achieve that future vision have been briefly discussed. These strategies are narrative reasoning and active judgement. These forms of reasoning serve to enlarge clinicians' stock of tacit knowledge and expand their expertise.

REFLECTION POINT 3

- What have you learned about the place of action and narrative from this chapter?
- What have you learned about your own reasoning and practice? Do you have ideas or aims for changing how you reason and act in your practice?
- How do you think the context or situation of the client and the professional(s) affects reasoning and requires variation in reasoning from one client to another?
- Do you think that the interpretation of narrative and action as dimensions of clinical reasoning are applicable across different professions?

A suggested task: Write your own therapeutic short story from your experience as a healthcare professional, and reflect on how and what you learn from this activity (a) reveals your past and present practice story and (b) might impact on your future practice story.

REFERENCES

Buchler, J., 1955. Nature and Judgement. Columbia University Press, New York, NY.

Bruner, J., 1986. Actual Minds, Possible Worlds. Harvard University Press, Cambridge, MA.

Bruner, J., 1990. Acts of Meaning. Harvard University Press, Cambridge, MA.

Bruner, J., 1996. The Culture of Education. Harvard University Press, Cambridge, MA.

Carr, D., 1986. Time, Narrative, and History. Indiana University Press, Bloomington, IN.

Carrithers, M.B., 1992. Why Humans Have Cultures. Oxford University Press, Oxford.

Csikszentmihalyi, M., 1975. Beyond Boredom and Anxiety: The Experience of Play in Work and Game. Jossey-Bass, San Francisco, CA.

Dray, W., 1954. Explanatory narrative in history. Philos. Q. 23, 15–27.

Frankenberg, R., 1993. Risk: anthropological and epidemiological narratives of prevention. In: Lindenbaum, S., Lock, M. (Eds.), Knowledge, Power and Practice: The Anthropology of Everyday Life. University of California Press, Berkeley, CA, pp. 219–242.

Good, B., 1994. Medicine, Rationality, and Experience: An Anthropological Perspective. Cambridge University Press, New York, NY.

Hunt, L., 1994. Practicing oncology in provincial Mexico: a narrative analysis. Soc. Sci. Med. 38, 843–853.

Hunter, K.M., 1991. Doctors' Stories: The Narrative Structure of Medical Knowledge. Princeton University Press, Princeton, NJ.

MacIntyre, A., 1981. After Virtue: A Study in Moral Theory. University of Notre Dame Press, Notre Dame, IN.

Mattingly, C., 1991. The narrative nature of clinical reasoning. Am. J. Occup. Ther. 45, 998–1005.

Mattingly, C., Fleming, M.H., Gillette, N., 1997. Narrative explorations in the tacit dimension: bringing language to clinical practice. Nordiske Udkast 1, 65–77.

Mattingly, C., 1998a. Healing Dramas and Clinical Plots: The Narrative Structure of Experience. Cambridge University Press, Cambridge, MA.

Mattingly, C., 1998b. In search of the good: narrative reasoning in clinical practice. Med. Anthropol. Q. 12, 273–297.

Mattingly, C., 2004. Performance narratives in clinical practice. In: Hurwitz, B., Greenhalgh, T., Skultans, V. (Eds.), Narrative Research in Health and Illness. Blackwell, London, UK, pp. 73–94.

Mattingly, C., 2007. Acted narratives: from storytelling to emergent dramas. In: Clandinin, D.J. (Ed.), Handbook of Narrative Inquiry: Mapping a Methodology. Sage Publications, Thousand Oaks, CA, pp. 405–425.

Mattingly, C., 2008. Reading minds and telling tales in a cultural borderland. Ethos 36, 181–205.

Mattingly, C., 2010. The Paradox of Hope: Journeys Through a Clinical Borderland. University of California Press, Berkeley, CA.

Mattingly, C., 2014. Moral Laboratories: Family Peril and the Struggle for a Good Life. University of California Press, Berkeley, CA.

Mattingly, C., Fleming, M.H., 1994. Clinical Reasoning: Forms of Inquiry in a Therapeutic Practice. FA Davis, Philadelphia, PA.

Nussbaum, M., 1990. Love's Knowledge. Oxford University Press, New York, NY.

Polanyi, M., 1966. The Tacit Dimension. Doubleday, Garden City, NY.

Ricœur, P., 1980. Narrative time. In: Mitchell, T.J. (Ed.), On Narrative. University of Chicago Press, Chicago, IL, pp. 165–186.

Ricœur, P., 1984. Time and Narrative, vol. 1. University of Chicago Press, Chicago, IL.

Schön, D.A., 1983. The Reflective Practitioner: How Professionals Think in Action. Basic Books, New York, NY.

THE LANGUAGE OF CLINICAL REASONING

STEPHEN LOFTUS ■ JOY HIGGS

CHAPTER AIMS

The aims of this chapter are to:

■ look at clinical reasoning and its communication through the frame of language,

■ examine three key devices of language in relation to clinical reasoning: metaphor, narrative and rhetoric and

■ consider the implications of using these devices on the acts, experience and sense making involved in clinical reasoning.

KEY WORDS

Metaphor

Narrative

Rhetoric

INTRODUCTION

In this chapter, we examine the role of language in clinical reasoning. We consider that attention to this aspect of clinical reasoning can help all healthcare professionals come to a deeper understanding of what clinical reasoning is. An awareness of how language works in practice can help novices master the intricacies of clinical reasoning. This awareness can also help teachers develop appropriate pedagogies that can assist students to develop mastery of clinical reasoning.

An immediate problem with an approach based on language use is that we need first to dispel a commonly held myth. In the Western world, there is a widespread belief that language is nothing more than the representation of what is already 'out there' in the world. This is often called the representation view of language. This view oversimplifies things to the extent that it distorts how we can think about reality. Reality includes the clinical reality of our patients who come to us and expect us to understand their problems and deal with them.

A growing number of scholars have come to realize that language is far more complicated than the simple representation view. As Rorty once remarked, 'The world is out there, but descriptions of the world are not' (1989, p. 5). Rorty goes on to claim that we make up ways of describing the world that suit particular purposes of ours. For example, the way a clinical psychologist will use language to describe a patient with chronic pain will be quite different from the way a physician will use language to describe the same patient, even though both are being scientific and objective. Representation is just one of the functions of language, and there can be more than one valid way of representing something or someone. However, Wittgenstein (1958) pointed out there are many more functions of language besides representation that are just as important. For example, the following selection of 'language games' that Wittgenstein (1958) lists can all be relevant to the activity of clinical reasoning. They include describing the appearance of an object or giving its measurements, reporting an event, speculating about an event or forming and testing a hypothesis. These are language activities that include and go beyond mere representation, and they can all play a part in clinical reasoning. Wittgenstein's work has inspired other scholars, such as Gadamer (1989), who have deepened our understanding of how language works.

From the work of Gadamer (1989), we realize that language can also be about presentation and bringing things to our awareness in the first place. The ways in which we use language affect how we perceive the world around us, and this is just as true of clinical reasoning (Loftus, 2012). This view of clinical reasoning is interpretive and contrasts with the current and more widespread view that clinical reasoning is, or should be, regarded as a phenomenon of computational logic and symbolic processing, combined with probability mathematics and statistics. This is not to say that the mainstream approaches to clinical reasoning, such as information processing, are wrong but that there are alternative views that can be just as powerful and that can help us both theoretically and practically. This alternative view, based on language use, can sensitize us to important aspects of clinical reasoning that would otherwise be missed.

Many have argued, following Aristotle (1983, trans.), that thinking is the internalization of talk we have with others and that in learning to think we learn to have conversations with ourselves (Bakhtin, 1984; Toulmin, 1979; Vygotsky, 1986). According to this argument, we do not first have thoughts, which are then 'dressed up' in language. As Vygotsky (1986, p. 218) explained, 'Thought is not merely expressed in words: it comes into existence through them'. Language serves as a means of controlling what we think and how we communicate. To speak a particular language is to inhabit a particular 'way of being' (Wittgenstein, 1958). Language both shapes and limits how we construct our social realities (Higgs et al., 2004).

From this viewpoint, language is of primary importance for understanding the nature of thought. The underlying metaphors, the narrative formats and the persuasive ways in which we speak and write all play a role in our thinking and clinical reasoning. According to Vygotsky (1986), we learn at an early age to perceive the world as much through our language as through our eyes. Clinical reasoning is no exception. It is clear that language performs an integrative function. Other symbol systems and cognitive tools can have meaning because they are imbued with language and integrated within it. In the realm of clinical reasoning, there are

many symbol systems. These can include ECG traces, manual therapy symbols, dental notation, radiographs and MRI scans. Language, in Vygotsky's view, is the 'tool of tools' (Cole and Wertsch, 1996) that allows us to bring other symbol systems together into a meaningful whole.

There are several ways of looking at language use in clinical reasoning. In this chapter, we focus on a few of the better known. One example of language use is metaphor.

METAPHOR

Lakoff and Johnson (1980) claimed that thought and language are fundamentally metaphorical. Metaphor is not simply an embellishment of language exploited by writers and poets. It can be argued that language and thought are intensely and inherently metaphorical, and, because of this, metaphor use goes largely unnoticed as it is so completely natural to us. Metaphor is therefore a major means for constituting reality. The implication of this view is that we do not perceive reality and then separately interpret it and give it meaning. Once we acquire language, we perceive reality immediately through the lens of language. As Foss (2009) observed:

> *Metaphor is a basic way by which the process of using symbols to construct reality occurs. It serves as a structuring principle, focusing on particular aspects of a phenomenon and hiding others; thus, each metaphor produces a different description of the 'same' reality (p. 268).*

In recent years, there has been a growing recognition of the extent to which metaphor underlies scientific and medical practice and shapes the ways in which both healthcare professionals and their patients conceptualize their health problems and how they can be addressed (e.g., Reisfield and Wilson, 2004). One example of how different metaphors have shaped thinking in health care comes from the literature on the HIV/AIDS issue. See Case Studies 12.1 and 12.2.

REFLECTION POINT 1

What metaphors underpin clinical reasoning in your health profession? How are these metaphors helpful? What do they ignore or miss?

Metaphors in the Area of HIV/AIDS

Sherwin (2001) looked at the metaphors used by various interest groups in the HIV/AIDS issue, revealing how certain metaphors favour distinctive ways of thinking and showing that there are ethical implications arising from using particular metaphors. Sherwin argued that at one time epidemiologists favoured the metaphor 'AIDS is a lifestyle disease'. This encouraged them to pursue certain sorts of scientific practices such as looking for a multifactorial disease model, attending to some social conditions such as sexual orientation and patterns of drug use. However, the metaphor discouraged other lines of inquiry such as investigating homosexual behaviour in men who considered themselves to be heterosexual. The epidemiologists also resisted for some time the suggestion that a single causal virus might be responsible for AIDS. High-risk groups therefore became the focus of attention, instead of high-risk behaviour. Sherwin's opinion was that the underlying metaphor discouraged the epidemiologists from considering other ways of thinking about AIDS, and because they were so dominant in the field there was some delay before the medical establishment eventually accepted the viral cause of AIDS. The ethical implication is that the metaphors used might have resulted in unnecessary suffering of AIDS patients and infection of people who might otherwise have been alerted earlier to the dangers they faced. Another way of representing this is that the different metaphors encouraged healthcare professionals to tell particular stories/narratives about AIDS.

NEW METAPHORS IN CLINICAL REASONING

In recent years, there have been debates about other ways of reconceptualizing patient experiences; these debates include consideration of new metaphors that might be used to enrich our understanding of symptoms so that we can manage them better (Loftus, 2011). For example, pain has traditionally been regarded as a symptom, but there have been calls to reconceptualize pain as a disease entity in its own right (Siddall and Cousins, 2004). This debate is essentially about two metaphors we can use to think about pain – the older metaphor that represents pain as a symptom versus the newer metaphor that represents pain as a disease. Changing metaphors like this provides a 'reframing' in which the new metaphor offers a different way for interpreting and understanding patients and the problems they have. Conventionally, pathologies are seen as causes that produce effects that are called symptoms, such as pain. Following 'the body is a machine' metaphor, healthcare professionals have been taught that it is far more important to deal with the cause of a mechanistic problem rather than the effects.

Once the root cause of a mechanistic problem is dealt with, the effects tend to disappear. Because pain is seen as a 'mere' effect, it is often ignored while healthcare professionals focus their attention on finding and dealing with the causal pathology. As Siddall and Cousins (2004) point out, the result is that pain management is still very poor in the Western world. By trying to depict pain as a disease entity (a cause-effect mechanism in its own right), they are trying to reconceptualize pain as something that is more likely to attract the attention of healthcare professionals and be dealt with much more effectively.

A similar motive underlies the attempt to have pain recognized as the fifth vital sign, along with heart rate, respiratory rate, temperature and blood pressure (Berdine, 2002). There is frequently a requirement to observe and record vital signs in many hospital patients. If pain was included as a vital sign, then healthcare professionals would be required to routinely assess pain and document it. Presumably, pain management would then receive much more attention. Claiming that pain is a vital sign is a metaphorical switch that seeks to change thinking in an attempt to improve outcomes for patients.

CASE STUDY 12.2
Metaphors in Pain Management

Metaphors used in pain management can show how metaphor use affects clinical reasoning. A key metaphor underlying the biomedical model is 'the body is a machine'. This metaphor shapes the way many healthcare professionals think and is so widespread that many patients in Western societies also use this metaphor when thinking about their bodily problems (Hodgkin, 1985). The implication of this metaphor is that we can always, in principle at least, repair a broken machine. In acute care, this metaphor could be appropriate. For example, a patient with a toothache can go to a dentist who can provide a technical 'fix' in the form of fillings, root canal treatments or extractions. From this viewpoint, the body's technical problem is repaired, and the patient can go about his or her business. However, the metaphor frequently falls down in the chronic situation where repeated attempts at repair fail, resulting in frustration and disappointment for both patients and healthcare professionals. Often such patients are 'discarded' by the system as failed patients (Alder, 2003). This metaphor can also confuse healthcare professionals when they try to make sense of phenomena such as the placebo effect.

The placebo effect occurs when a beneficial effect is produced by a mechanism that is known to be technically ineffective. A well-known placebo example is pain relief from pills with no active ingredient. For healthcare professionals who restrict themselves to thinking with 'the body is a machine' metaphor, this makes little sense (Loftus, 2011). It is as if we took a malfunctioning car to a mechanic who used tools that do not work, and we then discover that the ineffective tools have repaired the problem. A way to understand what is happening in the placebo effect is to use different metaphors to conceptualize what is going on. Perhaps a more useful metaphor here would be 'pain is interpretation'. It is now widely accepted that pain is a subjective interpretation and that restricting ourselves to mechanistic thinking misses this interpretive element. Moerman (2002) spoke of the meaning effect. Placebos can work because of what they subjectively mean to us as people. Purely technical thinking prevents us from seeing that what experience means to us can profoundly alter how we perceive experiences like pain. This takes us back to the point made by Foss (2009) that metaphors can emphasize some aspects of a phenomenon but at the expense of hiding other aspects. 'The body is a machine' metaphor hides away the people who come to us as patients and seduces us into thinking of them only as machines to be mended.

Metaphors shape the way we think about health care in general terms, but they also shape the way healthcare professionals think through the individual problems of patients as they reason their way towards a diagnosis and treatment plan.

Much of the debate in the literature has been about which metaphors are closer to the 'truth'. In a sense, this debate is irrelevant. Metaphors cannot be true or false, but they can be more or less useful. What really matters in these debates is which metaphors are more useful and for whom. The overriding question is – what works for patients? How can we improve our clinical reasoning so that we get better results for patients? These questions emphasize the difference between medical science and medical practice. Medical practice is based on medical science, but the two are not identical. Whereas medical science, like all science, is concerned with the 'truth', medical practice is concerned with what works for patients. It is worth remembering the words of Rorty:

Human beings, like computers, dogs, and works of art, can be described in lots of different ways, depending on what you want to do with them – take them apart for repairs, reeducate them, play with them, admire them, and so on for a long list of alternative purposes. None of these descriptions is closer to what human beings really are than any of the others. Descriptions are tools invented for particular purposes, not attempts to describe things as they are in themselves, apart from any such purposes (Rorty, 1998, p. 28).

REFLECTION POINT 2

As we have seen, different metaphors provide the foundations for different descriptions. What matters is how well the descriptions (and their underlying metaphors) serve the purposes for which they are used. If the purpose is encouraging healthcare professionals to manage pain better, then describing pain as a disease or vital sign may well serve the purpose better than thinking of pain as a nerve signal or symptom. In this sense, the truth is irrelevant. The various descriptions healthcare professionals make of patients' problems are often in the form of narratives.

NARRATIVE

A major aspect of clinical reasoning is the construction of a narrative about a patient within the conceptual framework of a health profession and the specific context of the patient and the workplace. There is a growing realization of the importance of narrative in therapeutic encounters (e.g., Charon et al., 2017). The construction of a clinical narrative occurs in a manner that not only takes account of the past and present but also suggests the narrative trajectory that the patient's story might follow in the future, predisposing towards particular decisions about management. Such narratives can be

diagnostic, prognostic and therapeutic. See Case Studies 12.3 and 12.4.

REFLECTION POINT 3

What kinds of stories does your health profession use? How do these stories help your clinical reasoning?

RHETORIC

Rhetoric is the art of persuasive speaking or writing. A great deal of clinical reasoning is concerned with persuasion. Healthcare professionals need to persuade other people, such as funders, patients and their families and other clinicians, that a particular assessment and proposed course of action are both legitimate and sound. Above all, healthcare professionals have to persuade themselves. One medical student reflected on the importance of this issue when discussing how to cope with an inadequate clinical report from a colleague:

> *It's just being able to say what you find, and be able to say that … this person is in very dire straits. It's not making up stuff, but it's being able to present it in a convincing and competent manner that they [senior doctors] can say, 'All right, this requires my attention' (Loftus, 2006, p. 190).*

Another medical student described the feedback he received after reporting on a complex patient assessment conducted under examination conditions. The setting was an examination, and the two senior clinicians hearing the student's report knew exactly what was

---

CASE STUDY 12.3

Patient Narrative in Dentistry

A patient in her late teens presents to a dentist with a story of toothache at the back of the mouth that comes and goes spontaneously, is becoming more frequent and lasts longer each time it occurs. The dentist assesses the patient and reinterprets the patient's story in the professional discourse of dentistry and surgery. The reinterpreted narrative might then become a story of impacted wisdom teeth. This new story can be substantiated with scientific evidence in

the form of radiographs that show the offending teeth in their impacted position. The scientific evidence is given its meaning and importance by being integrated into the story of this patient's impacted wisdom teeth (Loftus and Greenhalgh, 2010). A major advantage of this professional reinterpretation is that the dentist's version has a narrative trajectory into the future. This narrative trajectory gives meaning to the whole episode.

CASE STUDY 12.4

Patient Narrative in Rehabilitation

Sometimes the meaning given by this narrative trajectory can be crucial. One of the best examples of this comes from the work of a rehabilitation centre in which a patient recovering from a head injury is introduced to the centre by an occupational therapist and shown where the various therapeutic activities will take place (Mattingly, 1994). The therapeutic activities, however, are not introduced simply as activities. As Mattingly points out, there is a deliberate effort by the occupational therapist to outline to the patient how the activities can be used so that he can

eventually leave and move on to a life beyond therapy. Mattingly's point is that without this narrative trajectory, there is a risk that the patient would find the therapy meaningless and might not collaborate with treatment. This is another situation in which the meaning of the clinical situation can have a dramatic effect on what happens and how well patients do. It is also clear from this example that the healthcare professional has to persuade the patient to accept this narrative trajectory.

---

wrong with the patient, along with all the comorbidities and how they complicated management. They told the student: 'you're very organized but you've got to get to the point now and tell us to where you want to go. You should be a bit more specific' (Loftus, 2006, p. 154).

Reflecting on this exchange, the student realized that the examiners wanted him to be more persuasive and lead them more convincingly to a definitive diagnosis and course of action. They wanted to hear a more persuasive story that worked towards a clear goal at the end. This is an important aspect of medical practice. In many countries, senior doctors cannot physically see all the patients nominally in their care. They rely on junior doctors doing assessments and giving reports. The senior doctors want to be able to make decisions based on these reports, and therefore they depend on junior doctors persuading them that the assessment has been done thoroughly and can be relied on. Senior doctors themselves confirm this insight.

> The trainees [junior doctors] need to learn that [they have to] cut down the amount of information to a manageable summary for your colleagues ... and for yourself because ... at the end of the day ... you have to be able to isolate them [important findings] and make a decision on them (Loftus, 2006, p. 193).

This ability is both a narrative and a rhetorical skill. In constructing a clinical report, a healthcare professional

is justifying a claim about a patient. The justification is supported by arguments that depend on the context of that patient and that will stand up to reasonable criticism. As Perelman (1982, p. 162) argued, 'As soon as a communication tries to influence one or more persons, to orient thinking ... to guide their actions, it belongs to the realm of rhetoric'.

There is frequently uncertainty in clinical reasoning, uncertainty that is associated not with self-doubt or the inability to make sound decisions but rather with the 'greyness' or complexity of practice situations, the variability of patient's or client's needs and the presence in many situations of various acceptable solutions (e.g., management strategies). And, when there is uncertainty, judgements must be made in light of all the information available for that case. This is not done mathematically or statistically but persuasively and argumentatively. This is the essence of rhetoric and of pragmatism – not the abandonment of logic or professional judgement but the incorporation of these into the intensely practical and human world of health care.

Consider the use of language devices in reasoning using Case Study 12.5.

REFLECTION POINT 4

Does Joe's story reflect your experience of framing and presenting your reasoning? What sort of language devices do you use to make sense of your reasoning and communicate it?

CASE STUDY 12.5

Joe's Story

Joe was getting used to working as a physiotherapist in an interprofessional pain management clinic. He wrote quickly as he summarized the assessment of his last patient. Although the assessment had taken 1 hour and the patient had lots of problems, he knew that he would only get about 1 minute to report on this patient at the case conference with the other healthcare professionals who had also seen the patient that day. He was mastering the art of confining his report to the key findings that the rest of the team would find useful. He realized that there would be some overlap with the doctor's report, and he would need to avoid repetition. On reflection, he realized that the rest of the team questioned him now far less than they did when he first started work there. They were clearly learning to trust his judgement.

One of his key findings was that the patient strongly believed that her ongoing pain meant that there was continuing injury. This was why the patient was so reluctant to move. If their management was to be successful, it would need to include a strong educational element in the treatment plan. They would need to persuade the patient to think about the pain differently. He realized just how much his own thinking had changed through working in the clinic. Most of the therapy they offered was designed to get patients to move away from thinking of their bodies as broken machines and instead to work on ways of managing their chronic pain. The underlying message of the therapy was that 'life is a journey', and they could provide patients with the means of moving on with that life, despite chronic pain.

CHAPTER SUMMARY

Using language as a theoretical lens allows us to see clinical reasoning in a very different way compared with the mainstream views such as hypothetico-deductive reasoning, information processing or evidence-based practice. This is not to deny the importance of the mainstream views but to point out that we can integrate them into a more coherent, and more cohesive, whole by seeing the role they play in the overall language game of clinical reasoning. The information from the evidence base, like all relevant information about a patient, has to be integrated into the narratives we construct about our patients, and this is done persuasively.

REFLECTION POINT 5

How can we use the ideas in this chapter to improve the teaching of clinical reasoning to students?

REFERENCES

Alder, S., 2003. Beyond the Restitution Narrative. PhD thesis. University of Western Sydney, Sydney, NSW.

Aristotle, 1983. (trans.) Aristotle's Physics i, ii, trans. W. Charlton. Oxford University Press, Oxford, UK. (originally published c. 400 bc).

Bakhtin, M., 1984. Problems of Dostoevsky's Poetics. University of Minnesota Press, Minneapolis, MN.

Berdine, H.J., 2002. The fifth vital sign: cornerstone of a new pain management strategy. Dis. Manage. Health Out. 10, 155–165.

Charon, R., DasGupta, S., Hermann, N., et al., 2017. The Principles and Practice of Narrative Medicine. Oxford University Press, New York, NY.

Cole, M., Wertsch, J.V., 1996. Beyond the social-individual antimony in discussions of Piaget and Vygotsky. Hum. Devel. 39, 250–256.

Foss, S.K., 2009. Rhetorical Criticism: Exploration and Practice, fourth ed. Waveland Press, Long Grove, IL.

Gadamer, H.G., 1989. Truth and Method, second ed. Continuum, New York, NY.

Higgs, J., Andresen, L., Fish, D., 2004. Practice knowledge: its nature, sources and contexts. In: Higgs, J., Richardson, B., Abrandt Dahlgren, M. (Eds.), Developing Practice Knowledge for Health Professionals. Butterworth-Heinemann, Edinburgh, pp. 51–69.

Hodgkin, P., 1985. Medicine is war: and other medical metaphors. Br. Med. J. 291, 1820–1821.

Lakoff, G., Johnson, M., 1980. Metaphors We Live By. University of Chicago Press, Chicago, IL.

Loftus, S., 2006. Language in Clinical Reasoning: Learning and Using the Language of Collective Clinical Decision Making. PhD thesis. The University of Sydney, Sydney, NSW. Available from: http://ses.library.usyd.edu.au/handle/2123/1165.

Loftus, S., 2011. Pain and its metaphors: a dialogical approach. J. Med. Human. 32, 213–230.

Loftus, S., 2012. Rethinking clinical reasoning: time for a dialogical turn. Med. Educ. 46, 1174–1178.

Loftus, S., Greenhalgh, T., 2010. Towards a narrative mode of practice. In: Higgs, J., Fish, D., Goulter, I., et al. (Eds.), Education for

Future Practice. Sense Publishers, Rotterdam, The Netherlands, pp. 85–94.

Mattingly, C., 1994. The concept of therapeutic 'emplotment'. Soc. Sci. Med. 38, 811–822.

Moerman, D., 2002. Meaning, Medicine and the Placebo Effect. Cambridge University Press, Cambridge, UK.

Perelman, C., 1982. The Realm of Rhetoric, trans. W. Kluback. Notre Dame University Press, Notre Dame, IN.

Reisfield, G.M., Wilson, G.R., 2004. Use of metaphor in the discourse on cancer. J. Clin. Oncol. 22, 4024–4027.

Rorty, R., 1989. Contingency, Irony and Solidarity. Cambridge University Press, Cambridge, UK.

Rorty, R., 1998. Against unity. Wilson Q. 22, 28–39.

Sherwin, S., 2001. Feminist ethics and the metaphor of AIDS. J. Med. Philos. 26, 343–364.

Siddall, P., Cousins, M., 2004. Persistent pain as a disease entity: implications for clinical management. Anesth. Analges. 99, 510–520.

Toulmin, S., 1979. The inwardness of mental life. Crit. Inq. 6, 1–16.

Vygotsky, L.S., 1986. Thought and Language, trans. A. Kozulin. MIT Press, Cambridge, MA (originally published 1962).

Wittgenstein, L., 1958. Philosophical Investigations, trans. GEM Anscombe. third ed. Prentice Hall, Upper Saddle River, NJ (originally published 1953).

13

EVIDENCE-BASED PRACTICE AND CLINICAL REASONING
In Tension, Tandem or Two Sides of the Same Coin?

ALIKI THOMAS ■ MEREDITH YOUNG

CHAPTER AIMS

The aims of this chapter are to:

■ explore relationships and differences between clinical reasoning and evidence-based practice and

■ consider the implications of adopting different approaches to understanding these relationships.

KEY WORDS

Evidence-based practice
Clinical reasoning

ABBREVIATIONS/ ACRONYMS

EBP Evidence-based practice
EBM Evidence-based medicine

INTRODUCTION

Evidence-based medicine (EBM) and clinical reasoning are distinct but interrelated concepts and have evolved in relatively parallel literatures. Several definitions of EBM have emerged over the years sparked largely by differences in disciplinary and professional perspectives. One of the earliest and most commonly used definitions of EBM described 'the conscientious, explicit and judicious use of current best evidence in making decisions about the care of individual patients. The practice of evidence-based medicine means integrating individual clinical expertise with the best available external clinical evidence from systematic research' (Sackett et al., 1996, p. 71). In parallel to an evolution of the concept of EBM, we have also seen an evolution in language surrounding the concept – with professions such as nursing and rehabilitation adopting terms such as evidence-based practice (EBP) (Bennett and Bennett, 2000) or evidence-based health care (EBHC) (Hammell, 2001) to reflect a broader application of this concept across health professions. For the purposes of this chapter, we will use the term EBP to reflect the multiple dimensions of the concept.

The formalized steps involved in the EBP process include 1) posing a clinical question, 2) searching the literature, 3) appraising the literature, 4) considering research evidence in clinical decision making and 5) reviewing the procedure and outcome of the EBP process (Sackett et al., 1996; Sackett et al., 2000). See Fig. 13.1.

Conceptualizations and ensuing refinements of the concept of EBP have since expanded to include consideration for the sociohistorical, political, professional, economic and institutional contexts (Banningan and Moores, 2009) (Fig. 13.2). Further considerations can include explicit integration of the mandate of the healthcare organization, a role for community involvement and potential limitations imposed by organizational and resource constraints. This apparent evolution in what EBP 'is' or represents is in large part a result of decades of debate about the merits of the EBP approach to decision making (Dijkers et al., 2012; Greenhalgh et al., 2015). A number of debates have been centralized around disagreements regarding the meaning and significance of 'evidence' and the implications associated with clinical decision making 'based' on evidence in

contrast to clinical decisions 'informed by' evidence (Wyer and Silva, 2009).

The literature has been rich with discussions regarding the value of EBP and its corresponding epistemological foundations (Bennett et al., 2003; Djulbegovic et al., 2009; Hammell, 2001). It is beyond the scope of this chapter to delve into, or preferentially support, one particular viewpoint over another; sophisticated debates have already taken place across many other disciplines and professions. The disputes and deliberations notwithstanding, EBP is regarded as an integral and necessary component of clinical decision making (Sackett et al., 2000; Salmond, 2013).

Clinical reasoning carries its own set of definitional challenges. There is an abundance of literature on clinical reasoning across disciplines, professions and methodological traditions, and clinical reasoning is considered core to the practice of health practitioners (Higgs et al., 2008; Schell, 2009). Though not as overtly contentious as the definition of EBP, there is little agreement about what is specifically meant by

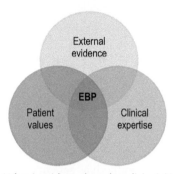

Fig. 13.1 ■ What is evidence-based medicine? (Adapted from Sackett, D.L., Rosenberg, W.M., Gray, J.A., Haynes, B.R., Richardson, S.W., 1996. Evidence based medicine: what it is and what it isn't. BMJ 312, 71–72.)

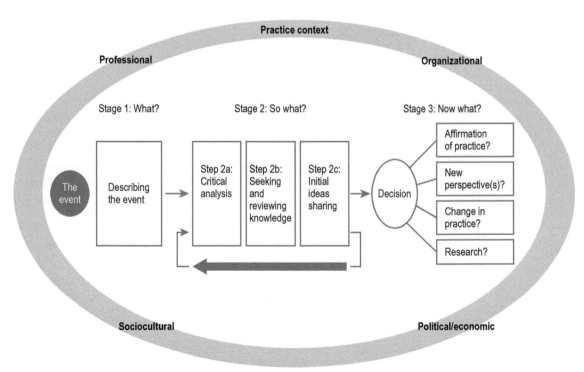

Fig. 13.2 ■ Model of professional thinking. (From Banningan, K., Moores, A., 2009. A model of professional thinking: integrating reflective practice and evidence based practice. Can. J. Occup. Ther. 76, 342–350, with permission.)

the term 'clinical reasoning' or what it entails (Durning et al., 2013). Considered as the backbone of professional practice (Higgs et al., 2008; Mattingly, 1991), clinical reasoning has been defined as an outcome, a means to an end and a process that results in diagnosis and treatment (Eva, 2005).

REFLECTION POINT 1

To you, is clinical reasoning an outcome, a process, a means to an end or something else?

Clinical reasoning and EBP have, for the most part, existed in parallel bodies of literature attempting to describe the practice of health professionals and suggest areas of improvement. Although both literatures house independent debates regarding how a clinician should 'best solve' a clinical case and discuss areas for better patient outcomes and how best to support clinical decisions, little work has engaged directly with both concepts to identify areas of similarity or overlap. With these historically siloed areas of work, important questions have remained underaddressed. Here, we propose to delve into the potential relationships between EBP and clinical reasoning. We will engage with the conceptual arguments that one is a precursor, component, or vehicle for the other. The purpose of this chapter is not to provide a 'right' answer to these questions but, rather, to explore these distinctions. In this chapter, we will summarize appropriate frameworks or theories relevant to the relationship between EBP and clinical reasoning, to consider potential unintended consequences of adopting a specific stance about their relationship, to discuss how these different interplays between EBP and clinical reasoning might manifest in clinical practice and to identify areas rich for future research.

The chapter is organized in three sections, each representing a different stance regarding the relationship between clinical reasoning and EBP. Within each section, we pose a series of questions for reflection. The first section explores *EBP as a contributor to the process of clinical reasoning*. Drawing from the literature on the theoretical and philosophical tenets of EBP, we present circumstances in which EBP could be considered a contributor to the overarching process of clinical reasoning and potential downstream consequences of this conceptualization. Then we discuss implications for healthcare professionals who may be situated within

this perspective and present unanswered questions for reflection and future research.

In the second section, we explore the premise that *EBP is the way in which clinical reasoning unfolds – or should unfold*. In this section, we draw primarily from the clinical reasoning literature to highlight how this relationship may or may not hold true depending on the chosen theoretical perspective informing clinical reasoning. We conclude the section with potential downstream consequences, implications for practitioners and future areas for research.

The final section considers the proposition that *EBP and clinical reasoning are different words/frames for the 'same thing'*. We begin this section by presenting the multiple possible conceptualizations of evidence and propose that 'evidence' is more than knowledge generated through empirical research. As with the first two sections, we explore potential downstream consequences of this approach and what this may mean for a practicing health professional with a focus on issues of professional autonomy and discuss avenues for future research.

SECTION 1: EVIDENCE-BASED PRACTICE IS A CONTRIBUTOR TO CLINICAL REASONING

Clinical reasoning has been proposed to encompass all cognitive and environmental factors that lead to, support and shape a final decision – whether about a diagnosis or treatment plan (Durning et al., 2013). If clinical reasoning reflects an overarching set of approaches or processes that are a 'means to an end', then it stands to reason that EBP could be considered within the 'laundry list' of approaches or processes that lead to, support or shape a final clinical decision. As mentioned in the introduction to this chapter, there is an abundance of literature that converges on the notion that EBP is an approach to clinical decision making. It is considered an approach, not the only approach (Haynes, 2002). Whether one is referring to Sackett's earlier definition of EBP (Sackett et al., 1996) or to the one represented in a recently revised transdisciplinary model by Banningan and Moores (2009), EBP emphasizes the interaction of three main factors: the best available evidence, input from the patient regarding his or her care and the clinician's experience and professional expertise (Craik and Rappolt, 2003; Thomas and Law,

2013). Fig. 13.1 is a traditional representation of EBP, and in this Venn diagram, the clinical decision making lies in the middle – it is a result of the contribution of, and the interactions between, its three main components. There is no implied weight or size associated with each component, leaving one to presume that a clinical decision is the result of equal interdependent contributions from each of the three components. Though this equitable balance of sources of information may be the case in some clinical situations, there is a paucity of research to substantiate such an interpretation.

REFLECTION POINT 2

How does this interpretation align with your view of the relationship between EBP and clinical reasoning?

The notion of balancing multiple sources of information (Yousefi-Nooraie et al., 2007) puts the onus and focus on the reasoning of the individual clinician. Much of the debate surrounding the EBP movement has been attributed to the implicit value judgement that an evidence-based approach to any clinical decision is only as good as the clinician who is responsible for balancing the multiple sources of evidence – of evaluating the available scientific evidence, considering it in light of the patient's personal and unique circumstances and balancing the unique expertise of the clinician.

Haynes et al. (2002) suggested that 'evidence does not make decisions, people do'. If one accepts this premise, then it follows that most, if not all, clinicians who find themselves in a situation of having to deliberately and consciously combine formal research evidence, patient preferences and a knowledge base derived from their own experience are engaging in a particular form of clinical reasoning. The use of and reliance on information are predominantly for the end goal of making a clinical decision.

Combining various sources of data, making sense of the evidence and considering the patient's unique situation and goals for treatment would require that the clinician engage in clinical reasoning. In the absence of a reasoning process, it would seem reasonable to suggest that the various knowledge sources are discrete pieces of information without a unifying purpose and with limited meaning. If one accepts that clinical reasoning is a large collection of approaches and strategies used to reach a clinical decision, then it follows that

EBP represents one approach to reaching that decision and is one strategy among other strategies or approaches such as, for example, nonanalytic reasoning (Kulatunga-Moruzi et al., 2001), reliance on heuristics (Kahneman, 2011), mobilization of illness scripts (Charlin et al., 2007) and reflective practice (Kinsella, 2007).

Studies of experienced clinicians in rehabilitation contexts who embrace and apply EBP have shown that the patient is at the centre of all decisions (Craik and Rappolt, 2006; McCluskey et al., 2008; Thomas and Law, 2013; Thomas et al., 2012). Although the available scientific evidence is used to inform assessment choices and treatment interventions, findings from these studies suggest that the reasoning involved in the decision-making process is largely influenced by a deep desire and motivation to improve patient outcomes (Thomas et al., 2012). The scientific evidence in these circumstances is one 'tool' in a clinician's repertoire. If EBP is one approach to clinical reasoning, and formal scientific evidence is one component of that process, it follows that other component 'pieces' such as clinical experience, patients' wishes, organizational mandates and professional culture are likewise significant and valued contributors to the reasoning process. In this conceptualization of evidence as a contributor, these components are equally valued, recognized and rewarded.

If we adopt the view the EBP is one among many means by which to reach a clinical decision, then several downstream consequences may become apparent (Box 13.1).

REFLECTION POINT 3

What would happen to the role of the medical scholar described in the CanMeds framework (Frank et al., 2015, p. 24) as 'physicians who demonstrate a lifelong commitment to excellence in practice through continuous learning and by teaching others, evaluating evidence, and contributing to scholarship' or the medical expert described 'as a physician who provides high-quality, safe, patient-centred care, physicians draw upon an evolving body of knowledge, their clinical skills, and their professional values' given this perspective?

Similarly, in another health profession – occupational therapy – the scholarly practitioners are defined as individuals who 'bases their work on the best evidence from research, best practices, and

BOX 13.1

DOWNSTREAM CONSEQUENCES OF THE VIEW THAT EBP IS A CONTRIBUTOR TO THE PROCESS OF CLINICAL REASONING

- EBP is one among many, not 'first among equals'. Therefore it isn't the 'best' way of reasoning, only one of many approaches to reasoning.
- If EBP isn't 'the best kind' of reasoning, but rather only one kind of reasoning, how do we decide what the 'best' way to treat someone is? How do we develop decision algorithms or practice guidelines for best practice if EBP is just 'one way' of reasoning?
- EBP may undervalue 'evidence' that is not generated through empirical research. If EBP is only one potential approach to reasoning, what would the downstream consequences be for health professions education?
- The perspective that EBP is one contributor, or potential approach to clinical reasoning, may be both empowering and validating for clinicians. It supports the notion that there is a multiplicity of information and knowledge sources, factors that influence the reasoning process and different 'means to an end'. This perspective allows

for recognition of the value of professional experience and clinicians' ability to make thoughtful decisions, some informed by best available scientific evidence, others not. Further, this perspective aligns well with what it means to be a healthcare professional. Healthcare professionals have the autonomy to exercise judgement about how they make decisions (Cruess and Cruess, 2008), what information sources they draw from to come to those decisions and under what circumstances they will resort to scientific evidence to support a clinical decision.

- Finally, this perspective suggests that complex health issues experienced by human beings with unique backgrounds and lived experiences cannot ultimately be reduced to problems that can and must be solved with the application of the best available scientific evidence.

---

experiential knowledge. Practitioners evaluate the effectiveness, efficiency, and cost-effectiveness of client services and programs. Occupational therapists engage in a lifelong pursuit to continuously maintain and build personal expertise. A commitment is demonstrated to facilitate learning and contribute to the creation, dissemination, application, and translation of knowledge' (Canadian Association of Occupational Therapists, 2012, p. 3).

If we accept that EBP is one way, not the way, of engaging in clinical reasoning, how do we simultaneously encourage and promote the development of the scholarly practitioner?

Areas for Future Research

Accepting that EBP *is as a contributor to the process of clinical reasoning*, we are left with questions that we hope will stimulate discussion among our colleagues in the scholarly and clinical communities and present these as suggestion of areas for future research.

1. If EBP is one among many strategies, we need to better understand how evidence is used and/or mobilized during the decision-making process. It is possible that the process of evoking the evidentiary base for a clinical decision has become

automatic. If so, a clinician would not necessarily be engaging in the traditional evidence-based approach to practice with its corresponding five steps. In other words, EBP would not manifest as typically represented in the EBP literature. Is the practitioner still engaging in EBP? Or is he or she engaging in nonanalytic reasoning? What are the implications for education and continuing profession development – both in terms of process and practice change?

2. If we consider that 'using evidence' can be done automatically, this may necessitate some conceptual reframing of the traditional understanding of EBP and the coordination with other clinical reasoning concepts such as nonanalytic reasoning.

3. What is the relative contribution of the scientific evidence to clinical reasoning, regardless of nomenclature? Some work has suggested the role of basic science in reasoning through novel problems (Woods et al., 2006); however, little is known regarding the extent to which clinicians evoke the evidence in a conscious or a more automatized process during decision making. In what kind of clinical situations would conscious reliance on scientific evidence be most effective? How should this be communicated to learners

and novice clinicians who, for the most part, have been trained in an era of very formalized and stepwise EBP?

4. Knowledge translation researchers are tasked with bridging research to practice gaps to ensure the most recent relevant evidence is being utilized to make clinical decisions (Graham et al., 2006). If EBP is viewed as a contributor or one of many possible approaches or strategies for clinical reasoning, what does this mean for the practice of and research on knowledge translation, which predominantly emphasizes the dissemination and utilization of research evidence?

SECTION 2: EVIDENCE-BASED PRACTICE IS THE WAY IN WHICH CLINICAL REASONING UNFOLDS OR SHOULD UNFOLD

The assumption underlying this conceptualization is that EBP is how clinical reasoning is manifested. It suggests that clinical reasoning takes the form of EBP, and as such, clinical reasoning is, and becomes a part of, clinicians' decision-making process. This conceptualization also assumes that all clinical decisions are, or ought to be, based on evidence. Thus 'evidence' of good clinical reasoning is through the 'doing' of EBP. In this case if one accepts that EBP leads to better patient care

and improves transparency, accountability and value, as has been suggested in the literature (Emparanza et al., 2015), then EBP is the way we 'should' make decisions about clinical care. Consequently, if clinical reasoning is 'best' manifested as EBP, it shouldn't be 'one of the ways to do it' but rather a 'first among equals' way of reasoning.

Consider three distinct instances of decision making. A physician must order and justify the use of a series of diagnostic tests for acute onset of abdominal pain; a healthcare team must decide if a patient arriving in the emergency department with debilitating headaches needs immediate hospitalization; an occupational therapist considers how to provide psychosocial support for a young mother newly diagnosed with multiple sclerosis who is caring for her 3-month-old infant. Existing scientific evidence has informed the development of care algorithms or contributed to practice guidelines concerning the most appropriate use of health resources. Does the 'stepwise' separation of scientific evidence from practice-based tools such as guidelines automatically divorce the enactment of these decisions from a frame of evidence-based tools? If good clinical reasoning is embodying the spirit (rather than solely the stepwise approach) of EBP, then reliance on guidelines for good practice or care algorithms could be considered a manifestation of EBP. We reflect on this stance in the following case study.

CASE STUDY 13.1

Julie is a physiotherapist working in an inpatient rehabilitation centre specializing in musculoskeletal conditions. She is asked whether Mrs. Jones, her 79-year-old recently widowed patient with a new onset of falls, is a suitable candidate for an outpatient falls-prevention program offered in the community. Knowing that Mrs. Jones lives alone, that she has limited social support and is at risk for recurrent falls, Julie discusses the benefits of the program with Mrs. Jones and suggests that they look into transportation services. In this example, Julie is not formally searching for scientific research and not engaging in the 'stepwise' approach to EBP, nor is she appraising papers for their quality or relevance to Mrs. Jones' situation. She is, however, drawing from her practice knowledge

of the effectiveness of fall-prevention programs to help her in suggesting and promoting the program to her patient. Most importantly, her 'clinical decision' is very much influenced by her in-depth knowledge of the lived experience and situation that her patient finds herself in. She 'knows' that a recently widowed older adult with limited social support may isolate herself by fear of being a burden on her family or putting herself at greater risk for falling by venturing out of her home more often. Yet Mrs. Jones refuses to participate. Her decision to forego the fall-prevention program is further justified given her limited access to transportation services to the community centre where the program is being offered.

This sophisticated and presumably rapid decision-making process rests upon Julie's extensive knowledge base of the effectiveness of fall-prevention interventions for community dwelling seniors, the functional outcomes following falls and injuries and the typical developmental features of the aging process. Could Julie's decision about recommending the fall-prevention program be made without evoking the scientific literature? In other words, could Julie conclude that this would be a beneficial program for her patient without having to go through the full formal EBP stepwise process?

We suggest that it is indeed possible, particularly given the more modern broad definitions of EBP, and we posit that this situation occurs frequently. This scenario suggests that Julie is balancing various sources of knowledge and evidence. She is, therefore,

engaging in EBP and is likely to be demonstrating good clinical reasoning. This reflects the notion that EBP is the way in which clinical reasoning does or should unfold.

What are the possible downstream consequences of this view of EBP (Box 13.2)?

Areas for Future Research

If we accept that *EBP is the way in which clinical reasoning unfolds or should unfold,* we propose the following questions for discussion and future research.

1. If EBP and clinical reasoning are interdependent, efforts should be directed towards merging the areas of compatibility across these two areas. More specifically, if we adhere to the notion that clinical reasoning is best enacted through EBP, then are

---

BOX 13.2

DOWNSTREAM CONSEQUENCES OF THE VIEW THAT EBP IS THE WAY IN WHICH CLINICAL REASONING UNFOLDS OR SHOULD UNFOLD

- If EBP is the means by which clinical reasoning should unfold, what happens to the construct of clinical reasoning in the absence of a concrete final decision? Does clinical reasoning need the decision-making framework of EBP to 'exist' or to manifest itself? If one answers yes, how do we avoid a potential slippery slope whereby every decision, made under every possible circumstance, for all patients, in all contexts must by definition be made as a result of consulting or evoking the scientific evidence of some kind to be considered the result of 'good' clinical reasoning? This perspective suggests that without a decision being made, or without an evidence base to draw from, there is no evidence of clinical reasoning. Anything that is not EBP is suboptimal or inadequate clinical reasoning. If EBP is manifested in a less than ideal manner, is enacted ineffectively or leads to the wrong decision for a given patient in a given situation and context, then is this evidence of poor clinical reasoning?

- EBP, as defined in the literature and taught in many health professions education programs, is a deliberate, conscious process. If we accept the view that EBP is how clinical reasoning unfolds, then it follows that understanding, valuing and teaching reasoning modes that are not perfectly conscious, structured, reportable and teachable become challenging at best and likely become devalued as reasoning processes.

- If we accept a broad definition of EBP in which scientific evidence, experiential knowledge and patient preferences are valued, the assumed necessary reasoning processes include the collection of 'evidence', the interpretation of that evidence and the balancing of that evidence across the three components of Fig. 13.1. If this is the interpretation of EBP being adopted, we assume that the framework of EBP is how reasoning 'should' unfold, then applying an EBP frame to the study of clinical reasoning may actually provide a more concrete structure through which to study the relatively nebulous concept of clinical reasoning.

- Finally, one could speculate that a consequence of disregarding contributors other than EBP approaches to clinical reasoning could result in devaluing professional expertise, which in turn can lead to professional dissatisfaction and clinician resentment towards efforts aimed at promoting EBP. Indeed, there are many lessons learned from earlier studies exploring attitudes towards EBP. Earlier studies showed clinicians' less than favourable perceptions of and attitudes towards EBP were in part a result of an overemphasis on scientific evidence to the detriment of professional experience and expertise and the role that clinical reasoning plays in decision making (Dubouloz et al., 1999).

there particular conceptualizations of clinical reasoning (Young et al., in press) that are more amenable to the valuing of evidence and the consideration for EBP as a means to enact clinical reasoning? If such a conceptualization does not exist, could the health professions education community benefit from multidisciplinary efforts towards developing one?

2. If we agree that without EBP there is no clinical reasoning, how do we avoid the potential negative effect on the autonomy and professional experience of clinicians and/or their profession? If clinical reasoning is a careful balancing of the evidentiary sources in Fig. 13.1, would it be possible to consider the de-professionalization or atomization of clinical practice? How would this view affect the many other roles expected of a healthcare practitioner such as effective communication or advocacy or the dynamic adapting of a management plan in situation such as when a clinician is attending to a patient's distress or fear? Or when a clinician is interacting with individuals experiencing life-altering health challenges? Moments and interactions that strengthen the therapeutic relationship could be said to allow for a deeper connection if for no other reason than to create a strong therapeutic bond. Are we losing a part of what it means to be a healthcare professional? These are building blocks for many successful clinician–patient interactions. And what if this view succeeds in alienating clinicians by undervaluing clinical decisions that are meant to deepen the therapeutic bond?

3. If EBP is how clinical reasoning unfolds, do we need to understand 'the balancing' of different sources of (potentially conflicting) evidence? If this is how clinicians 'should' reason, should we try to understand EBP as an overarching process or frame for clinical reasoning?

4. If EBP is the larger or overarching concept, does this mean that it loses some of its precision inherent in some of the earlier models of a deliberate stepwise structure? As an overarching concept it becomes more flexible, allowing for latitude and what it attempts to achieve. However, does it also deserve more attention regarding its potential complexity?

REFLECTION POINT 4

How does this interpretation match your view of the relationship between EBP and clinical reasoning?

SECTION 3: EVIDENCE-BASED PRACTICE AND CLINICAL REASONING ARE DIFFERENT WORDS/FRAMES FOR THE 'SAME THING'

Are EBP and clinical reasoning different sides of the same coin? In this last stance regarding the relationship between the two processes, we propose that both clinical reasoning and EBP are approaches to clinical decision making representing means to arriving at a clinical decision. EBP combines evidence, patients' input and clinician experience, suggesting that these are, as mentioned earlier, interacting with the purpose of making a final decision.

Clinical reasoning, though a fragmented literature, has also been discussed as a means to an end, a process used to establish a diagnosis to decide on and implement the best possible course of action (Eva, 2005). Although clinical reasoning has been informed by a variety of theories, stances and perspectives, a common theme among these approaches has been the notion that clinical reasoning produces diagnoses, management plans or investigative plans – that it ends in a decision (Durning et al., 2013; Eva, 2005; Young et al., in press). Viewed in this way, clinical reasoning and EBP are both processes or approaches used to come to a decision, whether that decision is about a diagnostic test, a discharge date, admitting a patient to hospital or assessing an older adult's competence to care for himself or herself. Though the components or nature of these processes is not trivial or inconsequential given that they likely contribute to the end goal (i.e., clinical decisions), they may take a 'backseat' to the actual decision.

Alternately, clinical reasoning and EBP could be two different families of approaches to the study of how clinical decisions are made – with different areas of focus, importance and value stances as to what are important contributors to the process of generating a clinical decision and shaping the research within each field. Clinical reasoning and EBP have emerged from different disciplinary areas; clinical reasoning emerged primarily from cognitive science and psychology and

> **BOX 13.3**
>
> **DOWNSTREAM CONSEQUENCES OF THE VIEW THAT EBP AND CLINICAL REASONING ARE DIFFERENT WORDS/FRAMES FOR THE 'SAME THING'**
>
> ▪ Accepting this view suggests that the component processes are less important than the quality of the eventual outcome – as long as a decision is made, how the individual 'got there' is not as important. We propose that this has potentially precarious implications for teaching and assessment, particularly given the increasing attention to assessing process of learning and outcomes (Bransford et al., 2000; National Research Council, 2001).
> ▪ If EBP and clinical reasoning are indeed two different sides of the same coin but remain largely in different research silos, we are not advancing the knowledge base nor well situated to move our field(s) forward. We may actually be failing to clarify concepts that may reflect only linguistic differences rather than conceptual ones.

EBP from epidemiology, and as such, may have concretized different areas of focus or importance for the same set of processes. Although this interpretation remains speculative, and likely contentious, it is an area for future research. Consider the downstream consequences of this view (Box 13.3).

REFLECTION POINT 5

How does this interpretation match your view of the relationship between EBP and clinical reasoning?

Areas for Future Research

If we agree that *EBP and clinical reasoning are different words/frames for the 'same thing'*, we propose the following questions for reflection and discussion.

1. We propose that the research community should find areas of overlap, similarity and differences across these bodies of work to deepen our understanding of these key principles.
2. What main messages do we want to send to educators and scholars who teach, assess and study decision making in and out of the classroom?
3. If EBP and clinical reasoning are a set of processes, what cues would be available to us to see

'high-quality reasoning or decision making' whether labelled as clinical reasoning or EBP?
4. How can we best design teaching, assessment and continuing professional development activities to align with, and to promote EBP and clinical reasoning?

CHAPTER SUMMARY

This chapter presents three different stances regarding the relationship between clinical reasoning and EBP. We have deliberately not chosen to privilege one of these views. Rather, we have presented them critically, considering practice, education and research implications. We invite you to reflect on your own stance to the relationship, areas of overlap and areas of differentiation between these two concepts.

REFLECTION POINT 6

Do the arguments presented in this chapter reflect your current stance on the relationship between EBP and clinical reasoning? Do they prompt you to consider a new stance? What implications arising from this discussion might lead you to make a change in your practice?

REFERENCES

Banningan, K., Moores, A., 2009. A model of professional thinking: integrating reflective practice and evidence based practice. Can. J. Occup. Ther. 76, 342–350.

Bennett, S., Bennett, J.W., 2000. The process of evidence-based practice in occupational therapy: informing clinical decisions. Aust. Occup. Ther. J. 47, 171–180.

Bennett, S., Tooth, L., McKenna, K., et al., 2003. Perceptions of evidence based practice: a survey of occupational therapists. Aust. Occup. Ther. J. 50, 13–22.

Bransford, J.D., Brown, A., Cocking, R., 2000. How People Learn: Brain, Mind, Experience, and School. National Academies Press, Washington, DC.

Canadian Association of Occupational Therapists, 2012. Profile of practice of occupational therapists in Canada 2012. Viewed 1 June 2017. Available from: https://www.caot.ca/document/3653/2012otprofile.pdf.

Charlin, B., Boshuizen, H.P., Custers, E.J., et al., 2007. Scripts and clinical reasoning. Med. Educ. 41, 1178–1184.

Craik, J., Rappolt, S., 2003. Theory of research utilization enhancement: a model for occupational therapy. Can. J. Occup. Ther. 70, 266–275.

Craik, J., Rappolt, S., 2006. Enhancing research utilization capacity through multifaceted professional development. Am. J. Occup. Ther. 60, 155–164.

Cruess, R.L., Cruess, S.R., 2008. Expectations and obligations: professionalism and medicine's social contract with society. Perspect. Biol. Med. 51, 579–598.

Dijkers, M.P., Murphy, S.L., Krellman, J., 2012. Evidence-based practice for rehabilitation professionals: concepts and controversies. Arch. Phys. Med. Rehabil. 93 (Suppl. 8), S164–S176.

Djulbegovic, B., Guyatt, G., Ashcroft, R., 2009. Epistemologic inquiries in evidence-based medicine. Cancer Control 16, 158–168.

Dubouloz, C.J., Egan, M., Vallerand, J., et al., 1999. Occupational therapists' perceptions of evidence-based practice. Am. J. Occup. Ther. 53, 445–453.

Durning, S.J., Artino, A.R., Jr., Schuwirth, L., et al., 2013. Clarifying assumptions to enhance our understanding and assessment of clinical reasoning. Acad. Med. 88, 442–448.

Emparanza, J.I., Cabello, J.B., Burls, A.J., 2015. Does evidence-based practice improve patient outcomes? An analysis of a natural experiment in a Spanish hospital. J. Eval. Clin. Pract. 21, 1059–1065.

Eva, K.W., 2005. What every teacher needs to know about clinical reasoning. Med. Educ. 39, 98–106.

Frank, J., Snell, L., Sherbino, J., 2015. CanMEDS 2015 Physician Competency Framework. Royal College of Physicians and Surgeons of Canada, Ottawa.

Graham, I.D., Logan, J., Harrison, M.B., et al., 2006. Lost in knowledge translation: time for a map? J. Contin. Educ. Health Prof. 26, 13–24.

Greenhalgh, T., Snow, R., Ryan, S., et al., 2015. Six 'biases' against patients and carers in evidence-based medicine. BMC Med. 13, 200.

Hammell, K.W., 2001. Using qualitative research to inform the client-centered evidence-based practice of occupational therapy. Br. J. Occup. Ther. 64, 228–234.

Haynes, R.B., 2002. What kind of evidence is it that evidence-based medicine advocates want health care providers and consumers to pay attention to? BMC Health Serv. Res. 2, doi:10.1186/1472-6963-2-3.

Haynes, R.B., Devereaux, P.J., Guyatt, G.H., 2002. Clinical expertise in the era of evidence-based medicine and patient choice. ACP J. Club 136, A11–A14.

Higgs, J., Jones, M., Loftus, S., et al. (Eds.), 2008. Clinical Reasoning in the Health Professions, third ed. Elsevier, Edinburgh.

Kahneman, D., 2011. Thinking, Fast and Slow. Doubleday, Toronto, Canada.

Kinsella, E.A., 2007. Embodied reflection and the epistemology of reflective practice. J. Philos. Educ. 41, 395–409.

Kulatunga-Moruzi, C., Brooks, L.R., Norman, G.R., 2001. Coordination of analytic and similarity-based processing strategies and expertise in dermatological diagnosis. Teach. Learn. Med. 13, 110–116.

Mattingly, C., 1991. What is clinical reasoning? Am. J. Occup. Ther. 45, 979–986.

McCluskey, A., Home, S., Thompson, L., 2008. Becoming an evidence-based practitioner. In: Law, M., MacDermid, J. (Eds.), Evidence-Based Rehabilitation: A Guide to Practice, second ed. Slack, Thorofare, NJ, p. 35.

National Research Council, 2001. Implications of the new foundations for assessment design. In: Pellegrino, J.W., Chudowsky, N.Glaser, R. (Eds.), Knowing What Students Know: The Science and Design of Educational Assessment. National Academies Press, Washington, DC, pp. 176–219.

Sackett, D.L., Rosenberg, W.M., Gray, J.A., et al., 1996. Evidence based medicine: what it is and what it isn't. BMJ 312, 71–72.

Sackett, D.L., Straus, S.E., Richardson, W.S., et al., 2000. Evidence-Based Medicine: How to Practice and Teach EBM, second ed. Churchill Livingstone, Edinburgh.

Salmond, S.W., 2013. Finding the evidence to support evidence-based practice. Orthop. Nurs. 32, 16–22.

Schell, B.A.B., 2009. Professional reasoning in practice. In: Crepeau, E.B., Cohn, E.S., Schell, B.A.B. (Eds.), Willard and Spackman's Occupational Therapy, tenth ed. Lippincott Williams & Wilkins, Philadelphia, PA, pp. 314–327.

Thomas, A., Law, M., 2013a. Research utilization and evidence-based practice in occupational therapy: a scoping study. Am. J. Occup. Ther. 67, e55–e65.

Thomas, A., Saroyan, A., Lajoie, S.P., 2012. Creation of an evidence-based practice reference model in falls prevention: findings from occupational therapy. Disabil. Rehabil. 34, 311–328.

Woods, N.N., Neville, A.J., Levinson, A.J., et al., 2006. The value of basic science in clinical diagnosis. Acad. Med. 81, 124–127.

Wyer, P.C., Silva, S.A., 2009. Where is the wisdom? A conceptual history of evidence-based medicine. J. Eval. Clin. Pract. 15, 891–898.

Young, M., Dory, V., Lubarsky, S., et al., in press. How different theories of clinical reasoning influence teaching and assessment. Acad. Med.

Yousefi-Nooraie, R., Shakiba, B., Mortaz-Hedjri, S., et al., 2007. Sources of knowledge in clinical practice in postgraduate medical students and faculty members: a conceptual map. J. Eval. Clin. Pract. 13, 564–568.

14

METHODS IN THE STUDY OF CLINICAL REASONING

JOSE F. AROCHA ▪ VIMLA L. PATEL

CHAPTER AIMS

This chapter aims to:

▪ provide a description of the most used methods for the investigation and assessment of clinical reasoning,

▪ classify such methods in terms of their nature and unit of analysis and

▪ show how the methods can be of utility for the study of clinical reasoning.

KEY WORDS

Clinical reasoning (CR)

Thinking

Quantitative methods

Qualitative methods

INTRODUCTION

Methods for the study of clinical reasoning are often selected based on the philosophical outlook considered by the researcher. Philosophically, quantitative methods are said to be characteristic of a positivist methodological approach to research, which posits the essentiality of quantifiable behaviour in the conduct of scientific research. In turn, qualitative methods are often based on a philosophy that proposes the constructive nature of human thought and action. Despite the difference in outlook, there has been a recent push to investigate thinking within a framework that forgoes to some extent the philosophical chasm between quantitative and

qualitative research, while adopting a more pragmatic approach to research. From our view, this situation has positively affected the study of clinical reasoning. Indeed, its study in the fields of health has positively changed in recent years. Some of the major changes are the following:

First, some theories, notably dual-process theory (Croskerry, 2009), have become widely used to guide research studies and to explain cognitive processes, such as problem solving and reasoning. Second, new and not so new methodologies have been introduced and applied to the investigation of such processes, which promise to better elucidate what goes on when a clinician interprets a patient problem. Third, the traditional and clearly delineated distinction between quantitative and qualitative research methods has become fuzzy (Haig, 2013), as new research increasingly makes use of both approaches in clinical reasoning investigations (e.g., Rice et al., 2014). Fourth, although in previous years the study of clinical reasoning was mostly focussed on medical tasks, there has been increasing research in other health fields, such as occupational therapy (Cramm et al., 2013), physiotherapy (Langridge et al., 2015) and nursing (Stec, 2016).

Methods of investigation of clinical reasoning can be grouped into those that look at outcomes to hypothesize the underlying cognitive processes and those that explore the processes of reasoning themselves. We found it useful to classify methodologies as quantitative or qualitative to the extent to which they generate numerical or verbal/gestural data. Also, some can be aggregated into statistics, while others are less suitable for aggregation. Specific studies can, of course, vary and use quantitative methods to identify average differences between groups together with qualitative methods to characterize individual performance (Patel et al., 2001). This chapter is devoted to the study of clinical reasoning as an individual process, leaving out methods designed to capture clinical reasoning as it occurs in teams or work groups (e.g., Patel et al., 2013).

QUANTITATIVE METHODS

Quantitative methodologies for investigating clinical reasoning have been used in various clinical problems. One of them is the study of diagnosis in perceptual tasks, such as x-ray or dermatological image interpretation (Jaarsma et al., 2015; Norman et al., 1992), where study participants are shown a series of slides after which they are asked to interpret or recall the information of the visual material. A goal of this research is to show how variations in the participants' performance (e.g., assessed through verbal recall) relate to variations on the experimental conditions (e.g., types of stimuli). These data are then quantified, using descriptive statistics and subjected to standard statistical analysis (e.g., null-hypothesis testing). These methods have also been employed to compare clinical performance by groups with different levels of expertise (Norman et al., 2007). The study of group differences serves to estimate population parameters. However, quantitative methods can also be used for investigating individuals (Runkel, 1990), although unfortunately little use has been made of such methods for this purpose. Next, we cover specific quantitative techniques recently applied to the study of clinical reasoning.

The Script Concordance Test

The Script Concordance (SC) test has gained considerable attention in recent years (Charlin et al., 2007). The test, theoretically based on script theory (Schmidt and Rikers, 2007), poses that clinicians develop increasingly coherent knowledge structures, called scripts, as their experience increases from students to seasoned practitioners (Schmidt and Rikers, 2007). The test is also informed by dual-process theory. As clinicians' expertise increases in a given health field, they also develop two distinct thinking processes: 'analytical', which is slow, effortful and more characteristic of novices and 'nonanalytical', which is fast, subconscious and more characteristic of experts.

The SC test (Charlin et al., 2000; Lubarsky et al., 2013) is a psychometrically validated written instrument particularly designed to assess clinical reasoning. The test is normally developed with the help of a group of experts, who generate vignettes describing clinical cases and provide interpretations of the cases. The vignettes should allow for different interpretations to reflect the various expert judgements and should not assume a single correct answer but alternative interpretations based on the response variations found among the experts who developed the vignettes. The interpretation selected by most experts is taken to be the 'best' answer, although other responses are also considered to be reasonable. After a case is introduced, a series of questions with several hypotheses below are presented. The questions are of the form 'If you were thinking of [e.g., diagnosis, investigation, treatment] and then you find a new [sign or symptom], your diagnosis becomes more or less likely [selected on a scale ranging from −2 to +2]?'. By presenting the case in partial form, adding new information at a time and asking whether the selected hypothesis becomes more or less likely, the test can capture parts of the reasoning process. The SC test has been applied successfully in several health settings (e.g., Carrière et al., 2009; Kazour et al., 2017). Its relative ease makes the SC test an appealing way of studying clinical thinking. Computerized or online forms of the test are likely to make it even easier (Sibert et al., 2002). However, researchers should be aware of some validity and reliability concerns with the standard application and interpretation of SC test results (Lineberry et al., 2013).

The Repertory Grid Technique

The repertory grid technique was developed by George Kelly (1991) to elicit and examine the personal constructs (e.g., personal beliefs) people use when interpreting a problem or situation. The theory posits that people interpret the world around them much like a scientist, generating hypotheses to understand and predict events. Kelly viewed personal constructs as existing along a bipolar dimension, where one construct was conceived in relation to its opposite, for instance, viewing a problem along the dimension of 'easy' versus 'difficult'. Thus one assumption is that people's personal constructs can be elicited by placing them at some distance between two poles of the dimension. A benefit of the repertory grid is that it can be quantified and statistically analyzed at the individual level.

The method has been applied to the study of clinical reasoning (Kuipers and Grice, 2009a, 2009b). Kuipers and Grice (2009a) illustrate the use of the technique by analyzing an interview with an expert occupational therapist. The expert's constructs were elicited from a vignette describing a patient suffering from a neurological problem and a question, called 'element', (e.g., 'what is the first thing you attend to when you see the client?'), which prompted the expert to generate a series of personalized questions regarding a therapy session. These 'elements' were then used to assist the expert in eliciting the polar constructs along which each element was situated within a numbered grid (Box 14.1). For instance, the expert in the study judged the element mentioned earlier to exist between 'assess functional issues' and its polar opposite 'reason and determine action' by numbering the element along a scale, e.g., with 5, if closest to the emerging construct and 1, if closest to the opposite construct (Kuipers and Grice, 2009a, pp. 280–281).

The method provided both qualitative data (from the interview) and quantitative data (from completing the grid). By applying a statistical method for finding clusters along dimensions in the data, called principal component analysis (PCA), it was possible to identify two components, labelled 'therapist role' and 'practice scope', which accounted for 83% of the variance in the expert's responses. Another study (Kuipers and Grice, 2009b) expanded the use of the repertory grid interview to explore differences between novice and expert occupational therapists before and after introducing a protocol designed to guide the process of clinical reasoning in cases of 'upper limb hypertonia'. The research

showed differences between the groups: the novices' reasoning significantly changed their approach to be consistent with the protocol, while experts did not. Although the repertory grid technique has not been extensively used, it is a promising theoretically based method for the study of clinical reasoning. A basic introduction to the use of repertory grid can be found in Pollock (1986).

Neuro-Imaging Methods

Recently researchers have looked at clinical reasoning processes using neuro-imaging methods (Chang et al., 2016; Durning et al., 2012, 2013b, 2016). The major aim of this kind of research is to uncover the brain structures that underlie the processes of reasoning and thinking. Basically, the method consists of carrying out one or more reasoning tasks while the study participant is in the functional magnetic resonance imaging (fMRI) scanner. The method has been applied to identify the neural structures involved in analytic and nonanalytic reasoning (Durning et al., 2015); memory structure and flexibility in thinking and the differences between experts and novices (Durning et al., 2016); the differences involved in answering questions versus thinking 'aloud' (Durning et al., 2013a); and clinical problem solving and recall by medical students (Chang et al., 2016).

REFLECTION POINT 1

Some scientists and philosophers maintain that the key to understanding human reasoning is by uncovering the neural processes underlying thinking, and others maintain that many different approaches are needed to understand reasoning.

Multiple-choice questions (e.g., items from the US medical licensing examination) are often used during the scanning process, although concurrent and retrospective protocols also have been employed (Durning et al., 2016). In a typical study, Durning et al. (2015) made use of dual-process theory as an explanatory framework and fMRI to investigate nonanalytic reasoning and thinking efficiency of internal medicine interns (novices) and board-certified internists (experts). The method used involved presenting a series of timed multiple-choice questions (e.g., 60 seconds for reading and 7 seconds for answering) to the participants, which they had to answer by pressing a button while they

---

BOX 14.1
SCRIPT CONCORDANCE

Although the Script Concordance test is an outcome measure, the partial presentation of data allows a reasonable representation of the reasoning process. The repertory grid is based on the idea that people generate personal constructs as scientists generate hypotheses to interpret the world.

were in the scanner. After providing the responses, the participants were allowed some time to reflect on their answers, which was done to assess analytic reasoning. The results showed that although sharing a great deal of neural activation (e.g., in brain areas responsible for pattern recognition), novice and expert physicians also demonstrated some differences in the brain areas involved and in reasoning efficiency. Although the results of fMRI may be sometimes difficult to interpret, the method shows encouraging applicability to the study of clinical reasoning in controlled situations (Box 14.2).

Eye Tracking

Eye-tracking technology has become more available, less intrusive, smaller and simpler to use. A benefit of eye-tracking technology is that it precisely measures gaze behaviour (e.g., number, location and duration of eye fixations) providing evidence of the information that the clinician can focus attention on. Today's eye-tracking technology consists of nonintrusive small cameras that capture infrared light reflected on the cornea. Several eye-tracking studies have been recently conducted to investigate clinical reasoning (Blondon et al., 2015), where the method has been combined with concurrent or retrospective verbal protocols. The vast majority of the studies to date have been conducted in visual domains, such as radiology (Krupinski, 2010),

to identify the location of lesions or in the utilization of information technology (Tourassi et al., 2013). A review of the literature by Blondon et al. (2015) identified 10 studies that in various degrees can shed light on the process of clinical thinking. In one study, Tourassi et al. (2013) investigated the diagnostic accuracy in the processing of mammographies within a novice-expert paradigm. They showed that decision making in diagnostic accuracy could be predicted by the patterns of gaze behaviour, which suggests that eye-tracking may be a valid indicator of clinical reasoning.

QUALITATIVE METHODS

Verbal Protocols

The methods described in this section vary widely in terms of their origins and applications and cover concurrent (Fonteyn et al., 1993; Lundgrén-Laine and Salanterä, 2010) and retrospective (Elstein, 2009; Elstein et al., 1978) protocols. The more commonly used methods are the think-aloud and the explanation protocols. The first originates in the study of problem solving and computer simulation of thought (Elstein et al., 1978; Simon, 1993); the second originates in the analysis of text comprehension (Kintsch, 1998). In both cases, the researcher uses verbalizations as data, without involving introspection. That is, research participants are asked to verbalize their thoughts without 'theorizing' about their thinking. Examples of verbal report analyses can be found in Ericsson and Simon (1992) and Arocha et al. (2005).

Think-Aloud Protocol and Analysis

Think-aloud is still an extensively used technique for the study of clinical reasoning (Lee et al., 2016; Lundgrén-Laine and Salanterä, 2010). This is not surprising given the difficulties of investigating cognitive processes

---

BOX 14.2
CR MEASURES

Clinical reasoning can be investigated with outcome and process measures. Using more than one kind of measure ensures a more complete description of clinical reasoning. Diverse measures involving biological, behavioural and cognitive have been developed.

CASE STUDY 14.1

Investigation of Reasoning Strategies

A researcher is interested in assessing physiotherapy students' clinical reasoning skills. She knows that there are several methods of doing this because she is familiar with outcome-based performance measures, but she would like to understand the different

strategies that students use to arrive at the solution of a patient problem. If the physiotherapist aims at capturing the actual process of reasoning, what quantitative method is the most useful to meeting his or her aims?

without making use of verbal data. As in many other methods, think-aloud protocols are based on a theory, in this case, the information processing model of Newell and Simon (1972). The method, to be applied successfully, needs a period of training before it can be used to collect data and requires study participants to follow some stringent criteria. The criteria pertain to the type of task that should be used, the kinds of instruction given to study participants and their familiarity with the task. Although criticisms have been raised against the method, e.g., the potential effect of the verbalization itself on the thought processes, it has been found to produce a reasonable description of the underlying thinking process (e.g., Durning et al., 2013b).

In typical think-aloud research, clinicians are presented with a patient problem, frequently in written vignettes. A vignette may contain anything from a single sentence to a whole patient record including the clinical interview, the physical examination results and the laboratory results. The clinician is asked to read the information and verbalize whatever thoughts come to mind. If he or she pauses for a few seconds, the experimenter intervenes with questions such as 'What are you thinking about?' or, more appropriately, with demands such as 'Please, continue', which encourages the clinician to carry on talking without introspecting. A detailed and lengthy description is provided by Ericsson and Simon (1992), although shorter introductions have been published (e.g., Lundgrén-Laine and Salanterä, 2010).

Once the protocol has been collected, it is subjected to an analysis aimed at uncovering the cognitive processes and the information that were used. The analysis of the protocol is then compared with a reference or domain model of the task to be solved. This model is frequently taken either from an expert collaborator in the study or from printed information about the topic, such as textbooks or scholarly expositions. For instance, in an earlier paper, Kuipers and Kassirer (1984) used a model of the Starling equilibrium mechanism, which was compared with the clinician's protocol. Patel et al. (Arocha et al., 2005; Patel et al., 1994) also used a reference model of the clinical problem generated by exceptional practitioners, which serves as a standard for comparison with the obtained protocol. More recently, researchers in fields other than medicine have proposed (Lundgrén-Laine and Salanterä, 2010) and

used the think-aloud method (Lee et al., 2016). In a recent study (Lee et al., 2016), a group of nurses were given two scenarios describing patients with complex chronic diseases and were prompted to think aloud while interpreting the problem. The protocols were used to develop a detailed model of the nurses' reasoning process. Other researchers have used the think-aloud method in combination with other techniques. For instance, Power et al. (2016) used the method in tandem with the SC test. Also, Durning et al. (2013a) combined its use with fMRI imaging, and Balsev et al. (2012) had clinicians at different levels of expertise think aloud while solving diagnostic problems in paediatric neurology using eye-tracking technology.

Explanation Protocols

Explanation protocols are a form of retrospective protocol in which people are asked to explain a case to the researcher while the person is being audio-recorded. The explanation protocol is based on a number of assumptions (Arocha et al., 2005). First, information, such as a clinical case description, is processed serially. The information generated from a clinical problem passes through working memory first and then is linked later to information in long-term memory, which provides context for interpretation. Second, the temporal sequence in an explanation protocol follows that of the underlying reasoning, in the sense that ideas that are verbalized first are processed first. Third, although the clinical problem may be the same, the reasoning strategies and the final response (e.g., final diagnosis) vary because people process clinical information at several levels of generality, from the very specific symptom level to the general diagnostic level. Research shows that the expertise of the clinician is the critical factor in determining the level of generality at which the clinical case is processed. Finally, both reasoning strategies and inferences used during clinical reasoning are a function of the clinician's domain-specific prior knowledge.

In practice, the explanation protocol method involves asking research participants to explain the pathophysiology of a case. The transcription of the recorded session is analyzed using propositional analysis, which represents the propositional structure of the explanation. Analysis consists of several steps: 1) segment the recorded protocol into clauses; 2) identify the propositions, or

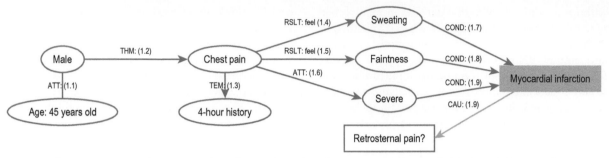

Fig. 14.1 ■ Network representation of propositional analysis generated from a clinician's verbal protocol.

idea unit, in each clause; and 3) connect the propositions to reveal the overall semantics of the protocol. A semantic network can be developed from the list of propositions by representing concepts as nodes and relations as links between nodes. Fig. 14.1 shows a network representation of a propositional analysis generated from a clinician's verbal protocol. The oval nodes indicate patient-presented data, the green box indicates suggested diagnosis and the white box indicates generated hypothetical symptom. The links indicate the direction of reasoning. The links from data to diagnosis refers to data-driven reasoning, and the link (in green) from diagnosis to hypothesis indicates hypothesis-driven reasoning. The text over the links designates semantic markers, e.g., ATT: attribute; CAU: cause; and COND: conditional. The resulting network is a connected conceptual that represents the information used and the process of reasoning the clinician goes through. The method has been used to investigate patterns of explanations in novices and experts (Patel et al., 1994).

Video Data Collection and Analysis

Videotaping and video analysis can be very useful methodological tools for the study of behaviour and cognition. There are various uses of video-based data collection. A video camera can be used to capture the stimulus material, such as patient simulation, and a video monitor can be used to present material to the study participants (Durning et al., 2012). Video can also be used as a data collection tool, where the video camera is positioned externally to the study participant, e.g., for analyzing gestures, or can be used mounted on the participant's head (Pierce, 2005) to analyze the problem from the participant's point of view. It is especially the second use of video data collection that

is more useful to the study of clinical reasoning (Unsworth, 2001b), especially when combined with concurrent or retrospective protocols (Box 14.3).

A benefit of video data is that they can capture the context of reasoning. In fact, one may argue that videotaping and analysis allow for a more complete characterization of cognitive processing, by providing extra nonverbal information, such as gestures, movements and gazes, which complements the information obtained from verbal protocols. Video data are helpful in analyzing tasks designed to externalize someone's thought processes, for instance in physical therapy. In such tasks, both verbalizations and physical actions (e.g., pointing, gazing) can be analyzed in a more complete fashion. Video recording has been used in several health disciplines, such as kinesiology, to conduct computer-based analysis of movements, or speech therapy, to analyze language production problems (Pierce, 2005), among others.

Several studies have been conducted in the health sciences using video recording and analysis (Bailliard, 2015). Roots et al. (2016) investigated osteopaths' clinical reasoning while assessing patients with low back pain. The session was recorded of the interaction between

Choosing Method(s)

A nurse administers a written test to research participants in a study. The nurse could not obtain think-aloud data because of some reasons related to the investigation itself, but the nurse would like to understand the knowledge participants' use during reasoning. Given those aims, what qualitative method among the ones presented is the most suitable to answer the nurse's question?

---

the health practitioner and the patient. After the session finished, the therapist was asked to watch the recording while commenting on the session. This part was audio-recorded for later analysis. Research from the point of view of the study participant has been conducted by Unsworth (2001b). In a study of expert and novice occupational therapists (Unsworth, 2001a), a small camera was strapped around the therapist's head and used to record a typical therapy session with a client. The therapists did not need any time for practice because the head-mounted camera did not disturb their normal work. After the session, the therapists were asked to think aloud while the recording of the session was being shown on a monitor to facilitate recall.

Video data analysis methods vary (Bailliard, 2015), ranging from qualitative to quantitative, the selection of which depends on the theoretical framework used, the objectives of the research and the nature of the data (Derry et al., 2010). Thematic or behavioural analyses exist, both top-down (i.e., categories are generated in advance) or bottom-up (i.e., coding is generated inductively from the data). These analyses can be carried out with the help of video software, which is commercially available.

CONCLUSION

The panorama of current research methods for the study of clinical reasoning has changed a great deal. First, methodological pluralism is now a common occurrence in research studies. Although one may argue that a methodological fragmentation still exists, it is inspiring to see different methods used in single clinical reasoning studies. The distinction between quantitative and qualitative research methods is now less important as researchers make use of think-aloud in tandem with eye fixations, fMRI, video recording, repertory grids and the SC test. This way, data can be collected and analyzed that integrate numerical information with qualitative

descriptions, which facilitates the comprehension of what goes on during clinical reasoning at several levels, from the purely behavioural, to the cognitive, to the neural. Although early research into clinical reasoning was somewhat characterized by methodological isolation, new methods and techniques have become increasingly used to capture different aspects of the same phenomenon. Approaching the study of clinical reasoning from different perspectives and integrating methods in single studies may facilitate a more complete understanding of the underlying processes and the settings where reasoning is deployed. Second, although not covered in this chapter, other major changes have occurred in the way clinical sciences are practiced that may require methodological approaches that permit a fresh look at the processes of reasoning. Clinical reasoning can be considered, in the case of medicine for instance, as thinking through the various aspects of patient care to make a decision about the diagnosis or the therapeutic management of patient problems. This includes history-taking, physical examination, ordering laboratory and ancillary tests and making evidence-based patient management plans.

The increasing amount of research in allied health areas, such as nursing, occupational therapy, social work and physical therapy, has extended the scope of clinical reasoning to a variety of tasks not typically thought within its purview. Furthermore, given the considerable variety of these tasks, clinical reasoning can no longer be considered as a characteristic of the single individual only, as it is being increasingly done by teams and collaborative groups often through technological means, such as the electronic health record and decision support systems. The nature itself of clinical reasoning may need to be reconsidered and tackled with new eyes with the help of novel methods that can capture, holistically, the interactive processes generated by clinicians, patients and technology.

CHAPTER SUMMARY

In this chapter we have presented:

- a description of selected methods for the investigation of clinical reasoning in the health professions,
- examples of their use in research on clinical decision making and thinking in medical and other healthcare settings and
- comments about future methods and their potential integration to provide a more complete picture of the process of clinical reasoning.

REFLECTION POINT 2

Consider what research questions you might pose if you were planning to research clinical reasoning. What methods would be useful for researching these questions?

REFERENCES

Arocha, J.F., Wang, D., Patel, V.L., 2005. Identifying reasoning strategies in medical decision making: a methodological guide. J. Biomed. Inform. 38, 154–171.

Bailliard, A.L., 2015. Video methodologies in research: unlocking the complexities of occupation. Can. J. Occup. Ther. 82, 35–43.

Balslev, T., Jarodzka, H., Holmqvist, K., et al., 2012. Visual expertise in paediatric neurology. Eur. J. Paediatr. Neurol. 16, 161–166.

Blondon, K., Wipfli, R., Lovis, C., 2015. Use of eye-tracking technology in clinical reasoning: a systematic review. Stud. Health Technol. Inform. 210, 90–94.

Carrière, B., Gagnon, R., Charlin, B., et al., 2009. Assessing clinical reasoning in pediatric emergency medicine: validity evidence for a Script Concordance Test. Ann. Emerg. Med. 53, 647–652.

Chang, H.J., Kang, J., Ham, B.J., et al., 2016. A functional neuroimaging study of the clinical reasoning of medical students. Adv. Health Sci. Educ. Theory Pract. 21, 969.

Charlin, B., Boshuizen, H.P., Custers, E.J., et al., 2007. Scripts and clinical reasoning. Med. Educ. 41, 1178–1184.

Charlin, B., Roy, L., Brailovsky, C., et al., 2000. The Script Concordance test: a tool to assess the reflective clinician. Teach. Learn. Med. 12, 189–195.

Cramm, H., Krupa, T., Missiuna, C., et al., 2013. Broadening the occupational therapy toolkit: an executive functioning lens for occupational therapy with children and youth. Am. J. Occup. Ther. 67, e139–e147.

Croskerry, P., 2009. Clinical cognition and diagnostic error: applications of a dual process model of reasoning. Adv. Health Sci. Educ. Theory Pract. 14, 27–35.

Derry, S.J., Pea, R.D., Barron, B., et al., 2010. Conducting video research in the learning sciences: guidance on selection, analysis, technology, and ethics. J. Learn. Sci. 19, 3–53.

Durning, S.J., Artino, A.R., Beckman, T.J., et al., 2013a. Does the think-aloud protocol reflect thinking? Exploring functional neuroimaging differences with thinking (answering multiple choice questions) versus thinking aloud. Med. Teach. 35, 720–726.

Durning, S.J., Artino, A.R., Boulet, J.R., et al., 2012. The impact of selected contextual factors on experts' clinical reasoning performance (does context impact clinical reasoning performance in experts? Adv. Health Sci. Educ. Theory Pract. 17, 65–79.

Durning, S.J., Costanzo, M., Artino, A.R., et al., 2013b. Functional neuroimaging correlates of burnout among internal medicine residents and faculty members. Front. Psychiatry 4, 131–136.

Durning, S.J., Costanzo, M.E., Artino, A.R., et al., 2015. Neural basis of nonanalytical reasoning expertise during clinical evaluation. Brain Behav. 5, e00309.

Durning, S.J., Costanzo, M.E., Beckman, T.J., et al., 2016. Functional neuroimaging correlates of thinking flexibility and knowledge structure in memory: exploring the relationships between clinical reasoning and diagnostic thinking. Med. Teach. 38, 570–577.

Elstein, A.S., 2009. Thinking about diagnostic thinking: a 30-year perspective. Adv. Health Sci. Educ. Theory Pract. 14 (Suppl. 1), 7–18.

Elstein, A.S., Shulman, L.S., Sprafka, S.A., 1978. Medical Problem Solving: An Analysis of Clinical Reasoning. Harvard University Press, Cambridge, MA.

Ericsson, K.A., Simon, H.A., 1992. Protocol Analysis: Verbal Reports as Data, Revised Edition. MIT Press, Cambridge, MA.

Fonteyn, M.E., Kuipers, B., Grobe, S., 1993. A description of think aloud method and protocol analysis. Qual. Health Res. 3, 430–441.

Haig, B.D., 2013. The philosophy of quantitative methods. In: Little, T.D. (Ed.), The Oxford Handbook of Quantitative Methods, vol. 1. Oxford University Press, New York, pp. 7–31.

Jaarsma, T., Jarodzka, H., Nap, M., et al., 2015. Expertise in clinical pathology: combining the visual and cognitive perspective. Adv. Health Sci. Educ. Theory Pract. 20, 1089–1106.

Kazour, F., Richa, S., Zoghbi, M., et al., 2017. Using the Script Concordance Test to evaluate clinical reasoning skills in psychiatry. Acad. Psychiatry 41, 86–90.

Kelly, G., 1991. The Psychology of Personal Constructs. Routledge in association with the Centre for Personal Construct Psychology, London.

Kintsch, W., 1998. Comprehension: A Paradigm for Cognition. Cambridge University Press, Cambridge, MA.

Krupinski, E.A., 2010. Current perspectives in medical image perception. Atten. Percept. Psychophys. 72, 1205–1217.

Kuipers, K., Grice, J.W., 2009a. Clinical reasoning in neurology: use of the repertory grid technique to investigate the reasoning of an experienced occupational therapist. Aust. Occup. Ther. J. 56, 275–284.

Kuipers, K., Grice, J.W., 2009b. The structure of novice and expert occupational therapists' clinical reasoning before and after exposure to a domain-specific protocol. Aust. Occup. Ther. J. 56, 418–427.

Kuipers, B., Kassirer, J.P., 1984. Causal reasoning in medicine: analysis of a protocol. Cogn. Sci. 8, 363–385.

Langridge, N., Roberts, L., Pope, C., 2015. The clinical reasoning processes of extended scope physiotherapists assessing patients with low back pain. Man. Ther. 20, 745–750.

Lee, J., Lee, Y.J., Bae, J., et al., 2016. Registered nurses' clinical reasoning skills and reasoning process: a think-aloud study. Nurse Educ. Today 46, 75–80.

Lineberry, M., Kreiter, C.D., Bordage, G., 2013. Threats to validity in the use and interpretation of script concordance test scores. Med. Educ. 47, 1175–1183.

Lubarsky, S., Dory, V., Duggan, P., et al., 2013. Script concordance testing: from theory to practice: AMEE guide no. 75. Med. Teach. 35, 184–193.

Lundgrén-Laine, H., Salanterä, S., 2010. Think-aloud technique and protocol analysis in clinical decision-making research. Qual. Health Res. 20, 565–575.

Newell, A., Simon, H.A., 1972. Human Problem Solving. Prentice-Hall, Englewood Cliffs, NJ.

Norman, G.R., Coblentz, C.L., Brooks, L.R., et al., 1992. Expertise in visual diagnosis: a review of the literature. Acad. Med. 67 (Suppl. 10), S78–S83.

Norman, G.R., Young, M., Brooks, L., 2007. Non-analytical models of clinical reasoning: the role of experience. Med. Educ. 41, 1140–1145.

Patel, V.L., Arocha, J.F., Leccisi, M.S., 2001. Impact of undergraduate medical training on housestaff problem-solving performance: implications for problem-based curricula. J. Dent. Educ. 65, 1199–1218.

Patel, V.L., Arocha, J.F., Kaufman, D.R., 1994. Diagnostic reasoning and medical expertise. Psychol. Learn. Motiv. 31, 137–252.

Patel, V.L., Kaufman, D.R., Kannampallil, T.G., 2013. Diagnostic reasoning and decision making in the context of health information technology. Rev. Hum. Fact. Ergonom. 8, 149–190.

Pierce, D., 2005. The usefulness of video methods for occupational therapy and occupational science research. Am. J. Occup. Ther. 59, 9–19.

Pollock, L.C., 1986. An introduction to the use of repertory grid technique as a research method and clinical tool for psychiatric nurses. J. Adv. Nurs. 11, 439–445.

Power, A., Lemay, J.F., Cooke, S., 2016. Justify your answer: the role of written think aloud in script concordance testing. Teach. Learn. Med. 23, 1–9.

Rice, K.L., Bennett, M.J., Clesi, T., et al., 2014. Mixed-methods approach to understanding nurses clinical reasoning in recognizing delirium in hospitalized older adults. J. Contin. Educ. Nurs. 45, 136–148.

Roots, S.A., Niven, E., Moran, R.W., 2016. Osteopaths' clinical reasoning during consultation with patients experiencing acute low back pain: a qualitative case study approach. Int. J. Osteopath. Med. 19, 20–34.

Runkel, P.J., 1990. Casting Nets and Testing Specimens: Two Grand Methods of Psychology, second ed. Praeger, New York, NY.

Schmidt, H.G., Rikers, R.M., 2007. How expertise develops in medicine: knowledge encapsulation and illness script formation. Med. Educ. 41, 1133–1139.

Sibert, L., Charlin, B., Corcos, J., et al., 2002. Assessment of clinical reasoning competence in urology with the script concordance test: an exploratory study across two sites from different countries. Eur. Urol. 41, 227–233.

Simon, H., 1993. The human mind: the symbolic level. Proc. Am. Philos. Soc. 137, 638–647.

Stec, M.W., 2016. Health as expanding consciousness: clinical reasoning in baccalaureate nursing students. Nurs. Sci. Q. 29, 54–61.

Tourassi, G., Voisin, S., Paquit, V., et al., 2013. Investigating the link between radiologists' gaze, diagnostic decision, and image content. J. Am. Med. Inform. Assoc. 20, 1067–1075.

Unsworth, C.A., 2001a. The clinical reasoning of novice and expert occupational therapists. Scand. J. Occup. Ther. 8, 163–173.

Unsworth, C.A., 2001b. Using a head-mounted video camera to study clinical reasoning. Am. J. Occup. Ther. 55, 582–588.

Section 3

COLLABORATIVE AND TRANSDISCIPLINARY REASONING

15

COLLABORATIVE DECISION MAKING IN LIQUID TIMES

FRANZISKA TREDE ■ JOY HIGGS

CHAPTER AIMS

The aims of this chapter are to:

■ consider the importance of our liquid times for decision making,

■ support critical social science as a basis for collaborative decision making and

■ encourage practitioners to develop, critically, their own collaborative decision-making practices.

KEY WORDS

Collaborative decision making

Clinical reasoning

Critical social science

INTRODUCTION

Healthcare practice is rapidly changing with advances in technology in a globalized world. The way we practice, communicate and relate to each other is relentlessly changing and with it the way we make decisions. Decision making in healthcare practice is an important clinical reasoning process and issue. It has impact on efficiency and consequences for effectiveness.

In a simple (science-driven) world, healthcare practitioners would make expert decisions based on scientific empirico-analytical evidence that promises the best health outcomes. In this world, patients would concur with the expert decision and carry out the behaviours required. This vision portrays decision making from a biomedical model perspective, where the roles of patients and healthcare practitioners are clearly defined.

Decision making affects not only patients, their families and carers but also healthcare teams and services. Furthermore, decision making occurs within sociopolitical contexts. Decisions about postsurgery treatment in a first-world country with free healthcare insurance looks different from that of developing countries. Further, the decision-making process needs to include economic, educational, cultural, ethical and material considerations. Whose interests are being considered? Whose interests prevail? What role is played by hospital budgets, bed occupancy, views about good health and the pursuit of a quality life? What else should be included that enables responsible, morally justifiable, productive and effective decisions? In this chapter, we focus on collaborative decision making and explore the new conditions of decision-making processes in liquid times (or times of rapid change, where the only real constant is change itself), discuss conceptual perspectives and principles of collaborative decision making and report on a critical practice perspective on collaborative decision making. See later in the chapter for further discussion on liquid times.

NEW CONDITIONS OF DECISION-MAKING PROCESSES IN LIQUID TIMES

Decision making is part of everyday healthcare practice. Many decisions can be made in a largely routine manner and require little conscious effort such as how to greet a patient, position oneself in relation to a patient, read progress notes and so on. In relation to sharing decision-making processes with patients and others, this was not routinely part of traditional health care. Today in thinking about shared decision making, a number of considerations arise. What questions should be asked? How can we encourage patients to reveal their expectations, hopes and fears? What label should be used to describe a diagnosis? What treatment options should be discussed? All these questions relate to providing a context and boundaries for shared discussions.

The way decisions are made affects patients' motivation, persistence with treatment, sense of ownership, control and perceptions of healthcare outcomes. The more patients are involved and participate in the decision-making process, the more likely they are to be well informed, involved, satisfied and feeling valued (Trede and Higgs, 2003). It is equally likely that healthcare practitioners who enable collaboration come to understand their patients better, practice person-centred care more deeply and role-model respect and curiosity more authentically.

Many factors support the case for collaboration in decision making, and these factors have been well documented (Elwyn et al., 2012; Lin and Fagerlin, 2014; Matthias et al., 2013). These include ethical issues related to quality of life, end-of-life decisions, legal issues regarding informed consent, patient's rights for self-determination, patient safety, culturally appropriate care and valuing of diversity. Many patient complaints about health care relate to dissatisfaction with communication aspects of health care including poor communication skills of healthcare practitioners and breakdowns in communication. Potentially, collaborative decision-making processes could be a means of overcoming some of the causes of poor communication. Collaboration and communication are considered as important as delivering quality health care. These expectations are influenced by such factors as changing attitudes to health and patients' rights, increasing cultural diversity of concepts of what constitutes good health, advocacy of community support and patient groups, increasing litigiousness, improved patient education, increased access to healthcare information via the Internet and organizing of self-help groups online.

The world of healthcare practices and systems has been evolving over the centuries and continues to do so. However, over the past decade and with the arrival of mobile technology, health care, including conditions for practicing and collaborating in health care, has changed radically. As Floridi (2015, p. 131) argued, our thinking, doing and relating 'is fluidly changing in front of our eyes and under our feet, exponentially and relentlessly'. The new ways of practicing that are fast, public and open, made possible by digital and mobile technologies, have made the old way of doing things redundant because they no longer suit these new conditions. These changes bring with them the increasing contestation of the notion and superiority of 'the knowledge expert'. The role of privileged and restricted knowledge owned by individuals and professional groups that underpinned decision making (performed by experts for their clients) needs to be rethought. We live in transitional times, where it remains unclear what knowledge, practices and structures will be redundant, what will persist and what new will emerge. In short, we live in uncertain, ambiguous times.

Zygmunt Bauman (2012) coined the concept of 'liquid times' to give expression to the current times we live in. He makes two key points about his term 'liquid times'. Liquid times are marked by rapid change, where the only constant is change itself. The changes we are experiencing are much more fundamental and rapid than ever before. The term 'liquid times' describes how the concept of time has quickened. Knowledge, practice and structures liquefy before they have had time to solidify. Bauman explains that old, solidified ways of doing are no longer working, but new ways of doing have not yet been established, and there is no clarity in where new directions lead. The focus is now on immediacy, on short-term outcomes and instant impact. Holding on to old ideas and long-term commitments can be seen as being outdated. Thus standing still or slowing down is seen as a risk in liquid times. In this context, long-term thinking and long-term goals have collapsed and have been replaced by strategies that focus on being agile and keeping up with the latest developments.

The second assertion Bauman makes is his observation of a separation between power and politics. The regard for knowledge is decreasing, giving way to feeling. We live in postfactual times, where it is increasingly difficult to distinguish between real and fake news. The idea of hard facts is changing to notions of fluid facts where new insights are generated more rapidly. The lifespan of knowledge is shortening more than ever before. We need to rethink how we interact with knowledge and news. This weakens certainty, control and authority. It also can undermine agency and confidence. The rapid developments in digital and mobile technologies provide a clear illustration of Bauman's argument. With digital and mobile technologies, boundaries are blurring between professions and laity, between personal and professional, and between producer and consumer of services.

In this context, predictability and certainty are increasingly unattainable. We have given up on modernity – the quest for certainty and control – and now live in liquid modernity, the acknowledgement of the need to align with complexity, diversity and ambiguity. Bauman (2012) describes liquid modernity as a world where '[e]verything could happen yet nothing can be done with confidence and certainty'. Liquid times remind us to stay humble. It is important to be mindful that not everything is liquid. Liquidity on its own would be meaningless. It becomes meaningful only in an interdependent relationship with solidity, where one without the other could not exist (Bauman, 2012). Not everything is fluid, and not everything is solid. Without understanding and appreciating the role of solidity, it would be impossible to understand and appreciate liquidity. Both provide opportunities and barriers, and weighing up both enables deliberate professional decision making.

Liquid times can be threatening, but there are positive effects to living and working in liquid times, especially when it comes to collaborating in decision making. It makes collaboration an imperative. In an increasingly complex and diverse healthcare landscape, collaborative decision making seems a desirable and productive way to proceed. It brings people together and engages with diversity. Healthcare models with strong and closed borders and rigid roles are no longer conducive to timely, safe and effective healthcare delivery. Instead, complex and global health problems and rich human diversity are in a state of constant increase that cannot rest secure in the context of a single discipline, one healthcare model or one school of thought alone, as such rigidity cannot provide the answers and solutions.

Instead, interdisciplinary, collaborative decision-making practices are needed in liquid times.

REFLECTION POINT 1

How have you experienced liquid times? Have you encountered systems that are too rigid and unchangeable to cope with liquidity in healthcare contexts?

CONCEPTUAL PERSPECTIVES AND PRINCIPLES OF COLLABORATIVE DECISION MAKING

Readiness for Collaborative Decision Making Is Not a Given

It cannot be taken for granted that patients (and clients) will be ready for and agree to participating in clinical decision-making processes or share in the responsibilities for clinical decision-making outcomes. Therefore practitioners need to check on patients' readiness and willingness to collaborate in decision making about their health care.

Patients enter healthcare situations with a wide range of preparedness for the events that will unfold during their journey of ill health or disability and limited preparedness (usually) for the processes and opportunities for decision making they will encounter. They may or may not have had time to investigate the nature of their condition or its medical management, to prepare mentally, physically or emotionally for the health situation they are facing and to develop a position on what they want or hope their health outcome to be. In addition, they commonly do not have the relevant medical knowledge or expertise to understand adequately the nature of the condition, its treatment options and potential health outcomes.

Agreement to Participate in Collaborative Decision Making Needs to Be Checked via Informed Consent

Agreements (to participate and agreements about outcomes) need to be checked because patients may only indicate implicit agreement through apparent compliance with treatment or healthcare programs. Practitioners need to consider whether agreements are real rather than apparent and genuinely collaborative rather than a matter of compliance in the face of unbalanced power. To do this, practitioners need to ensure an authentic collaborative decision-making process is enabled, taking complex factors into consideration.

Many Factors Influence Patients' Agreements About Decisions – Yes May Not Mean (Informed) Yes

When it comes to the point of agreeing with a healthcare professional or healthcare team in decision making, the patient's agreement could be influenced by many 'entry' factors. Any agreement or otherwise could also be influenced by factors within the communication or interaction, such as the relationship built with the practitioner(s), language or cultural familiarity or barriers, aspects of behaviour such as intentions, motivations and practitioners' practice models (e.g., biomedical, biopsychosocial and emancipatory models). In addition, decision-making processes are influenced by professional authority, professional roles and expectations held by professional groups and the community.

Agreement May Be Apparent and Unchallenged Rather Than Genuine and Empowered

When clinicians and patients share the same values, intentions and interests, agreement is more likely. However, agreement or compliance that is unarticulated or unquestioned may not be true agreement at all. It is tempting to assume that patients adopt the role that practitioners assign to them, without checking with patients either at the point of decision making or during subsequent treatment programs whether these roles are acceptable in terms of both ability and choice. Are patients reporting honestly on their perceptions of progress or their pain levels and so on? Considering a critical perspective to decision making reminds us that commonality of values and interests between patients and practitioners should not be taken for granted.

CONCEPTUAL MODELS OF SHARED DECISION MAKING

The traditional way of decision making that was entrusted to expert practitioners no longer fits the new conditions where patients are not only encouraged but frequently expected to participate in their treatment

decisions (Lin and Fagerlin, 2014). Today is the time to reframe the notion of decision-making experts to include practitioners *and* patients. Most of the literature on decision making has a tendency to use the term 'shared decision making' but then discusses a great diversity of decision-making processes that range from paternalistic to informed decision making (Lin and Fagerlin, 2014). Makoul and Clayman (2006), in a systematic review of the literature on shared decision making, found great fluidity in what was understood by the term, ranging from clinician-led decision making across a spectrum to patient-led decision making. The authors listed essential elements of shared decision making: defining the problem, presenting the options, identifying patient values and preferences and doctor knowledge, and clarifying understanding. This checklist reflects the transactional procedures in decision making. Although this is a useful start, it falls short of considering contexts and deep-rooted motivations for collaborating.

Matthias et al. (2013) argued that shared decision making cannot be discussed out of context and requires consideration of the entire patient encounter and particularly the nature of the patient–practitioner relationship. Mulley et al. (2012) asserted that excluding patients from decision making can be the reason for misdiagnoses. And Charles et al. (1997) summed it up succinctly in the subtitle of their seminal paper 'It takes at least two to tango'. What the literature is pointing to is the importance of integrating various interests and motivations that influence the reasoning behind decision making. To this end, it is useful to consider a series of questions that helps clarify assumptions about decision making and how knowledge is generated (Edwards et al., 2004).

REFLECTION POINT 2

Clarifying assumptions about decision making
- When is it appropriate to be practitioner-centred, and when is it appropriate to be patient-centred?
- Who has permission to define the problem?
- Who is authorized to identify and legitimize what all the options are?
- How are patients invited and encouraged to share their values?
- Whose understanding needs clarification?
- What counts as knowledge and evidence?

THE PRIMACY OF INTERESTS: A CRITICAL MODEL FOR COLLABORATIVE DECISION MAKING

In Chapter 4, we discussed the work of Habermas (1972), who developed a theory of knowledge and human interest (1972). Interests are the motivations, intentions and goals that guide behaviours. Of Habermas' three interest categories (technical, practical and emancipatory) we see emancipatory interests as most relevant to the liberatory goals mentioned earlier that are linked to genuine patient-collaborative clinical decision making. Fig. 15.1 illustrates the extreme ends of the various interests that shape practice models.

Many scholars have delineated the dualism between practitioner-centred and patient-centred care (e.g., Arnetz et al., 2004; Lin and Fagerlin, 2014), leaving the reader and practitioner appreciating differences between these terms but not helping them to communicate and transcend this dualism. A critical perspective in this context starts with critical self-awareness of what motivates professional bias, professional authority and professional roles, and it illuminates the various interests and interpretations underpinning practice approaches, especially those interests that pursue and drive power rather than reason. For example, adopting a critical perspective means seeking first to understand the historical and social factors and influences that have led practice to be accepted and valued the way it is (in a given context) and then to challenge and change this practice with the goal of emancipating those who are restricted or disempowered by it. Within this framework, practitioner-centred practice is typically practice that favours technical rationalism and privileges those in power (commonly the practitioners), whereas in truly (critical) patient-centred practice the practitioner seeks to share knowledge and power with the patient and to respect the input the patient can make to clinical decision making and healthcare management. Box 15.1 presents arguments in favour of adopting a critical perspective on collaborative decision making.

Collaboration is based on the conviction that inclusiveness and critical self-reflection produce better outcomes for patients than empirico-analytical precision. Collaborative decision making is based on inclusive evidence that entails embracing uncertainty and recognizing diversity of patients, clinicians and therapeutic environments (Jones et al., 2006). A critical approach helps practitioners to become conscious of their interests and choices in decision making because hidden agendas and bias are made explicit.

We see collaborative decision making as a strategy enabling practitioners to liberate themselves from unnecessary constraints to work authentically with patients to empower patients to reclaim responsibility for their

Unconscious	Known
Tacit	Knowing
Minimal capacity development	Explicit capacity development
Detached from self	Being self
Safe replication	Calculated risk
Single perspective	Multiple perspectives
Telling	Listening and responding

Practice interests

Technical	Practical	Emancipatory

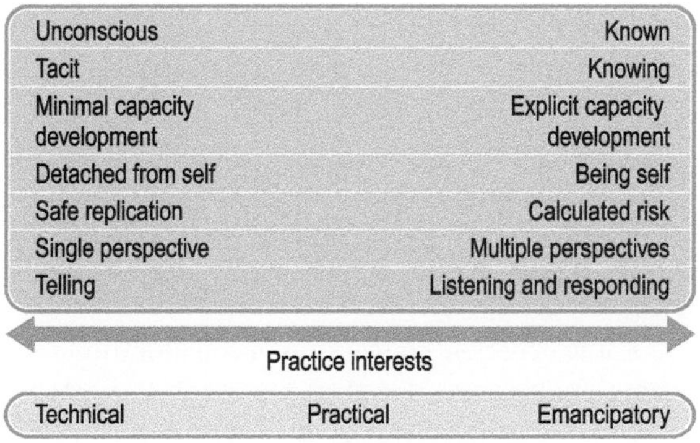

Fig. 15.1 ■ Practice approaches.

BOX 15.1
ADOPTING A CRITICAL PERSPECTIVE IN COLLABORATIVE DECISION MAKING

When adopting a critical perspective in collaborative decision making, remember the following:

■ Not all parties involved in the decision-making process necessarily share the same values, intentions and interests about health beliefs and health behaviours. Decisions need to be negotiated free of coercion and power imbalances.

■ Decision-making roles of practitioners and patients are dynamic and change as the health condition of patients progresses from acute, life-threatening to subacute and chronic conditions. Therefore, it is important to make conscious choices about which approach to decision making is appropriate.

■ Patients are increasingly better informed, and they (or at least many of them) want to know their options and be involved in decision making and self-management.

■ Given appropriate opportunity and inclusive environments, most patients can be empowered to collaborate in decision making and have a say in their health management.

health, autonomy, dignity and self-determination. The intention of collaboration in critical practice is to engage in dialogue and to democratize roles. Collaboration starts with critique, scepticism and curiosity to deepen understanding and to identify the scope of common ground for change. In our work, we have found that critique of decision making focussed on four closely interrelated dimensions:

- capacity for critical self-reflection,
- rethinking professional roles,
- rethinking professional power relations and
- rethinking rationality and professional practice knowledge.

REFLECTION POINT 3

In what ways do you see collaborative decision making as liberating for practitioners and patients?

OPERATIONALIZING COLLABORATIVE DECISION MAKING

In Chapter 4, we reported on five prototypes (the uninformed, the unconvinced, the contemplators, the transformers and the champions) that represented the way the participants in a research project (Trede, 2008) engaged (or did not engage) with a critical perspective in their practice. Here we take each of these prototypes in turn and consider their implications for collaborative decision making.

The Uninformed

In Franziska's research (Trede, 2008), the *uninformed* were participants who were not aware of conceptual ideas of a critical practice perspective, their own interests and how those interests influenced their decisions; they often said they did not know what their patients really wanted and what their goals were. The uninformed group's practice interests were blurred. Practitioners did not think in terms of models or interests but reacted to presenting challenges. There seemed to be a lack of reflexivity. The uninformed had unknowingly adopted the mainstream approach to decision making. However, there was a tendency towards technical rather than emancipatory interests. One participant learned about collaborative reasoning

---

BOX 15.2
BEING UNINFORMED

The penny dropped for me only after 10 years of clinical experience. I had [a patient with] an above-knee amputation, and he had a prosthesis. He walked perfectly in the gym. I had him walk without a limp. I was really pleased with all this. Then I met him downtown in the shopping centre: he had his knee locked, he was walking on the inner quarter of his foot, foot stuck out at right angle, and he was perfectly happy. I stood and looked at him and thought 'I can make you walk perfectly without a limp, but you don't want to do that'. And you know when he came to treatment he would do it, but obviously he wasn't feeling safe, and he didn't want to do it that way and that is that. I think I wanted him to do what I wanted. I was trying to be a perfectionist. And it has also to do with all the other physiotherapists. They are checking on you that you are doing it all properly. (Jill)

---

by reflecting upon a critical incident that made her question the way she tended to make clinical decisions (Box 15.2).

Seeing her patient mobilizing in a nonideal way but with confidence and seeing him integrated into social community life made Jill start to question her goal-setting practices and her professional interests. Why should she make patients walk without a limp if all they wanted was to walk safely? Jill became aware of clashes between professional and patient goals. She was aware of peer expectations, and she felt pressured to comply with the professional physiotherapy culture. Collaborative decision making is influenced not only by the stakeholders of decisions but also by the practice culture and the workplace environment.

The Unconvinced

Dorothy, who fitted the *unconvinced* prototype, equated collaboration with compliance. She felt that patients had to understand physiotherapy reasoning, but she did not think that physiotherapists had to understand the way patients reasoned. She did not challenge the biomedical interests that influenced the way she reached decisions (Box 15.3).

Dorothy experienced working in collaboration with patients as positive. However, her understanding of collaboration was narrowly defined because she limited the patients with whom she chose to collaborate. She

BOX 15.3
BEING UNCONVINCED

Giving the patients options is definitely making them feel more in control, and you get a better response out of them. They don't just feel like sitting there having things done to them. They are having a bit more of a say what is happening to them. So it is good for both. (Dorothy)

BOX 15.4
BEING A CONTEMPLATOR

Doing-to patients saves lives and prevents complications. Doing-to is simple and straightforward. It means following my duty of care. In acute [settings], you focus on biomedical signs, and you cannot always develop a relationship with the human being. In chronic settings, you have time to develop a professional/personal relationship. In long-term rehabilitation, you need to consider the human being more. It is more relaxing, working slower with patients. (Petra)

noticed that patients who shared her values and expectations made her more relaxed, and she was able to give them choice. These patients did not challenge her practice. What Dorothy described as collaboration was patient compliance. With difficult patients, she felt she chose to be more forceful.

She categorized patients who did not agree with her as difficult people with stubborn personalities. It appeared that either patients worked with her, or she had to use professional power to get patients to comply. She did not acknowledge her motivations and interests, and she did not practice self-critique.

The Contemplators

The *contemplators* struggled with the concept of collaboration and patient emancipation. They interpreted collaboration as allowing patients to dominate them, and they rejected this approach to decision making. However, they could see some benefits in trying to work with patients by 'making practice suitable to the patient's background, as much as their biomedical illnesses allowed'.

Petra understood collaborative decision making as persuading patients to adopt the physiotherapist's perspective. It was not based on egalitarian, equal terms; the biomedical perspective prevailed unchallenged. Petra's practice values remained firmly grounded in the acute medical model despite appreciation of patients' individual fears and needs. Petra believed that once patients were familiar with their acute conditions, they could be empowered to take more control and determine their own treatment routine in consultation (Box 15.4).

This quote succinctly describes the attitude of the contemplators, who saw collaboration as optional and not suitable in some settings. The attitude was that practitioners have permission to assume professional power over their patients because of their professional status and knowledge. That is, they considered that professional relationships in the healthcare context start with uneven power relationships, where practitioners have more power than patients. When the participants were asked to rethink and democratize their relationships with patients, the implication was that patients had to be taken more seriously as people with a role to play in clinical decision making and self-management. In exploring collaboration, the participants were challenged to listen critically to patients and develop open dialogue with patients.

The Transformers

The *transformers* trialled democratizing their relationships with patients; they were willing to challenge their use of professional power. Jocelyn, for example, became more attentive to interests and to her patients' expectations of physiotherapy. She found that some patients had clear expectations and knew what they wanted. When comparing these with her own professional expectations and goals, Jocelyn experienced conflict. She described an incident with an 80-year-old patient who could not carry her shopping home but otherwise was able to be fully independent. Jocelyn noted the decreased range of motion in her shoulder joint, and she wanted to work first on increasing range of motion and then on strengthening muscles. However, her patient was not interested in increasing range of motion (Box 15.5).

In this situation, Jocelyn appeared comfortable to go with her patient's goals. Her decision was influenced by her patient's age. Had her patient been younger, she might have insisted on improving range of motion as well. Jocelyn made decisions in the context of her

---

BOX 15.5
BEING A TRANSFORMER

I could see that [this] patient was not interested in my plan. I thought this wasn't particularly functional [wanting to increase strength before increasing range of motion], but she was able to do everything: cook, clean and so on. The only thing she couldn't do was go shopping because she couldn't carry anything. So, that was really glaring in my face. This is what she wants to do. I am not sure if I always pick that up. (Jocelyn)

BOX 15.6
BEING A TRANSFORMER

I want to learn from patients so that I can improve my own skills. I think that every treatment session is a learning session for me. I learn from my patients. (Corinne)

BOX 15.7
BEING A CHAMPION

Is physiotherapy a social science? To me it is, and my colleagues will hit me over the head. I think there are the arts and the sciences. It is somewhere between the two. You have to oscillate all the time to facilitate an outcome for the patient. So I have this pulling force in me all the time. I value the scientific and searching for the evidence, but I am worried about the patient. (Raymond)

BOX 15.8
BEING A CHAMPION

You cannot tell a teenager to stop smoking. You need to look at their social issues. I practice physiotherapy like that. First [I consider] scientific knowledge and then social beliefs and patient knowledge. (Raymond)

---

patient's age and function and with a critical stance to self. She was willing to reconsider, in this situation. However, generally speaking, Jocelyn was not content to allow patients to lead treatment plans unconditionally.

Corinne displayed a capacity for critical self-reflection in relation to her issues around professional authority and power relations. Corinne had over 30 years of clinical experience, and her area of expertise was outpatient physiotherapy. She questioned her practice and viewed each treatment as a learning process for herself and her patients (Box 15.6).

Corinne learned to recognize that she was not the only expert or the professional who should know all the answers. She could appreciate that patients had relevant knowledge as well. Corinne learned to reframe herself as a facilitator of collaborative decision making. She not only transformed her approach to practice and her view of herself as a professional, but she also learned about practice as a collaborative transformation.

The Champions

Participants who had operationalized collaborative decision making and endorsed the values of inclusion and power sharing were labelled *champions* or advocates of the critical social science approach. These participants were skeptical and critical of professional authority that was taken for granted and automatically assumed.

Raymond, one of this group, saw himself as a scientist, a critical self-reflector and a patient collaborator (Box 15.7).

Raymond saw himself as integrating biomedical facts with patients' perceptions of their healthcare needs and condition. He defined his practice as 'doing qualitative medicine'. He recognized that a collaborative approach to decision making did not exclude propositional or scientific knowledge, but it also required nonpropositional knowledge to achieve emancipatory outcomes. Champions do not make decisions without continually checking their impact with individual patients; they regard patients as social, cultural and political human beings (Box 15.8).

In analyzing the interviews with the champion group, a number of factors that indicated participants' capacity or inclination for participating in collaborative decision making were identified. These included:

- appreciating patients' perspectives (e.g., fear, lack of knowledge),
- becoming self-aware of personal bias,
- actively providing opportunities for patients to participate,
- being willing to reconsider treatment choices,
- exploring options with patients,
- establishing reciprocal relationships (by being open and enabling patients to be open),

- facilitating a reciprocal process of teaching and learning from each other and
- recognizing clearly the values that inform decision making.

The champions in this study (Trede, 2008) used their human agency to facilitate change in their patients. They can be described as deliberate professionals (Trede and McEwen, 2016); they were aware of self, their patients and the context around them, they weighed up possibilities and made a decision together with their patients and shared responsibilities for the consequences of these decisions.

CHAPTER SUMMARY

In this chapter we have done the following:

- We discussed the new conditions, diverse interests and fluid roles and contexts of practitioners and patients and the complex processes that need to be meaningfully integrated in collaborative decision-making processes in these liquid times.
- We identified a series of questions for clarifying assumptions about decision making.
- We demonstrated the central importance of adopting a critical perspective on collaborative decision making.
- We illustrated various operationalizations of collaborative decision-making practices.

REFLECTION POINT 4

Can you see yourself as a practitioner in any of these prototypes? Where do you think students and experts fit into this set? What do you see as the implications for collaborative decision making?

REFERENCES

Arnetz, J.E., Almin, I., Bergström, K., et al., 2004. Active patient involvement in the establishment of physical therapy goals: effects on treatment outcome and quality of care. Adv. Physiother. 6, 50–69.

Bauman, Z., 2012. Liquid Modernity. Polity Books, Cambridge, UK.

Charles, C., Gafni, A., Whelan, T., 1997. Shared decision-making in the medical encounter: what does it mean? (or it takes at least two to tango). Soc. Sci. Med. 44, 681–692.

Edwards, I., Jones, M., Higgs, J., et al., 2004. What is collaborative reasoning? Adv. Physiother. 6, 70–83.

Elwyn, G., Frosch, D., Thomson, R., et al., 2012. Shared decision making: a model for clinical practice. J. Gen. Intern. Med. 27, 1361–1367.

Floridi, L., 2015. Hyperhistory and the philosophy of information policies. Philos. Technol. 25, 129–131.

Habermas, J., 1972. Knowledge and Human Interest. Heinemann, London, UK.

Jones, M., Grimmer, K., Edwards, I., et al., 2006. Challenges in applying best evidence to physiotherapy. Internet J. Allied Health Sci. Pract. 4.

Lin, G.A., Fagerlin, A., 2014. Shared decision making: state of the science. Circ. Cardiovasc. Qual. Outcomes 7, 328–334.

Makoul, G., Clayman, M.L., 2006. An integrative model of shared decision making in medical encounters. Patient Educ. Couns. 60, 301–312.

Matthias, M.S., Salyers, M.P., Frankel, R.M., 2013. Re-thinking shared decision making: context matters. Patient Educ. Couns. 91, 176–179.

Mulley, A.G., Trimble, C., Elwyn, G., 2012. Stop the silent misdiagnosis: patients' preferences matter. BMJ 345, e6572.

Trede, F.V., 2008. A Critical Practice Model for Physiotherapy: Developing Practice Through Critical Transformative Dialogues. VDM Verlag Dr Müller, Saarbrücken, Germany.

Trede, F., Higgs, J., 2003. Re-framing the clinician's role in collaborative clinical decision making: re-thinking practice knowledge and the notion of clinician–patient relationships. Learning Health Soc. Care 2, 66–73.

Trede, F., McEwen, C., 2016. Scoping the deliberate professional. In: Trede, F., McEwen, C. (Eds.), Educating the Deliberate Professional: Preparing for Emergent Futures. Springer, New York, NY.

16

ETHICAL REASONING

IAN EDWARDS ▪ CLARE DELANY

CHAPTER AIMS

The aims of this chapter are to:

- outline the Ethical Reasoning Bridge model,
- explain the relationship between normative and nonnormative ethics and
- present the relationship among individual ethical reasoning, social ethical reasoning and moral agency.

KEY WORDS

The Ethical Reasoning Bridge
Normative and nonnormative ethics
Individual and social ethical reasoning
Moral agency

ABBREVIATIONS/ ACRONYMS

ER Bridge Ethical Reasoning Bridge
ACFI Aged Care Funding Instrument

INTRODUCTION

Ethics is essentially concerned with how people should conduct themselves in particular social roles and practices (Purtilo, 2005). In health care, ethics has to fulfil two quite different and sometimes competing tasks (Komesaroff, 2008). First, it has a regulatory role in ensuring that widely agreed-upon and expected standards of professional behaviour, including the ethical conduct of healthcare practitioners, are adhered to. These ethical standards are expressed in professional codes of conduct, compliance with which is overseen by professional associations and boards (Hugman, 2005). A second less visible task of ethics, as suggested by Komesaroff (2008, p. xiii), is subversive in that it questions the prevailing values and conditions in which an ethical issue arises and is played out and the assumptions and motives, which influence people (healthcare practitioners and nonpractitioners alike) to act and behave as they do. This second task of ethics also seeks to understand a person's moral agency (or capacity to act). And this involves an understanding of the choices - or lack of them – that people have, or perceive that they have, in various situations or dilemmas (Edwards et al., 2011).

Although both share the care of the patient as an ultimate goal, the first task of ethics is normative as it is concerned with 'what ought to happen', and the second is nonnormative and focusses on 'what actually happens'. Between 'what ought to happen' and 'what actually happens' in the care of the patient, there is a moral landscape that is often uncertain and difficult for practitioners to negotiate. It is a terrain that is continually being reshaped by changing societal values, patterns of healthcare practice and funding models (Delany et al., in press; Edwards, 2016). Ethical reasoning refers to the thinking and decision-making processes by which the practitioner evaluates what takes place between 'what ought to happen' and 'what actually happens' for the purpose of an ethical response.

169

In the previous edition, we presented an ethical reasoning and decision-making model called the Ethical Reasoning Bridge (ER Bridge) (Edwards and Delany, 2008). This model was originally derived from research of the decision making of expert physical therapists, which was described as dialectical insomuch as it moved between, and expressed, different conceptions of knowledge (Edwards et al., 2004). The ER Bridge model aims to assist the ethical problem solver to both recognize and engage with the different conceptions of normative and nonnormative ethics.

On the normative ethics side of the ER Bridge (Fig. 16.1), the professional world of the healthcare practitioners, are universal ethical principles (beneficence, nonmaleficence, respect for autonomy and justice – Beauchamp and Childress, 2009) that have traditionally underpinned professional codes of conduct. It has been widely argued that this approach to ethics, also known as 'third-person' ethics (Mattingly, 2012), expresses the deductive and rationalist methods of scientific problem solving because it privileges the application of universal or generalizable rules and principles in predicting what impartial 'outcomes' should be in particular ethical dilemmas (Callahan, 2003; Fox, 1994; Komesaroff, 2008; Mattingly, 2012; MacIntyre, 2007).

On the nonnormative side of the ER Bridge, the site of others (patients, carers and the community), is a method of inquiry called narrative reasoning that is concerned with understanding the lived experience of people, their sense of identity and their moral strivings in particular contexts. Narrative reasoning has as its

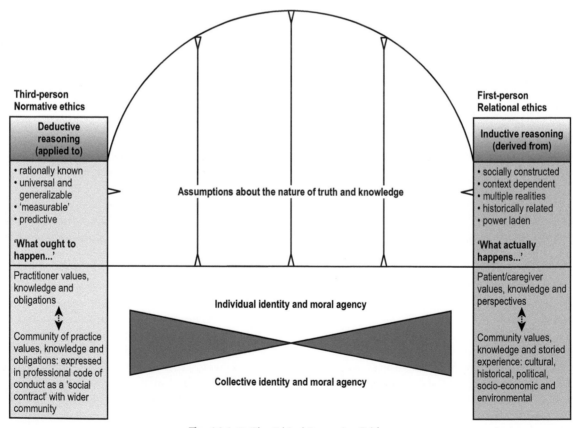

Fig. 16.1 ■ The Ethical Reasoning Bridge.

theoretical basis that we are 'self-interpreting creatures' (Taylor, 1985b) who make sense of our lives and form identities, and therefore purpose, via the construction (and ongoing 'reconstruction') of our narratives (Ricoeur, 2006). Understanding what is morally at stake for people in their moral struggles in various contexts has been termed first-person ethics (Mattingly, 2012) and requires a recognition of multiple and socially constructed realities in our relationships with others (see Fig. 16.1).

The ER Bridge model of ethical reasoning, as a means of inquiry and analysis, is not unlike a mixed-methods research approach. A hallmark of mixed-methods research is that the different paradigms of inquiry, somewhat counterintuitively, inform each other *during* the conduct of the research and not just at its conclusion when making sense of findings (Burke et al., 2007). We would make the same kind of claim with respect to the ER Bridge: namely, that moving between and engaging different paradigms of inquiry and reasoning - crossing 'the bridge' – yields richer insights regarding the nature of the ethical issue and the relationships between various factors and social actors involved in it than via one method alone (Edwards, 2016; Swisher et al., 2012).

In this revised chapter, we wish to reassert the relevance of the ER Bridge model and argue that it has utility for the ethical problem solver in being able to span a morally diverse and changing healthcare terrain. Like any model, it aims to represent important concepts or ideas and their relationships. However, we acknowledge a need to further explain aspects of the ER Bridge model that were either unelaborated or unexplained in the previous edition. In this chapter, we focus on healthcare practitioners who, in intentionally crossing and recrossing the ER Bridge, are able to nurture moral agency in themselves and others. We structure this focus by: a) discussing the rationale for the relationship between normative and nonnormative ethical reasoning, arguing that it is a mutually informing interaction; b) describing how, when the practitioner 'crosses' and 'recrosses' the ER Bridge, there is both an individual *and* a social reasoning process; and c) examining the relationship between the moral identity and moral agency of practitioners as a means of discovering ethical possibilities, with others, in difficult and ambiguous ethical scenarios.

THE ETHICAL REASONING BRIDGE

Normative and Nonnormative Ethics

Students in the various healthcare disciplines are commonly taught versions of patient interviewing and physical examination (previously known as subjective and objective assessments) that are relevant to the 'diagnostic' and therapeutic practices of their discipline. Healthcare students have often learned, whether educators intended it or not (Shepard and Jensen, 1990), that 'to be objective' and to avoid 'subjective bias' are the preeminent perceptual postures of the problem solver. The desire for 'objectivity' has also permeated ethical reasoning models in health care (Callahan, 2003; Komesaroff, 2008). The hegemony of data that is 'objective' over that which is 'subjective' is gradually changing as the utility of collaborative goal setting and incorporating the 'patient's point of view' is increasingly valued (Reunanen et al., 2016). Notwithstanding this, 'being objective' remains relevant for particular instrumental problem solving and procedural tasks in health care. However, it is not the clear-cut problem solving posture that it might seem, particularly if one applies the notion to one's dealing with others (Mattingly, 2014; Zahavi, 2005).

Thomas Nagel (1989), in his philosophical treatise, 'The view from nowhere', stated that the problem of objectivity was, 'how to combine the perspective of a particular person inside the world with an objective view of that same world, the person and his viewpoint included' (Nagel, 1989, p. 3). Even with his particular interest in the physical sciences and proclivity towards 'objectivity', Nagel conceded that for a person who is trying to make sense of what he or she sees before him or her, pure 'objectivity' is not possible, because in looking at the world, 'However often we may step outside ourselves, something will have to stay behind the lens, something in us will determine the resulting picture' (p. 68). Nagel therefore proposed the need for a 'double vision', where we see the world 'from nowhere' (unbiased and objective) while at the same time we see the world 'from here' (our own perspective) (p. 86). To see the world 'from nowhere', however, is to arguably neutralize both our own and others' perspectives, neither achieving objectivity nor further insight into understanding how either party experiences the world (Volf, 1996). Reinforcing this idea, Gallagher and Zahavi

(2007) state (we have added the terms 'objective' and 'subjective'):

> *There is no pure third-person (objective) perspective, just as there is no view from nowhere. … This is not to say that there is no third-person (objective) perspective, but merely that such a perspective is exactly a perspective from somewhere … it emerges out of the encounter between at least two first-person (subjective) perspectives; that is, it involves intersubjectivity (Gallagher and Zahavi, 2007, p. 40).*

Intersubjectivity, as an encounter between different perspectives, supports the idea that we see the world not as a view from nowhere but from 'here' (our own) and from 'there' (others' perspectives) (Taylor, 1985a). This is a rationale for the ER Bridge. The practitioner crosses from 'here' (his or her own professional and/ or personal perspectives) to 'there' (the perspectives of others – patients/carers/other healthcare workers). And so, although the theoretical underpinnings on the ER Bridge relating to research paradigms may suggest a dichotomy between objectivity and subjectivity, we propose that it is conceptually more helpful to think of this 'crossing' in terms of reasoning with either a normative or a nonnormative intentionality.

'Intentionality' is a term from phenomenology (Larkin et al., 2011). It does not refer to a practical intention to 'do something' but instead refers to the proposition that we have a conscious relationship with an object – externally or in mind or memory – about which we interpret and develop meaning (Greenfield and Jensen, 2010, p. 1190). For example, when engaged in diagnostic or procedural clinical reasoning, the healthcare practitioner adopts what might be termed a 'normatively oriented intentionality.' That is, when listening to and examining a patient, the practitioner looks for what he or she already recognizes, in terms of what he or she considers as significant towards forming some kind of diagnosis or other evaluation of the patient. A doctor looks, therefore, for the signs and symptoms of a particular disease entity. This leads to a categorization and ordering of the features of a presentation, with an emphasis on recognizing what is known and what – in a normative sense – is expected or ought to be found (Edwards et al., 2011; Kahneman, 2011).

A normative intentionality with respect to ethical reasoning would see a similar framing and categorizing of an ethical scenario or dilemma via certain recognizable features or categories – at least to the practitioner – in terms of injunctions of a code of conduct or particular ethical principle (Callahan, 2003). Read Case Study 16.1 to see how physiotherapy student, Theresa, initially frames the ethical dilemma involving her patient Coral.

The Social Formation of Ethical Reasoning

On each side of the ER Bridge are represented relationships between individuals and communities (see Fig. 16.1). There is a relationship between individual

---

CASE STUDY 16.1

Ethical Reasoning

Theresa is a final-year physiotherapy student on clinical placement at an aged care residential facility. This facility offers a range of healthcare services to both its residents and its home-based clients, including physiotherapy, podiatry, occupational therapy, dietetics, speech pathology, social work and nursing.

Coral is a 62-year-old woman who had a right-sided stroke some 9 months previously that left her with left-sided hemiparesis. Before the stroke, she lived independently with her husband of 35 years and did most of the housework. She also took care of her two young grandchildren (3 and 5 years of age) on a regular basis and was an active member at her local Rotary club. She had been assessed by an Aged Care Assessment Team (ACAT) and deemed to be 'high care' using the Resident Classification Scale. Based on this assessment, and the fact that her husband, John, was not able to assume the responsibility of caring for her at home, Coral was admitted into this

Ethical Reasoning (Continued)

care facility. It had been a difficult decision about which both Coral and John were still grieving.

The ACAT assessment had also determined that Coral needed two heavy 'assists' and a lifter to get her in and out of the bed. However, Coral had also engaged in rehabilitation at the facility, and there were slow but demonstrable changes towards more independence and increased function. Theresa (the physical therapy student) was asked to visit Coral to provide physiotherapy treatment. After her assessment, she concluded that although it was true that Coral still required some assistance, it was clear she no longer needed the lifter to transfer in and out of the bed. She also found that Coral was teary and emotional, especially when she talked about her life before the stroke. She felt the stroke had rendered her useless, and she felt like a burden to her family now. She wanted to get better but felt it was better for everyone if she stayed in the residential facility. John was a supportive husband and carer. He was also present at this session, and he, too, became emotional when recalling their life together before her stroke. However, he also expressed anger and frustration at the time and delay it took for a lifter to be organized every time Coral wanted to get out of bed. John said that this just seemed to further reinforce how Coral felt about herself.

In addition to physiotherapy, Coral was also receiving visits from occupational therapy and speech pathology. In a case meeting with the nursing home administrator, Theresa, the occupational therapist and speech pathologist, stated that Coral was progressing quite well in particular areas of function and may need another assessment by ACAT. The administrator was reluctant to proceed. To Theresa's surprise, Bev, her physiotherapy clinical supervisor, also seemed to drag her feet in the discussion. Later, Bev discreetly told Theresa about the nursing home's precarious financial position. Not needing a lifter would change Coral's care level and therefore reduce the funding they were receiving for Coral. Bev admitted that this was not an ideal situation, but they were having to maximize funding opportunities with respect to the residents, wherever possible, to keep their jobs and the facility open. It was a difficult balance, she explained.

Theresa is an inexperienced practitioner but enters this scenario as someone with 'fresh' eyes. From her professional training, she already has acquired a strong sense of the philosophy of physiotherapy, which is to assist people to maximize their physical capacities and functioning for better participation in the activities that they value in their lives. Theresa judges that this professional obligation is being compromised in Coral's overall care. It is because she has also acquired normative ethical knowledge in learning about ethical principles and professional codes of conduct that Theresa is sensitized to what she has witnessed in Coral and John's situation, recognizing this as being unethical. More specifically, she is able to say that respect for Coral's autonomy or, to put it another way, Coral's right (together with John) to make significant decisions in her own health care is not being upheld.

A nonnormative intentionality concerns 'recognition' of another kind. It focusses less on the 'what' of an ethical problem and more on the motives and choices of those involved in it. Theresa has noted the apparent frustration of participants in this scenario that arises for different reasons. Coral is feeling useless and that she is a burden to everyone. Her partner, John, is angry and frustrated because of the strict implementation of the regime concerning the use of the lifter. He believes that it is demeaning to Coral and further contributes to her sense of being a burden to everyone. Theresa's physiotherapy clinical supervisor, Bev, does not dispute Theresa's (or John's) analysis of the situation. She does provide, in an embarrassed, almost defeated manner, an explanation of why things are currently as they are. What was initially a definable ethical issue in normative terms now seems to be more like a spider web in which people are each caught and held between competing interests.

practitioners and their own professional communities of practice. Patients and carers are also members of the various contexts and communities in which they live their lives. Finally, there is also a relationship between healthcare practitioners and the workplaces or institutions in which they work. This leads to the idea of individuals as members of various cultures, each one having a shared set of beliefs and practices, however explicitly or implicitly these may be recognized. We focus here on healthcare practitioners in workplace cultures and the formation of ethical behaviour in these cultures. The ethical reasoning of an individual is always constructed with 'reference to some defining communities' (Mattingly, 2014, p. 22). Taylor (1989) illustrates the dialectical nature of the individual and the social in the formation of moral identity when he writes 'one cannot be a self on one's own' (p. 36). Ethical reasoning is likewise both an individual and a social (or public) phenomenon.

A number of healthcare scandals have recently been reported (Box 16.1) where formal inquiries into what went wrong later found that it was not the actions of one particular individual or practitioner that led to the malpractice. Instead, these inquiries found, in each example, a complicity among practitioners that was termed by one inquiry as 'a culture of acceptance' and by another as 'systemic failure'. Practitioners had either become resigned to current practices or had become

---

BOX 16.1
ETHICAL SCENARIOS AND 'CULTURES OF ACCEPTANCE'

'Bloodgate'
- http://www.smh.com.au/rugby-union/union-news/doctor-ashamed-of-role-in-fake-blood-scandal-20100825-13qwe.html
- Bacchus Marsh Community Hospital – 11 preventable neonatal deaths
- http://www.abc.net.au/news/2016-06-08/review-finds-11-baby-deaths-avoidable-at-djerri-warrh-health/7492030

Incorrect results for prostate cancer
- http://www.abc.net.au/news/2016-04-03/cancer-pathology-blunder-false-positive-sacking/7295132
- Underdosing of chemotherapy for cancer patients
- http://www.abc.net.au/news/2016-10-31/chemotherapy-inquiry-to-hear-about-culture-of-acceptance/7978548

---

desensitized to their ethical obligations, allowing them to turn 'a blind eye' to what was going on.

Theresa decides to share her sense of ethical distress with a mentor, while maintaining confidentiality (see Case Study 16.2).

Theresa's conversation with her mentor raises the notion of moral agency or a person's capacity to act for the good in a situation. In terms of the Ethical Reasoning Bridge, by paying attention to 'what actually happens', as suggested by her mentor, via a self-expressed narrative (or lived experience), rather than via *a priori* normative ethical principles, Theresa begins to recognize and then exercise her moral agency. Ricoeur (2006) expresses this as being able to connect oneself to an experience and one's own actions in it and in doing so make oneself the 'author' of an ethical response. Although it is still not clear to Theresa what she 'ought to do' in this situation, she now understands that there are also other 'moral agencies' to be considered in this scenario, each with a willingness *or* capability to act that is yet to be determined.

Theresa takes what she has learned from adopting a nonnormative intentionality back to the 'site' of her professional knowledge base and decision-making responsibilities: the side of the ER Bridge where 'what ought to happen' is waiting for a response. But this normative 'what ought to happen' does not necessarily now offer the same conception of the scenario that it did before the first crossing of the ER Bridge. It is now less amenable to a prescriptive and individual solution, and more requires a negotiated and cultural change, in concert with others. It is also a necessary step, rather than an end in itself, because it is ultimately important 'to know not about *actuality* but about *possibility*' (Lear, 2006, cited in Mattingly, 2014, p. 28 – our emphasis).

Possibilities of 'what is the good' in a situation may arise from among a range of different perspectives and interests. The capability theory of justice proposed by Amartya Sen (2009), and further developed by Martha Nussbaum (2011), proposes that it is not sufficient for healthcare professions and practitioners to provide the conditions – via universal ethical principles or moral rules – by which the freedoms, personal autonomy and right to fairness for patients and others are respected. We need to be equally concerned with people's *actual* capabilities to exercise or act upon these things towards what they consider as important for their lives

CASE STUDY 16.2

Truth and Ethics

Theresa angrily expresses her feelings about her experience, 'The truth needs to be told about this situation!'

Her friend listens and responds, 'Yes, but whose truth?'

'What do you mean whose truth?' replies Theresa, suppressing a certain agitation at the question.

'Well, the way you are talking suggests that this is only one 'truth' or interpretation of what is happening when in fact there are multiple 'truths' in this scenario. Each person involved here has a particular perspective that influences their actions'.

'But surely' exclaims Theresa, 'the only perspectives that really count are those of Coral and John, and they are the ones we should be really listening to and acting upon'.

'You may well be right' replies the friend, 'but the fact is that this is not happening, regardless of whether it ought to. And so, although I agree with you that this resident's autonomy is not being fully respected, in order for there to be any meaningful change in this place, there has to be an understanding of everyone's choices in the situation – real or perceived – and who or what constrains those choices. Theresa, you have found yourself in 'a culture of acceptance'.

'What do you mean by 'culture of acceptance?' asks Theresa, calling upon her reserves of patience.

'Just that this ethical issue you have come across requires the assent – tacit or otherwise – and complicity of more than one person for it to be perpetrated. For there to be any change, you are going to have to understand why this "culture of acceptance" has come into being. Cultures tend to "happen" over time without explicit decision making or intention. Getting people to speak about their particular situation and how they see the situation helps open up this "culture" for examination. Sharing your dilemma with someone else – like me – was a good start'.

'And another thing, you could also find out more about the Aged Care Funding Instrument (ACFI) and how it is intended to work. I can assure you that what you are witnessing is not just happening where you are doing your placement. The claims made by aged care units on the high care needs of residents[1] have exceeded budgetary expectations. After you do that, you might be able to work out what other conversations and actions are possible. If you are still interested in working in the aged care field, you are going to need to come to grips with the way in which funding models and budgetary pressures influence behaviour and practice'.

[1]See https://agedcare.health.gov.au/tools-and-resources/aged-care-funding-instrument-acfi-reports

(Nussbaum, 2011; Sen, 2009). And this requires a public form of ethical reasoning and decision making that allows people to understand and act upon what they value in given situations (Sen, 2009).

Moral Identity and Agency

The question remains: How does a healthcare practitioner generate moral agency to act for the good in a workplace culture mediating ethical misconduct, where the wielding of power and rank by some persons over others may largely extinguish it? In such situations, the practitioner's capacity to critically reason and then act cannot be separated from his or her sense of a moral self (Ruitenberg, 2011).

How we understand 'our moral self' (or moral identity), according to the ancient Greek philosopher Aristotle, will determine the extent to which we can 'act for the good' (Mattingly, 2014). We, therefore, turn to a brief discussion of contemporary virtue ethics where the question concerning 'who we are' has become 'how we claim to know who we are' (Frank and Jones, 2003).

Two directions have arisen in the scholarship reinterpreting Aristotle's philosophy. One direction included philosophers such as Martin Heidegger, Alasdair MacIntyre, Iris Murdoch, Martha Nussbaum, Paul Ricoeur and Charles Taylor who, although not homogenous in their explanations of morality, nevertheless share a claim that a moral decision or action cannot be determined through some universal set of rules, procedures or reasoning processes derived from an Archimedean or 'third-person position'. The second direction is found in poststructuralism and the work of Foucault and Derrida (among others), who, in large part, agree with the first group discussed earlier, that what is 'moral' in a society is 'dependent upon the cultivation of virtues that are developed in and through social practices' (Mattingly, 2012, p. 164).

Foucault examined the social practices through which people create (or have created for them) their sense of who they are (Frank and Jones, 2003, p. 179). In doing so, he uncovered the surreptitious, often damaging and unjust ways that moral claims were made about those with mental health problems, those who were prisoners and (particularly relevant for medicine) those who were considered 'deviant', all as part of '"rehabilitative" practices that constructed those very same categories and created new forms of knowledge that defined them' (Mattingly, 2012, p. 163); the so-called shaping of 'docile bodies' under the 'clinical gaze'(Foucault, 1991). The overuse of psychotropic medication has been likened to this (De Bellis, 2006). He further demonstrated the role of social structures and discourse in shaping what is even understood as moral. And, for Foucault, this inevitably involved the exercise of power (Frank and Jones, 2003). In his later work, Foucault drew on Aristotelian ideas to offer a recognition of moral practices that he termed 'self-care' or 'self-cultivation' (of virtue) but warned that it can end up as 'no more than (or less than) practices of normalization of a particular regime of truth' (Mattingly, 2012, p. 173). And so, for Foucault, first-person ethics is the subjective work produced by (moral) agents to conduct themselves in accordance with their inquiry about what a good life is (Fassin, 2012, p. 7), and human agency is defined in terms of 'one's awareness of the nature of one's conformity (or not) to certain discursive practices rather than the efforts of particular individuals in particular circumstances' (Mattingly, 2012, p. 175).

Others have questioned whether Foucault's conclusions regarding the power of discourse to subjugate people collectively in particular social practices need also mean rejecting the idea of an individual moral agent who is able to develop a 'hermeneutic understanding of truth as self-interpretations' (Taylor, 1985b, p. 385). Such a hermeneutic-oriented, first-person ethics

draws on the phenomenological construct of intentionality (discussed earlier), where our understanding of reality 'out in the world' presents itself to us only in our engagement with it (Mattingly, 2012). Aristotle believed that 'the self' is 'grounded in capabilities for experiencing the world' (Baracchi, 2008, p. 2). Similarly, Ricoeur (1992) has argued that our moral identity is a narrative identity, where we make sense of ourselves only in and through our involvement with others and through the exercise of our capabilities. We do not simply enact a role, function or practice that has been assigned to us (in contrast to Foucault's ideas) but are capable of initiating new actions and choices (Ricoeur, 2006).

In summary, and without fully reconciling these two broad directions in virtue ethics, a view of moral identity and agency arises in which the power of discourse to subjugate people and the way they think, as outlined by Foucault, is acknowledged. That is, social practices – of which health care is one – are inevitably and thoroughly permeated by the use of power by some over others (see De Bellis, 2010; Parker, 2007, for discourses in aged care in Australia). However, at the same time, we concur with Ricoeur, Taylor, Sen and Nussbaum that individuals are capable of self-interpretation and, arising from that, therefore capable of choice and action. In Case Study 16.3, Theresa speaks once more with her clinical supervisor, Bev. Although she does not have much power as a student, in either the relationship or the aged care facility, she does exercise the moral agency that she has.

In her discussion with Bev, Theresa is able to name the complicity that enables this ethical scenario to continue, with its effects on residents such as Coral and her partner, John. From being tacit and unexpressed as an ethical issue, it begins to be articulated. To that extent, this is a movement towards public or social ethical reasoning. The exercise of moral agency by one party (student Theresa) leads, in this case, to the facilitation of moral agency in another, her clinical supervisor, Bev. Although there is usually a significant power and rank differential between a student and supervisor, nevertheless, it is one among others in this scenario – for example, between John and the nursing staff, between Bev and her manager, June. We want to suggest that the power in such relationships is not so fixed that capability for moral action is not possible. Theresa's overture to Bev may not

CASE STUDY 16.3

A Second Conversation Between Theresa and Bev

'Bev, thanks for agreeing to meet with me once more. I have looked at the way the ACFI works, and I can understand how, from a funding perspective, it may be better financially for the unit to maximize impairments of residents. However, I am still concerned that this approach is having a negative effect on residents. In particular, Coral's activity and participation capabilities are being held back by the reluctance to review the use of a lifter for every transfer. I find it really hard to face John and justify its use, when he is so frustrated and angry about it, and when I really think that there is potential for her to be able to transfer safely without it'.

'I have been here for 11 years now, Theresa. Over that time, I have seen how funding to run this place became more and more precarious. It got to the stage where the organization was laying off staff and our positions were in jeopardy. My partner and I still have a mortgage – it wasn't easy. I think with the ACFI model, we were thrown something of a lifeline. And maybe there is now some kind of overly strong grasp on this lifeline – I don't know. I will say that I hadn't realized quite how upset John was about Coral and the lifter. You must not have a very good opinion of me.'

'Well, I think what worries me, Bev – apart from Coral and John's situation – is that I am discovering an unwanted truth about the extent to which I am able to practice my profession in an ethical way. And that is, a growing realization that other things outside my own knowledge, skills and values influence what I do as a physiotherapist with people, more than I would have ever believed'.

'You do learn not to be naïve in this work, Theresa. But ... on the other hand, I don't want to lose sight of why I entered aged care work either. I think that there may still be some in our organization who remain caught in our traditional identity as a nursing home and aren't willing to recognize the more recent focus on the rehabilitative work we undertake with residents – you know, the idea that they can actually improve. I think we should get another review done of Coral and her level of care. I will have to speak with June – she has lots of pressures on her – but the satisfaction of the residents and families is an important part of our ongoing viability – and accreditation – too. I am not sure, but maybe we need to have some sort of in-service staff session about these issues'.

---

always 'work' as a conflict resolution 'method' or lead to a particular outcome.

Occasionally workplace cultures can become so entrenched in ethical misconduct and resistant to change that moral agency must take the form of becoming a whistleblower.[i] However, our focus here is in recognizing and working in less extreme cases. In the way that Theresa approaches this conversation, we see that it does provide space for Bev to engage in self-interpretation and consider her own moral identity and choices. And from this, Bev may, in turn, choose to similarly converse with other staff, including her boss, June, about Coral and John's situation.

A single conversation does not represent a complete resolution of this ethical dilemma. However, it is a step toward 'critiquing' a culture. Possibilities will need to be explored by the various parties at the local level (i.e., in addressing Coral and John's situation); at the institutional level (i.e., recognizing what is happening at the facility and engaging staff perspectives regarding what may be possible as a response); and finally, at wider policy levels (i.e., how the company running this unit together with the wider Aged Care industry, and professional associations, and providing feedback to government regarding the efficacy of funding models such as ACFI). Such actions will only be achieved when those involved in this scenario realize their own moral agency.

The ER Bridge (see Fig. 16.1) represents how one's moral identity, as an individual, is shaped in and by

---

[i]For example, Bundaberg Hospital: http://www.abc.net.au/news/2005-06-23/whistleblower-nurse-fronts-bundaberg-hospital/1599220

our relationships with others in the various communities (practice, workplace and societal) to which we belong. Moral agency is therefore partly a function of how we see or interpret ourselves in relation to others in these communities. Individuals have capabilities to act 'for the good' in their communities – of whatever kind – to the point where a community might then reexamine their own collective sense of identity and purpose.

CHAPTER SUMMARY

In this chapter, we have outlined an ethical reasoning model termed the Ethical Reasoning Bridge. This model aims to assist the practitioner to negotiate the sometimes difficult moral terrain between the normative 'what ought to happen …' and nonnormative 'what actually happens…'. When the practitioner 'crosses' the ER Bridge, he or she explores the relationship between normative ethics and nonnormative ethics such that the value of each is further enriched by the ethical insights provided by the other.

We have also outlined how, in crossing the ER Bridge, there is also a movement between individual ethical reasoning and social or public ethical reasoning. Social reasoning allows for the examination of relations between various parties – sometimes presenting as cultures – as factors that influence or constrain choice. Understanding people's choices (or their perception of them) helps understand their sense of moral agency.

Finally, we have proposed that ethical reasoning cannot be separated from the moral identity of the problem solver. One's moral identity is formed, in part, through the relationships an individual has with others, and this, in turn, influences a sense of moral agency.

REFLECTION POINT 1

Think of an ethical scenario that you have either observed or been involved in at your workplace (or on placement).

1. How might using the ER Bridge, with normative and nonnormative ethical analyses of the case, inform your response to both the ethical issue and the other persons involved?
2. What communication skills might you need for your intended response to become an action?
3. How does your ethical response relate to your professional identity and role?

REFERENCES

Baracchi, C., 2008. Aristotle's Ethics as First Philosophy. Cambridge University Press, Cambridge, MA.

Beauchamp, T.L.C., Childress, J.F., 2009. Principles of Biomedical Ethics, sixth ed. Oxford University Press, New York, NY.

Burke Johnson, R., Onwuegbuzie, A., Turner, L., 2007. Toward a definition of mixed methods research. J. Mix Methods Res. 1, 112–133.

Callahan, D., 2003. Principlism and communitarianism. J. Med. Ethics 29, 287–291.

De Bellis, A., 2006. Behind open doors: a construct of nursing practice in an Australian residential aged care facility, PhD thesis. Flinders University, Adelaide, VIC.

De Bellis, A., 2010. Australian residential aged care and the quality of nursing care provision. Contemp. Nurse 35, 100–113.

Delany, C., Edwards, I., Fryer, C., In press. How physical therapists perceive, interpret and respond to the ethical dimensions of practice: a qualitative study. Physiother. Theory Pract.

Edwards, I., 2016. The moral experience of the patient with chronic pain. In: van Rysewyk, S. (Ed.), Human Meanings of Pain. Springer International Publishing, New York, NY, pp. 195–210.

Edwards, I., Delany, C., 2008. Ethical reasoning. In: Higgs, J., Jones, M.A., Loftus, S., et al. (Eds.), Clinical Reasoning in the Health Professions, third ed. Elsevier, Edinburgh, pp. 279–289.

Edwards, I., Delany, C.M., Townsend, A.F., et al., 2011. Moral agency as enacted justice: a clinical and ethical decision-making framework for responding to health inequities and social injustice. Phys. Ther. 91, 1653–1663.

Edwards, I., Jones, M.A., Carr, J., et al., 2004. Clinical reasoning strategies in physical therapy. Phys. Ther. 84, 312–335.

Fassin, D., 2012. Introduction: toward a critical moral anthropology. In: Fassin, D. (Ed.), Toward a Critical Moral Anthropology. Wiley-Blackwell, Oxford, UK, pp. 1–17.

Foucault, M., 1991. Discipline and Punish. Penguin Books, London, UK.

Fox, R., 1994. The entry of U.S. bioethics into the 1990's: a sociological analysis. In: Dubose, E.R., Hamel, R., O'Connell, L.I. (Eds.), A Matter of Principles? Ferment in US Bioethics. Trinity Press International, Valley Forge, PA, pp. 21–71.

Frank, A., Jones, T., 2003. Bioethics and the later Foucault. J. Med. Human. 24, 179–186.

Gallagher, S., Zahavi, D., 2007. The Phenomenological Mind: An Introduction to Philosophy of Mind and Cognitive Science. Routledge, London, UK.

Greenfield, B.H., Jensen, G.M., 2010. Understanding the lived experiences of patients: application of a phenomenological approach to ethics. Phys. Ther. 90, 1185–1197.

Hugman, R., 2005. New Approaches in Ethics for the Caring Professions. Palgrave Macmillan, New York, NY.

Kahneman, D., 2011. Thinking, Fast and Slow. Farrar, Straus and Giroux, New York, NY.

Komesaroff, P., 2008. Experiments in Love and Death: Medicine, Postmernism, Microethics and the Body. Melbourne University Press, Melbourne, VIC.

Larkin, M., Eatough, V., Osborn, M., 2011. Interpretative phenomenological analysis and embodied, active, situated cognition. Theory Psychol. 21, 318–337.

MacIntyre, A.C., 2007. After Virtue: A Study in Moral Theory, third ed. University of Notre Dame Press, Notre Dame, IN.

Mattingly, C., 2012. Two virtue ethics and the anthropology of morality. Anthropol. Theory 12, 161–184.

Mattingly, C., 2014. Moral Laboratories: Family Peril and the Struggle for a Good Life. University of California Press, Oakland, CA.

Nagel, T., 1989. The View From Nowhere. Oxford University Press, New York, NY.

Nussbaum, M., 2011. Creating Capabilities: The Human Development Approach. The Belknap Press of Harvard University Press, Cambridge, MA.

Parker, D., 2007. The discourses of death and dying in residential aged care facilities in Australia. In: Abstracts Supplement, DDD8: The Social Context of Death, Dying & Disposal Conference 2007. DDD8: 8th International Conference on the Social Context of Death, Dying and Disposal, 12–15 September, Bath, UK, p. S68.

Purtilo, R., 2005. Ethical Dimensions in the Health Professions, fourth ed. Saunders, Philadelphia, PA.

Reunanen, M.A., Talvitie, U., Jarvikoski, A., et al., 2016. Client's role and participation in stroke physiotherapy encounters: an observational study. Eur. J. Physiother. 18, 210–217.

Ricoeur, P., 1992. Oneself as Another. University of Chicago Press, Chicago, IL.

Ricoeur, P., 2006. Capabilities and rights. In: Nebel, M., Sagovsky, N. (Eds.), Transforming Unjust Structures: The Capability Approach. Springer, Dordrecht, The Netherlands, pp. 17–26.

Ruitenberg, C., 2011. The empty chair: education in an ethic of hospitality. Philos. Educ. 28–36.

Sen, A., 2009. The Idea of Justice. The Belknap Press of Harvard University Press, Cambridge, MA.

Shepard, K., Jensen, G., 1990. Physical therapist curricula for the 1990's: educating the reflective practitioner. Phys. Ther. 70, 566–577.

Swisher, L.L., van Kessel, G., Jones, M.A., et al., 2012. Evaluating moral reasoning outcomes in physical therapy ethics education: stage, schema, phase, and type. Phys. Ther. Rev. 17, 167–175.

Taylor, C., 1985a. Philosophy and the Human Sciences: Philosophical Papers, 2. Cambridge University Press, Cambridge, MA.

Taylor, C., 1985b. Connelly, Foucault, and truth. Polit. Theory 13, 377–385.

Taylor, C., 1989. Sources of the Self: The Making of the Modern Identity. Harvard University Press, Cambridge, MA.

Volf, M., 1996. Exclusion and Embrace: A Theological Exploration of Identity, Otherness and Reconciliation. Abingdon Press, Nashville, TN.

Zahavi, D., 2005. Subjectivity and Selfhood: Investigating the First Person Perspective. MIT Press, Cambridge, MA.

17

SHARED DECISION MAKING IN PRACTICE

CINDY COSTANZO ▪ JOY DOLL ▪ GAIL M. JENSEN

CHAPTER AIMS

The aims of this chapter are to:

▪ identify key attributes of shared decision making (SDM) in practice,

▪ recognize organizational characteristics that support and facilitate SDM and

▪ describe practice strategies that lead to successful outcomes when engaged in SDM.

KEY WORDS

Shared decision making

Decision making

Interprofessional teams

ABBREVIATIONS/ ACRONYMS

EHR Electronic health record

IPE Interprofessional education

IPCP Interprofessional collaborative practice

IPDAS International Patient Decision Aids Standards Collaboration

IP-SDM Interprofessional Shared Decision Making

SDM Shared decision making

INTRODUCTION

Health and well-being rely on the ability of a patient to make good decisions every day and over time.

Healthcare providers often express frustration by the lack of engagement patients hold in the healthcare process and their own well-being. Yet healthcare systems and cultures clearly do not consistently support collaborative decision making of healthcare team members with patients. Shared decision making (SDM) offers an avenue to address the disconnects in care by engaging patients in collaboration with healthcare professionals in making informed healthcare decisions. In addition to identifying and describing the processes and best practices of SDM, the chapter will discuss the importance of organizational culture in the influence of the adoption and sustainability of SDM. In addition, SDM models, measurement tools and decisional aids that augment SDM in practice will be shared. This chapter promotes the use of interprofessional, team-based practices and a patient-centred SDM model to ultimately improve clinical outcomes of care.

SHARED DECISION MAKING

Historically, decision making between healthcare professionals and patients has followed three definitive models: paternalism, consumerism and SDM (Fig. 17.1). A paternalistic model occurs when a provider or healthcare team makes the primary decisions and choices *for* the patient. A consumerist informative model occurs when the consumer makes a decision *without* involvement of a provider or healthcare team (Charles et al., 1997). SDM occurs *with* the involvement of patients, providers and interprofessional team members in the decision-making process. SDM is defined as 'an approach where

181

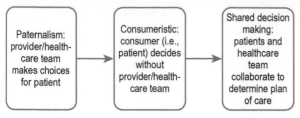

Fig. 17.1 ■ Patient decision-making approaches.

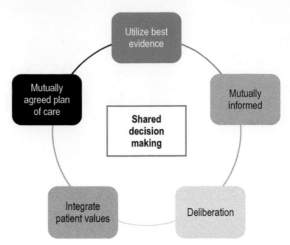

Fig. 17.2 ■ Components of shared decision making.

clinicians and patients share the best available evidence when faced with the task of making decisions, and where patients are supported to consider options, to achieve informed preferences' (Barr et al., 2014).

SDM is best practice and should be mainstreamed, but its implementation and execution continue to be challenging (Müller et al., 2016). Informed consent, informed choice, consumer rights, patient-centred care and chronic illnesses with a lifetime management approach have accelerated the shift from the once dominant paternalistic approach to SDM (Charles et al., 1997). SDM provides a forum for the healthcare team to involve the patient and family as part of the team. Today's complexity of care reinforces the need for SDM and requires that the interprofessional team become adept at utilizing this approach. As health care moves towards interprofessional collaborative practice, it is critical that patients and families are valued members of this team (Interprofessional Education Collaborative, 2016).

Attributes of Shared Decision Making

In SDM, the perspectives of the patient and/or family are valued as they collaborate with the healthcare team to make decisions about care (Interprofessional Education Collaborative, 2016). For SDM to be successful, several important actions are required. In SDM, interprofessional team members and patients must acknowledge that a decision should be made utilizing the best evidence, are mutually informed with an understanding of the decision's risks and benefits, hold a period of deliberation and incorporate the patient's values and preferences as the team and patient arrive at a mutually agreed-upon care plan (Charles et al., 1997; Légaré et al., 2010; Légaré and Witteman, 2013; Sepucha et al., 2016) (Fig. 17.2). Gravel et al. (2006) also acknowledge that SDM relies on provider

motivation and the experience of positive outcomes of SDM experienced by both the clinicians and patients involved. Although patients and healthcare team members often speak different languages, health literacy and the healthcare team's ability to provide health information in a manner that supports the patient's capacity to make an informed shared decision are vital (Edwards et al., 2009).

SDM is not necessarily a natural process for the healthcare team. Légaré and Witteman (2013) identify three elements that are critical for SDM, including recognition that a decision needs to occur, knowledge of evidence-based practice and ensuring that the patients' values are part of the decision-making process. Although SDM has been particularly addressed as a role for physicians, all members of the healthcare team can assist and be involved in SDM. Makoul and Clayman (2006) provide an integrative model that identifies essential elements of SDM. These elements include the following:

- The problem is defined by patients and providers.
- Options are presented with supportive physician knowledge and recommendations.
- Benefits and risks are discussed.
- Patient values and preferences are included.
- The ability for the patient to follow through with the plan is discussed.
- There is an opportunity for any reclarification.
- The decision is made or deferred.
- Follow-up is organized.

Barriers to Shared Decision Making

Overcoming barriers to SDM can facilitate its adoption and use across healthcare settings. Historically, healthcare decisions were made utilizing a paternalistic approach, and this continues across many healthcare settings today. As with any change in healthcare delivery, barriers exist in the implementation of SDM. When it comes to the healthcare team, barriers can occur with or between individual practitioners and could include differences in healthcare knowledge, attitudes or beliefs that are not supportive of SDM and lack of agreement among team members when making a decision (Légaré et al., 2008, 2013). Similar to the barriers seen in implementing interprofessional care, SDM faces challenges when healthcare team members do not dedicate time to discuss the processes of SDM. Lack of investment of time in identifying the processes of SDM leads to discrepancies in how decisions are made, which may cause conflict among the team members and the patient. Healthcare team members must commit to SDM and not let issues like individual practitioners' lack of motivation or self-confidence interfere with SDM (Légaré et al., 2008).

SDM may also be a challenge when patients are not interested in being part of the decision process. Depending on differences in culture and health beliefs, some patients may find the process of being asked to engage in SDM uncomfortable and countercultural. These beliefs can act as barriers to the successful implementation of SDM. Beyond providers and patients, systemic barriers exist for SDM, including time constraints, lack of resources to support SDM, reimbursement concerns and lack of organizational support. Some barriers may not actually exist but may be perceived to occur, such as lack of support for SDM by the healthcare system or healthcare team; such support and relevant infrastructure for implementation of SDM are necessary at team and organizational levels (Légaré et al., 2008).

REFLECTION POINT 1

How do these barriers for SDM apply to your practice?

Shared Decision Making in Practice

SDM in practice environments calls upon healthcare teams to take on a healing- and wellness-oriented approach rather than a scientific approach based on cure and pathology. Such an approach recognizes not only *scientific* evidence but also human perspectives and aspirations in healthcare decisions. The first step in implementing SDM is ensuring that all healthcare team members are educated and understand how to engage in SDM. Team members must address their own professional socialization issues and enculturation, including attitudes of paternalism and power that often influence the patient, family and team. Next, healthcare team members need to become comfortable with uncertainty, which will help them assist patients to recognize that much of health care includes varied levels of uncertainty that can be uncomfortable for all involved. Yet SDM offers an avenue for addressing uncertainly and further dialogue by all stakeholders, including patients, families and members of the healthcare team. Ultimately, addressing uncertainty and encouraging further dialogue in an open and honest forum can facilitate positive healthcare decisions (Braddock 2012).

Cultural Influences: Individual and Organizational on Shared Decision Making

Individual cultural beliefs and values have an influence on SDM. Healthcare providers' norms, language and practices are formed and framed within a cultural perspective that is unique to each individual and profession (Pecukonis et al., 2008). Both patients and healthcare professionals hold cultural beliefs and stereotypes about each other. Recognizing how beliefs and perceptions are formed about other people, professions and the roles that (healthcare) professionals play are important all of these factors directly affect the development and implementation of SDM practices. Realizing the opportunities and challenges created by professionalism and intercultural interactions with the patient is important and helps identify opportunities and barriers to communication and collaboration with patients. This, in turn, helps ensure that SDM promotes optimal health outcomes (Légaré et al., 2008). Barriers between patients and providers can lead to medical errors, poor patient outcomes, decreased patient satisfaction and health disparities (Nelson, 2002).

Organizations are composed of individuals with beliefs, values and practices that are unique to each person but which unite and represent the overall organizational culture. Leadership, operational procedures and processes, care practices and employee behaviours are influenced by the organizational culture. Shared decision-making processes are congruent with organizational cultures that demonstrate strong, mutually respectful relationships between the patient, care providers and interprofessional healthcare team. An organization that adopts and supports a shared relationship model (i.e., relational coordination, relational coproduction and relational leadership) contributes to operational success and positive outcomes for the organization (Gittell et al., 2012; Moreau et al., 2012). Adopting SDM principles can help interprofessional teams by supporting a shared mental model that has been identified as a strategy for success among interprofessional teams (Ginsburg and Tregunno, 2005). Fortunately, many of the SDM practice environment and organizational culture issues can be addressed simultaneously with interprofessional collaborative practice development.

CASE STUDY 17.1

Shared Decision Making

Tom, a 45-year-old construction worker, has an appointment at a recently opened ambulatory care clinic in his neighbourhood. When making his appointment, Tom reported he experienced a fall a couple days ago hurting his wrist and ankle. During the phone call for the appointment, the front desk staff asked Tom to begin thinking about options for his care and his priorities. The front desk scheduler explains to Tom that the clinic uses a healthcare team, and he may be seen by multiple professionals to address his issues, and patients are a valued member of this team. She indicates Tom will have an active role in deciding his care.

After arriving for the appointment, the front desk receptionist reiterates to Tom that he will see a team and that at the clinic patients are encouraged to voice their desires for their care. Once Tom is checked in, the medical assistant brings him back to an examination room to get a brief history and also learns that he recently lost his job as a construction worker. The medical assistant encourages Tom to share this with the provider and also documents it in the electronic health record. During the patient interview, the medical assistant observes and notes that some cuts Tom received from the fall do not look well cleaned. The medical assistant mentions this to Tom, and Tom asks what he could do to keep them clean. At this request, the medical assistant cleans the cuts and educates Tom how to properly keep the wounds clean. Before departing the examination room, the medical assistant encourages Tom to ask questions during his visit and share how he wants his care delivered. The medical assistant enters the ambulatory care pod, where clinicians can speak openly about patients, and shares information from the brief patient history.

As a result of previous physician visits, Tom believes that he will just be getting some medication and sent on his way. He does not realize that behind the doors of his room, there is a large team of medical professionals collaborating to meet all of his needs. Tom is also viewed as a valued member of this team who will be asked to help make decisions regarding his care. The healthcare team, including Tom, is committed to engaging patients in their health care and value-shared decision making as part of patient care. The team is composed of a medical assistant, medical resident, occupational therapist, pharmacist, physical therapist, psychologist, public health nurse, radiological technician and social worker. The team holds the value that all members of the team, including the patient, can speak up and advocate for the patient. Patients are informed about the opportunity to be engaged in their care and encouraged to engage in SDM as part of the team. The psychologist acts as the team coach supporting the team and its members, ensuring that the team works effectively. He or she ensures that the patient is included and is a facilitator for SDM among the team and the patient. The team engages in 'huddles' twice a day, where team members identify clinic issues for each session followed by a previsit planning session, where the healthcare team reviews the patient caseload for the session. When a patient's case is considered complex, any team member can identify the individual for case review at the weekly interprofessional care planning meeting.

The medical resident enters the room after being briefed by the medical assistant. She reviews with

Shared Decision Making (Continued)

Tom the concerns the medical assistant reported. Upon this review, the medical resident informs Tom that she wants him involved with deciding the next steps in his care. Tom tells her his priority is his wrist, but he is very concerned that if it is broken he will not have insurance for follow-up. The medical resident acknowledges this fear and tells Tom she would recommend a radiograph to determine whether it is broken. She would also like him to visit with the social worker to discuss options for job opportunities and insurance coverage. She would recommend a prescription of an antibiotic for his cuts because of risk for infection. Tom reports he would like to first determine whether his wrist is broken with a radiograph. He feels this is a good first step.

Upon exiting the examination room, the medical resident with physician supervision identifies that she and Tom identified the following priorities:

- radiograph of wrist to determine potential fracture,
- prescription for antibiotic to address potential infection in his cuts and
- referral to social work to address recent job loss.

The resident knows he has access to many resources on the healthcare team but also recognizes that Tom is feeling very overwhelmed from the fall and his job loss. The medical resident proceeds to review all the options with the patient including inviting him to attend the interprofessional team meeting later that week. Tom gets a little teary eyed, admitting to the resident that with his job loss, he will soon lose health insurance coverage. He is anxious about accessing other services because of cost. The resident recommends that because of the acuteness of his wrist injury, a radiograph is highly recommended at the appointment. He encourages Tom to take a moment to consider his options and leaves the examination room.

Tom decides that he would like the radiograph and to visit with the social worker. Because of transportation issues, he does not feel he can come back to the clinic for the interprofessional team meeting but is willing to have the team discuss options and have the social worker follow up with him.

When the healthcare team meets to discuss Tom's case, the medical resident reports concern for Tom, including the possibility of developing depression because of his recent job loss. The team decides that the social worker will contact Tom to discuss his options, especially related to his wrist fracture confirmed via the radiograph.

Because of the collaboration of the interprofessional team and efforts to engage Tom in SDM, the healthcare team is able to work with him to identify his prioritized needs that include finding a new job, which is identified as a priority by both Tom and the healthcare team.

REFLECTION POINT 2

What attributes of SDM and key elements of organizational culture contributed to a collaborative team approach in this case?

Interprofessional Collaborative Practice and Shared Decision Making

When the Core Competencies for Interprofessional Collaborative Practice (IPCP) were released in 2011, these competencies provided a foundation for a larger discussion about interprofessional education and practice (Interprofessional Education Collaborative, 2011, 2016). Healthcare professions exhibit many differences, including their professional cultures, but they have one thing in common: their caring for the patient and family. Despite their differences, all healthcare professionals identify with 'a sense of shared purpose to support the common good in healthcare, and reflect a shared commitment to creating safer, more efficient and more effective systems of care' (Interprofessional Education Collaborative, 2011, p. 17). The intent of interprofessional collaboration is that clinicians work 'deliberatively' together with the patient and family to provide optimal health care. Based on the principles and values of IPCP, healthcare professionals must learn to work in teams to collaborate 'with others through shared problem-solving and SDM, especially in circumstances of uncertainty' (Interprofessional Education Collaborative, 2011, p. 24). Despite extensive literature supporting SDM as a valuable approach for the patient and single physician, emerging models for SDM with the interprofessional care team are increasingly supported as a means of helping the team engage in collaborative patient-centred care planning (Légaré et al., 2010).

Implementation of the Interprofessional Shared Decision-Making (IP-SDM) Model

Légaré et al. (2010, 2011a, 2013) implemented and tested a IP-SDM model. They found the model useful and easy to understand for team members during the implementation phase of SDM. The authors report that the model served as an excellent guide, enhanced the team's understanding of the conceptual foundation of the SDM process and enhanced collaboration within the interprofessional team. Having a team member enact the role of a decisional coach has been found to be a successful strategy during the implementation process of IP-SDM (Shunk et al., 2014). Decision coaches can be any one of multiple team members who helps the patient, family and healthcare team members reach a decision based on the principles of SDM. Coaches help the team engage in effective SDM by overseeing the process and providing feedback to team members. Through this process, team members develop in their abilities with SDM. Decision coaches can be members of the healthcare team who agree to take on this additional role to support the interprofessional healthcare team. The IP-SDM model with six process steps is outlined in Table 17.1.

Although there are limitations identified in using the IP-SDM model, Yu et al. (2014) identified that these limitations can be resolved by a deliberative interprofessional team that is engaged in respectful communication. The challenges with implementing interprofessional collaborative practice have been well documented and are no different from the support needed for SDM in the interprofessional team. Barriers to SDM for the interprofessional team include issues with knowledge of IP-SDM and patient-centred care among team members, team performance norms, individual team members' attitudes and perceptions towards IP-SDM, external factors like reimbursement and organizational support by leadership (Chong et al., 2013). Clinicians may have differing opinions of how much patients should be involved in SDM. Yet IP-SDM can be supported and facilitated through training of team members, establishing team commitments among team members and organizational support. The barriers and supports for both SDM and interprofessional care align. Overall, in order for SDM to be successful in the interprofessional care model, the healthcare team has to work through the basic principles of team development to ensure that power dynamics are conducive to SDM and essentially work towards becoming a high-performing, *collaborative*

TABLE 17.1
Interprofessional Shared Decision-Making Model

Steps	Description
1. Patient presents (at the healthcare centre), and a decision needs to be made	'professionals share their knowledge and understanding of the options with the patient while recognizing equipoise* and the need for a decision' (Légaré et al., 2011b, p. 21). *a balance of forces or interests
2. Exchange of information	'The health professional(s) and the patient share information about the potential benefits and harms of the options, using educational material, patient decision aids, and other evidence-based resources' (Légaré et al., 2011b, p. 22).
3. Value clarification	Clarifying values by all involved in the decision-making process.
4. Feasibility of options	The healthcare team has a good understanding of options available to the patient.
5. Decision	Team members agree upon a decision.
6. Support patient	Healthcare team members support the patient revisiting the decision as needed.

REFLECTION POINT 3

Why is SDM a challenge in comparison to traditional approaches to clinical reasoning? What teaching and learning strategies might be most effective to help develop SDM commitment and abilities? How do you think EHR might facilitate SDM?

REFERENCES

Archer, N., Fevrier-Thomas, U., Lokker, C., et al., 2011. Personal health records: a scoping review. J. Am. Med. Inform. Assoc. 18, 515–522.

Barr, P.J., Thompson, R., Walsh, T., et al., 2014. The psychometric properties of CollaboRATE: a fast and frugal patient-reported measure of the shared decision-making process. J. Med. Internet Res. 16, e2.

Bouniols, N., Leclère, B., Moret, L., 2016. Evaluating the quality of shared decision making during the patient-carer encounter: a systematic review of tools. BMC Res. Notes 9, 382.

Braddock, C., 2012. Supporting shared decision making when clinical evidence is low. Med. Care Res. Rev. 70 (Suppl. 1), 129S–140S.

Charles, C., Gafni, A., Whelan, T., 1997. Shared decision-making in the medical encounter: what does it mean? (or it takes at least two to tango). Soc. Sci. Med. 44, 681–692.

Chong, W., Aslani, P., Chen, T., 2013. Multiple perspectives on shared decision-making and interprofessional collaboration in mental healthcare. J. Interprof. Care 27, 223–230.

Cox, C., White, D., Abernethy, A., 2014. A universal decision support system: addressing the decision-making needs of patients, families, and clinicians in the setting of critical illness. Am. J. Resp. Crit. Care Med. 190, 366–373.

Davis, S., Roudsari, A., Raworth, R., et al., 2017. Shared decision-making using personal health record technology: a scoping review at the crossroads. J. Am. Med. Inform. Assoc. Available from:: https://doi.org/10.1093/jamia/ocw172.

Edwards, M., Davies, M., Edwards, A., 2009. What are the external influences on information exchange and shared decision-making in healthcare consultations: a meta-synthesis of the literature. Patient Educ. Couns. 75, 37–52.

Epstein, R., Street, R., 2011. Shared mind: communication, decision making, and autonomy in serious illness. Ann. Fam. Med. 9, 454–461.

Ginsburg, L., Tregunno, D., 2005. New approaches to interprofessional education and collaborative practice: lessons from the organizational change literature. J. Interprof. Care 19 (Suppl. 1), 177–187.

Gittell, J., Godfrey, M., Thistlethwaite, J., 2012. Interprofessional collaborative practice and relational coordination: improving healthcare through relationships. J. Interprof. Care 27, 210–213.

Gravel, K., Légaré, F., Graham, I., 2006. Barriers and facilitators to implementing shared decision-making in clinical practice: a systematic review of health professions perceptions. Implement. Sci. 9, 1–16.

Hauser, K., Koerfer, A., Christian, K., et al., 2015. Outcome-relevant effects of shared decision making: a systematic review. Dtsch. Arztebl. Int. 112, 665–671.

International Patient Decision Aids Standards Collaboration (IPDAS), n.d. Viewed 7 April 2017. Available from: http://ipdas.ohri.ca.

Interprofessional Education Collaborative, 2011. Core Competencies for Interprofessional Collaborative Practice: Report of an Expert Panel. Interprofessional Education Collaborative, Washington, DC.

Interprofessional Education Collaborative, 2016. Core Competencies for Interprofessional Collaborative Practice: Report of an Expert Panel. Interprofessional Education Collaborative, Washington, DC.

Kasper, J., Hoffmann, F., Heesen, C., et al., 2012. MAPPIN'SDM: the multifocal approach to sharing in shared decision making. PLoS ONE 7, 123.

Körner, M., Ehrhardt, H., Steger, A., 2013. Designing an interprofessional training program for shared decision making. J. Interprof. Care 27, 146–154.

Leader, A., Daskalakis, C., Braddock, C.H., et al., 2012. Measuring informed decision making about prostate cancer screening in primary care. Society for Medical Decision Making 32, 327–336.

Légaré, F., Witteman, H., 2013. Shared decision making: examining key elements and barriers to adoption into routine clinical practice. Health Aff. (Millwood) 32, 276–284.

Légaré, F., Ratté, S., Gravel, K., et al., 2008. Barriers and facilitators to implementing shared decision-making in clinical practice: update of a systematic review of health professionals' perceptions. Patient Educ. Couns. 73, 526–535.

Légaré, F., Ratté, S., Stacey, D., et al., 2010. Interventions for improving the adoption of shared decision making by healthcare professionals. Cochrane Database Syst. Rev. (5), CD006732.

Légaré, F., Stacey, D., Brière, N., et al., 2011a. A conceptual framework for interprofessional shared decision making in home care: protocol for a feasibility study. BMC Health Serv. Res. 11, 23.

Légaré, F., Stacey, D., Brière, N., et al., 2013. Healthcare providers' intentions to engage in an interprofessional approach to shared decision-making in home care programs: a mixed methods study. J. Interprof. Care 27, 214–222.

Légaré, F., Stacey, D., Pouliot, S., et al., 2011b. Interprofessionalism and shared decision-making in primary care: a stepwise approach towards a new model. J. Interprof. Care 25, 18–25.

Légaré, F., Turcotte, S., Robitaille, H., et al., 2012. Some but not all dyadic measures in shared decision making research have satisfactory psychometric properties. J. Clin. Epidemiol. 65, 1310–1320.

Makoul, G., Clayman, M., 2006. An integrative model of shared decision making in medical encounters. Patient Educ. Couns. 60, 301–312.

McDonald, H., Charles, C., Gafni, A., 2011. Assessing the conceptual clarity and evidence base of quality criteria/standards developed for evaluating decision aids. Health Expect. 17, 232–243.

Moreau, A., Carol, L., Dedianne, M., et al., 2012. What perceptions do patients have of decision making (DM)? Toward an integrative patient-centered care model: a qualitative study using focus-group interviews. Patient Educ. Couns. 87, 206–211.

Müller, E., Hahlweg, P., Scholl, I., 2016. What do stakeholders need to implement shared decision making in routine cancer care? A qualitative needs assessment. Acta Oncol. (Madr) 55, 1484–1491.

Nelson, A., 2002. Unequal treatment: confronting racial and ethnic disparities in health care. J. Natl Med. Assoc. 94, 666–668.

Oshima Lee, E., Emanuel, E.J., 2013. Shared decision making to improve care and reduce costs. N. Engl. J. Med. 368, 6–8.

Pecukonis, E., Doyle, O., Bliss, D., 2008. Reducing barriers to interprofessional training: promoting interprofessional cultural competence. J. Interprof. Care 22, 417–428.

Ruland, C., Bakken, S., 2002. Developing, implementing, and evaluating decision support systems for shared decision making in patient care: a conceptual model and case illustration. J. Biomed. Informat. 35, 313–321.

Scholl, I., Kriston, L., Dirmaier, J., et al., 2012. Development and psychometric properties of the shared decision making questionnaire-physician version (SDM-Q-Doc). Patient Educ. Couns. 88, 284–290.

Sepucha, K., Borkhoff, C., Lally, J., et al., 2013. Establishing the effectiveness of patient decision aids: key constructs and measurement instruments. BMC Med. Inform. Decis. Mak. 13 (Suppl. 2), S12.

Sepucha, K., Breslin, M., Graffeo, C., et al., 2016. State of the science: tools and measurement for shared decision making. Acad. Emerg. Med. 23, 1325–1331.

Shunk, R., Dulay, M., Chou, C., et al., 2014. Huddle-coaching. Acad. Med. 89, 244–250.

Tinetti, M.E., Fried, T.R., Boyd, C.M., 2012. Designing health care for the most common chronic condition—multimorbidity. JAMA 307, 2493–2494.

Yu, C., Stacey, D., Sale, J., et al., 2014. Designing and evaluating an interprofessional shared decision-making and goal-setting decision aid for patients with diabetes in clinical care: systematic decision aid development and study protocol. Implement. Sci. 9, 16.

18

USING DECISION AIDS TO INVOLVE CLIENTS IN CLINICAL DECISION MAKING

LYNDAL TREVENA ■ KIRSTEN MCCAFFERY

CHAPTER AIMS

The aims of this chapter are to:

- introduce the principles of shared decision making and the potential role of patient decision aids,
- define the types of clinical decisions that are best suited to the use of patient decision aids,
- outline the evidence for the effectiveness of patient decision aids on involving patients in clinical decisions,
- outline the International Patient Decisions Aids Standards (IPDAS) and how they can be used to assess the quality of patient decision aids,
- introduce emerging evidence on team-based decision making in health care and
- introduce emerging evidence on involvement of patients with lower health literacy.

KEY WORDS

Decision aids

Patient involvement

The evidence-base

Quality standards

ABBREVIATIONS

IPDAS International Patient Decision Aids Standards

SDM Shared decision making

RCT Randomized controlled trial

INTRODUCTION

Shared decision making (SDM) is a process by which a healthcare decision is made collaboratively among a patient, healthcare professionals and others. It has also been described as 'collaborative deliberation' (Elwyn et al., 2014) with one of the key components of this process being to ensure that both knowledge and power are shared between the healthcare professional and the patient (Joseph-Williams et al., 2014). This is an important and effective strategy for involving clients in decisions about their health care.

Increasingly, client involvement is being included in policies such as the US Affordable Care Act and the UK's 'No decision about me without me' report (Department of Health, 2011). Similarly, Canada, France, Germany, Netherlands and Australia all have policies and patient charters that include greater client involvement in healthcare decisions. There are many different strategies and tools that can be used to facilitate this process (Hoffmann et al., 2014), but arguably the most studied of these (and the focus of this chapter) are patient decision aids.

WHAT IS A PATIENT DECISION AID?

The International Patient Decision Aids Standards (IPDAS) Collaboration (Trevena et al., 2013) defines decision aids as "evidence-based tools designed to help patients to participate in making specific and deliberated choices among healthcare options" (Trevena et al., 2013, n.p.). They are intended to supplement (rather than replace) conversations with healthcare professionals, and they generally will:

1. 'Explicitly state the decision that needs to be considered;
2. Provide evidence-based information about a health condition, the options, associated benefits, harms, probabilities and scientific uncertainties;
3. Help patients to recognize the values-sensitive nature of the decision and to clarify, either implicitly or explicitly, the value they place on the benefits and harms. (To accomplish this, patient decision aids may describe the options in enough detail that clients can imagine what it is like to experience the physical, emotional and social effects and/or guide clients to consider which benefits and harms are most important to them)' (Stacey et al., 2014, n.p.).

Patient decision aids are different to patient education materials because they aim to personalize the decision for the individual patient and facilitate patient involvement rather than simply provide explanatory information about diseases and their management. Decision aids are designed to provide a balanced and neutral presentation of the options in healthcare decisions.

Such aids may be concise or detailed; they can be provided in hard copy or online; they may include videos and/or graphics; and they can be used within or outside the health consultation. Many of them are based on theoretical frameworks (Fig. 18.1).

WHEN SHOULD YOU CONSIDER USING A DECISION AID?

Decision aids are one way that patients can be involved in their healthcare decisions. It is not practical (or even necessary) to use a patient decision aid in every health decision, but we know that patients tend to want a more active role in certain decision types. These include:

1. decisions relating to preventive health care,
2. situations with potential negative future consequences, e.g., chronic diseases,
3. decisions where evidence is lacking or uncertain and
4. decisions involving potential side effects, e.g., immunization, antihypertensive therapy (Müller-Engelmann et al., 2013).

For some decisions, there is clear evidence that a test or treatment should be recommended. Its benefits clearly outweigh any harms, and it may be lifesaving. The healthcare worker has an obligation to recommend such treatment and to ensure that the patient's consent is valid. In other words, an evidence-based recommendation is made *and* the patient is made aware of the likelihood of benefits and harms. Even with this 'consider a recommendation' approach (Entwistle et al., 2008), some patients will remain uncertain and want more detailed information (Waller et al., 2012). A decision aid may be a very well-received option in such cases (see Case Studies 18.1 and 18.2).

There are also many decisions in which we should recommend against a test or treatment because it may cause significant harm with little or no benefit. The

---

CASE STUDY 18.1

Bowel Cancer Screening

Many countries around the world have national screening programs for bowel cancer. There is good evidence that biennial faecal occult blood testing (FOBT) every 2 years has a modest effect on reducing the incidence and mortality of bowel cancer, but there are risks associated with colonoscopies arising from positive results – true and false (Hewitson et al., 2007). Governments have therefore invested in FOBT screening programs and offer the test to people in the target age range. A UK study showed that the majority of the British public (84%) preferred an expert recommendation about bowel cancer screening, but they also wanted to be informed about the benefits and risks.

Conversely, around 16% people prefer to weigh up the benefits and harms for themselves (Waller et al., 2012).

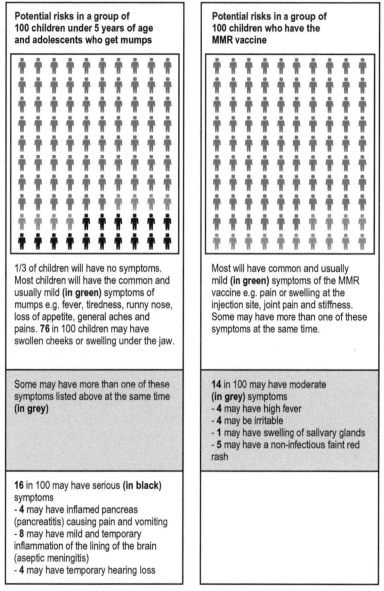

Potential risks in a group of 100 children under 5 years of age and adolescents who get mumps

1/3 of children will have no symptoms. Most children will have the common and usually mild **(in green)** symptoms of mumps e.g. fever, tiredness, runny nose, loss of appetite, general aches and pains. **76** in 100 children may have swollen cheeks or swelling under the jaw.

Some may have more than one of these symptoms listed above at the same time **(in grey)**

16 in 100 may have serious **(in black)** symptoms
- **4** may have inflamed pancreas (pancreatitis) causing pain and vomiting
- **8** may have mild and temporary inflammation of the lining of the brain (aseptic meningitis)
- **4** may have temporary hearing loss

Potential risks in a group of 100 children who have the MMR vaccine

Most will have common and usually mild **(in green)** symptoms of the MMR vaccine e.g. pain or swelling at the injection site, joint pain and stiffness. Some may have more than one of these symptoms at the same time.

14 in 100 may have moderate **(in grey)** symptoms
- **4** may have high fever
- **4** may be irritable
- **1** may have swelling of salivary glands
- **5** may have a non-infectious faint red rash

Fig. 18.1 ■ Excerpt from MMR (Measles, Mumps and Rubella) Decision Aid. (From Leask, J., Wallace, C., Trevena, L., Jackson, C., Shouri, S., 2009. MMR decision aid, http://www.ncirs.edu.au/consumer-resources/mmr-decision-aid/, with permission.)

healthcare worker in this case has a duty of care to explain this for patient safety. An example of this type of decision is not ordering x-rays for people with acute nonspecific low back pain (provided they do not have any 'red flag' symptoms or signs). Imaging provides no benefit to these patients but exposes them to unnecessary radiation and financial costs (Maher et al., 2016).

Patient decision aids are most commonly used when there is equipoise (a trade-off between benefits and harms) and where patient preferences have an important role to play. There may be a number of reasonable options to choose from, and the individual patient may place importance on particular factors such as side effects, efficacy and financial costs (Box 18.1).

CASE STUDY 18.2

Measles Vaccination

The World Health Organization estimates that around 17 million lives have been saved since 2000 as a result of childhood vaccination. Although there are rare serious consequences of vaccination, the benefits of vaccination substantially outweigh the harms. Most parents are accepting of the recommendation to vaccinate their children against measles, but some have concerns and are not accepting. In these cases, patient decision aids can be a useful way to involve parents in decisions through clarifying what's important to them and providing balanced information about the consequences of vaccinating or not vaccinating. In fact, a randomized controlled trial (RCT) of a patient decision aid with parents who were vaccine-hesitant showed that those receiving the decision aid were more likely to vaccinate their children than those who received a government-developed leaflet (Shourie et al., 2013). The web-based tool was also likely to be cost effective (Tubeuf et al., 2014).

BOX 18.1

EXAMPLES OF CLINICAL DECISIONS POTENTIALLY SUITED FOR DECISION AIDS

Choosing treatment for:
- early-stage prostate cancer (surgery vs radiotherapy vs active surveillance),
- knee osteoarthritis (pharmacological vs nonpharmacological),
- quitting smoking (pharmacological vs nonpharmacological) and
- mild-moderate depression (antidepressant vs psychological vs both).

For example, when smokers want to quit, they have the choice of a number of options for smoking cessation – 'no treatment', nicotine replacement patches/gum and prescription medications. Some smokers will prefer to quit with the assistance of nicotine replacement therapy, and others will choose 'no treatment' when provided with the evidence for benefits and harms of each option. A recent RCT of a smoking-cessation decision aid app showed a significant increase in continuous abstinence after 6 months compared with a traditional patient education app. Allowing patients to choose an option that aligns with their personal goals, values and circumstances in this way can result in better health outcomes (BinDhim et al., 2014; Müller-Engelmann et al., 2013).

HOW DO DECISION AIDS WORK?

The most recent update of the Cochrane systematic review of patient decision aids includes 105 RCTs and shows that they significantly increase patients' knowledge and that patients are more likely to make a decision that is concordant with their personal values. Decision aids improve patients' accuracy of risk perception, reduce decisional conflict and increase patient involvement. These findings appear to be similar regardless of whether the decision aid is used within or outside the healthcare consultation (Stacey et al., 2014). It is important to ensure that within the clinical reasoning process, decision points are identified and the need for a tool is assessed. It is also important to find the right tool for the situation. This involves being sure that the tool is relevant to your patient's context.

REFLECTION POINT 1

Some questions to ask yourself are:
Question: What type of patient is the decision aid designed for?
Rationale: Applying evidence across different population groups needs caution. The rate of a particular outcome can change in certain patient subgroups (e.g., age, family history, ethnicity and social circumstances can all have an effect).
Question: What health decision is the tool designed for?

Rationale: It is important to ensure that the tool aligns with the decision facing your patient.

Question: Are the options relevant to the patient's context?

Rationale: Some treatments may not be available or affordable in particular contexts.

WHAT MAKES A 'GOOD' DECISION AID?

The IPDAS Collaboration published a series of articles in 2013 detailing the evidence supporting their standards (Volk et al., 2013). As more patient decision aids are being developed, it is becoming increasingly difficult for healthcare workers and patients to be sure of the quality of these tools. The IPDAS series of manuscripts summarizes the evidence for decision aid developers and users when appraising the quality of tools (Box 18.2).

Unfortunately, many patient decision aids have been developed for research purposes and have not subsequently been made available to the public. In addition, many have been published and not updated with the latest evidence. A small audit of the Ottawa A to Z Inventory of Patient Decision Aids (Ottawa Hospital Research Institute, n.d.[a]) found that only one-half had provided references for the evidence used or the date they were last updated (Montori et al., 2013). It has been suggested that evidence-based systematic reviews should be updated every 2 to 5 years (Shojania et al., 2007). Thus, when looking for a decision aid, use it with caution if it is more than 5 years old and has not been updated. It may also be necessary to supplement a decision aid with locally relevant information about costs, resources and accessibility for particular treatment options. These issues can be important to decision making with clients but are less frequently included in published decision aids (McCurtin and Clifford, 2015). Similarly, the role of patient stories and experiences within decision aids has been controversial, with insufficient evidence to support their inclusion routinely (Bekker et al., 2013).

Disclosure of conflicts of interest is another important quality issue for patient decision aids. A recent analysis of disclosure policies among 25 organizations that develop patient decision aids showed that only 6 of the 12 who responded had any written policy of disclosure (Elwyn et al., 2016). Similar problems with lack of disclosure have been highlighted for clinical practice guidelines (Norris et al., 2011). It is important to consider the developers of a decision aid and whether there could be potential conflicts of interest.

It has been suggested that patient decision aid certification is a mechanism for addressing some of these quality issues. The IPDAS Collaboration has developed a set of minimum standards for patient decision aid certification to address this need, identifying 6 items that confirm that a tool 'qualifies' as a decision aid; 10 items for use in 'certification'; and 28 'quality' criteria that will strengthen a decision aid but whose omission does not create a high risk for harmful bias (Joseph-Williams and Newcombe et al., 2014).

An analysis of 30 decision aids from the Cochrane review were scored against these items and found that most met the qualifying criteria but only three met the proposed certification threshold (Durand et al., 2015). Most of these omissions were from a lack of update policy and disclosure of funding sources. The Washington Health Care Authority (n.d.) has implemented a certification process from 2016 that calls for submission four times per year, sends submissions for independent

---

BOX 18.2

SOME FACTORS RELEVANT TO THE QUALITY OF PATIENT DECISION AIDS

1. What was the development process?
2. Are there any relevant conflicts of interest, and have they been disclosed?
3. Are all the options set out clearly?
4. Is the information evidence-based?
5. Is the information presented in a balanced way?
6. Are the quantitative outcomes of the options presented clearly?
7. Can patient values be clarified?
8. Is the decision aid accessible to people across the health literacy spectrum?

Adapted from the IPDAS series of manuscripts in BioMedCentral (see Volk, R.J., Llewellyn-Thomas, H., Stacey, D., Elwyn, G., 2013. Ten years of the International Patient Decision Aid Standards Collaboration: evolution of the core dimensions for assessing the quality of patient decision aids. BMC Med. Inform. Decis. Mak. 13[suppl. 2], S1).

review, an opportunity for improvement after review and a requirement for recertification every 2 years.

REFLECTION POINT 2

Consider the following issues in choosing a patient decision aid:

- Who developed the decision aid, and have potential conflicts of interest been disclosed?
- When was the decision aid last updated?
- Using the IPDAS checklist, how does the decision aid score?

WHERE CAN YOU FIND PATIENT DECISION AIDS?

Although you can search on the Internet for patient decision aids, this often results in poor-quality resources and a maze of different alternatives that are hard to make sense of. Increasingly, reputable decision aid developers and groups worldwide are publishing their tools on the Internet. Box 18.3 provides a short list of some to consider.

A major equity issue at present is the restriction of access to patient decision aids. Some developers require

---

BOX 18.3
EXAMPLES OF PATIENT DECISION AID DEVELOPER WEBSITES

Agency for Healthcare Research and Quality
- http://www.effectivehealthcare.ahrq.gov/index.cfm/tools-and-resources/patient-decision-aids/
- Cincinnati Children's Hospital Anderson Center Decision Aids
- https://www.cincinnatichildrens.org/service/j/anderson-center/evidence-based-care/decision-aids

Mayo Clinic Decision Aids
- http://shareddecisions.mayoclinic.org/decision-aid-information/decision-aids-for-chronic-disease/
- Med-Decs
- http://www.med-decs.org

The Option Grids Decision Aids
- http://optiongrid.org/option-grids/current-grids
- Ottawa Health Research Institute Inventory A–Z
- https://decisionaid.ohri.ca/index.html
- Université Laval Decision Boxes
- http://www.decisionbox.ulaval.ca/index.php?id=810&L=2

---

membership of a particular health insurance agency. Some have restricted access to country-specific IP addresses, and others require payment to access.

WHAT IS THE BEST WAY TO INVOLVE CLIENTS IN USING DECISION AIDS?

There does not appear to be any difference in the effect of patient decision aids whether they are used *within* or *outside* the healthcare consultation (Stacey et al., 2014). However, we do know that healthcare professional endorsement of decision aids has a positive effect on patient involvement (Légaré et al., 2014). It is also important to clarify how *much* involvement patients want in each health decision and to clearly separate 'deliberation' from 'determination' (Politi et al., 2013). Earlier in this chapter, we introduced the term 'collaborative deliberation', which involves exchanging knowledge, eliciting what is important to the patient, communicating about options, engaging patients in discussion and finding out what role they would like to play in the final decision. We also highlighted that many patients would prefer a recommendation *but also want to know their options and their benefits and harms.* More informed patients are also more likely to want involvement in decisions, and most patients (regardless of demographic characteristics) want to be offered choices about their care and asked about their preferences (Politi et al., 2013). Having done this, some will defer the actual decision (i.e., 'determination') to the healthcare professional or others. In other words, the preference for involvement needs to be informed by the deliberative process (Politi et al., 2013).

WHAT SHOULD I DO IF I CANNOT FIND A RELEVANT DECISION AID?

If a specific decision aid cannot be found, you can either use a 'generic' decision support tool such as the one available from the Ottawa Hospital Research Institute (n.d.[b]). This guide is designed to help people with any personal or social decision; it is available in a version that might also include family members or others. It has been translated into French, Swedish, Dutch, Danish, Spanish German and Japanese. This website also has an online tutorial about how to use

ask the 3 questions:

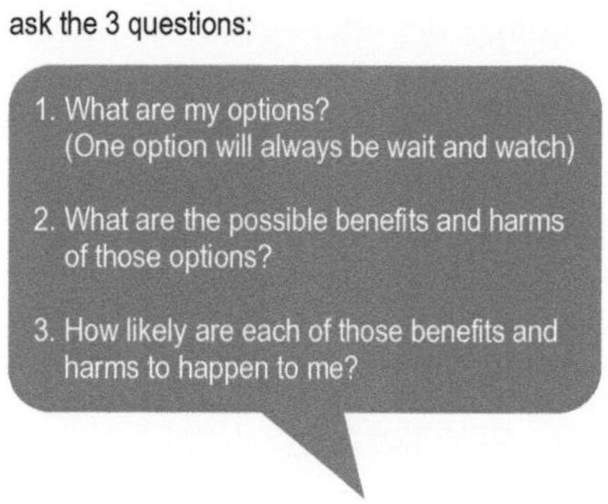

1. What are my options?
   (One option will always be wait and watch)

2. What are the possible benefits and harms
   of those options?

3. How likely are each of those benefits and
   harms to happen to me?

Fig. 18.2 ■ Three questions that patients can ask. (From Ask Share Know, n.d., The Ask Share Know project, www.askshare-know.com.au, with permission)

these generic tools in coaching someone through a decision.

Another way to approach collaborative deliberation when a patient decision aid is not available is to use a simple question framework to encourage patients to be involved in decisions. Patients who are trained to ask these three questions are more likely to be actively involved in their healthcare decisions and more likely to have a discussion about the harms and benefits of treatment options (Shepherd et al., 2011) (Fig. 18.2).

HOW CAN THE HEALTH TEAM PLAY A ROLE?

Despite the fact that there is an increasing emphasis on multidisciplinary teams in health care, there has been very little work on how SDM and patient decision aids might fit within this context. Two reviews of theories of interprofessional SDM highlighted the argument that very few make explicit the roles of team members in decision making and that family members are often subsumed into the patient role (Lewis et al., 2016; Stacey et al., 2010). For example, cancer multidisciplinary team meetings are variable in their involvement of patients, families and primary care professionals, and patients find the challenges of seeking second opinions to be particularly difficult (Hamilton et al., 2016).

There has been very limited research into how nonmedical members of the healthcare team can include shared decision making as part of their daily clinical practice. Supporting patients' involvement in their health care to the extent they would like should be part of all healthcare interactions. Relevant patient decision aids can be used and adapted in many encounters with allied healthcare professionals, although implementation to this extent is not yet routine.

The implementation of SDM has been sporadic and often dependent on 'champions' at the institution. It is important to consider the workflow of the clinic and the patient journey as they navigate across the healthcare team. Involving teams in the design of SDM implementation plans is vital. In the future, we will hopefully see patient preferences and decisions shared across the healthcare team to ensure a more consistent and seamless experience (Lloyd et al., 2013).

CAN PATIENT DECISION AIDS BE USED TO INVOLVE FAMILY MEMBERS AND CARERS?

Some patient decision aids have been developed to take into account that there may need to be a surrogate decision maker for the patient who is not able to give informed consent. This can include situations such as end-of-life care for unconscious patients, care decisions for patients with dementia or children who are not legally old enough to give informed consent. There are also situations such as pregnancy-related decisions in which any woman may wish to take into account the preferences of her partner. There are also some patients who simply prefer to involve their family or others in a healthcare decision, and healthcare professionals should take this into consideration whenever possible. Patients with lower levels of literacy appear to prefer greater involvement and consultation with family and others. A study of 73 men and women living in Australia with varying educational and functional health literacy showed that patients with lower education levels described how relatives and friends sought information on their behalf and played a key role in their decisions (Smith et al., 2009). However, all levels of literacy consistently saw the practitioner–patient relationship as being key to their involvement regardless of family roles. It is therefore important for healthcare professionals to balance and negotiate the preference for family involvement alongside the integrity of the relationship with the individual patient.

Consider the following questions:

- What other members of the healthcare team are involved in your patient's healthcare decision and its implementation? How do you ensure relevant communication with them?
- To what extent does your patient want family members involved in this decision? How is that best done?
- How would you be able to discern your patient's preferences for other team and family member involvement in decisions? Who will make the decisions, and how will the decisions be made?

CAN PATIENTS FROM VULNERABLE POPULATIONS BENEFIT FROM USING PATIENT DECISION AIDS?

At the beginning of this chapter, we outlined the principle that SDM is a process requiring an exchange of power within the clinician–patient communication (Joseph-Williams et al., 2014) and that the use of patient decision aids is an effective way to increase patient involvement resulting in better knowledge, understanding of risks and benefits and making decisions that are values-concordant.

A subanalysis of the Cochrane systematic review of patient decision aids has shown that patients who had a lower baseline knowledge level had a greater effect from the decision aids than those with higher knowledge at baseline. In other words, there is the potential to reduce the socioeconomic knowledge gap through the use of such tools.

Health literacy has been described as having 'functional', 'critical' and 'communicative' components (Nutbeam, 2000). The IPDAS criteria include the recommendation to consider literacy and numeracy in decision aid development. There is a growing body of evidence that patients with lower literacy do want involvement in healthcare decisions, but they are more likely to confer with family and friends and also to rely on the opinion of their healthcare worker in doing so (Smith et al., 2009).

A review of patient decision aids for lower-literacy populations concluded that although there are few studies where research has been conducted, findings

are encouraging (McCaffery et al., 2013). One trial of a patient decision aid for lower-literacy participants did show an increase in knowledge and informed choice compared with standard information, suggesting that they have potential for increasing patient involvement in decision making across all literacy levels (Smith et al., 2010).

CHAPTER SUMMARY

- Patient decision aids are useful tools to engage patients in healthcare decisions.
- Healthcare professional endorsement of SDM is important for patient engagement in collaborative deliberation.
- Most patients would like to know there is a choice, know what their options are and be asked about their preferences.
- Patients' preferences for involvement in determination (i.e., making the choice) may mean that they defer this to others such as their healthcare professional.
- Patient involvement in healthcare decisions can occur without a patient decision aid and is feasible and appropriate for patients from a range of demographic backgrounds.
- Healthcare teams with the patient as a member are likely to be the future face of shared decision making.

Consider your daily work as a clinician.

- Do you involve patients in decisions about their health care? Why or why not?
- How do you currently do this?
- What tools could you use to increase patient involvement in these decisions?

REFERENCES

Ask Share Know, n.d. The Ask Share Know project. Viewed 28 March 2017. Available from: www.asksharethnow.com.au.

Bekker, H.L., Winterbottom, A.E., Butow, P., et al., 2013. Do personal stories make patient decision aids more effective? A critical review of theory and evidence. BMC Med. Inform. Decis. Mak. 13, S9.

BinDhim, N.F., McGeechan, K., Trevena, L., 2014. Assessing the effect of an interactive decision-aid smartphone smoking cessation application (app) on quit rates: a double-blind automated randomised control trial protocol. BMJ Open 4, e005371.

Department of Health, 2011. Liberating the NHS: no decision about me, without me: further consultation on proposals to secure shared decision making. Department of Health, London, UK.

Durand, M.A., Witt, J., Joseph-Williams, N., et al., 2015. Minimum standards for the certification of patient decision support interventions: feasibility and application. Patient Educ. Couns. 98, 462–468.

Elwyn, G., Dannenberg, M., Blaine, A., et al., 2016. Trustworthy patient decision aids: a qualitative analysis addressing the risk of competing interests. BMJ Open 6, e012562.

Elwyn, G., Lloyd, A., May, C., et al., 2014. Collaborative deliberation: a model for patient care. Patient Educ. Couns. 97, 158–164.

Entwistle, V.A., Carter, S.M., Trevena, L., et al., 2008. Communicating about screening. BMJ 337, a1591.

Hamilton, D.W., Heaven, B., Thomson, R.G., et al., 2016. Multidisciplinary team decision-making in cancer and the absent patient: a qualitative study. BMJ Open 6, e012559.

Hewitson, P., Glasziou, P., Irwig, L., et al., 2007. Screening for colorectal cancer using the faecal occult blood test, Hemoccult. Cochrane Database Syst. Rev. (1), CD001216.

Hoffmann, T.C., Légaré, F., Simmons, M.B., et al., 2014. Shared decision making: what do clinicians need to know and why should they bother? Med. J. Aust. 201, 35–39.

Joseph-Williams, N., Elwyn, G., Edwards, A., 2014. Knowledge is not power for patients: a systematic review and thematic synthesis of patient-reported barriers and facilitators to shared decision making. Patient Educ. Couns. 94, 291–309.

Joseph-Williams, N., Newcombe, R., Politi, M., et al., 2014. Toward minimum standards for certifying patient decision aids: a modified Delphi Consensus Process. Med Decis Making. 34, 699–710.

Leask, J., Wallace, C., Trevena, L., et al., 2009. MMR decision aid. Viewed 28 March 2017. Available from: http://www.ncirs.edu.au/consumer-resources/mmr-decision-aid/.

Légaré, F., Stacey, D., Turcotte, S., et al., 2014. Interventions for improving the adoption of shared decision making by healthcare professionals. Cochrane Database Syst. Rev. (9), CD006732.

Lewis, K.B., Stacey, D., Squires, J.E., et al., 2016. Shared decision-making models acknowledging an interprofessional approach: a theory analysis to inform nursing practice. Res. Theory Nurs. Pract. 30, 26–43.

Lloyd, A., Joseph-Williams, N., Edwards, A., et al., 2013. Patchy 'coherence': using normalization process theory to evaluate a multi-faceted shared decision making implementation program (MAGIC). Implement. Sci. 8, 102.

Maher, C., Underwood, M., Buchbinder, R., 2016. Non-specific low back pain. Lancet 389, 736–747.

McCaffery, K.J., Holmes-Rovner, M., Smith, S.K., et al., 2013. Addressing health literacy in patient decision aids. BMC Med. Inform. Decis. Mak. 13 (Suppl. 2), S10.

McCurtin, A., Clifford, A.M., 2015. What are the primary influences on treatment decisions? How does this reflect on evidence-based practice? Indications from the discipline of speech and language therapy. J. Eval. Clin. Pract. 21, 1178–1189.

Montori, V.M., LeBlanc, A., Buchholz, A., et al., 2013. Basing information on comprehensive, critically appraised, and up-to-date syntheses of the scientific evidence: a quality dimension of the International Patient Decision Aid Standards. BMC Med. Inform. Decis. Mak. 13 (Suppl. 2), S5.

Müller-Engelmann, M., Donner-Banzhoff, N., Keller, H., et al., 2013. When decisions should be shared: a study of social norms in medical decision making using a factorial survey approach. Med Decis Making. 33, 37–47.

Norris, S.L., Holmer, H.K., Ogden, L.A., et al., 2011. Conflict of interest in clinical practice guideline development: a systematic review. PLoS ONE 6, e25153.

Nutbeam, D., 2000. Health literacy as a public health goal: a challenge for contemporary health education and communication strategies into the 21st century. Health Promot. Int. 15, 259–267.

Ottawa Hospital Research Institute, n.d.(a). Ottawa A to Z inventory of patient decision aids. Viewed 28 March 2017. Available from: https://decisionaid.ohri.ca/AZinvent.php.

Ottawa Hospital Research Institute, n.d.(b). Patient decision aids: Ottawa personal decision guides. Viewed 28 March 2017. Available from: https://decisionaid.ohri.ca/decguide.html.

Politi, M.C., Dizon, D.S., Frosch, D.L., et al., 2013. Importance of clarifying patients' desired role in shared decision making to match their level of engagement with their preferences. BMJ 347, f7066.

Shepherd, H.L., Barratt, A., Trevena, L.J., et al., 2011. Three questions that patients can ask to improve the quality of information physicians give about treatment options: a cross-over trial. Patient Educ. Couns. 84, 379–385.

Shojania, K.G., Sampson, M., Ansari, M.T., et al., 2007. How quickly do systematic reviews go out of date? A survival analysis. Ann. Intern. Med. 147, 224–233.

Shourie, S., Jackson, C., Cheater, F.M., et al., 2013. A cluster randomised controlled trial of a web based decision aid to support parents decisions about their child's Measles Mumps and Rubella (MMR) vaccination. Vaccine 31, 6003–6010.

Smith, S.K., Dixon, A., Trevena, L., et al., 2009. Exploring patient involvement in healthcare decision making across different education and functional health literacy groups. Soc. Sci. Med. 69, 1805–1812.

Smith, S.K., Trevena, L., Simpson, J.M., et al., 2010. A decision aid to support informed choices about bowel cancer screening among adults with low education: randomised controlled trial. BMJ 341, c5370.

Stacey, D., Légaré, F., Col, N.F., et al., 2014. Decision aids for people who are facing health treatment or screening decisions. Cochrane Database Syst. Rev. (1), CD001431, doi:10.1002/14651858.CD001431.pub5.

Stacey, D., Légaré, F., Pouliot, S., et al., 2010. Shared decision making models to inform an interprofessional perspective on decision making: a theory analysis. Patient Educ. Couns. 80, 164–172.

Trevena, L.J., Zikmund-Fisher, B.J., Edwards, A., et al., 2013. Presenting quantitative information about decision outcomes: a risk communication primer for decision aid developers. BMC Med Inform Decis Mak. 13 (Suppl. 2), S7.

Tubeuf, S., Edlin, R., Shourie, S., et al., 2014. Cost effectiveness of a web-based decision aid for parents deciding about MMR vaccination: a three-arm cluster randomised controlled trial in primary care. Br. J. Gen. Pract. 64, e493–e499.

Volk, R.J., Llewellyn-Thomas, H., Stacey, D., et al., 2013. Ten years of the International Patient Decision Aid Standards Collaboration: evolution of the core dimensions for assessing the quality of patient decision aids. BMC Med. Inform. Decis. Mak. 13 (Suppl. 2), S1.

Waller, J., Macedo, A., von Wagner, C., et al., 2012. Communication about colorectal cancer screening in Britain: public preferences for an expert recommendation. Br. J. Cancer 107, 1938–1943.

Washington Health Care Authority, n.d. Patient decision aid certification process. Viewed 28 March 2017. Available from: http://www.hca.wa.gov/assets/program/sdm_cert_overview .pdf.

19

CLINICAL DECISION MAKING, SOCIAL JUSTICE AND CLIENT EMPOWERMENT

DEBBIE HORSFALL ■ DIANE TASKER ■ JOY HIGGS

CHAPTER AIMS

The aims of this chapter are to:

■ examine connections between clinical decision making (from person to system levels) in relation to social justice and empowerment,

■ reflect on the meaning of social justice and how it can be incorporated into health care and

■ promote reflection on practices in this arena.

KEY WORDS

Social justice

Empowerment

INTRODUCTION

A child born today in Japan, for example, can expect to live to 82 years of age on average, whereas it is unlikely that a newborn infant in Zimbabwe will reach his or her 34th birthday. Extreme deprivation in health is still widespread. Resolving this predicament of major health improvement in the midst of deprivation is one of the greatest global challenges of the new millennium (Ruger 2004).

The picture of a person's health cannot be complete without consideration and full acknowledgement of his or her place within the society in which he or she lives. Accordingly, the best outcomes for that person can only be achieved if we adjust the processes of decision making and action in health care in relation to that person's place in his or her society. Rather than expecting people with many personal and social differences to fit into standard healthcare services and systems, such adjustments can result in enhancing the efficacy of individual and societal health outcomes and producing more equitable and just health care for all.

The gross inequalities in health that we see within and among countries present a challenge to the world. That there should be a spread of life expectancy of 48 years among countries and 20 years or more within countries is not inevitable. A burgeoning volume of research identifies social factors at the root of much of these inequalities in health. Social determinants are relevant to communicable and noncommunicable disease alike (Marmot, 2005).

Many healthcare providers relate real-life stories of their sadness and frustration in dealing with healthcare issues arising from social problems. Clients also relate how they suffer from the effects of social and economic inequality, which exacerbates any health issues they may want or need to address. In the following case study, the cascading effect of life events can be seen to overwhelm a young mother and, as a result, her children.

SOCIAL DETERMINANTS OF HEALTH

Talking of social justice and client empowerment means that as practitioners we should see people as social beings, located within sociocultural contexts, relationships and systems, which work together in myriad ways (Lutfey Spencer and Grace, 2016), materially affecting people's physical, emotional, mental and spiritual health.

CASE STUDY 19.1

Social Influences on Health

Sally is being treated for clinical depression. She has spent significant periods of time in institutionalized care settings for people who have mental health issues. She has seen two psychiatrists and attended a number of group therapy programs aimed at helping her set achievable life goals including finding meaningful work. Her two children are currently cared for by their grandmother as Sally has been unable to provide a stable home environment for them. Sally left her physically abusive husband when her second child was 2 years of age. She had no paid employment and was unable to secure rental accommodation as the family had been blacklisted by real estate agents as a result of the damage to property caused by her husband in previous rentals. She now sleeps between two of her friends' houses. She has become significantly overweight, a common side effect of the medication she has been prescribed. This has led to a further decrease in her self-esteem and has made it more difficult for her to be physically active. Her GP (general practitioner or primary care provider) has just told her that she is now prediabetic and must lose weight.

As illustrated in the earlier example, it is clear that homelessness, unemployment, intimate partner abuse, loss and grief and health interventions themselves have affected Sally's current mental and physical health. Additionally, the sociocultural factors of gender and class have an already deep effect: You are more likely to experience intimate partner violence if you are a girl or woman. Women are more likely to be the primary carer for young children or to be in part-time or casual work, thus affecting their economic security and access to, and treatment within, appropriate healthcare contexts.

These outcomes are also determined by class and gender (Lutfey Spencer and Grace, 2016; Solar and Irwin, 2010). Clinicians make gender-based decisions, albeit perhaps unconsciously, by making more sophisticated and determined efforts for men than women, even when they present with the same health condition. Society still gives more support to men when it comes to salary levels, employment and promotion but also, in health care, in the need to help men return promptly to well-being and employment to 'take care of their families'. Female partners are expected to take on the main work of child care to accommodate this male privileging. Women who are ill are also more likely to be expected to carry on their family roles and their healthcare actions and responsibilities (for themselves and their children). This is particularly exacerbated if the woman does not have extended family support or is a single parent. Women are also more likely to be diagnosed as mentally ill when their real diagnosis is more to do with the experience of abuse or being excluded from access to material resources, such as somewhere to live (Alvarez-Dardet and Ruiz, 2000).

A World Health Organization (WHO) Commission completed by the Women and Gender Equity Knowledge Network concluded that:

Gender inequality damages the health of millions of girls and women across the globe. It can also be harmful to men's health despite the many tangible benefits it gives men through resources, power, authority and control. These benefits to men do not come without a cost to their own emotional and psychological health, often translated into risky and unhealthy behaviours, and reduced longevity. Taking action to improve gender equity in health and to address women's rights to health is one of the most direct and potent ways to reduce health inequities overall and ensure effective use of health resources (Sen and Östlin, 2007, p. xii).

The provision of health services and healthcare relationships also occurs within a complex sociocultural context. For example, there is a large body of evidence that demonstrates how perceived social worth affects what health conditions are researched, what drugs get developed and how clinicians diagnose, treat and follow up patients (Australian Institute of Health and Welfare, 2016; Marmot et al., 2008; Wallerstein et al., 2011). Perceived social worth is determined by a number of factors such as employment status, relationship status, how a person physically presents in terms of body shape and clothing, if he or she has a drug and alcohol dependency or if he or she is part of the welfare system. These factors have been shown to construct what is known as provider and system bias. Taken to extremes, Sudnow (1967) found that '[o]verall, the lower the social standing of a patient, the lower the likelihood that the staff would exhaust all resuscitative options to save him or her. In many instances, patients of low social viability were declared dead in advance of their actual death' (as quoted by Timmermans, 1998, in Lutfey Spencer and Grace, 2016, p. 108). A follow-up study by Timmerman (1998) revealed that resuscitation of people with drug and alcohol abuse histories was affected by staff's negative attitudes to that history – in contrast to resuscitations performed on people they knew to have greater community standing. Whether we like it or not, at times, treatment decisions and applications are based on stereotypes, prejudices and resulting acts of discrimination by providers and clinicians across the spectrum of health services.

REFLECTION POINT 1

Consider your own clinical work experience. How have you encountered decision making or healthcare actions that demonstrate discrimination or lack of consideration of sociocultural differences among patients? Perhaps you have experienced such actions yourself as a patient or healthcare professional. How have these affected your approach to clinical decision making?

Let's go back to Sally for a moment. If Sally were an indigenous person, her access to fair and equitable treatment would typically be further compounded, and her current health status would probably be even worse. In Australia, it is well recognized that the mental, spiritual and physical health of the indigenous peoples of this country is considerably worse than that of the nonindigenous population; it is also well recognized that Aboriginal and/or Torres Strait Islander people are among the most disadvantaged indigenous peoples in the developed world (World Health Organization, 2008). They experience lower levels of access to health services, and when they do access services, they are more likely to be hospitalized for treatment than the nonindigenous population (Australian Institute of Health and Welfare,

2016). Although hospitalization may appear to be positive and supportive, it fails to consider cultural concerns like family support and emotional stress at isolation. Dispossession, racism and lack of basic human rights directly affect mental, physical and spiritual well-being and health (Australian Bureau of Statistics, 2013; Australian Indigenous HealthInfoNet, 2016; United Nations Development Programme, 2003). Such inequalities generate a relationship of complex, compounding issues, which materially present in and on people's minds, spirits and bodies when they encounter the healthcare professional.

[T]he social problems of the contemporary world walk into the clinician's office every day. The mundane details of the social determinants of health are writ small in our daily encounters with patients (The Editors, 2006, p. 2).

Another such example comes from Canada. Adelson (2005) investigated health care in the First Nations (indigenous Canadian) populations and reported on the disproportionate burden of ill health and social suffering of these peoples. She argued '[i]n analyses of health disparities, it is as important to navigate the interstices between the person and the wider social and historical contexts as it is to pay attention to the individual effects of inequity' (p. S46). Browne and Fiske (2001, p. 126) examined mainstream healthcare encounters from the perspective of First Nations women from a reserve community in northwestern Canada. The resulting narratives 'revealed that women's encounters were shaped by racism, discrimination and structural inequities that continue to marginalize and disadvantage First Nations women. The women's health care experiences have historical, political and economic significance and are reflective of wider postcolonial relations that shape their everyday lives'.

The situation of refugees is an extreme case of sociopolitical effects on health and well-being. Sharara and Kanj (2014, n.p.) draw attention to the health effect of Syria's ongoing civil war that has 'displaced 6.5 million Syrians, left hundreds of thousands wounded or killed by violence, and created a vacuum in basic infrastructures that will reverberate throughout the region for years to come. Beyond such devastation, the civil war has introduced epidemics of infections that have spread through vulnerable populations in Syria and neighboring countries'. According to El-Khatib et al. (2013), around 3% of the world's population (214 million people) has, for various reasons, crossed international borders. They draw attention to Syria, which has, since March 2011, experienced a state of political crisis and instability resulting in an exodus of more than 1 million Syrian refugees to neighbouring countries (Lebanon, Jordan, Turkey, Egypt and North Africa). They call for the international community to support Syrian refugees and their host governments. The United Nations High Commissioner for Refugees (UNHCR) (2011) contends that refugee resettlement has the potential to serve as 'an important expression of international solidarity and responsibility sharing', providing international protection 'to meet the specific needs of vulnerable persons whose life, liberty, safety, health, or other fundamental rights are at risk in the country where they have sought refuge' (UNHCR 2011, from Ostrand 2015 p. 267).

Health practitioners, governments and nations must recognize that social relations, structures and histories are different for all groups and affect our health and well-being, our access to and treatment within the health system and the decisions made by governments, health-care organizations and professionals within that system. Social and economic inequity means that those who are disadvantaged experience disability, illness and death disproportionately more than people lucky enough to be protected by their social and economic situation. The study of these social determinants of health includes the conceptual and operational frameworks of the health system itself.

If we are to achieve fair and just access to, and treatment within, healthcare systems and by healthcare professionals, then it is important to acknowledge the relationship among perceived social worth, health status and treatment. We need to work against discrimination and prejudice at systemic and individual levels. Understanding health and well-being from a social justice perspective can help healthcare professionals uncover hidden assumptions and resulting discriminatory interactions that result in systems and provider bias.

REFLECTION POINT 2

What part has social justice played in your thinking about health care? Consider the concept and practice of duty of care. This is part of the core rhetoric, socialization and education of healthcare professionals. How much of our health care – at individual, organizational and national levels of provision – embodies social justice as part of our duty of care to the individuals and societies we claim to provide this care for?

SOCIAL JUSTICE

So what do we mean by a social justice framework, and what does it mean to work within such a framework? First, it means accepting that injustices do exist and that these affect people's health and well-being. It also means understanding that structural and everyday violence exists and that this too affects people's health and well-being, be it racism, homophobia, ableism or small acts of discrimination because a person does not meet our own moral standards. It means taking into account people's biopsychosocial contexts: where they live, the work (or lack of work) they do, the lives they lead, their histories and their place with/in sociocultural contexts. It means seeing Sally as more than a person needing to lose weight but as someone who needs help and support to find a secure place to live and work to pay the bill. And, it means working with her so that she can live with her own children. On a larger scale, it may mean putting money into researching drugs that do not cause weight gain for people who have depression. This is just one example of a healthcare strategy that might help one problem but cause others – and the patient 'just has to live with it'. How do we take these strategies into account in our clinical reasoning?

Hixon et al. (2013) argue that healthcare professionals must both recognize and understand that health is a fundamental human right and that healthcare professionals must pursue the goal of health for all, not just good health for some and not so good health for others. This stance is seen as quite radical in some countries, such as the United States, at present, but it nonetheless is an important aspirational goal for all:

A commitment to social justice requires that we not limit our sense of justice simply to the more equitable provision of health care to those who are ill, but demands that we examine injustices in the distribution of health and the underlying reasons for unjust burdens of illness. (Hixon et al. 2013, pp. 161–162)

This argument draws upon sociological and social psychological understandings of health and illness and the broader sociohistorical determinants of these. Known as social medicine, social epidemiology, or the social model of health, it is a potentially powerful corrective to the more recent reductionist approach to people where medical care has often been reduced to 'efficient business practices [which] treat disease as though only isolated organ systems of sick individuals are involved' (Hixon et al. 2013, p. 163).

If we adopt a social justice orientation and accept that health is a social phenomenon and that we live in a word riddled with social injustices such as systemic marginalization and oppression, then we can privilege social concerns (see also Nikhil and Patel, 2015). This means that in our practice we understand that supporting Sally to achieve more control and self-determination in her life may be as, if not more, effective than putting her on a weight management program or that helping Sally lose weight will not be effective in the long run if she continues to be marginalized. A social justice orientation also means that we see gender-based violence as causal in Sally's current health and well-being status. This is quite a challenge to conventional thinking, where we treat the patient and the 'problem' they are immediately presenting with. Marginalized and oppressed people suffer the most in terms of health trajectories and treatment, and many people who suffer from certain health conditions are further oppressed and discriminated against, for example, those with mental illness or drug dependency. The World Health Organization Commission on Social Determinants of Health has articulated these relationships in its comprehensive assessment of global health inequities (Marmot et al., 2008). These ongoing and compounding injustices contribute to both the health and well-being of individuals or groups and also contribute to research priorities, health treatment availability and everyday interactions within the system.

REFLECTION POINT 3

Do you have a viewpoint on social determinants of disease? Perhaps your education has led you to adopt a purely biomedical model of health and illness or a wellness model. Perhaps you work in a primary or tertiary healthcare setting or in community-based health care. Where does health as a social phenomenon fit into your current healthcare model and practice?

There are two main branches of social justice that are relevant to consider here: distributive justice (Rawls, 1971) and deliberative justice (Young, 1990), and both can, and probably should, coexist. *Distributive justice* is primarily concerned with fair and equitable distribution of resources. In democratic nations, governments and systems are held responsible for this. The assumption is that everyone is entitled to basic human rights and a minimum standard of social goods and opportunities to achieve those social goods. This position is strongly embedded in many patient charters in hospitals; for instance, see Box 19.1. Within this distributive justice framework, each person is expected to be treated equally,

---

BOX 19.1
PATIENT CHARTERS

Patient charters are statements by organizations (healthcare providers) pertaining to rights and responsibilities. The content of these charters varies. Ideally, they encompass rights and responsibilities for patients, the public and staff. An example of this is provided by the Mater Hospital, Queensland (http://www.mater.org.au/Home/For-Patients-and-Visitors/Patient-rights-and-responsibilities). In summary it states:

Mater respects your right to receive healthcare services. We are committed to provide exceptional, patient-focused, high-quality and safe healthcare. To provide such care, a partnership between patients, carers and families and healthcare providers is essential. The Mater Patient Charter addresses rights and responsibilities with regard to access, safety, respect, communication, participation, privacy and comment. The Patient Charter explains what you can expect from us and what we expect from you as we strive to provide you with the best possible care.

Such charters potentially provide many benefits and simultaneously raise serious issues. For instance, charters of health responsibilities raise ethical tensions, such as whether patients' responsibility for their own health might deny them health care (Schmidt, 2007).

For further reading, see Darzi A., 2007. Our NHS, our future: NHS next stage review—interim report. Department of Health, London, UK.

and everyone is expected to be afforded the same degree of fairness, respect and dignity.

Deliberative justice enhances and extends distributive justice by exploring and understanding notions of social worth and the processes that enable individuals and groups to be valued, or devalued, within society and in everyday interactions. This is then extended to understand how social worth is perpetuated through marginalization, domination and exclusion from decision-making processes, sedimenting both advantage and disadvantage in our social systems and everyday lives (McLaughlin, 2009). Taking these two ideas together, the focus is then on putting in place laws, policies and practices to:

- distribute the goods, resources and opportunities in society fairly,
- challenge the processes that enable and perpetuate the domination and advantage of certain groups of people and their values, beliefs and behaviours and
- champion equity, self-determination, interdependence and social responsibility of marginalized groups and individuals (Aldorondo, 2007).

These are not new ideas, but they do call for new practices and decision-making processes and behaviours in health care. Public health and health promotion, social work, radical psychiatry, critical public health or the new public health – critical psychology and liberation psychology – are all areas of clinical practice that have been leading the way in professional and systems change. Some branches of nursing and nursing scholarship have also embraced such ideas:

We have come to realize that our nursing scholarship needs to look beyond individual experiences of health and illness to encompass the social foundations that determine health status to a large extent … Influenced by the realization of a society structured by discrimination and inequities, as well as legislated and public health policies that mandate equitable and accessible health care, nursing scholarship has begun to examine the role of the profession in fostering social justice (Kirkham and Anderson, 2002, p. 2).

However, our experience is that this movement is frustratingly slow. One reason for this is that the health system itself is embedded in a larger social system, which struggles to realize social equity and justice. Another reason is the lack of social justice education and training for healthcare professionals and that current professionals find it difficult to make the link between social justice and their own individual practice. Many professionals seem unaware of their own taken-for-granted assumptions about the causes of health and well-being and their own place in perpetuating or challenging the status quo. Vera and Speight (2003) offer a useful set of guiding principles to synthesize deliberative social justice and professional practice. Although they focus on psychology and counselling, the synthesis is a useful one to consider across the health professions. They argue for an emancipatory practice, both as process and outcome, stating that '[i]dentifying the philosophies and professional roles that will most effectively promote the healthy development and well-being of oppressed groups is our ethical and moral obligation' (2003, p. 270). Many of their guidelines echo what we have already discussed in this chapter in terms of holistic respectful approaches and understanding that health and illness are as much outcomes of social contexts and social worth as biology. What they add are some direct strategies that professionals can adopt in their practices.

Other strategies inform day-to-day interactions with clients and patients and include not overemphasizing *individual* determination, as this is maintaining the status quo; using interventions that change individuals and social systems; engaging in community outreach such as facilitating support and care networks, and identifying community strengths and developing partnerships. They believe that 'the professional's expertise may be better applied by helping to organize (e.g., encouraging the creation of, or joining with, grass-roots community organizations) or advocate (e.g., facilitating contacts with community leaders, policy makers, legislators, etc.) within the community' (Vera and Speight 2003, p. 265).

The Royal Australian College of General Practitioners (RACGP), in its 2016 curriculum guidelines for the education and training of Australian GPs in terms of Aboriginal and Torres Strait Islander peoples, wholeheartedly embraced the same guiding principles as discussed by Vera and Speight, firmly placing GPs at the forefront of the struggle for social justice. They state that a partnership approach (in terms of 1:1 interactions and between communities of clients and communities of practice) is more likely to lead to successful outcomes and that implementing a model of holistic health care that addresses the social determinants of health and the right to self-determination is essential. This change in current practice and decision making can be achieved, they believe, by the provision of education and training that promote relevant knowledge, skills and attitudes that enable respectful and appropriate treatment of people and the ability to advocate for health equity and associated health outcomes. Furthermore, by enacting the principles of deliberative justice, Aboriginal and Torres Strait Island peoples can be centrally involved in the development and delivery of such education and training (RACGP, 2016). This, we would argue, could be applied to all health education and training and all disadvantaged groups in our societies. All health and allied healthcare professionals need to have the knowledge and skills needed to provide holistic and useful care that does not perpetuate the current advantage/disadvantaged dichotomy.

EMPOWERMENT

The World Health Organization Commission on Social Determinants of Health, referred to previously, calls for a global movement to address health inequities through political, civic and personal empowerment (Marmot et al., 2008). An understanding of the theory and application of empowerment is central to both the development of knowledge, skills and attitudes to advocate for, and operationalize, social justice in our healthcare interactions and systems and also to understand why this is, in fact, so difficult to realize. Central to empowerment is the concept of decision making by the people whose health we are talking about. This position has been taken up strongly by the disability sector with the slogan 'nothing about us without us' being an international rallying cry. This slogan foregrounds the notion that people with disabilities, who are routinely and systematically disempowered and marginalized, know what is best for them and must be included at all levels of decision making about their lives (Charlton, 2000).

The implementation of such an idea has proved problematic because it requires a redistribution of power

to the benefit of disadvantaged groups, especially in decision making (Labonte, 1994). This is challenging for healthcare professionals and the health system, as most health systems are hierarchical and authoritarian in nature and are designed with little or no participatory space for individuals and groups, other than those already in control (Pulvirenti et al., 2014). And although much policy rhetoric supports such ideas (e.g., Australia's National Chronic Diseases Strategy, where Principle 2 concerns growing a person's control over their own health) when it comes to policy implementation, support dwindles as those with the power cry 'but we know best'. So, for example, if Sally was given control over deciding where she would like the health resources currently allocated to her to be spent, she might say securing somewhere to live, or having a mental health peer support person to work with to problem-solve everyday life, or any number of things that she believes would be useful for her health. If you asked her current GP to decide, he or she might say a series of dietitian appointments and attending a group-based weight-loss program.

The term 'empowerment' is problematic and has historically been poorly defined (Finfgeld, 2004). It also presupposes the existence of a disempowered individual or group, which many challenge. However, a social justice and human rights–based approach to health empowerment is concerned with enabling disadvantaged and marginalized groups, who by definition *are* disempowered, to have the greatest control possible over their own health and the factors that influence their health. Conducive social conditions and practices that facilitate meaningful empowerment must be designed and operationalized to enable people to have a significant input into their own treatment and establishing the priorities of the system and advocating for resources. Empowering people by redesigning systems and practices will have a material effect on that group's health and well-being and is vital to influencing the social determinants of health and reducing health inequality. Empowerment understood in this way means a whole-of-systems approach where health interventions go beyond the clinic and into the community (Keleher, 2007; Greenhalg, 2009, in Pulvirenti et al., 2014, p. 306). It means professional, political and structural change, redistribution of resources and individual behaviour change by practitioners to tackle social injustice effectively.

Such individual professional behaviour change may be seen in the model of Mindful Dialogical Relationships, enacted by community-based therapists for people with physical and cognitive impairments, where 'some of the most efficient and effective ways to meet their clients' complex needs are informal, fluid, organic and often not preprogrammed' (De Bortoli et al., 2017, p. 102). This could include therapist participation in community-based sports organizations or liaison with local schools, councils or government departments with the aim of developing avenues of empowerment for people with impairments who can then more fully participate in their own local communities. Community activities can then become the inclusive living space needed for everyone living within that community. Such professional and personal efforts necessarily take place *within* communities, often where the professionals and clients involved may live together in the same community, allowing ongoing mindful, engaged and responsive relational development among people, first to include a person with special needs but gradually expanding community responses to become commonplace for other people within these communities.

In the area of mental health, the relatively new implementation of the Recovery Model provides one example in which a whole of systems approach is being taken. The recovery movement has grown from recognition that people who have a mental illness want to be empowered (Leamy et al., 2011). This means that they want service providers to view them as whole people and to work collaboratively with them towards goals, discussing options and choices with respect. Here decision making and provision of treatment are also relationship based, promoting trust and empowering people with choice and control. Systems and procedures recognize that even those with complex needs have capacities, resilience and insight. There is recognition that these people are the experts in their own lives and illness. Care plans must be developed with the service users accepted as self-determining agents with rights, choice and expertise (Horsfall et al., 2016; Slade et al., 2012). This, we argue, is one such model that could inform the operationalizing of a social justice and empowerment framework across all health systems and domains.

CHAPTER SUMMARY

Vogel (2010, p. 109) argues that if we 'scratch the surface of recent healthcare reform' we will likely to find a commitment to 'patient-centred care', but we need to note that 'beyond a general promise to put patients at the heart of health care decision-making, most nations are still in the early stages of defining concrete parameters for the delivery of patient-centred care'. At the heart of patient-centred care is patient empowerment and a commitment to genuine social justice and decision making that both champions and enables these processes and outcomes.

The need for a social justice framework or perspective arises from the recognition that:

- health and illness are determined socially and biologically,
- health and illness are distributed inequitably throughout society and
- access to fair and equitable treatment for illness is often determined by perceived social worth and social positioning.

REFLECTION POINT 4

Where do we go from here – as practitioners, patient advocate groups, educators, researchers, healthcare systems and society? What is your view?

REFERENCES

Adelson, N., 2005. The embodiment of inequity: health disparities in Aboriginal Canada. Can. J. Public Health 96 (Suppl. 2), S45–S61.

Aldorondo, E., 2007. Advancing Social Justice Through Clinical Practice. Routledge, London, UK.

Alvarez-Dardet, C., Ruiz, M.T., 2000. Rethinking the map for health inequalities. Lancet 356, S36.

Australian Bureau of Statistics, 2013. Australian Aboriginal and Torres Strait Islander health survey: first results, Australia, 2012–13, table 19 (data cube). Australian Bureau of Statistics, Canberra, ACT.

Australian Indigenous HealthInfoNet, 2016. Summary of Aboriginal and Torres Strait Islander health, 2015, Australian Indigenous ealthInfoNet, Perth, WA.

Australian Institute of Health and Welfare (AIHW), 2016. Healthy futures: Aboriginal community controlled health services report card 2016, cat. no. IHW 171. AIHW, Canberra, ACT.

Browne, A.J., Fiske, J., 2001. First nations women's encounters with mainstream health care services. West. J. Nurs. Res. 23, 126–147.

Charlton, J.I., 2000. Nothing About Us Without Us: Disability, Empowerment and Oppression. University of California Press, Oakland, CA.

Darzi, A., 2007. Our NHS, our future: NHS next stage review—interim report. Department of Health, London, UK. Viewed 1 June 2017. Available from: <www.dh.gov.uk>.

De Bortoli, T., Couch, B., Tasker, D., 2017. Therapy tales. In: Tasker, D., Higgs, J., Loftus, S. (Eds.), Mindful Dialogues in Community-Based Healthcare. Sense Publishers, Rotterdam, The Netherlands.

El-Khatib, Z., Scales, D., Vearey, J., et al., 2013. Syrian refugees, between rocky crisis in Syria and hard inaccessibility to healthcare services in Lebanon and Jordan. Confl. Health 7, 18–21.

Finfgeld, D.L., 2004. Empowerment of individuals with enduring mental health problems: results from concept analyses and qualitative investigations. ANS Adv. Nurs. Sci. 27, 44–52.

Hixon, A.L., Yamada, S., Farmer, P.E., et al., 2013. Social justice: the heart of medical education. Soc. Med. 7, 161–168.

Horsfall, D., Carrington, A., Paton, J., 2016. Stories of recovery from the bush: unravelling mental illness, self and place, research report. Western Sydney University, Sydney, NSW. Viewed 1 June 2017. Available from: <http://researchdirect.uws.edu.au/islandora/object/uws:35379>.

Keleher, H., 2007. Empowerment and health education. In: Keleher, H., MacDougall, C., Murphy, B. (Eds.), Understanding Health Promotion. Oxford University Press, Melbourne, VIC.

Kirkham, S.R., Anderson, J.M., 2002. Postcolonial nursing scholarship: from epistemology to method. ANS Adv. Nurs. Sci. 25, 1–17.

Labonte, R., 1994. Health promotion and empowerment: reflections on professional practice. Health Educ. Q. 21, 253–268.

Leamy, M., Bird, V., Le Boutillier, C., et al., 2011. Conceptual framework for personal recovery in mental health: systematic review and narrative synthesis. Br. J. Psychiatry 199, 445–452.

Lutfey Spencer, K., Grace, M., 2016. Social foundations of health care inequality and treatment bias. Annu. Rev. Sociol. 42, 101–120.

McLaughlin, A.M., 2009. Clinical social workers: advocates for social justice. Adv. Soc. Work 10, 51–68.

Marmot, M., 2005. Social determinants of health inequalities. Lancet 365, 1099–1104.

Marmot, M., Friel, S., Bell, R., et al., 2008. Closing the gap in a generation: health equity through action on the social determinants of health. Lancet 372, 1661–1669.

Nikhil, A., Patel, N.A., 2015. Health and social justice: the role of today's physician. AMA J. Ethics 17, 894–896.

Ostrand, N., 2015. The Syrian refugee crisis: a comparison of responses by Germany, Sweden, the United Kingdom, and the United States. J. Migr. Hum. Secur. 3, 255–279.

Pulvirenti, M., McMillan, J., Lawn, S., 2014. Empowerment, patient centred care and self-management. Health Expect. 17, 303–310.

Rawls, J., 1971. A Theory of Justice. Harvard University Press, Cambridge, MA.

Royal Australian College of General Practitioners (RACGP), 2016. RACGP curriculum for Australian general practice: curriculum for Australian general practice 2016, Melbourne, VIC, RACGP. Viewed 28 June 2017. Available from: <https://www.racgp.org.au/Education/Curriculum>.

Ruger, J.P., 2004. Health and social justice. Lancet 364, 1075–1080.

Schmidt, H., 2007. Patients' charters and health responsibilities. Br. Med. J. 335, 1187.

Sen, G., Östlin, P., 2007. Unequal, unfair, ineffective and inefficient gender inequity in health: why it exists and how we can change it. Final report to the WHO Commission on Social Determinants of Health, Women and Gender Equity Knowledge Network. Viewed 1 June 2017. Available from: <http://cdrwww.who.int/social_determinants/resources/csdh_media/wgekn_final_report_07.pdf>.

Sharara, S.L., Kanj, S.S., 2014. War and infectious diseases: challenges of the Syrian Civil War. PLoS Pathog. 10, e1004438.

Slade, M., Adams, N., O'Hagan, M., 2012. Recovery: past progress and future challenges. Int. Rev. Psychiatry 24, 1–4.

Solar, O., Irwin, A., 2010. A conceptual framework for action on the social determinants of health: social determinants of health, Discussion paper 2 (policy and practice). World Health Organization, Geneva, Switzerland. Viewed 1 June 2017. Available from: <http://www.who.int/sdhconference/resources/ConceptualframeworkforactiononSDH_eng.pdf?ua=>.

Sudnow, D., 1967. Passing on: The Social Organization of Dying. Prentice Hall, Englewood Cliffs, NJ.

The Editors, 2006. Introducing social medicine. Soc. Med. 1, 1–4.

Timmermans, S., 1998. Social death as a self-fulfilling prophecy: David Sudnow's 'passing on' revisited. Sociol. Q. 39, 453–472.

United Nations Development Programme, 2003. Human development reports 2003. Viewed 27 October 2003. Available from: <http://hdr.undp.org/en/content/human-development-report-2003>.

United Nations High Commissioner for Refugees (UNHCR), 2011. UNHCR Resettlement Handbook. UNHCR, Geneva, Switzerland.

Vera, E.M., Speight, S.L., 2003. Multicultural competence, social justice, and counseling psychology: expanding our roles. Couns. Psychol. 31, 253–272.

Vogel, L., 2010. International patient charters are often nonbinding or feature fuzzy metrics. CMAJ 182, doi:10.1503/cmaj.109-3342.

Wallerstein, N.B., Yen, I.H., Syme, S.L., 2011. Integration of social epidemiology and community-engaged interventions to improve health equity. Am. J. Public Health 101, 822–830.

World Health Organization, 2008. Closing the gap in a generation: health equity through action on the social determinants of health. Commission on social determinants of health final report, executive summary. WHO, Geneva, Switzerland. Viewed 1 June 2017. Available from: <www.who.int/social_determinants/thecommission/finalreport/en/index.html>.

Young, I.M., 1990. Justice and the Politics of Difference. Princeton University Press, New York, NY.

20

CLINICAL DECISION MAKING ACROSS ORTHODOX AND COMPLEMENTARY MEDICINE FIELDS

SANDRA GRACE ▪ STEPHEN LOFTUS

CHAPTER AIMS

The aims of this chapter are to:

▪ discuss the implications for mainstream allopathic practitioners of the widespread use of complementary medicine among their patients,

▪ discuss the practice of person-centred care that takes into account patients' illness experiences and values their healthcare preferences,

▪ explore alternative ways of thinking through clinical problems and provide specific examples and

▪ explore strategies for integrating alternative ways of thinking that combine the strengths of both mainstream allopathic medicine and complementary and alternative medicine.

KEY WORDS

Complementary and alternative medicine

Allopathic medicine

Integrative medicine

Evidence-based medicine

Practice-based evidence

ABBREVIATIONS/ ACRONYMS

CAM Complementary and alternative medicine

INTRODUCTION

The goal of clinical reasoning of all healthcare professionals is to identify and articulate patients' health needs and to use specialized knowledge and skills to work out ways to help patients achieve optimal health. To state this seems straightforward and obvious, but it can be problematic. This is because in developed countries the dominant healthcare system is Western medicine, often referred to as allopathic medicine. It has been characterized as biomedical, pathology-driven, cure- or disease-oriented, based on the scientific method and using evidence that is predominantly empirical-analytical (Capra, 1983; Hawk, 2005; Hayes, 2007). Foucault (1994) discussed the rise of allopathic medicine in terms of the 'clinical gaze' that focusses on a pathological view of the body, usually a dead body rather than a living person. From this allopathic viewpoint, health is seen simplistically as the absence of pathology. Once some pathology has been identified and removed, it is assumed that a patient is then automatically healthy. The problem is that this biomedical view has great difficulty articulating health and well-being. If we view health and the illness experience from other perspectives, it is clear that there are far more complex issues than a biomedical view assumes. For example, health, from the patient's viewpoint, has been described as a sense of 'homelike being in the world' (Svenaeus, 2000).

Mainstream allopathic medicine is not naturally disposed to take the patient's viewpoint into account,

211

as pathology does not need to know anything about a patient's sense of 'being at home in the world'. This may be one reason why complementary and alternative medicine (CAM) approaches to health care are so popular with patients and people who are well. Advocates of CAM approaches claim that CAM practitioners pay far more attention to what the patient feels and says about his or her health (Berger et al., 2012). One way of summarizing these differences is to say that allopathic medicine has a disease focus (what the pathologist looks at), and CAM approaches focus on the illness experience (what the patient goes through). Likewise, allopathic medicine has tended to assume that health is simply absence of pathology, whereas CAM pays far more attention to developing the wellness of patients. There is often a much greater holistic view in CAM. As Reeve (an allopathic doctor) puts it:

There is evidence within the complementary and alternative medicine (CAM) literature of individuals undertaking sophisticated and multidimensional assessments of health status and need. For some, explanations of 'dis-ease' within CAM frameworks make more sense of individual illness experiences than a pathological account. CAM users are not simply dissatisfied with conventional medicine, but make sophisticated assessments of their health needs and the appropriate therapeutic approach needed to address them, drawing on a range of knowledges to support this process (Reeve, 2010, p. 6).

Clinicians' views of legitimate health care are shaped by their education, personal experiences and their own health beliefs, which may be different from those of their patients. The diversity of views means that patients are often willing to call on a surprising range of what they see as health-promoting strategies, including self-directed activities like physical exercise, meditation and CAM. CAM encompasses a broad domain of healing resources and approaches along with their accompanying theories, evidence and beliefs. The range of therapies is wide. Some of the most popular are acupuncture, chiropractic, homoeopathy, Western herbal medicine, naturopathy, massage therapy, hypnotherapy, traditional Chinese medicine and osteopathy. Many patients are enthusiastic about the use of CAM products like herbal

and homoeopathic medicines and nutritional supplements (Armstrong et al., 2011; Reid et al., 2016).

A significant step forward in our understanding of the prevalence of CAM occurred when Eisenberg et al. (1993) published a paper on the use of unconventional medicine in the United States. This paper reported that one-third of adults in the United States had used at least one unconventional therapy in the previous year, bringing into sharp focus 'one of the most important health consumer trends of the 20th century' (Andrews, 2004, p. 226). Similar growth in CAM use has been observed in other developed countries (Williamson et al., 2008). For example, it is estimated that over two-thirds of Australians use CAM, with AUD $4 billion national annual 'out-of-pocket' expenditure (Xue et al., 2007). It is also known that consumers often use CAM in conjunction with other health-promoting strategies, yet most patients do not tell their medical doctors (Eisenberg et al., 2001). Some studies have reported that fewer than 10% of women ask their doctor's advice about using CAM during pregnancy (Forster et al., 2006; Holst et al., 2009). Failure to disclose the totality of their health care to their health practitioners could be detrimental to patients who may be ill-informed about safety risks associated with combining some herbal medicines and prescribed drugs. *Hypericum perforatum* (St. John's wort), for example, has been shown to reduce pharmaceutical effectiveness in a range of different drug classes (Hennessy et al., 2002; Mills and Bone, 2005; Pfrunder et al., 2003). A patient taking warfarin is at risk for increased bleeding if he or she is also taking gingko biloba, and a patient on hypoglycaemic therapy who takes Korean ginseng (Panax ginseng) is at risk for inadvertently altering his or her blood glucose levels (Harris et al., 2015).

Given that such a large proportion of the population in Western countries uses CAM, it is important that allopathic medical practitioners have some understanding of all the health measures taken up by their patients. Even if the medical practitioners are opposed to CAM, they need to know something about the CAM services or products that their patients are using. Clinicians owe it to their patients' health to be conversant with issues associated with the combination of CAM and allopathic medicine (Phelps, 2001). Beyond this, it can also be argued that all clinicians need to find and use anything and everything that can reasonably be expected to help their patients achieve optimal health (Saper, 2016), and this may include CAM. Person-centred care demands that clinicians focus on the patient, on the patient–practitioner relationship and on what works best for a particular patient at a particular time. Such a focus renders applying labels like 'allopathic medicine' and 'CAM' irrelevant (Cohen, 2004; Eisenberg, 1997).

> *Ultimately, medicine has a single aim: to relieve human suffering. When measured against this benchmark, different therapies can be seen as either effective or ineffective rather than 'orthodox' or 'unorthodox'. No single professional group has ownership of health, and the best healthcare requires a multidisciplinary approach (Cohen 2004, p. 646).*

Person-centred care also requires doctors to acknowledge and work with their patients' preferences for health care. As patients gain greater knowledge of, and agency in, managing their health care, it is important to work with what patients know and want. Moreover, being aware of CAM approaches can give clinicians new ways of thinking through clinical problems.

ALTERNATIVE WAYS OF THINKING THROUGH CLINICAL PROBLEMS

Practicing person-centred care means taking patients' use of CAM into account, valuing their healthcare choices and being informed about them. This could mean that clinicians may have to learn different ways of thinking through clinical problems, based on CAM or collaborating with CAM practitioners in various ways.

The dominant model of clinical reasoning in allopathic medicine is based on a technical rational approach that is grounded in biomedical science. The current dominance of evidence-based medicine is a good example of this technical rational approach. However, it is often forgotten that David Sackett, one of the pioneers of evidence-based medicine, made it clear that good clinical decision making required the integration of the best available evidence together with the expertise and experience of the clinician and the wishes and values of the patient (Sackett et al., 2000). If the patient is a passionate believer in the benefits of CAM, then this needs to be part of the clinical decision making that

occurs. Because the technical rational approach has a poor vocabulary for articulating both the personal experience of clinicians and the wishes and value systems of patients, these aspects of clinical decision making are often ignored. This is a major reason for integrating the humanities and social sciences into the curriculum of many health professions. These disciplines have vocabularies and discourses that can enable health professions to think through these wider aspects of health care. In the same way, it can be argued that CAM approaches also open up our thinking about what our patients want, need and value so that we can adopt more than one perspective in our attempts to understand and help them.

In Western medicine, biomedical and/or biopsychosocial practice models predominate, demonstrating the primacy granted to biomedical evidence. By contrast, CAM practitioners draw on a range of different practice models. For example, in homoeopathy most practitioners identify spiritual and energetic dimensions in a metaphysical model of diagnosis and treatment. Traditional Chinese medicine (TCM) interprets channels of energy or life force (Qi) as they traverse the body in 12 meridians. The underlying concepts of TCM are illustrated in Box 20.1.

Other CAM practices have evolved distinctive models of practice to assess and treat their patients. Australian osteopaths and naturopaths, for example, tend to see

---

BOX 20.1
UNDERLYING CONCEPTS OF TRADITIONAL CHINESE MEDICINE (NATIONAL CENTER FOR COMPLEMENTARY AND INTEGRATIVE HEALTH, 2013)

- The human body is a miniature version of the larger, surrounding universe.
- Harmony between two opposing yet complementary forces, called Yin and Yang, supports health, and disease results from an imbalance between these forces.
- Five elements—fire, earth, wood, metal and water—symbolically represent all phenomena, including the stages of human life, and explain the functioning of the body and how it changes during disease.
- Qi, a vital energy that flows through the body, performs multiple functions in maintaining health.

patients with complex problems who do not easily fit conventional disease patterns (Licciardone et al., 2005; Orrock, 2009). Such practitioners have had to be inventive and willing to embrace a wide range of aetiological and treatment possibilities. For example, in osteopathy, patients are initially assessed for red flags, but if a patient is deemed suitable for osteopathic care, attempts are made to make sense of the patient information by considering a range of practice models. Subjective information collected from patients and objective data from tests and examinations are considered in a context of connected functioning body systems, including biomechanical, biopsychosocial, energy-expenditure, neurological, nutritional and respiratory-circulatory (Table 20.1). It is worth noting that osteopathic medicine is now accepted as mainstream healthcare practice in some countries such as the United States.

Bortoft (2012) refers to *diversity in unity* to emphasize the multiplicity of parts that underpins a holistic view of the world. CAM approaches offer a way to be holistic and at the same time make the most of diverse approaches. Another CAM approach is that of energetic or vibrational medicine that takes account of critical events in the patient's life reasoning that emotional trauma may affect the patient's physical health. An 'energetic healer' described her diagnostic process in the following example:

A patient came in. She had had ulcerative colitis for 10 years. She was 26. It started at 16. She had medical treatment, but it was getting worse, not responding. Before it started, she was fine. I said, 'What happened at 16?' She broke down crying, and she told me the whole story. Her grandmother was a control freak, commanding the whole household, having arguments with everyone. And she said, 'I had a big argument with my grandmother one night, and the next day my grandmother suicided'. So she took all the guilt. Guilt effects the large intestine. I used psychotherapy because that's the quickest way to deal with this, and then we did acupuncture. Ten years of treatment and nobody had asked her what happened at the time her troubles started. Nobody checked why she had the problem. They were just treating the symptoms (CAM practitioner).

INTEGRATING ALTERNATIVE WAYS OF THINKING WITH THE THINKING OF MAINSTREAM ALLOPATHIC MEDICINE

Fundamental differences between the underlying philosophies of allopathic medicine and CAM are cited by many as the main barrier to their integration. These

TABLE 20.1	
Diagnostic Models Used in Osteopathic Medicine (Kuchera and Kuchera, 1994)	
Biomedical	Consideration of signs and symptoms in the context of defined diseases and a need for referral for further medical assessment and management (red flags). This is similar to any primary care practitioner.
Biomechanical	Assessment of the health of the musculoskeletal system, including how the structure (posture) and function are integrated. This is similar to other manual medicine practices and is primarily a mechanical/orthopaedic approach.
Biopsychosocial	Consideration of the psychosocial factors influencing the patient's health, including relational, occupational and financial, and the need for multidisciplinary care. (Mainstream allopathic medicine is now starting to adopt a more biopsychosocial position.)
Energy expenditure	Assessment of whether the patient has optimal energy utilization and consideration of issues that may affect the healing process (e.g., relatively minor mechanical or immune dysfunctions).
Neurological	Assessment of function in the central, peripheral and autonomic nervous systems and the relationship of those systems to all tissues of the body.
Nutritional	Foundational dietary analysis for signs of deficiency or suboptimal nutritional status.
Respiratory/circulatory	Examination of the respiratory mechanism–ensuring that the function of breathing is optimal. Assessment of all tissues of the body for full blood supply and drainage. Assessment of the structural and functional relationship between the two systems.

differences include the traditional reductionist, mechanistic approach of biomedicine as opposed to the more biocultural approach of CAM. Allopathic medicine has a focus on eliminating the disease-producing agent as opposed to CAM's focus on encouraging the innate ability of the human body to restore itself to health, and although allopathic medicine tends to have a focus on disease, CAM's focus is more on wellness (Capra, 1983; Nahin and Straus, 2001). If one adopts a strictly allopathic pathological focus, then all CAM approaches are likely to be dismissed as unsound and unscientific. However, there are now attempts to reconcile CAM approaches with allopathic medicine, evident strongly in the integrative medicine movement that is expanding globally.

MODELS OF INTEGRATION

Three different relationships between allopathic medicine and CAM have been described: pluralism, harmonization and full integration (Lewith and Bensoussan, 2004) (Fig. 20.1).

Pluralism

Pluralism refers to contrasting systems operating alongside one another with mutual respect but little or no interaction. Given the unbridgeable epistemological (i.e., knowledge determination) differences that are sometimes described between CAM and allopathic medicine, this model of parallel systems seems realistic and achievable even for the allopathic practitioners who are opposed to CAM.

Harmonization

In this model, allopathic medicine and CAM practitioners work together but with no predetermined agenda or bias. Referral may occur between systems but does not need to be the result of a planned collaboration. Such an arrangement has been described by many CAM practitioners working in allopathic medical centres (Grace, 2009; Hunter, 1993). They have described moving from 'in principle approval' to acceptance as the medical practitioners became aware of their skills and scopes of practice. In such cases, medical practitioners have come to understand and appreciate the therapeutic

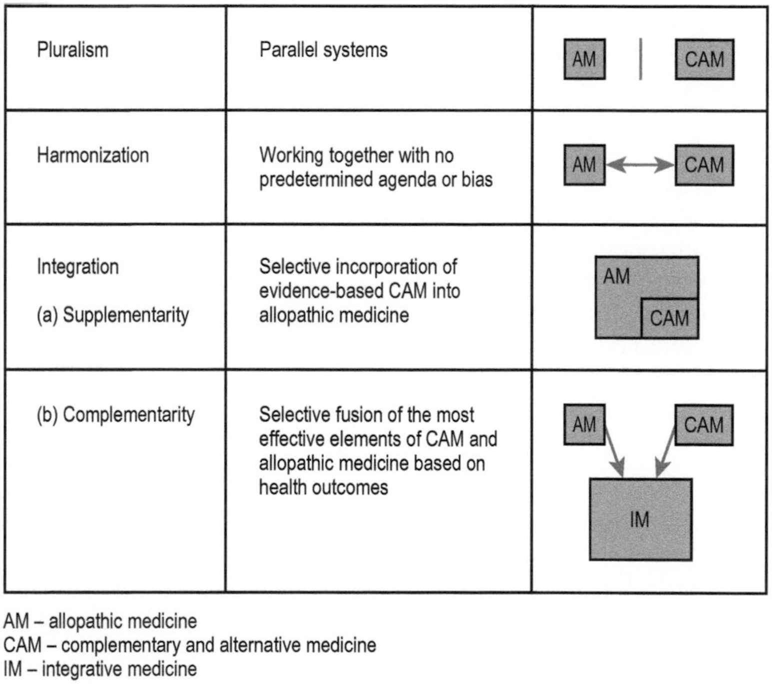

Pluralism	Parallel systems	AM ǀ CAM
Harmonization	Working together with no predetermined agenda or bias	AM ←→ CAM
Integration (a) Supplementarity	Selective incorporation of evidence-based CAM into allopathic medicine	AM / CAM
(b) Complementarity	Selective fusion of the most effective elements of CAM and allopathic medicine based on health outcomes	AM CAM → IM

AM – allopathic medicine
CAM – complementary and alternative medicine
IM – integrative medicine

Fig. 20.1 ■ Models of integration.

benefits of CAM practices. These CAM practitioners have become part of the healthcare team without any formal collaboration.

Integration

Within the model of integration, there are two dominant submodels in the literature:

1. *Selective incorporation of evidence-based CAM into allopathic medicine*
   Integrative practice in which allopathic medical practitioners act as primary contact clinicians (with subsequent referral to other providers) appears to be a common practice model in many areas (Grace and Higgs, 2010; Hollenberg, 2006; Shuval et al., 2002). In this model, allopathic medical practitioners are responsible for diagnosis and coordination of healthcare plans. The Australian Government's Enhanced Primary Care system, for instance, recognizes this model in its subsidizing of chiropractic, osteopathy, podiatry, psychology and other allied health treatments for patients with chronic health conditions. Subsidies are available only if the services are part of enhanced care plans and are supervised by allopathic medical practitioners (Health and Aged Care, 2004).
2. *Selective fusion of the most effective elements of both CAM and allopathic medicine based on health outcomes*
   The ideal model described by Lewith and Bensoussan (2004) is a selective fusion of the most effective elements of CAM and allopathic medicine for the optimal health outcomes for patients. Both biomedical evidence and clinical efficacy are valued. In this model, CAM and allopathic medicine are seen as complementary, and CAM practitioners and members of the allopathic medical profession become coworkers with equal input and standing.

INTEGRATED CLINICAL REASONING

There is increasing recognition that some allopathic clinicians readily embrace complementary approaches and have been extensively educated in both allopathic and CAM approaches (Loftus, 2009). The usual practice is to follow standard allopathic protocols with all patients to begin with and ensure there is no pathology (red flags) that should be dealt with by conventional means. There is a clear preference for using the strengths of allopathic medicine to begin with. If there are no red flags or if allopathic medicine fails, as it can do, especially in some chronic conditions such as chronic pain, these clinicians may then resort to a CAM approach. For example, one allopathic doctor who had extensive training and experience of acupuncture spoke in terms of taking one thinking hat off and putting on another (S. Loftus, 2006, pers. comm.). This same doctor also related that while undergoing the training in acupuncture, he and his other medical colleagues would regularly try to 'translate' what they were seeing and doing in the acupuncture clinic into allopathic terms. After several months of trying this, they eventually gave up and concluded that this translation was not realistic. The two ways of conceptualizing the body, health and disease were essentially incompatible. However, this did not dissuade these clinicians from using both allopathic medicine and acupuncture. This can be seen as a form of practicing the pluralism mentioned earlier. The two forms are happily used side by side but are not integrated in any deep way.

REFLECTION POINT 1

Reflection on clinical reasoning of a general medical practitioner who practices both allopathic medicine and CAM:

'I'm certainly aware of the idea that certain facts, certain concepts derive from homoeopathic ideas and certain others derive from what is common mainstream medical thinking. Within my mind these are contained within one sphere of understanding of the world. It's not so much a matter of jumping from one to the other as it is trying to appreciate what that globe actually is from any particular vantage point I happen to be looking at it from, and then comparing in my mind which pathways are going to be most useful at that point in time. Some of the more difficult decisions are to do with if I follow one route, if I give this patient an antibiotic now, how will that influence the information gathering that I need to prescribe a homoeopathic remedy that I've been trying to offer for some time? I'm trying to project outcomes based on different interventions and what's going to be most useful for the patient using different possible ways of going about it and whether it's reasonable, perhaps, to use both systems of medicine at the same time. One has to think about a number of factors in making that decision – whether the patient's going to be in close contact with you, how that influences what the best thing to do is. It's rare that the different interventions open to me are in direct competition. It's more a matter of trying to decide what's going to be most useful at any point in time.'

Readers – What do you think of these arguments and approaches?

An important challenge facing clinicians in the future is to explore ways in which allopathic medicine and CAM might become integrated in a rigorous manner that respects the strengths of both without jeopardizing the rational foundations of either. It is said we live in a postmodern world, and perhaps the integration of CAM is part of what it means to have postmodern health care. Modernism is the view, now largely discredited, that there is only one (scientific) way to view anything. This view is exemplified in health care by the dominance of biomedical allopathic medicine. A postmodern view accepts that there can be multiple perspectives on anything. The inadequacies of allopathic medicine are evident in the dissatisfaction that many people experience with conventional health care in general and its failure to provide satisfactory solutions to chronic conditions in particular. This is one of the main reasons why so many people turn to CAM. The other big reason, of course, is that patients want to actively pursue a wellness agenda in their health care and lifestyles. Therefore, we need to find new ways of conceptualizing and carrying out the care we provide.

One step that has been taken in this direction is the development of practice-based evidence. Clinicians can develop new knowledge from their experience of practice itself. There is a realization that the balance between theory and practice is not all one way (that is, from theory to practice) but can be bidirectional. This raises the important questions of how evidence from practice can be theorized, how it is theorized in different systems of thought, and how these systems of thought can inform each other.

We can take some lessons from the literature on communities of practice. There are well-known cases where people have had the courage and insight to be boundary crossers between different communities of practice. For example, Erwin Schrödinger (1947) wrote a book that brought together physicists and biologists, two groups who previously had little in common. Schrödinger was able to persuade the two groups that they did in fact have a great deal in common, and his work is now seen as the start of a new and very successful community of practice, that of molecular biology. Perhaps what we need now are people who are well informed about allopathic medicine and CAM and who can explore ways to bridge the gaps between them. Even if no new community of practice is formed, there is always the chance of cross-fertilization of ideas to the benefit of all concerned. The integrated clinical reasoning they undertake will emphasize holism and multiple ways of thinking and knowing together with what the patient values and brings to the clinical encounter (Fig. 20.2).

CHAPTER SUMMARY

In this chapter, we have explored a number of arguments:

■ The attraction of CAM to health consumers has been attributed to its much more holistic approach to health care than the more narrow and

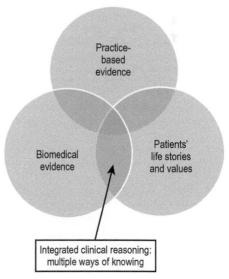

Fig. 20.2 ■ Integrated clinical reasoning.

conventional pathological account of diseases found in allopathic medicine. CAM can focus more on a patient's sense of 'dis-ease'.

■ CAM offers alternative ways of clinical reasoning and thinking through clinical problems.

■ Despite traditional epistemological differences, various collaborations between allopathic medicine and CAM have been developed in many Western countries. Such collaborations provide opportunities to create new practice knowledge, out of which can arise new practice epistemologies based on understanding of how this practice knowledge arises, is used and is developed. Individual clinicians within these collaborations both acquire practice knowledge and contribute to it.

■ A distinctive characteristic of the clinical reasoning and practice epistemology of integrative medicine is the emphasis on holism and multiple ways of thinking and knowing together with what the patient values and brings to the clinical encounter.

REFERENCES

Andrews, G.J., 2004. Sharing the spirit of the policy agenda? Private complementary therapists attitudes towards practising in the British NHS. Complement. Ther. Nurs. Midwifery 10, 217–228.

Armstrong, A., Thiebaut, S., Brown, L., 2011. Australian adults use complementary and alternative medicine in the treatment of chronic illness: a national study. Aust. N. Z. J. Public Health 35, 384–390.

Berger, S., Braehler, E., Ernst, J., 2012. The health professional-patient-relationship in conventional versus complementary and alternative medicine: a qualitative study comparing the perceived use of medical shared decision-making between two different approaches of medicine. Patient Educ. Couns. 88, 129–137.

Bortoft, H., 2012. Taking Appearance Seriously: The Dynamic Way of Seeing in Goethe and European Thought. Floris Books, Croydon.

Capra, F., 1983. Turning Point. HarperCollins, London.

Cohen, M., 2004. CAM practitioners and 'regular' doctors: is integration possible? Med. J. Aust. 180, 645–646.

Eisenberg, D., 1997. Advising patients who seek alternative medical therapies. Ann. Intern. Med. 127, 61–69.

Eisenberg, D., Kessler, R.C., Foster, C., et al., 1993. Unconventional medicine in the United States: prevalence, costs and pattern use. N. Engl. J. Med. 328, 246–252.

Eisenberg, D., Kessler, R., Van Rompay, M., et al., 2001. Perceptions about complementary therapies relative to conventional therapies among adults who use both: results from a national survey. Ann. Intern. Med. 135, 344–351.

Forster, D., Denning, A., Wills, G., et al., 2006. Herbal medicine use during pregnancy in a group of Australian women. BMC Pregnancy Childbirth 6, doi:10.1186/1471-2393-6-21.

Foucault, M., 1994. The Birth of the Clinic: An Archaeology of Medical Perception. Pantheon Books, New York.

Grace, S., 2009. Integrative Medicine in Australian Health Care: A New Direction for Primary Health Care. Vdm Verlag Dr. Müller, Saarbrücken, Germany.

Grace, S., Higgs, J., 2010. Interprofessional collaborations in integrative medicine. J. Altern. Complement. Med. 16, 1185–1190.

Harris, T., Grace, S., Eddey, S., 2015. Adverse events from complementary therapies: an update from the natural therapies workforce survey. J. Aust. Trad. Med. Soc., Part 2, 21, 162–167.

Hawk, C., 2005. When worldviews collide: maintaining a vitalistic perspective in chiropractic in the postmodern era. J. Chiropr. Humanit. 12, 2–7.

Hayes, C., 2007. Back pain: new paradigms in community care, Sydney general practitioner conference and exhibition primary care. Sydney GPCE Primary Care, 24.

Health and Aged Care, 2004. Promoting More Coordinated Care: Enhanced Primary Care: Building Better Care. Australian Government Department of Health and Ageing, Canberra.

Hennessy, M., Kelleher, D., Spiers, J.P., et al., 2002. St John's Wort increases expression of P-glycoprotein: implications for drug interactions. Br. J. Clin. Pharmacol. 53, 75–82.

Hollenberg, D., 2006. Uncharted ground: patterns of professional interaction among complementary/alternative and biomedical practitioners in integrative health care settings. Soc. Sci. Med. 62, 731–744.

Holst, L., Wright, D., Nordeng, H., et al., 2009. Use of herbal preparations during pregnancy: focus group discussion among expectant mothers attending a hospital antenatal clinic in Norwich, UK. Complement. Ther. Clin. Pract. 15, 225–229.

Hunter, A., 1993. Working in a multidisciplinary clinic: the pleasures and the pitfalls, Address to the Complementarity in Health Conference. Complement. Health Users Group, 36–43.

Kuchera, W., Kuchera, M., 1994. Osteopathic Principles in Practice. Greyden Press, Columbus.

Lewith, G.T., Bensoussan, A., 2004. Complementary and alternative medicine—with a difference. Med. J. Aust. 180, 585–586.

Licciardone, J., Brimhall, A., King, L., 2005. Osteopathic manipulative treatment for low back pain: a systematic review and meta-analysis of randomised controlled trials. BMC Musculoskel. Disord. 6, 43.

Loftus, S., 2009. Language in Clinical Reasoning: Towards a New Understanding. VDM Verlag, Saarbrucken.

Mills, S., Bone, K., 2005. The Essential Guide to Herbal Safety. Elsevier Health Science, St. Louis, MO.

Nahin, R.L., Straus, S.E., 2001. Research into complementary and alternative medicine: problems and potential. BMJ 322, 161–164.

National Center for Complementary and Integrative Health, 2013. Traditional Chinese medicine: in depth. US Department of Health and Human Services. Viewed 7 September 2016. Available from: https://nccih.nih.gov/health/whatiscam/chinesemed.htm.

Orrock, P., 2009. Profile of members of the Australian Osteopathic Association: part 1—the practitioners. Int. J. Osteopath. Med. 12, 14–24.

Pfrunder, A., Schiesser, M., Gerber, S., et al., 2003. Interaction of St John's Wort with low-dose oral contraceptive therapy: a randomized controlled trial. Br. J. Clin. Pharmacol. 56, 683–690.

Phelps, K., 2001. AMA discussion paper: complementary medicine. J. Austr. Integr. Med. Soc. 4.

Reeve, J., 2010. Interpretive medicine: supporting generalism in a changing primary care world. Royal College of General Practitioners, Occasional paper 88.

Reid, R., Steel, A., Wardle, J., et al., 2016. Complementary medicine use by the Australian population: a critical mixed studies systematic review of utilisation, perceptions and factors associated with use. BMC Complement. Altern. Med. 16, 176.

Sackett, D.L., Straus, S.E., Richardson, W.S., et al., 2000. Evidence-based Medicine: How to Practice and Teach EBM. Churchill Livingstone, Edinburgh.

Saper, R., 2016. Integrative medicine and health disparities. Global Adv. Health Med. 5, 5–8.

Schrödinger, E.C., 1947. What Is Life? The Physical Aspect of the Living Cell. Cambridge University Press, Cambridge.

Shuval, J.T., Mizrachi, N., Smetannikov, E., 2002. Entering the well-guarded fortress: alternative practitioners in hospital settings. Soc. Sci. Med. 55, 1745–1755.

Svenaeus, F., 2000. The Hermeneutics of Medicine and the Phenomenology of Health: Steps Towards a Philosophy of Medical Practice. Kluwer Academic, Dordrecht.

Williamson, M., Tudball, J., Toms, M., et al., 2008. Information Use and Needs of Complementary Medicines Users. National Prescribing Service, Sydney.

Xue, C., Zhang, A., Lin, V., et al., 2007. Complementary and alternative medicine use in Australia: a national population-based survey. J. Altern. Complement. Med. 13, 643–650.

Section 4 CLINICAL REASONING AND THE PROFESSIONS

21

CLINICAL REASONING IN MEDICINE

ALAN SCHWARTZ ■ OLGA KOSTOPOULOU

CHAPTER AIMS

The aims of this chapter are to:

■ describe the process of diagnostic reasoning in medicine,

■ compare problem-solving and decision-making approaches to research on clinical reasoning and diagnostic error,

■ introduce dual-process models of reasoning and

■ explain educational implications of dual-process theory.

KEY WORDS

Decision making

Problem solving

Dual-process theory

Bayes' theorem

Hypothesis testing

Pattern recognition

ABBREVIATIONS/ ACRONYMS

EBM Evidence-based medicine

INTRODUCTION

How do physicians solve diagnostic problems? What is known about the process of diagnostic clinical reasoning? Why might a diagnosis be missed? In this chapter, we sketch our current understanding of answers to these questions by reviewing the cognitive processes and mental structures employed in diagnostic reasoning in clinical medicine. We will not consider the parallel issues of selecting a treatment or developing a management plan. For theoretical background, we draw upon two approaches that have been particularly influential in research in this field: problem solving and decision making.

Problem-solving research has usually focussed on how an ill-structured problem situation is defined and structured (normally by generating a set of diagnostic hypotheses) and is exemplified in the work of Elstein et al. (Elstein, 2009; Elstein et al., 1978), Bordage et al. (e.g., Bordage, 1994) and Norman (2005). Psychological decision research (also known as 'behavioural decision making') has typically looked at factors affecting diagnosis or treatment choice in well-defined, tightly controlled situations, as illustrated in the work of Kahneman et al. (Kahneman et al., 1982), Kahneman (2003) and Schwartz and Bergus (2008). A common theme in both approaches is that human rationality is limited or 'bounded'. Nevertheless, researchers within the problem-solving paradigm have concentrated on identifying the strategies of experts in a field of medicine, with the aim of facilitating the acquisition of these strategies by learners. Behavioural decision research, on the other hand, contrasts human performance with a normative statistical model of reasoning under uncertainty. It illuminates cognitive processes by examining people's inherent reasoning tendencies (cognitive heuristics) and the associated reasoning errors (cognitive biases) to which even experts are not immune. As a way of improving human reasoning, this literature concentrates on debiasing and decision aids.

A COMMON BASIS: DUAL-PROCESS THEORY

Both medical problem-solving and decision-making research have adopted dual-process or 'two systems' accounts of cognition described (with variations in details) by Kahneman (2003), Stanovich and West (2000) and, perhaps most accessibly, by Kahneman (2011). These accounts posit two distinct cognitive systems or types of processing. System 1 is a fast, automatic and intuitive mode of thinking that shares similarities with perception. Judgements made using System 1 take advantage of the power of pattern recognition, emotional cues and a set of cognitive heuristics and are susceptible to associated biases and the effect of the emotional state of the judge and emotional content of the judgement. System 1's accuracy is contingent on interactions among the features of the task and the judge's prior experiences and memories. System 2 is a slow, effortful, analytic mode that applies rules in an emotionally neutral manner (Fig. 21.1, from Kahneman, 2003). When appropriate data are available, System 2 yields the most normatively rational reasoning, but it is easily disrupted by high cognitive load. Therefore both systems can lead to error under different conditions. Dual-process theory is broadly accepted among psychologists, with variations

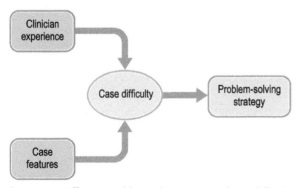

Fig. 21.1 ■ Effect on problem-solving strategy of case difficulty, clinician experience and case features. (From Kahneman, D., 2003. Maps of bounded rationality: a perspective on intuitive judgement and choice. In: Frangsmyr, T. (Ed.), Les Prix Nobel: The Nobel Prizes 2002. Stockholm, Sweden, Almqvist & Wiksell International, pp. 416–499, with permission from The Nobel Foundation.)

focussing on when and how the two systems activate and interact with one another, differences in how experts and novices rely on each system and conditions under which each system is expected to provide better performance.

REFLECTION POINT 1

Reasoning operates simultaneously through dual processes: a fast, intuitive process (System 1) and a slow, analytical process (System 2).

PROBLEM SOLVING: DIAGNOSIS AS HYPOTHESES GENERATION AND SELECTION

To solve a clinical diagnostic problem means first to recognize a malfunction and then to set about tracing or identifying its causes. The diagnosis is thus an explanation of disordered function and, where possible, a causal explanation.

In most cases, not all of the information needed to identify and explain the situation is available in the early stages of the clinical encounter. Physicians must outline potential diagnoses (a 'differential diagnosis'), consider their likelihood and severity and decide what information to collect, which aspects of the situation need attention and what can be safely set aside. Thus data collection is both sequential and selective. Experienced physicians often go about this task almost automatically, sometimes very rapidly; novices are slower and collect more information. There are several likely reasons for this. For example, novices may generate more diagnostic hypotheses on average than experts, or they may generate less appropriate diagnostic hypotheses that do not help them reduce the 'problem space' quickly; they may experience greater uncertainty and think that more information may reduce this; or they may lack efficient strategies for information search.

THE HYPOTHETICO-DEDUCTIVE METHOD

Early Hypothesis Generation and Selective Data Collection

In their pioneering studies on clinical reasoning, Elstein et al. (1978) found that diagnostic problems are solved by a process of generating a limited number of hypotheses, or problem formulations, early in the workup and using them to guide subsequent data collection and integration. Each hypothesis can be used to predict what additional findings ought to be present if it were true. The workup is then a guided search for these findings; hence, the method is hypothetico-deductive and based on System 2 processes. Elstein et al. ascertained the universality of the hypothetico-deductive method in diagnostic problem solving: Novices and experienced physicians alike attempt to generate hypotheses to explain clusters of findings, although the content of the experienced group's productions is of higher quality.

Other clinical researchers have concurred with this view (Kuipers and Kassirer, 1984; Nendaz et al., 2005). It has also been favoured by medical educators (e.g., Kassirer and Kopelman, 1991), but the emergence of dual-process theory has redirected interest towards System 1 processes in hypothesis generation, with many authors and practitioners claiming that they lead to better diagnosis, at least in expert clinicians.

Data Collection and Interpretation

Data obtained must be interpreted in the light of the hypotheses being considered. A clinician could collect data quite thoroughly but could nevertheless ignore, misunderstand or misinterpret a significant fraction. In contrast, a clinician might be overly economical in data collection but could interpret whatever is available quite accurately. Elstein et al. (1978) found no statistically significant association between thoroughness of data collection and accuracy of data interpretation. Although studies based on medical record reviews have often attributed diagnostic failures to inadequate data collection (e.g., Singh et al., 2007), experimental research has not found a strong association between thoroughness of data collection and accurate judgement or diagnosis (Kostopoulou et al., 2017a).

Investigators in the problem-solving tradition have asked study participants to think aloud while problem solving and have then analyzed their verbalizations and their data collection (Elstein et al., 1978; Kostopoulou et al., 2017b; Nendaz et al., 2005; Neufeld et al., 1981). Considerable variability in acquiring and interpreting data has been found, increasing the complexity of the research task.

Consequently, some researchers switched to controlling the data presented to participants, to concentrate on data interpretation and problem formulation (e.g., Kuipers et al., 1988). Controlling the presentation of data facilitates analysis at the price of fidelity to clinical realities. This strategy is the most widely used in current research on clinical reasoning, the shift reflecting the influence of the paradigm of decision-making research. Sometimes clinical information is presented sequentially to participants so that the case unfolds in a simulation of real time, but the participant is given few or no options in data collection (e.g., Kostopoulou et al., 2012; Nurek et al., 2014). The analysis can focus on memory organization, knowledge utilization, data interpretation or problem representation (e.g., Bordage, 1994; Groves et al., 2003). In other studies, clinicians are given all the data at once and asked to make a diagnostic or treatment decision (e.g., Sirota et al., 2017). Weiner et al. (Weiner et al., 2010, 2013) used unannounced standardized patients (actors presenting as patients incognito to physicians) and real patients carrying concealed audio recorders to demonstrate several important features of diagnostic decision making. These included failure to probe for information and identify diagnoses based in patient context rather than physiology (Weiner et al., 2010, 2013) and greater attention to case features identified by physician activity rather than those features revealed spontaneously by patients (Schwartz et al., 2016).

Case Specificity

Problem-solving expertise varies greatly across cases and is highly dependent on the clinician's mastery of the particular domain. Differences among clinicians are to be found more in their understanding of the problem and their problem representations rather than in the reasoning strategies employed (Elstein et al., 1978). Thus it makes more sense to talk about reasons for success and failure in a particular case than about generic traits or strategies of expert diagnosticians.

REFLECTION POINT 2

Reasoning depends on knowledge and the structure of knowledge in memory. General 'reasoning skills' may result in different outcomes depending on the experiences stored in the reasoner's memory.

DIAGNOSIS AS CATEGORIZATION OR PATTERN RECOGNITION

The finding of case specificity also challenged the hypothetico-deductive model as an adequate account of the process of clinical reasoning. Patel et al. (e.g., Eva et al., 1998; Groen and Patel, 1985) pointed out that the clinical reasoning of experts in familiar situations frequently does not display explicit hypothesis testing. It is rapid, automatic and often nonverbal.

Expert reasoning in familiar situations looks more like a System 1 process of pattern recognition or direct automatic retrieval from a well-structured network of stored knowledge (Groen and Patel, 1985). Because experienced clinicians have a better sense of clinical realities and the likely diagnostic possibilities, they can also more efficiently generate an early set of plausible hypotheses to avoid fruitless and expensive pursuit of unlikely diagnoses. The research emphasis thus shifted from the problem-solving process to the organization of knowledge in the long-term memory of experienced clinicians. Unlike hypothetico-deduction, pattern recognition and matching approaches do not require, or assume, that causal reasoning takes place. Expert–novice differences are partly explicable in terms of the size of the knowledge store of prior instances available for pattern recognition. This theory of clinical reasoning has been developed with particular reference to pathology, dermatology and radiology, where the clinical data are predominantly visual. Additionally, better diagnosticians are thought to have more diversified and abstract links between clinical features or aspects of the problem (Bordage, 1994). Experts in a domain are more able to relate findings to each other and to potential diagnoses and to identify what additional findings are needed to complete a picture (Elstein et al., 1993). These capabilities suggest that more experienced physicians are working with more abstract representations and are not simply trying to match a new case to a specific previous instance. However, such a matching process may still occur with simple cases (where there is a larger store of specific memories) or with cases that are somehow memorable, because matching would be quicker than abstraction.

MULTIPLE REASONING STRATEGIES

Norman et al. (1994) found that experienced physicians used a hypothetico-deductive strategy with difficult cases only. When a case is perceived to be less challenging, quicker and easier methods are used, such as pattern recognition or feature matching. Thus controversy about the methods used in diagnostic reasoning can be resolved by positing that the method selected depends on the perceived characteristics of the problem. Furthermore, there is an interaction between the clinician's level of skill and the perceived difficulty of the task (Elstein, 1994). Easy cases are solved by pattern recognition and going directly from data to diagnostic classification – what Groen and Patel (1985) called *forward reasoning*. Difficult cases need systematic hypothesis generation and testing. Whether a problem is easy or difficult depends in part on the knowledge and experience of the clinician who is trying to solve it (Fig. 21.2). At the same time, perceived difficulty can be manipulated: Mamede et al. (2008) suggested to study participants that some clinical cases had been previously seen by experienced physicians who had failed to diagnose them. The researchers found that cases perceived as difficult took longer to diagnose and were diagnosed more accurately than those perceived as straightforward. Using think-aloud strategies, they also found more frequent mentions of findings, causal mechanisms and diagnoses for the supposedly difficult cases, suggesting that participants were using an analytical rather than intuitive approach for those cases.

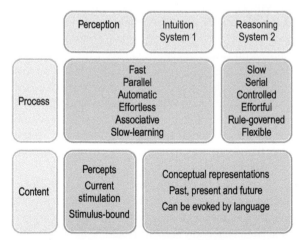

Fig. 21.2 ■ Characteristics of two cognitive systems for judgement. (From Kahneman, D., 2003. Maps of bounded rationality: a perspective on intuitive judgement and choice. In: Frangsmyr, T. (Ed.), Les Prix Nobel: The Nobel Prizes 2002. Stockholm, Sweden, Almqvist & Wiksell International, pp. 416–499, with permission from The Nobel Foundation.)

Dual-process accounts support the value of multiple reasoning strategies, particularly when different strategies (e.g., pattern recognition and hypothetico-deduction) may bring to bear the power of Systems 1 and 2, respectively.

DECISION MAKING: DIAGNOSIS AS OPINION REVISION

In the literature on medical decision making, reaching a diagnosis is conceptualized as a process of reasoning about uncertainty in a statistical manner and updating an opinion with imperfect information (the clinical evidence). As new information is obtained, the probability of each diagnostic possibility is continuously revised. Each posttest probability becomes the pretest probability for the next stage of the inference process. Bayes' theorem, the formal mathematical rule for this operation, states that the posttest probability is a function of two variables, pretest probability and the strength of the new diagnostic evidence. The pretest probability can be either the known prevalence of the disease or the clinician's belief about the probability of disease before new information is acquired. The strength of the evidence is measured by a *likelihood ratio*, the ratio of the probabilities of observing a particular finding in patients with and without the disease of interest. This framework directs attention to two major classes of errors in clinical reasoning: errors in a clinician's beliefs about pretest probability and errors in assessing the strength of the evidence. Bayes' theorem is a normative rule for diagnostic reasoning; it tells us how we *should* reason, but it does not claim that we actually revise our opinions in this way. Indeed, from the Bayesian viewpoint, the psychological study of diagnostic reasoning centres on errors in both components, which are discussed later in the chapter.

The revision of opinion, using Bayes' theorem, underlies teaching about diagnosis in evidence-based medicine (EBM) (Straus et al., 2010). A variety of paper and online tools and spreadsheets have been developed to provide decision support or simplify EBM calculations. A typical example is the graphical Bayesian nomogram, which permits quick calculation of posterior probabilities from prior probability and likelihood ratio information. Fagan (1975) published the best-known nomogram, which is widely available on a pocket-sized card. Schwartz (1998) provides a widely used online version.

A COMMON CHALLENGE: DIAGNOSTIC ERROR

Diagnostic error has attracted considerable interest in recent years due, in large part, to the patient safety movement. The US National Academy of Medicine (National Academies of Sciences, Engineering and Medicine, 2015) concluded that 'most people will experience at least one diagnostic error in their lifetime, sometimes with devastating consequences' (p. 1). Estimates of the number of deaths that might be a result of diagnostic errors are alarming (Graber, 2013).

CASE STUDY 21.1

Screening Mammography

Screening mammography for breast cancer has an overall likelihood ratio of about 9 for a positive test: The odds of breast cancer are about nine times higher in a woman with a positive mammogram than a woman with a negative mammogram (Breast Cancer Surveillance Consortium, 2013). How likely is it that an average adult woman who gets a positive mammogram actually has breast cancer? What if she is younger than 40 years of age? A Bayesian reasoner, considering a pretest breast cancer probability of 0.1% (1 breast cancer per 1000 women, or 1 : 999 odds),

should conclude that a woman with a positive mammogram will have about a 1% posttest probability of breast cancer. In a woman younger than 40 years of age, however, not only is the pretest probability lower than average (closer to .005%, or 5 breast cancers per 100,000 women), but the likelihood ratio of a positive test is lower (closer to 5). As a result, a positive test in a young woman suggests a 0.02% probability of breast cancer. How accurate was your estimate of the posttest probability, the pretest probability and the strength of the test?

Furthermore, in acute care settings such as general practice, accident and emergency and after-hours care, diagnostic error accounts for the majority of litigation cases (Gandhi et al., 2006; Silk, 2000).

Graber et al. define diagnostic error as a 'diagnosis that was unintentionally delayed (sufficient information was available earlier), wrong (another diagnosis was made before the correct one), or missed (no diagnosis was ever made), as judged from the eventual appreciation of more definitive information' (Graber et al., 2005, p. 1493). Similarly, and more concisely, Singh et al. (2014) define it as 'a missed opportunity to make a timely or correct diagnosis based on the available evidence'. The Committee of the National Academy of Medicine (National Academies of Sciences, Engineering, and Medicine, 2015) proposed a more patient-centred definition: 'the failure to (a) establish an accurate and timely explanation of the patient's health problem(s) or (b) communicate that explanation to the patient' (p. 85).

ERRORS IN HYPOTHESIS GENERATION AND RESTRUCTURING

Neither pattern recognition nor hypothesis testing is an error-proof strategy, nor is either always consistent with statistical rules of inference from imperfect information. Kassirer and Kopelman (1991) illustrated and discussed errors that can occur in difficult cases in internal medicine, and Graber et al. (2002) reviewed classes of error.

Because so much depends on the interaction between patient and clinician, prescriptive guidelines for the proper amount of hypothesis generation and testing are still unavailable for the student clinician and probably never will be. Perhaps the most useful advice is to emulate the hypothesis-testing strategy used by experienced clinicians when they are having difficulty, because novices will experience as problematic many situations that the former solve by routine pattern-recognition methods. In an era that emphasizes cost-effective clinical practice, routinely gathering data unrelated to diagnostic hypotheses should be discouraged.

Many diagnostic problems are so complex that the correct solution is not contained within the initial set of hypotheses. Restructuring and reformulating must occur through time, as data are obtained and the clinical picture evolves. Ideally, one might want to work purely inductively, reasoning only from the facts, but this strategy is never employed because it is inefficient and produces high levels of cognitive strain (Elstein et al., 1978). It is much easier to solve a problem where some boundaries and hypotheses provide the needed framework. On the other hand, early problem formulation may also bias the clinician's thinking (Voytovich et al., 1985). Errors in interpreting the diagnostic value of clinical information have been found by several research teams (Elstein et al., 1978; Kostopoulou et al., 2009).

ERRORS IN DATA INTERPRETATION

The most common error in interpreting findings is overinterpretation: Data that should not support a particular hypothesis, and that might even suggest that a new alternative be considered, are interpreted as consistent with hypotheses already under consideration (Elstein et al., 1978; Kostopoulou et al., 2009). The data best remembered tend to be those that support the hypotheses generated (Arkes and Harkness, 1980). Where findings are distorted in recall, it is generally in the direction of making the facts more consistent with typical clinical pictures. Positive findings are overemphasized, and negative findings tend to be discounted. From a Bayesian standpoint, these are all errors in assessing the diagnostic value of information, i.e., errors in subjective assessments of the likelihood ratio. These errors are thought to arise from an adaptive function: the need to keep problem representations simple enough to remain within the capacity of cognitive bounds (i.e., on working memory). Alternatively, decision makers need to find, or create, an alternative that is sufficiently superior to its competitors so that it can be defended from postdecisional challenges that occur to the decision maker or are posed by others (Svenson et al., 2009). Finally, according to theories of cognitive consistency, data interpretation errors may arise from an inherent need to avoid cognitive tension by forming coherent representations, where perceptions, beliefs, attitudes and feelings are all consonant with each other (Simon et al., 2004). Even when clinicians agree on the presence of certain clinical findings, wide variations have been found in the importance assigned to these findings in the course of interpreting their meaning.

Data interpretation errors occur not only postdiagnosis but also while clinical data are being evaluated before a final diagnosis. The latter phenomenon is known as 'predecisional information distortion' and has been observed and measured in a variety of judgement tasks (e.g., consumer, legal, political, investment, risk, medical) and with different populations, both lay and expert (see review by DeKay, 2015). Predecisional information distortion involves changing the value of incoming information to support the hypothesis or preference that is currently leading. It thus treats reasoning as bidirectional, from the observed data to an emerging hypothesis and from that hypothesis to any new data. From this point of view, predecisional information distortion is incompatible with the Bayesian approach that relies on the independence of the observed data from the prior hypothesis. Distortion of information can occur either by bolstering information in relation to the leading hypothesis or by denigrating information in relation to a trailing hypothesis. Two studies by Nurek et al. have found a tendency towards denigration in physicians' diagnostic judgements, i.e., undervaluing support for the trailing hypothesis, in comparison to unbiased evaluations of information by a control group (Nurek et al., 2014). Distortion is driven by the strength of belief in the initial diagnosis and, in turn, can maintain commitment to that diagnosis during the course of a diagnostic problem (Kostopoulou et al., 2012). Given that an initial hypothesis can bias judgement and lead to the wrong final diagnosis and decision (Kostopoulou et al., 2017b), we need to pay more attention to how physicians interpret information during the diagnostic process.

ERRORS IN PROBABILITY ESTIMATION

Many errors in probability revision result from reasoning tendencies, known as cognitive heuristics, which rely on the most salient and easily accessible information. These simple heuristics provide good estimates in most contexts but may yield systematic biases in others. For example, people are prone to overestimate the frequency of vivid or easily recalled events and to underestimate the frequency of events that are either very ordinary or difficult to recall (Tversky and Kahneman, 1981). As a result of this 'availability heuristic', clinicians may pursue investigations for rare but memorable diseases or injuries and may overlook more common explanations for the patient's symptoms. Memorability can be influenced by factors unrelated to probability, for example, high emotion (a missed diagnosis that led to patient death), novelty (an unusual presentation or disease), personal experience (it happened to me, to my family, to a friend, to a colleague), recency (a patient I saw yesterday) or a good story (patient surviving against all odds).

People also overestimate the frequency of events that fit their ideas of a prototypical or representative case (Tversky and Kahneman, 1974). When this 'representativeness heuristic' comes into play, the probability of a disease, given a finding (also known as the 'positive predictive value' of a finding), can be confused with the probability of a finding, given the disease (i.e., the 'sensitivity' of the finding).

Small probabilities tend to be overestimated, and large probabilities tend to be underestimated (Tversky and Kahneman, 1981). Cumulative prospect theory (Tversky and Kahneman, 1992) and similar theories provide formal descriptions of how people distort probabilities in risky decision making. The distortions are exacerbated when the probabilities are vague and not precisely known (Einhorn and Hogarth, 1986). Recent work in the science of emotion has also highlighted ways in which task-engendered emotions influence the estimation of probabilities and many other kinds of judgements (Lerner et al., 2015) (Box 21.1).

ERRORS IN PROBABILITY REVISION

Conservatism

In clinical case discussions, data are commonly presented sequentially. In this circumstance, people often fail to

---

BOX 21.1

SOME COMMON BIASES IN ESTIMATING PROBABILITY

- Overestimating probability of easily recalled events
- Overestimating probability of events that fit a perceived pattern
- Overestimating small probabilities
- Underestimating large probabilities
- Overconfidence in probability estimates

revise their diagnostic probabilities as much as they should, according to Bayes' theorem. This 'stickiness' has been called *conservatism* and was one of the earliest cognitive biases identified (Edwards, 1968). A heuristic explanation of conservatism is that people revise their diagnostic opinion up or down from an initial anchor, which is either given in the problem or subjectively formed. Final opinions are sensitive to the anchor, and the adjustment up or down from this anchor is typically insufficient, so the final judgement is closer to the initial anchor than Bayes' theorem would require (Tversky and Kahneman, 1974).

The effect of conservatism is compounded when, in collecting data, there is a tendency to seek information that confirms the current hypothesis rather than data that facilitate efficient testing of competing hypotheses. This tendency has been called 'pseudodiagnosticity' (Kern and Doherty, 1982) or 'confirmation bias'. Explanations, based on information-processing approaches to studying decision making, explain conservatism and confirmation bias in terms of how and in what order information is sampled from memory and the environment (Oppenheimer and Kelso, 2015).

Confounding Probability and Value of an Outcome

It is difficult for everyday judgement to keep separate accounts of the probability of a particular disease and the benefits that accrue from detecting it. Probability revision errors that are systematically linked to the perceived cost of mistakes demonstrate the difficulties experienced in separating assessments of probability from preferences or values (Poses et al., 1985), a phenomenon also known as 'value-induced bias'.

Base-Rate Neglect

The basic principle of Bayesian inference is that a posterior probability is a function of two variables, the prior probability and the strength of the evidence. Some studies have found that, unless trained to use Bayes' theorem and to recognize when it is appropriate, physicians are just as prone as anyone else to misusing or neglecting base rates in diagnostic inference (Elstein, 1988). Other studies, however, have failed to find evidence of base-rate neglect (Gill et al., 2005). In fact, in some clinical disciplines, such as general practice (family medicine), physicians are particularly sensitive to base-rate information (Sirota et al., 2017).

Order Effects

Bayes' theorem implies that, given identical information, clinicians should reach the same diagnostic opinion, regardless of the order in which information is presented. Order effects mean that final opinions are also affected by the order of presentation of information. Some studies have found primacy effects in diagnostic judgements (e.g., Nurek et al., 2014), and others have found recency effects (Bergus et al., 1995). In other words, the information presented early (or late) in a case is given more weight than information presented later (a primacy effect) (or earlier – a recency effect). Inconsistencies in the study results most likely stem from the different research methodologies and structure of the clinical cases employed. This, nevertheless, does not invalidate the general finding that order of information matters (Box 21.2).

EDUCATIONAL IMPLICATIONS

What can be done to help learners acquire expertise in clinical reasoning? Particularly in light of the two-system theory of cognition, we endorse the multiple reasoning strategies position espoused by both Norman and Eva (2010) and seek to identify educational implications from both intuitive and analytical models in problem solving and decision making.

PROBLEM SOLVING: EDUCATIONAL IMPLICATIONS

Even if experts in nonproblematic situations do not routinely generate and test hypotheses and instead retrieve a solution (diagnosis) directly from their

---

BOX 21.2
SOME COMMON BIASES IN REVISING PROBABILITIES

- Ignoring or overrelying on the initial probability
- Inadequate adjustment of initial probability
- Searching only for confirming evidence
- Interpreting neutral evidence as confirming evidence
- Confusing the seriousness of error (missing the disease) with the disease probability
- Greater attention to evidence presented early or late in the process

structured knowledge, they clearly do generate and evaluate alternatives when confronted with problematic situations. For novices, most situations will initially be problematic, and generating a small set of hypotheses is a useful procedural guideline. Because much expert hypothesis generation and testing are implicit, a model that calls it to the novice's attention will aid learning. The hypothetico-deductive model directs learners towards forming a conception of the problem and using this plan to guide the workup. This plan will include a set of competing diagnoses and the semantic relationships that facilitate separating between similar and different diagnostic candidates. This makes it possible to reduce unnecessary and expensive laboratory testing, a welcome emphasis in an era that stresses cost containment.

Clinical experience is needed in contexts closely related to future practice, because transfer from one context to another is limited. In one way, this phenomenon reinforces a very traditional doctrine in medical education: Practical arts are learned by supervised practice and rehearsal supplemented by didactic instruction. In another way, it conflicts with traditional training, because the model implies that trainees will not generalize as much from one context (say, hospitalized patients) to another (say, ambulatory patients) as has traditionally been thought.

For reasoners to generalize from specific exemplars to more abstract patterns, clinical experience must be reviewed and analyzed so that the correct general models and principles are abstracted from the experience. Well-designed educational experiences can facilitate the development of the desired cognitive structures. Given the emerging consensus about characteristics distinguishing experts from novices, an effective route to the goal would be extensive, focussed practice and feedback with a variety of problems (Eshach and Bitterman, 2003).

DECISION MAKING: EDUCATIONAL IMPLICATIONS

If expert clinicians are not consistent in their approach across cases, what can or should be taught to learners? In this section, we review some recent efforts to teach clinical decision making that have been strongly influenced by decision psychology principles and research results. Again, as dual-process theory has emerged as the dominant paradigm of judgement, medical educators

have begun to wrestle with its implications for education (Pelaccia et al., 2011).

Evidence-Based Medicine

EBM is particularly relevant for the diagnostic inference process discussed in this chapter because it is currently the most popular vehicle explicitly advocating a Bayesian approach to clinical evidence. Textbooks on EBM (e.g., Strauss et al., 2010) show how to use prevalence rates and likelihood ratios to calculate posterior probabilities of diagnostic alternatives (predictive value of a positive or negative test), and at least one recent study suggests that prevalence data may be readily available in the medical literature for inpatient adult medicine problems (Richardson et al., 2003). Formal statistical reasoning and decision analysis are likewise explained and advocated in an ever-growing number of works aimed at physicians (Kassirer and Kopelman, 1991; Lee, 2004; Mark, 2006; Sox et al., 1988). Decision theory, decision analysis and EBM seem to be on their way to becoming standard components of clinical education and training.

Decision Support Systems

Computer programs that run on microcomputers or in conjunction with electronic health records and can provide decision support have been developed. The role of these programs in medical education and in future clinical practice is still to be determined, but they hold out hope for addressing both cognitive and systemic sources of diagnostic error (Graber et al., 2002; Kostopoulou et al., 2017a). A recent metareview of systematic reviews of computer decision support systems found four significant challenges that remain for such systems to become more useful to physicians: improvement in knowledge representation, ability to update the system's knowledge to match advances in medicine, stronger interoperability with electronic health records and better matching of decision support tools with clinicians' cognitive workflow (Nurek et al., 2015).

Debiasing

A number of researchers have proposed methods for debiasing judgements without resorting to formal methods of probability estimation and revision (Morewedge et al., 2015; Mumma and Wilson, 1995). General debiasing methods include educating decision makers about common biases, encouraging them to consider information that is likely to be underweighted or over-looked, e.g., consider alternative hypotheses, consider the opposite and so on, and making decision makers more accountable for their decisions. Evidence for the effectiveness of debiasing strategies for diagnostic reasoning is mixed (Graber, 2003); however, a recent systematic review by Lambe et al. (2016) found two types to be the most promising in improving diagnostic accuracy: asking clinicians explicitly to consider alternative diagnoses, and guided reflection, i.e., using a structured process to reflect and reason. Guided reflection tended to improve diagnostic judgement relative to using intuition or first impressions, particularly in complex cases.

REFLECTION POINT 3

To reduce the chances of missing a diagnosis, 'consider the opposite': Think actively of other diagnostic alternatives. Consider case findings that do not support your current hypothesis or that also support other hypotheses.

Embracing System 1

Not all educators and researchers agree that intuition must result in biased diagnosis or that it is inferior to analytical reasoning. Some have sought to demonstrate the conditions under which System 1 judgements can be better than System 2 judgements and under which conditions intuition can be further improved.

In their review of heuristics in decision making, Gigerenzer and Gaissmeier (2011) identify fast-and-frugal trees as a valuable System 1 process that has received attention in diagnostic reasoning, both as a descriptive model of how physicians actually make diagnostic judgements and as a prescriptive approach to diagnosis that can outperform more complex, statistical clinical scoring rules, while being easier to apply. Research on fuzzy trace theory by Reyna et al. (see Blalock and Reyna, 2016) distinguishes between verbatim (System 2) and gist (System 1) encoding, retrieval and reasoning; research using the theory has demonstrated that reasoning from gist can lead to better decision making than reasoning from verbatim representations of the same problem (for a review, see Blalock and Reyna, 2016).

Hogarth (2001) called attention to the importance of the learning environment (particularly the quality of feedback and cost of error) in improving System 1 judgements. 'Kind' learning environments provide timely, accurate, relevant and informative feedback, thus enabling quick and accurate learning, especially if the outcome of an error is damaging. Short-term weather forecasting is the archetypal 'kind' learning environment. In contrast, in 'wicked' learning environments, feedback is incomplete, irregular or delayed, and outcomes cannot easily be attributed to specific events, i.e., there are confounders that make learning difficult. When the error cost is low, decision makers may develop unwarranted confidence, not realizing that they have learned the wrong lessons or drawn the wrong conclusions. Unfortunately, most clinical environments have more wicked than kind learning features. Norman and Eva (2010) nevertheless reviewed studies in diagnostic reasoning in which both experts and novices performed better and made fewer errors when explicitly instructed to use their experience (rather than analytical reasoning) and pointed out that intuitive reasoning should not be suppressed, even were it possible. They concluded that medical education should encourage both System 1 and System 2 judgement.

CHAPTER SUMMARY

- Research on the clinical reasoning of physicians has examined differences between expert and novice clinicians, psychological processes in judgement and decision making, factors associated with nonnormative biases in judgement, improving instruction and training to enhance acquisition of good reasoning and the development, evaluation and implementation of decision support systems and guidelines.

- Concerns about diagnostic error have become a motivating force in the study of clinical reasoning in medicine. Research in this area stands at the intersection of the interests of psychologists, medical sociologists, health policy planners, economists, patients and clinicians.

- The prevailing view of two parallel and interacting cognitive systems, one fast and intuitive, the other slow and deliberative, has led to increased focus on how to study and improve each system and its interaction.

REFERENCES

Arkes, H.R., Harkness, A.R., 1980. Effect of making a diagnosis on subsequent recognition of symptoms. J. Exp. Psychol. 6, 568–575.

Bergus, G.R., Chapman, G.B., Gjerde, C., et al., 1995. Clinical reasoning about new symptoms despite pre-existing disease: sources of error and order effects. Fam. Med. 27, 314–320.

Blalock, S.J., Reyna, V.F., 2016. Using fuzzy-trace theory to understand and improve health judgments, decisions, and behaviors: a literature review. Health Psychol. 35, 781–792.

Bordage, G., 1994. Elaborated knowledge: a key to successful diagnostic thinking. Acad. Med. 69, 883–885.

Breast Cancer Surveillance Consortium (BCSC), 2013. Performance measures for 1,838,372 screening mammography examinations from 2004 to 2008 by age—based on BCSC data through 2009, United States, National Cancer Institute. Viewed 16 February 2017. Available from: http://breastscreening.cancer.gov/data/performance/screening/2009/perf_age.html.

DeKay, M.L., 2015. Predecisional information distortion and the self-fulfilling prophecy of early preferences in choice. Curr. Dir. Psychol. Sci. 24, 405–411.

Edwards, W., 1968. Conservatism in human information processing. In: Kleinmuntz, B. (Ed.), Formal Representation of Human Judgement. Wiley, New York, NY, pp. 17–52.

Einhorn, H.J., Hogarth, R.M., 1986. Decision making under ambiguity. J. Bus. 59, S225–S250.

Elstein, A.S., 1988. Cognitive processes in clinical inference and decision making. In: Turk, D.C., Salovey, P. (Eds.), Reasoning, Inference, and Judgment in Clinical Psychology. Free Press, New York, NY, pp. 17–50.

Elstein, A.S., 1994. What goes around comes around: the return of the hypothetico-deductive strategy. Teach. Learn. Med. 6, 121–123.

Elstein, A.S., 2009. Thinking about diagnostic thinking: a 30-year perspective. Adv. Health Sci. Educ. Theory Pract. 14, 18.

Elstein, A.S., Kleinmuntz, B., Rabinowitz, M., et al., 1993. Diagnostic reasoning of high- and low-domain knowledge clinicians: a re-analysis. Med. Decis. Making 13, 21–29.

Elstein, A.S., Shulman, L.S., Sprafka, S.A., 1978. Medical Problem Solving: An Analysis of Clinical Reasoning. Harvard University Press, Cambridge, MA.

Eshach, H., Bitterman, H., 2003. From case-based reasoning to problem-based learning. Acad. Med. 78, 491–496.

Eva, K.W., Neville, A.J., Norman, G.R., 1998. Exploring the etiology of content specificity: factors influencing analogic transfer and problem solving. Acad. Med. 73 (Suppl. 10), S1–S5.

Fagan, T.J., 1975. Nomogram for Bayes' theorem. N. Engl. J. Med. 293, 257.

Gandhi, T.K., Kachalia, A., Thomas, E.J., et al., 2006. Missed and delayed diagnoses in the ambulatory setting: a study of closed malpractice claims. Ann. Intern. Med. 145, 488–496.

Gigerenzer, G., Gaissmaier, W., 2011. Heuristic decision making. Annu. Rev. Psychol. 62, 451–482.

Gill, C.J., Sabin, L., Schmid, C.H., 2005. Why clinicians are natural Bayesians. BMJ 330, 1080–1083.

Graber, M., 2003. Metacognitive training to reduce diagnostic errors: ready for prime time? Acad. Med. 78, 781.

Graber, M.L., 2013. The incidence of diagnostic error in medicine. BMJ Qual. Saf. 22 (Suppl. 2), ii21–ii27.

Graber, M.L., Franklin, N., Gordon, R., 2005. Diagnostic errors in internal medicine. Arch. Intern. Med. 165, 1493–1499.

Graber, M., Gordon, R., Franklin, N., 2002. Reducing diagnostic errors in medicine: what's the goal? Acad. Med. 77, 981–992.

Groen, G.J., Patel, V.L., 1985. Medical problem-solving: some questionable assumptions. Med. Educ. 19, 95–100.

Groves, M., O'Rourke, P., Alexander, H., 2003. The clinical reasoning characteristics of diagnostic experts. Med. Teach. 25, 308–313.

Hogarth, R.M., 2001. Educating Intuition. University of Chicago Press, Chicago, IL.

Kahneman, D., 2003. Maps of bounded rationality: a perspective on intuitive judgement and choice. In: Frangsmyr, T. (Ed.), Les Prix Nobel: The Nobel Prizes 2002. Almqvist & Wiksell International, Stockholm, Sweden, pp. 416–499.

Kahneman, D., 2011. Thinking, Fast and Slow. Farrar, Strous, & Giroux, New York, NY.

Kahneman, D., Slovic, P., Tversky, A. (Eds.), 1982. Judgement Under Uncertainty: Heuristics and Biases. Cambridge University Press, New York, NY.

Kassirer, J.P., Kopelman, R.I., 1991. Learning Clinical Reasoning. Williams & Wilkins, Baltimore, MD.

Kern, L., Doherty, M.E., 1982. 'Pseudodiagnosticity' in an idealized medical problem-solving environment. J. Med. Educ. 57, 100–104.

Kostopoulou, O., Mousoulis, C., Delaney, B.C., 2009. Information search and information distortion in the diagnosis of an ambiguous presentation. Judgm. Decis. Mak. 4, 408–418.

Kostopoulou, O., Porat, T., Corrigan, D., et al., 2017a. Diagnostic accuracy of GPs when using an early intervention decision support system: a high fidelity simulation. Br. J. Gen. Pract. 67, e201–e208.

Kostopoulou, O., Russo, J.E., Keenan, G., et al., 2012. Information distortion in physicians' diagnostic judgments. Med. Decis. Making 32, 831–839.

Kostopoulou, O., Sirota, M., Round, T., et al., 2017b. The role of physicians first impressions in the diagnosis of possible cancers without alarm symptoms. Med. Decis. Making 37, 9–16.

Kuipers, B.J., Kassirer, J.P., 1984. Causal reasoning in medicine: analysis of a protocol. Cogn. Sci. 8, 363–385.

Kuipers, B., Moskowitz, A.J., Kassirer, J.P., 1988. Critical decisions under uncertainty: representation and structure. Cogn. Sci. 12, 177–210.

Lambe, K.A., O'Reilly, G., Kelly, B.D., et al., 2016. Dual-process cognitive interventions to enhance diagnostic reasoning: a systematic review. BMJ Qual. Saf. 25, 808–820.

Lerner, J.S., Li, Y., Valdesolo, P., et al., 2015. Emotion and decision making. Annu. Rev. Psychol. 66, 799–823.

Lee, T.H., 2004. Interpretation of data for clinical decisions. In: Goldman, L., Ausiello, D. (Eds.), Cecil Textbook of Medicine, twenty-second ed. Saunders, Philadelphia, PA, pp. 23–28.

Mamede, S., Schmidt, H., Rikers, R., et al., 2008. Influence of perceived difficulty of cases on physicians' diagnostic reasoning. Acad. Med. 83, 1210–1216.

Mark, D.B., 2006. Decision-making in clinical medicine. In: Kasper, D.L., Braunwald, E., Fauci, A.S., et al. (Eds.), Harrison's Principles of Internal Medicine, sixtieth ed. McGraw-Hill, New York, NY.

Morewedge, C.K., Yoon, H., Scopelliti, I., et al., 2015. Debiasing decisions: improved decision making with a single training intervention. Policy Insights Behav. Brain Sci. 2, 129–140.

Mumma, G.H., Wilson, S.B., 1995. Procedural debiasing of primacy/anchoring effects in clinical-like judgements. J. Clin. Psychol. 51, 841–853.

National Academies of Sciences, Engineering, and Medicine, 2015. Improving Diagnosis in Health Care. The National Academies Press, Washington, DC.

Nendaz, M.R., Gut, A.M., Perrier, A., et al., 2005. Common strategies in clinical data collection displayed by experienced clinician-teachers in internal medicine. Med. Teach. 27, 415–421.

Neufeld, V.R., Norman, G.R., Feightner, J.W., et al., 1981. Clinical problem-solving by medical students: a cross-sectional and longitudinal analysis. Med. Educ. 15, 315–322.

Norman, G., 2005. Research in clinical reasoning: past history and current trends. Med. Educ. 39, 418–427.

Norman, G.R., Eva, K.W., 2010. Diagnostic error and clinical reasoning. Med. Educ. 44, 94–100.

Norman, G.R., Trott, A.L., Brooks, L.R., et al., 1994. Cognitive differences in clinical reasoning related to postgraduate training. Teach. Learn. Med. 6, 114–120.

Nurek, M., Kostopoulou, O., Delaney, B.C., et al., 2015. Reducing diagnostic errors in primary care: a systematic meta-review of computerized diagnostic decision support systems by the LINNEAUS collaboration on patient safety in primary care. Eur. J. Gen. Pract. 21 (Suppl.), 8–13.

Nurek, M., Kostopoulou, O., Hagmayer, Y., 2014. Predecisional information distortion in physicians' diagnostic judgments: strengthening a leading hypothesis or weakening its competitor? Judgm. Decis. Mak. 9, 572–585.

Oppenheimer, D.M., Kelso, E., 2015. Information processing as a paradigm for decision making. Annu. Rev. Psychol. 66, 277–294.

Pelaccia, T., Tardif, J., Triby, E., et al., 2011. An analysis of clinical reasoning through a recent and comprehensive approach: the dual-process theory. Med. Educ. Online 16, 5890.

Poses, R.M., Cebul, R.D., Collins, M., et al., 1985. The accuracy of experienced physicians' probability estimates for patients with sore throats: implications for decision making. JAMA 254, 925–929.

Richardson, W.S., Polashenski, W.A., Robbins, B.W., 2003. Could our pretest probabilities become evidence based? a prospective survey of hospital practice. J. Gen. Intern. Med. 18, 203–208.

Schwartz, A., 1998. Nomogram for Bayes' theorem. Viewed 16 February 2017. Available from: http://araw.mede.uic.edu/cgi-bin/testcalc.pl.

Schwartz, A., Bergus, G., 2008. Medical Decision Making: A Physician's Guide. Cambridge University Press, Cambridge, UK.

Schwartz, A., Weiner, S.J., Binns-Calvey, A., et al., 2016. Providers contextualise care more often when they discover patient context by asking: meta-analysis of three primary data sets. BMJ Qual. Saf. 25, 159–163.

Silk, N., 2000. What Went Wrong in 1000 Negligence Claims: Health Care Risk Report. Medical Protection Society, Leeds, UK, pp. 13–16.

Simon, D., Snow, C.J., Read, S.J., 2004. The redux of cognitive consistency theories: evidence judgments by constraint satisfaction. J. Pers. Soc. Psychol. 86, 814–837.

Singh, H., Meyer, A.N., Thomas, E.J., 2014. The frequency of diagnostic errors in outpatient care: estimations from three large observational studies involving US adult populations. BMJ Qual. Saf. 727–731.

Singh, H., Thomas, E.J., Khan, M.M., et al., 2007. Identifying diagnostic errors in primary care using an electronic screening algorithm. Arch. Intern. Med. 167, 302–308.

Sirota, M., Kostopoulou, O., Round, T., et al., 2017. Prevalence and alternative explanations influence cancer diagnosis: an experimental study with physicians. Health Psychol. 36, 477–485.

Sox, H.C., Jr., Blatt, M.A., Higgins, M.C., et al., 1988. Medical Decision Making. Butterworth-Heinemann, Boston, MA.

Stanovich, K.E., West, R.F., 2000. Individual differences in reasoning: implications for the rationality debate? Behav. Brain Sci. 23, 645–726.

Strauss, S.E., Glasziou, P., Richardson, W.S., et al., 2010. Evidence-Based Medicine: How to Practice and Teach It, fourth ed. Churchill Livingstone, London, UK.

Svenson, O., Salo, I., Lindholm, T., 2009. Post-decision consolidation and distortion of facts. Judgm. Decis. Mak. 4, 397.

Tversky, A., Kahneman, D., 1974. Judgement under uncertainty: heuristics and biases. Science 185, 1124–1131.

Tversky, A., Kahneman, D., 1981. The framing of decisions and the psychology of choice. Science 211, 453–458.

Tversky, A., Kahneman, D., 1992. Advances in prospect theory: cumulative representation of uncertainty. J. Risk Uncertain. 5, 297–323.

Voytovich, A.E., Rippey, R.M., Suffredini, A., 1985. Premature conclusions in diagnostic reasoning. J. Med. Educ. 60, 302–307.

Weiner, S.J., Schwartz, A., Sharma, G., et al., 2013. Patient-centered decision making and health care outcomes: an observational study. Ann. Intern. Med. 158, 573–579.

Weiner, S.J., Schwartz, A., Weaver, F.M., et al., 2010. Contextual errors and failures in individualizing patient care: a multicenter study. Ann. Intern. Med. 153, 69–75.

22 CLINICAL REASONING IN NURSING

BARBARA J. RITTER ■ MICHAEL J. WITTE

CHAPTER AIMS

The aims of this chapter are to:

- discuss theoretical perspectives pertaining to clinical reasoning,
- review studies relevant to understanding nurses' clinical reasoning,
- explore errors in diagnostic reasoning, implications and recommendations and
- highlight educational strategies to promote clinical reasoning.

KEY WORDS

Clinical reasoning
Clinical guidelines
Hypothetico-deductive model
Intuition
Pattern recognition
Skilled know-how

ABBREVIATIONS/ ACRONYMS

CT Critical thinking
EBP Evidence-based practice
EHR Electronic health record
H Hermeneutics
IOM Institute of Medicine

IPT Information Processing theory
PBL Problem-based learning

INTRODUCTION

Clinical reasoning represents the essence of nursing practice. It is intrinsic to all aspects of care provision and is critical to all forms of nursing education, practice and research. Knowledge about clinical reasoning is important for nursing education because education and teaching that are based on inappropriate or irrelevant models of reasoning can not only lead to wasted time and effort but also result in graduates who are ill-prepared to reason well in practice. Clinical reasoning is important for nursing practice. Patient care provision is becoming increasingly more complex and difficult. Nurses are assuming more responsibility with the emergence of nurse practitioners (NPs). There is, therefore, a need for sound reasoning skills to provide high-quality care with positive outcomes. It is also most important to avoid the costly, even deadly, mistakes that can occur from faulty reasoning and errors in decision making. An understanding of nurses' clinical reasoning is an important part of nursing research. There is a need to develop and test theories of nurses' cognitive processes and reasoning skills. Research is also needed to describe and explain the relationship between nurses' reasoning and patient outcomes. The results of this research can help nurses assume greater responsibility in the healthcare delivery system as we develop and improve nursing practice.

DEFINITION OF CLINICAL REASONING

The literature provides several definitions of nurses' clinical reasoning. For example, Gordon et al. (1994) saw nurses' reasoning as a form of clinical judgement that occurs in a series of stages: encountering the patient; gathering clinical information; formulating possible diagnostic hypotheses; searching for more information to confirm or reject these hypotheses; reaching a diagnostic decision; and determining actions. Ritter (1998) viewed clinical reasoning as a process involving inclusion of evidence to facilitate optimum patient outcomes. Using this logic, nurses' clinical reasoning is important in four ways:

1. Understanding the significance of data
2. Identifying and diagnosing actual or potential patient problems
3. Making clinical decisions to assist in problem resolution
4. Achieving positive patient outcomes

According to O'Neill et al. (2005), clinical decision making is a complex task geared towards the identification and management of patients' health needs that requires a knowledgeable practitioner combined with reliable information and a supportive environment. From this perspective, with experience, nurses can develop a method of reasoning that provides them with an 'intuitive grasp' of the whole clinical situation, without having to rely on the step-by-step analytic approach of the formal nursing process. These authors advocated a nursing curriculum that would include activities that would foster students' skills in intuitive judgement. Thus an understanding of nurses' reasoning and decision making is essential and fundamental to providing care.

THEORETICAL PERSPECTIVES

Several different theoretical perspectives have helped provide an understanding of nurses' clinical reasoning: information processing, decision analysis and hermeneutics.

Information Processing Theory

Information processing theory (IPT) was first described by Newell and Simon (1972) in their seminal work examining how individuals with a great deal of experience in a specific area (domain expertise) reasoned during a problem-solving task. A fundamental premise of Information Processing theory is that human reasoning consists of a relationship between an information processing system (the human problem solver) and a task environment (the context in which problem solving occurs). A postulate of this theory is 1) that there are limits to the amount of information that one can process at any given time, and 2) that effective problem solving is the result of being able to adapt to these limitations. Miller's (1956) earlier classic work had demonstrated that an individual's working, short-term memory can hold only 7 +/− 2 symbols at a time. However, a critique of Miller's work is that it focussed on the ability to remember random, meaningless facts. Newell and Simon (1972) showed that the capacity of short-term memory could be greatly increased by 'chunking' simple units into familiar and more meaningful patterns. Individuals with a great deal of knowledge and meaningful experience in a particular domain can more easily chunk information pertaining to that domain and thus can make more efficient use of their short-term memory during reasoning. Meaningful experience is crucial.

Another 'memory bank' identified by Newell and Simon (1972) was long-term memory, which has potentially infinite storage space for information. The theory proposes that information gained from knowledge and experience is stored throughout life in long-term memory and that it takes longer to access long-term memory information than the small amount of information temporarily stored in short-term memory. According to this theory, the information stored in long-term memory may need to be accessed by associating it with related information, which helps explain why experts reason so well within their own domain. Indeed, cognitive research has demonstrated that experts possess an organized body of domain-specific conceptual and procedural knowledge that can be easily accessed using reasoning strategies (heuristics) and specific reasoning processes that are gradually learned through academic learning and through clinical experience (Glaser and Chi, 1988; Joseph and Patel, 1990).

Decision Analysis Theory

Decision Analysis theory was introduced in medicine several decades ago as a method of solving difficult clinical problems. Decision Analysis theory methods include use of Bayes' theorem, use of decision trees, sensitivity analysis and utility analysis. Using the Decision Analysis theory involves mathematical formulas, tabular techniques, nomograms and computer programs. These techniques use the clinical data to calculate the probability of certain diagnoses and outcomes.

Several nursing studies have demonstrated the applicability of Decision Analysis theory to nurses' decision making. In her classic study examining the relationship between the expected value (anticipated outcome) that nurses assign to each of their outcomes and their ranking of nursing actions, Grier (1976) demonstrated that nurses select actions that are consistent with their expected values, which seems to support the use of decision trees in some instances of nurses' reasoning and decision making. Lipman and Deatrick (1997) found that NP students who used a decision tree made better decisions about diagnosis and treatment choices for both acute and chronic conditions. Lauri and Salantera (1995) studied decision-making models and the variables related to them. Findings were that the nature of nursing tasks and the context yielded the greatest difference in decision-making approach. Lewis (1997) found that conflict and ambiguity significantly increased task complexity. Therefore recommendations should consider task complexity during model design when developing decision models for use in nursing. Narayan et al. (2003) examined decision analysis as a tool to support an analytical pattern of reasoning; they found that decision analysis is especially valuable in difficult and complex situations when there are mutually exclusive options and there is time for deliberation. The reality is that in real-world practice there may not be time to work through a formal decision analysis. Formal decision analysis like this also assumes that the decision maker can gather all possible relevant information before making the final decision. This is in contrast to the use of heuristics and hermeneutics, which we consider next.

Hermeneutics and Heuristics

Hermeneutics is the art and study of interpretation. Hermeneutics should not be confused with heuristics or the use of cognitive shortcuts or rules of thumb. Heuristics can reduce the cognitive load and simplify the diagnostic reasoning process. Heuristics are often based on experience, patient characteristics and the context in which the patient presents. Good use of heuristics allows decisions to be made by gathering a limited amount of information, but this has to be information that is known to be relevant to the case. This is why past experience of similar cases matters. The past experience can help the nurse to judge what information might be most relevant. The intent of studies of nurses' reasoning, using heuristics, is to understand how nurses interpret the clinical world, including their reasoning as they make decisions about patient care. This means we can use a hermeneutic approach in these studies. Benner et al. (1992) used a hermeneutic approach to study the development of expertise in critical care nursing practice. Their findings indicated that nurses at different levels of expertise 'live in different clinical worlds, noticing and responding to different directives for action' (Benner et al., 1992, p. 13). Findings from a later study by the same authors (Benner et al., 1996) indicate that this clinical world is shaped by experience that teaches nurses to make qualitative distinctions in practice. They also found that beginner nurses were more task oriented, and those with more experience focussed more on understanding their patients and their illness states. Many studies of nurses' clinical reasoning have focussed on clinical judgement.

Clinical Judgement Studies

Nurses' clinical judgement represents a composite of traits that assists them in reasoning (Tanner, 1987). Benner et al. (1992), in their hermeneutic study, described characteristics of clinical judgement exhibited by critical care nurses with varying levels of practice experience when they reasoned about patient care. Characteristics of clinical judgement that were identified in the most experienced subjects included 1) the ability to recognize patterns in clinical situations that fit with patterns they had seen in other similar clinical cases, 2) a sense of urgency related to predicting what lies ahead, 3) the ability to concentrate simultaneously on multiple, complex patient cues and patient management therapies and 4) an aptitude for realistically assessing patient priorities and nursing responsibilities.

The characteristics of clinical judgement identified by Tanner (1987) and Benner et al. (1992) assist in our understanding of nurses' clinical reasoning by identifying and describing some of the cognitive traits or skills that nurses use during reasoning. Benner et al. (1996) and later Benner et al. (2011) in their subsequent work help further the theoretical understanding of nurses' judgement that is needed to improve educators' ability to teach their students to reason better and to provide nurses in practice with knowledge that will help them to solve problems and to make better decisions about patient care. In this later work, Benner et al. (2011) identified 'nine aspects of being and thinking like a nurse' (p. 9). They are as follows:

1. developing a sense of salience
2. situated learning and integrating knowledge acquisition and knowledge use
3. engaged reasoning-in-transition
4. skilled know-how
5. response-based practices
6. agency
7. perceptual acuity and interpersonal engagement with patients
8. integrating clinical and ethical reasoning
9. developing clinical imagination

REFLECTION POINT 1

The nine aspects of being and thinking like a nurse all stem from a critical thinking approach, which involves analysis, evaluation and synthesis of content. This approach can be fostered with student-centred learning activities, such as simulation, because they provide an opportunity for the theoretical memory to start to become 'muscle memory', or the movement from 'knowing that' to 'knowing how', according to Benner's 2015 Novice to Expert theory. Preceptorships with expert nurses, who exemplify the Bennerian qualities, are also powerful ways to expose novice nurses to role models who show what 'thinking like a nurse' means in the clinical setting.

Problem-Solving and Decision-Making Studies

One of the primary objectives of clinical reasoning is to make decisions to resolve problems. Thus research into nurses' problem solving and decision making provides understanding about the processes involved in their clinical reasoning. Problem-solving and decision-making studies can be regarded as a distinct body of

research that is separate from Decision Analysis theory and hermeneutic studies. The assumption in these studies is that one of the primary objectives of clinical reasoning is straightforward resolution of problems. A number of researchers have investigated the complexity of nurses' decision-making tasks from this perspective and have identified a range of reasoning strategies, including the hypothetico-deductive method, intuition and pattern recognition. Although there is frequently a focus on the healthcare professional making decisions alone, these studies sometimes do emphasize the importance of consultation with experienced colleagues, especially when still learning.

Intuition Studies

Several investigators have proposed that intuition is an important part of nurses' reasoning processes. A classic study that continues to guide nursing research on intuition was conducted by Pyles and Stern (1983) to explore the reasoning of a group of critical care nurses with varying levels of expertise. The investigators identified a 'gut feeling' experienced by the more seasoned nurse subjects, which they believed was just as important to nurses' reasoning about patient cases as their formal knowledge. Subjects said they used these gut feelings to temper information from specific clinical cues; they also emphasized the importance of previous clinical experience in developing intuitive skills. Rew (1990) demonstrated the important role that intuition played in nurses' reasoning and decision making. Subjects described their intuitive experiences as strong feelings or perceptions about their patients and about themselves and how they respond to their patients. These perceptions also involved anticipated outcomes that they sensed without going through an analytical reasoning process. Another perspective on intuition comes from Kahneman (2013), one of the pioneers of decision-making research, who proposed that intuition was nothing more or less than recognition, hence once again, the importance of experience.

Diagnostic Reasoning Studies

Ritter (2000) studied the combination of two models (Information Processing and Hermeneutics) to explain diagnostic reasoning. Although previous research related to clinical reasoning used either Information Processing or Hermeneutical models (Fig. 22.1 and Box 22.1), it

Information processing model

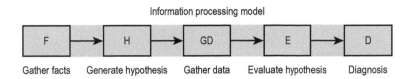

Gather facts   Generate hypothesis   Gather data   Evaluate hypothesis   Diagnosis

Hermeneutical model

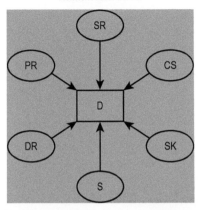

PR = pattern recognition; SR = similarity recognition; CS = common-sense understanding;
SK = skilled know-how; S = sense of salience; DR = deliberative rationality; D = diagnosis

Fig. 22.1 ■ Representation of the Information Processing and Hermeneutical model components.

BOX 22.1
HERMENEUTICAL MODEL DEFINITION OF TERMS (RITTER, 2000)

- **Common-sense understanding** is a common understanding in diverse situations of life in general.
- **Deliberative rationality** is the ability to change one's interpretation of a situation by considering other alternatives.
- **Pattern recognition** is the ability to recognize relationships among cues.
- **Sense of salience** is understanding certain events to be more important than others.
- **Skilled know-how** is independent of reliance on analytical thinking but rather involves processing numerous complex variables, simultaneously, in an unconscious, automatic, efficient manner knowing what to do, when to do it and how to do it to discern when particular findings might be relevant.
- **Similarity recognition** is the ability to recognize similarities with past experiences even if the current experience differs from the previous experience.

can be argued that neither model alone fully describes all components of diagnostic reasoning. The Ritter study systematically examined NPs' diagnostic reasoning using both models.

Findings suggest that both models operate among the 10 NPs who participated in this particular study (Ritter, 2000). The NPs used the Information Processing model 55% of the time and the Hermeneutical model 45% of the time.

Gathering data is a key aspect of clinical reasoning. It involves using the senses to purposefully collect specific meaningful information about a patient so that diagnostic meaning can be assigned to the information. The Ritter (2000) study makes it clear that the process of gathering data in generating a hypothesis is essential as the hypothesis is a tentative state that may be altered, confirmed or negated. Thus forming a tentative diagnosis is important to guard against prematurely closing the diagnostic reasoning process before considering an alternative diagnosis. In the Ritter study, expert NPs demonstrated skilled know-how when they meticulously gathered, and carefully acquired, the appropriate data to formulate a diagnosis. That NPs use a combination of both models (Fig. 22.2) is the most significant finding of this study. Expert NPs' diagnostic reasoning demonstrates an overlap and blending of each component. The two models of information processing and hermeneutics are quite different from the so-called dual-process theory of cognition.

The dual-process theory of cognition divides reasoning into System 1 and System 2 (Box 22.2). Pirret (2016) compared the diagnostic reasoning of 30 NPs and 16

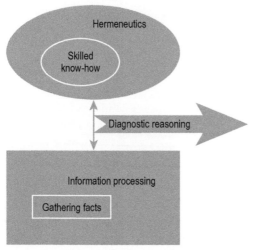

Fig. 22.2 ■ Blended Information Processing and Hermeneutical model.

BOX 22.2
DUAL PROCESSING

Intuitive (System 1) and analytic (System 2) processes; the degree to which each is used is dependent on the clinical situation.

■ **System 1 processes** (commonly referred to as heuristics such as intuition, gut feelings, pattern recognition) are fast and are used automatically when clinicians are involved in familiar case presentations. Cognitive load is reduced, and the diagnostic reasoning process is simplified. This enables clinicians to reach a diagnosis without proceeding with the time-expensive process of exploring unlikely 'differential' diagnoses.

■ **System 2 processes** (commonly referred to as hypothetico-deductive reasoning) are slower, logical, methodical and deliberative.

resident physicians engaging with a complex case, using dual-process theory.

The Pirret (2016) study revealed that NPs incorporated more System 1 (intuitive) processes in general compared with residents. However, the diagnostic reasoning style, use of either more analytical or more nonanalytical reasoning, was not related to the preferred diagnostic reasoning abilities of the participants. Findings indicated that both NPs and resident physicians used System 2 (analytic) processes when required. New or difficult cases triggered System 2 thinking. However, regardless of which clinical reasoning processes are used, diagnostic errors can occur (Institute of Medicine, 2015).

Diagnostic Errors in Clinical Reasoning and Preventing

In 2015, the Institute of Medicine (IOM) published a landmark study on diagnosis entitled 'Improving Diagnosis in Health Care'. The report noted that many patients will at some time experience one or more diagnostic errors including delayed or inaccurate diagnoses. According to the report, far too little attention has been paid to diagnostic errors, and if not addressed the incidence of these errors will likely become worse. To improve the situation, the report made eight recommendations (p. 306):

1. Facilitate more effective teamwork in the diagnostic process among healthcare professionals, patients and their families.
2. Enhance healthcare professional education and training in the diagnostic process.
3. Ensure health information technologies that support patients and healthcare professionals in the diagnostic process.
4. Develop and deploy approaches to identify, learn from and reduce diagnostic errors and near misses in clinical practice.
5. Establish a work system and culture that support the diagnostic process and improvements in diagnostic performance.
6. Develop a reporting environment and medical liability system that facilitate improved diagnosis through learning from diagnostic errors and near misses.
7. Design a payment and care delivery environment that supports the diagnostic process.

8. Provide dedicated funding for research on the diagnostic process and diagnostic errors.

REFLECTION POINT 2

Clinical reasoning assignments that teach the students an analytical approach to the patient encounter provide a greater understanding of safe diagnostic processes.

Informatics content that emphasizes a critical analysis of workflows enables students to identify inefficiencies and safety concerns in current care approaches. The informatics content also highlights how medical information systems, such as electronic health records (EHRs), are used to streamline communication of patient information and automate evidence-based practice and clinical decision tools. By understanding the way the EHR supports nursing, the student can maximize patient safety by correctly inputting patient data and utilizing the EHR's safety tools.

The Institute of Medicine emphasized the importance of development of sound data tools to examine diagnostic reasoning and errors. These tools should, and could, be used to evaluate current practices in the diagnostic process. The data could also be used to compare diagnostic decisions with clinical outcomes. Important developments that aid this work are the rapid improvements in information technology such as the growth in digital records. Using these new developments, some progress has been made in addressing systems causes of diagnostic error. Information technology has improved clinicians' ability to follow up on diagnostic tests in a timely fashion, which should reduce the incidence of delayed diagnoses. The development of an electronic workflow to standardize and improve communication among the team members could also reduce error. Del Fiol et al. (2008) and Zakim et al. (2008) claimed that diagnostic reasoning could be improved with electronic diagnostic decision support tools. For example, tools such as 'info-buttons' could be integrated into EHRs and provide direct links to relevant online clinical decision support (CDS) tools at the point of care.

CDS tools encompass a variety of information resources, such as online medical textbooks, and clinical practice guidelines that can enhance decision making in the clinical workflow. The aim is to close the gap between research and practice by providing clinicians with electronically communicated clinical knowledge and patient information at critical points in the diagnosis and treatment process. Evidence-based practice (EBP) has become the cornerstone strategy for clinicians to translate research findings into clinical practice. By incorporating scientific evidence and EBP into decision making, CDS can improve patient treatment. This facilitates diagnostic accuracy and more rational care with better outcomes. Thus it is essential that nursing curricula include activities that foster students' skills in diagnostic reasoning and are reflective of the realities encountered in actual practice, such as using modern technology on a regular basis.

Educational Focus on Clinical Reasoning

As noted, nurses increasingly need well-developed reasoning skills to assist them in understanding and resolving the complex patient problems encountered in practice. Barrows and Pickell (1991, p. 3) remind us that 'ambiguities and conflicting or inadequate information are the rule in medicine'. This is equally true in nursing, where dealing with complex patient problems with uncertain and unpredictable outcomes requires continual astute reasoning and accurate and efficient decision making. Thus the ability to think critically is essential. Lee et al. (2006) emphasize the importance of both cognitive and metacognitive skills, i.e., thinking about one's thinking, in clinical reasoning to promote the use of self-regulated learning and facilitate the development of critical thinking (CT) and reflective practice abilities. The cognitive skills that today's nursing students need to reason accurately and make decisions effectively in practice have prompted nurse educators to adjust their teaching methods. More creative teaching methods have been adopted that are designed to improve students' reasoning skills and furnish them with a repertoire of creative approaches to care (Norman and Schmidt, 1993).

Much of nursing education literature has begun to focus on ways to teach CT. Fonteyn and Flaig (1994) proposed using case studies to improve nursing students' reasoning skills by teaching them to identify potential patient problems, suggest nursing actions and describe outcome variables that would allow them to evaluate the effectiveness of their actions. Case studies provide the advantage of allowing nurse educators to give frequent feedback in the safe environment of simulation and to provide reality-based learning (Manning et al., 1995; Neill et al., 1997; Ryan-Wenger and Lee, 1997). Lipman and Deatrick (1997) found that beginning NP students tended to formulate diagnoses too early in the data-gathering phase, thus precluding consideration of all diagnostic options. When they used a case study approach incorporating algorithms to guide the decision-making process, students developed a broader focus, and diagnostic accuracy improved. To increase realism, case studies can be designed to provide information in chronological segments that more closely reflect real-life cases, in which clinical events and outcomes evolve over time (Fonteyn, 1991). Other methods that have been suggested by nurse educators to improve students' CT skills include conferences, computer simulations, clinical logs, collaboration, decision analysis, discussion, e-mail dialogue, patient simulations, portfolios, reflection, role modelling, role playing and writing position papers (Baker, 1996; Fonteyn and Cahill, 1998; Kuiper and Pesut, 2004; O'Neill et al., 2005; Todd, 1998; Weis and Guyton-Simmons, 1998; Wong and Chung, 2002).

O'Sullivan et al. (1997) indicated that teaching strategies that promote clinical reasoning are ones in which the educator designs classroom activities that explicitly engage the students in the activities of clinical reasoning. Paul and Heaslip (1995) advocated that students need to reason their way critically through nursing principles, concepts and theories frequently so that accurate application and transfer of knowledge occur in an integrated and intuitive way. Technological advances such as the Internet, with access to online video conferencing, journals, websites, interactive programs and distance learning, hold rich promise for promoting creative and effective teaching environments in addition to providing information sources (Fetterman, 1996). One learning activity that has proved popular for engaging students in clinical reasoning, with or without technology, is problem-based learning (PBL).

PBL was first developed in medicine but has now been adopted by many nursing programs. PBL develops students' ability to reflect frequently on their reasoning and decision making during patient care and leads to self-improvement through practice. Evidence exists that PBL significantly increases CT, clinical reasoning,

problem solving and transfer of knowledge gained (Norman and Schmidt, 1993). Once students have developed their reasoning skills in this manner, they can then apply them while caring for real patients in the clinical setting. Fonteyn and Flaig (1994) suggested teaching nursing students to reason and plan care in the same manner as practicing nurses. In practice, nurses first identify (from data initially obtained in report form and confirmed by patient assessment) the most important patient problems on which to focus during their nursing shift. Information from the patient, the family and other members of the healthcare team should be included in a plan of care that will assist in resolving the problems identified. As the shift progresses, nurses regularly evaluate and refine their plan of care based on additional data obtained from further patient assessment, additional clinical data and information from all individuals involved in carrying out the plan of care.

Durham et al. (2014) described teaching strategies to accelerate the development of student NP diagnostic reasoning. PBL was used to develop the hypothetico-deductive reasoning process in combination with assignments that fostered pattern recognition (a nonanalytical process), which effectively allowed NP students to experience the dual-process approach to diagnostic reasoning as used by NPs (see Case Study 22.1).

Videbeck (1997b) indicated that as well as being effectively taught, CT must be assessed in an appropriate manner. She pointed out that standardized paper-and-pencil tests are often selected as an evaluation measure because normative data are available and reliability has been established. However, none of the available instruments is specific to nursing, and there is no consistent relationship between scores on this type of test and CT. The use of faculty-developed instruments to assess student outcomes is strongly recommended. Course-specific measures, such as clinical performance criteria or written assignments, have the advantage of being specific to nursing practice. Videbeck (1997a) suggested that a model that integrates CT in all aspects of the program (definition, course objectives and evaluation) be used. Page et al. (1995) advocated the use of key feature problem (case scenario) examinations to assess clinical decision-making skills.

In the future, educators must strive to devise additional methods to develop and improve nurses' clinical

PBL and Dual Process Reasoning

Sonoma State University faculty applied the work of Durham et al. (2014) by using problem-based learning (PBL) cases that used the hypothetico-deductive and nonanalytical reasoning processes. Clinical case scenarios were presented to the students, and, with the assistance of the faculty, the students worked through each case. The faculty interaction during the case presentation also encouraged pattern recognition (a nonanalytical process) so reinforcing the dual-process model of diagnostic reasoning. Three cases were used that followed different paths. The clinical scenarios depicted various age groups and an increasing degree of complexity. The cases were presented as a chief complaint or symptom, and the students were asked to then interview the patient. The faculty encouraged the students to consider differential diagnoses early in the presentation of the case. The cases encouraged the students to consider all diagnoses, and, through the process, they were able to narrow down the possibilities and reach a most likely diagnosis. As the cases unfolded, further data gathering and clinical reasoning occurred, reinforcing the dual process of diagnostic reasoning. Students were positive about this approach to learning diagnostic reasoning. This process demonstrated a shift from the nursing model to the dual-process approach to diagnostic reasoning used by other healthcare professionals. This is important as transitioning from a nurse, where the diagnosis is known, to that of an NP, whose job is to diagnose, requires the development of expert diagnostic skills.

---

reasoning. Further changes will be required in the structure and function of nursing curricula. Students need to learn to improve the ways in which they identify significant clinical data and determine the meaning of data in regard to the problems of particular patients. They also need to learn how to reason about patient problems in ways that facilitate decisions about problem resolution.

Practice

The ultimate goal of both research and educational endeavours related to clinical reasoning in nursing is to improve nurses' reasoning in practice and, ultimately, to achieve more positive patient outcomes. Nurses' reasoning and interventions have a significant effect on patient outcomes (Fowler, 1994). We need to further explore the relationship between nurses' reasoning and patient outcomes, especially if nurses continue to extend their roles and take on more responsibility for deciding what care patients need. A major difficulty in demonstrating the influence of nurses' reasoning on patient outcomes is the complex nature of those outcomes. Outcomes span a broad range of effects, or presumed effects, that are influenced not only by nursing and other healthcare providers but by many other variables. These include time, environmental conditions, support systems and patient history.

Therefore continued development of decision support systems and expert systems to assist nurses in practice to make better clinical decisions and prevent diagnostic errors remains important. Expert system development began in research laboratories in the mid-1970s and was first implemented in commercial and practical endeavours in the early 1980s (Frenzel, 1987). Fonteyn and Grobe (1994) suggested that an expert system could be designed to represent the knowledge and reasoning processes of experienced nurses and could then be used to assist less experienced nurses to improve their reasoning skills and strategies. 'Illiad' is one such expert system case-based teaching program, which has been shown by Lange et al. (1997) to be effective in improving NP students' diagnostic abilities. Bowles (1997) claimed that expert system shells (computer systems that emulate the decision-making ability of a human expert) could be used in nursing. However, the nature of artificial intelligence and expert systems has changed in recent years with a move to machine learning. This change is showing great promise. Machine learning makes use of so-called 'big data'. There is a need to develop data sets that can link nursing decisions with patients' outcomes if these newer computer systems are to help nurses. More recently, Feldman et al. (2012) showed that a diagnostic decision support tool has a significant beneficial effect on the quality of first-year medicine residents' differential diagnoses and management plans. Recommendations were for further research to determine whether computer-based decision support tools with clinical workflows would facilitate improved diagnosis and more appropriate management at the point of care in healthcare settings.

Future Directions in Practice Related to Nurses' Clinical Reasoning

The relationship between nurses' reasoning and patient outcomes should receive greater attention in future research to demonstrate the important role that nurses play in healthcare delivery. There will be an increasing need to develop meaningful data sets related to patient outcomes. These data sets should allow us to record the actions that nurses commonly choose after reasoning about specific patient problems and relate these actions to intervention outcomes. Before the development of these data sets, the indicators of patient outcome that are related to nurses' reasoning and decision making need to be identified and described in a manner that facilitates their measurement. Computerized support systems will play an ever-increasing role in assisting nurses to reason, make decisions about appropriate nursing actions and evaluate their effect on patient outcome. Further studies are needed to evaluate the effect of these interventions on diagnostic error rates.

CHAPTER SUMMARY

In this chapter:

- Multiple theories have been discussed, including information processing, decision analysis and hermeneutics. These each contribute to how we can understand nurses' clinical reasoning, clinical judgement, problem solving and decision making and diagnostic reasoning.
- Research into the clinical reasoning of nurses has been explored. This research has often produced useful insights, but there is a need to build on this research.
- Ways to decrease diagnostic errors and improve clinical reasoning were explained. Recommendations proposed emphasize collaboration, communication, teamwork and decision support

modalities and teaching strategies that promote CT and clinical reasoning.

REFLECTION POINT 3

Multiple theoretical strategies can be employed such as simulations, role modelling, case studies and other in our curriculums to enhance clinical reasoning. Of these methods, PBL has been shown to facilitate application of acquired principles in the clinical arena. PBL combines problem-solving skills with didactic content within a clinical context that is organized to mimic the analytic reasoning process in clinical practice. Working through rich PBL cases helps students remember key information and see its application to real life. Looking to the future, further research on ways to promote CT and clinical reasoning is of importance.

REFERENCES

Baker, C.R., 1996. Reflective learning: a teaching strategy for critical thinking. J. Nurs. Educ. 35, 19–22.

Barrows, H.S., Pickell, G.C., 1991. Developing Clinical Problem-Solving Skills: A Guide to More Effective Diagnosis and Treatment. WW Norton, New York, NY.

Benner, P., 2015. Novice to expert: nursing theorist. Viewed 18 March 2017. Available from: http://nursing-theory.org/nursing-theorists/Patricia-Benner.php.

Benner, P., Hooper-Kyriakidis, P., Stannard, D., 2011. Clinical Wisdom and Interventions in Acute and Critical Care: A Thinking-in-Action Approach, second ed. Springer, New York, NY.

Benner, P., Tanner, C., Chesla, C., 1992. From beginner to expert: gaining a differentiated clinical world in critical care nursing. ANS Adv. Nurs. Sci. 14, 13–28.

Benner, P., Tanner, C., Chesla, C., 1996. Expertise in Nursing Practice: Caring, Clinical Judgment, and Ethics. Springer, New York, NY.

Bowles, K.H., 1997. The barriers and benefits of nursing information systems. Comput. Nurs. 15, 197–198.

Del Fiol, G., Haug, P.J., Cimino, J.C., et al., 2008. Effectiveness of topic-specific infobuttons: a randomized controlled trial. J. Am. Med. Inform. Assoc. 15, 752–759.

Durham, D., Fowler, T., Kennedy, S., 2014. Teaching dual-process diagnostic reasoning to Doctor of Nursing Practice students: problem-based learning and the Illness Script. J. Nurs. Educ. 53, 646–650.

Feldman, M.J., Hoffer, E.P., Barnett, G.O., et al., 2012. Impact of a computer-based diagnostic decision support tool on the differential diagnoses of medicine residents. J. Grad. Med. Educ. 4, 227–231.

Fetterman, D., 1996. Videoconferencing on-line: enhancing communication over the internet. Educ. Res. 24, 23–27.

Fonteyn, M., 1991. A descriptive analysis of expert critical care nurses' clinical reasoning, PhD thesis. University of Texas, Austin, TX.

Fonteyn, M.E., Cahill, M., 1998. The use of clinical logs to improve nursing students' metacognition: a pilot study. J. Adv. Nurs. 28, 149–154.

Fonteyn, M., Flaig, L., 1994. The written nursing process: is it still useful to nursing education? J. Adv. Nurs. 19, 315–319.

Fonteyn, M., Grobe, S., 1994. Expert system development in nursing: implications for critical care nursing practice. Heart Lung 23, 80–87.

Fowler, L., 1994. Clinical reasoning of home health nurses: a verbal protocol analysis, PhD thesis. University of South Carolina, Columbia, SC.

Frenzel, L., 1987. Understanding Expert Systems. Howard W Sama, Indianapolis, IN.

Glaser, R., Chi, M.T.H., 1988. Overview. In: Chi, M.T.H., Glaser, R., Farr, M.J. (Eds.), The Nature of Expertise. Lawrence Erlbaum, Hillsdale, NJ, pp. xv–xxviii.

Gordon, M., Murphy, C.P., Candee, D., et al., 1994. Clinical judgement: an integrated model. ANS Adv. Nurs. Sci. 16, 55–70.

Grier, M., 1976. Decision making about patient care. Nurs. Res. 25, 105–110.

Institute of Medicine, 2015. Improving diagnosis in health care. Viewed 18 March 2017. Available from: http://www.nationalacademies.org/hmd/Reports/2015/Improving-Diagnosis-in-Healthcare.aspx.

Joseph, G.M., Patel, V.L., 1990. Domain knowledge and hypothesis generation in diagnostic reasoning. Med. Decis. Making 10, 31–46.

Kahneman, D., 2013. Thinking Fast and Slow. Farrar, Strauss and Giroux, New York, NY.

Kuiper, R.A., Pesut, D.J., 2004. Promoting cognitive and metacognitive reflective reasoning skills in nursing practice: self-regulated learning theory. J. Adv. Nurs. 45, 381–391.

Lange, L.L., Haak, S.W., Lincoln, M.J., et al., 1997. Use of Illiad to improve diagnostic performance of nurse practitioner students. J. Nurs. Educ. 36, 35–45.

Lauri, S., Salantera, S., 1995. Decision-making models of Finnish nurses and public health nurses. J. Adv. Nurs. 21, 520–527.

Lee, J., Chan, A.C.M., Phillips, D.R., 2006. Diagnostic practise in nursing: a critical review of the literature. Nurs. Health Sci. 8, 57–65.

Lewis, M.L., 1997. Decision making task complexity: model development and initial testing. J. Nurs. Educ. 36, 114–120.

Lipman, L., Deatrick, J., 1997. Preparing advanced practice nurses for clinical decision making in specialty practice. Nurse Educ. 22, 47–50.

Manning, J., Broughton, V., McConnell, E., 1995. Reality based scenarios facilitate knowledge network development. Contemp. Nurse 4, 16–21.

Miller, G., 1956. The magical number seven, plus or minus two: some limits on our capacity to process information. Psychol. Rev. 63, 81–97.

Narayan, S.M., Corcoran-Perry, S., Drew, D., et al., 2003. Decision analysis as a tool to support an analytical pattern-of-reasoning. Nurs. Health Sci. 5, 229–243.

Neill, K., Lachat, M., Taylor-Panek, S., 1997. Enhancing critical thinking with case studies and nursing process. Nurse. Educ. 22, 30–32.

Newell, A., Simon, H.A., 1972. Human Problem Solving. Prentice-Hall, Englewood Cliffs, NJ.

Norman, G., Schmidt, H., 1993. The psychological basis of problem based learning: a review of the evidence. Acad. Med. 67, 557–565.

O'Neill, E.S., Dluhy, N.M., Chin, E., 2005. Modelling novice clinical reasoning for a computerized decision support system. J. Adv. Nurs. 49, 68–77.

O'Sullivan, P., Blevins-Stephens, W.L., Smith, F.M., et al., 1997. Addressing the National League for Nursing critical thinking outcome. Nurse. Educ. 22, 23–29.

Page, G., Bordage, G., Allen, T., 1995. Developing key-feature problems and examinations to assess clinical decision-making skills. Acad. Med. 70, 194–201.

Paul, R.W., Heaslip, P., 1995. Critical thinking and intuitive nursing practice. J. Adv. Nurs. 22, 40–47.

Pirret, A.A., 2016. Nurse practitioners' versus physicians' diagnostic reasoning style and use of maxims: a comparative study. J. Nurs. Pract. 12, 381–389.

Pyles, S., Stern, P., 1983. Discovery of Nursing Gestalt in critical care nursing: the importance of the Grey Gorilla syndrome. Image J. Nurs. Sch. 15, 51–57.

Rew, L., 1990. Intuition in critical care nursing practice. Dimens. Crit. Care Nurs. 9, 30–37.

Ritter, B., 1998. Why evidence-based practice? CCNP Conn. 11, 1–8.

Ritter, B., 2000. An analysis of expert nurse practitioners' diagnostic reasoning, PhD thesis. University of San Francisco, San Francisco, CA.

Ryan-Wenger, N., Lee, J., 1997. The clinical reasoning case study: a powerful teaching tool. Nurse Pract. 22, 66–70.

Tanner, C., 1987. Teaching clinical judgement. In: Fitzpatrick, J., Tauton, R. (Eds.), Annual Review of Nursing Research. Springer, New York, NY, pp. 153–174.

Todd, N., 1998. Using e-mail in an undergraduate nursing course to increase critical thinking skills. Comput. Nurs. 16, 115–118.

Videbeck, S., 1997a. Critical thinking: prevailing practice in baccalaureate schools of nursing. J. Nurs. Educ. 36, 5–10.

Videbeck, S., 1997b. Critical thinking: a model. J. Nurs. Educ. 36, 23–28.

Weis, P., Guyton-Simmons, J., 1998. A computer simulation for teaching critical thinking skills. Nurse. Educ. 23, 30–33.

Wong, T.K.S., Chung, J.W.Y., 2002. Diagnostic reasoning processes using patient simulation in different learning environments. J. Clin. Nurs. 11, 65–72.

Zakim, D., Braun, N., Fritz, P., et al., 2008. Underutilization of information and knowledge in everyday medical practice: evaluation of a computer-based solution. BMC Med. Inform. Decis. Mak. 8, 50.

23

CLINICAL REASONING IN PHYSIOTHERAPY

MARK JONES ▪ IAN EDWARDS ▪ GAIL M. JENSEN

CHAPTER AIMS

The aims of this chapter are to:

▪ discuss three important reasons why physiotherapists need to study and practice clinical reasoning,

▪ discuss three frameworks that can provide context and focus to the learning and practice of clinical reasoning in physiotherapy and

▪ discuss factors beyond cognitive processes that influence proficiency in clinical reasoning.

KEY WORDS

Evidence-informed practice

Human judgement

Errors in clinical reasoning

Fast and slow reasoning

Biopsychosocial framework

Clinical reasoning strategies

Hypothesis categories

Factors influencing clinical reasoning

ABBREVIATIONS/ ACRONYMS

CNS Central nervous system

ICF International Classification of Functioning, Disability and Health

INTRODUCTION

Two significant challenges to skilled clinical reasoning in physiotherapy practice since the last edition of this book have been the continued growth of research evidence clinicians are expected to know and use and the increased understanding in pain science; the latter has driven an increased emphasis on psychosocial assessment, pain education and cognitive-behavioural management (especially in, but not limited to, musculoskeletal practice). The political pressure to be 'research/evidence-based' is greater than ever. This is despite the plethora of systematic reviews now available concluding, more often than not, that there is insufficient high-level research to judge what managements are best. Pain science and chronic pain/disability research convincingly highlight the importance for physiotherapists to develop particular skills. These skills include psychosocial assessment for prediction of return to work and chronicity and psychologically informed management for already established 'chronic' presentations. Although formal education, in physiotherapy psychosocial assessment and management, is increasing, it is still arguably not well developed and often not well integrated into the clinical practice components of the curriculum. Psychosocial assessment and management, and similarly the clinical reasoning required for making judgements regarding psychosocial factor contribution to a patient's disability, are less formalized, less familiar and often seen as not as important as developing skills in physical assessment and management. Physiotherapy

247

'hands-on' procedural skills may be under threat from those who promote education (e.g., in pain management) as a replacement to established physical therapies rather than something that needs to be integrated with those same therapies (Edwards and Jones, 2013; Jull and Moore, 2012). Skilled clinical reasoning is more important than ever because of the external pressures for greater efficiency and quality patient outcomes. Within this context, research evidence should be seen as an important source of information and not a prescription.

WHY DO PHYSIOTHERAPISTS NEED TO STUDY AND PRACTICE CLINICAL REASONING?

Research Evidence Only Provides a Guide, Not a Prescription, to Practice

Despite its exponential growth over recent decades, our current body of research is far from conclusive in terms of sufficiently informing clinical decisions. Research is often insufficient to adequately guide therapists in their recognition and management of the multitude of patient problems we face (Jones et al., 2006; Mosely et al., 2014; Villas Boas et al., 2013). Further, the validity and status of what knowledge is actually derived from different populations within physiotherapy are often uncertain (Kerry et al., 2013).

Common limitations with physiotherapy effectiveness studies include high dropout rates or loss to follow-up, lack of blinding (patient, therapist, measurer), lack of random and concealed allocation to treatment arms, lack of adequate identification of population subgroups, artificial isolation of treatment interventions in determining their effect and lack of evidence of sustainable outcomes. As such, practicing clinicians face the daunting challenge of maintaining best practice based on best evidence when the evidence is still largely not available or is incomplete. Even when primary research studies (or systematic reviews) testing therapeutic interventions for the condition of interest are available, numerous issues must be considered for the clinician to have confidence in the applicability of the findings. These issues include whether or not their patient matches the population studied (often made difficult by lack of homogeneity of subjects and insufficient consideration of psychosocial variables) and

whether the intervention tested can be replicated. Very few studies provide sufficient detail and justification of the assessments and treatments to enable clinicians to replicate the assessments and management (educatively, behaviourally and humanistically) with confidence. The details needed include what precisely was done, including details of positions, dosage, sequence and progression; who treated the patients, including level of procedural competence; and what was the therapeutic environment, including associated explanations, instructions, verbal cues and advice. Application of this evidence to practice requires skilled clinical reasoning and judgement.

Human Judgement Is Prone to Error

Although inadequate knowledge understandably underpins errors of judgement, it is disconcerting to know that many errors in health- and nonhealth-related human judgement can be traced to the tendency for human bias (e.g., Hogarth, 2005; Kahneman et al., 1982; Lehrer, 2009; Schwartz and Elstein, 2008). Some examples, easily recognizable in clinical practice, include those in Box 23.1.

BOX 23.1
BIASES IN HUMAN JUDGEMENT

- The 'priming' influence of prior information (e.g., diagnosis provided in a referral, imaging findings, influence of a recent publication or course)
- 'Confirmation bias' or the tendency to attend to and collect data that confirm existing hypotheses
- 'Memory bias' of a spectacular successful outcome
- 'Overestimation of representativeness', as with the probability of a diagnosis given a finding being confused with the probability of a finding given a diagnosis (e.g., having a diagnosis of TB means there is a high probability you have a cough, but having a cough does not mean you have a high probability of having TB)
- 'Conservatism or stickiness', where initial impressions and hypotheses are not revised in the face of subsequent nonsupporting information
- 'Associative coherence', where we understandably attempt to provide coherent explanations of how signs and symptoms are associated

---

TB, Tuberculosis

Fast and Slow Reasoning in Physiotherapy Practice

Although thinking in clinical practice varies across therapists, three broad distinctions can be made. There are those who simply follow diagnostic/guideline prescriptions and uncritically administer treatment protocols as a technician (i.e., no clinical reasoning adaptation to the individual patient). There are those who make their own clinical judgements based on dominant features in a clinical presentation and use routine, habitual management strategies (i.e., 'fast' reasoning or forward reasoning). Finally, there are those who more holistically, reflectively and analytically examine and reason to understand their patients' full pain or disability experiences. The third group does this to adapt research/guideline evidence to collaboratively manage a patient's unique physical, psychosocial and environmental requirements (i.e., 'slow' reasoning or backwards reasoning). In reality, in addition to being holistic and collaborative in their reasoning (see Chapter 15), expert physiotherapists use a combination of fast and slow reasoning as required by the complexity and familiarity of the patient's unique clinical presentation and context. In his seminal text *Thinking, Fast and Slow,* Daniel Kahneman (2011) describes fast thinking as automatic, effortless first impressions and intuition (e.g., pattern recognition) and slow thinking as analytical deliberations requiring more attention, time and effort. Although shortcuts in thinking such as pattern recognition can be effective when working with very familiar presentations where little problem solving is required, errors are likely to occur if relied on in less familiar, more complex presentations.

Consider the scenario where a patient reports midthoracic pain consistently provoked after sitting slouched to eat lunch. Working on the premise that sustained flexion can strain spinal tissues leading to nociception, the physiotherapist deduces 'I've seen this before, the patient's midthoracic pain is caused by nociception associated with slouched sitting' and proceeds to postural assessment and advice. Although this inductive fast reasoning judgement certainly represents one plausible explanation to explore further, this patient actually had gallbladder disease with referred thoracic pain related to eating fatty foods at lunch, not slouched posture. Even when you consider patients with easily diagnosed problems and well-established management guidelines, their personal circumstances, goals and the extent of relevant impairments will be unique, requiring analysis and collaborative decisions beyond fast reasoning alone.

The greater the coherence of our fast reasoning impressions, the more likely we are to jump to conclusions without further slow reasoning analysis. Unfortunately, humans are prone to find and accept coherence on the basis of limited information. Kahneman (2011, p. 86) has characterized this trait, associated with many of our biases, as 'What You See Is All There Is'. There is an assumption or acceptance that the information at hand is all that is available. You build a story (explanation) from the information you have, and if it is a good, coherent story, you believe it. Paradoxically, coherent stories are easier to construct when there is less information to make sense of. Although overreliance on fast reasoning can clearly lead to errors, interestingly, research has demonstrated experts working with familiar problems function largely on pattern recognition (e.g., Boshuizen and Schmidt, 2008; Jensen et al., 2007; Kaufman et al., 2008; Schwartz and Elstein, 2008). Overanalysis also leads to errors in judgement (Lehrer, 2009; Schwartz and Elstein, 2008). The existence of our fast reasoning is obvious when you consider the large number of first-impression, fast-thinking judgements that lead up to, and inform, our understanding of the patient and his or her problems. These judgements include quick recognition of when a patient's telling of his or her story requires clarification; patient discomfort and emotions; observed postural, movement and control impairments; when a hands-on intervention requires mid-treatment adjustment and so on.

Openness to reflect on practice and recognition when an existing approach is inadequate are part of what has been described as 'adaptive expertise' (Cutrer et al., 2017). Successfully working with patients with complex presentations that fall outside what are typically uni-dimensional clinical guidelines requires a balance in fast and slow reasoning. There is a need to reframe the problem and combine this with an ability to adapt, explore and invent creative solutions. Clinicians have to be able to integrate and manage uncertainty as part of their clinical reasoning process (Cooke and Lemay, 2017). This requires critical thinking skills, as discussed later, but also creative or lateral thinking (de Bono,

2014). de Bono characterizes vertical thinking as logical, sequential, predictable thinking where the thinker aims to systematically make sense of all information. In contrast, lateral thinking involves restructuring and escaping from old patterns, looking at things in different ways and avoiding premature conclusions. Being able to reframe a problem and consider different perspectives requires first being able to recognize your own perspective or approach. For example, a student could be encouraged to conduct a review of patient progress and his or her reasoning through the problem. The student is explicitly asked to identify his or her dominant interpretation of the patient's diagnosis (e.g., pathology versus impairment, physical versus psychosocial) and the dominant approach he or she has been taking in management to date (e.g., passive or dynamic bias, bias to treating source versus contributing factors, bias to physical impairments versus psychosocial factors). It is difficult to think laterally/creatively if you cannot first recognize how you have been thinking and approaching the problem thus far. Once this is recognized, the student can then be encouraged to think more laterally about alternative interpretations of the patient's presentation and alternative management approaches.

REFLECTION POINT 1

Can you identify any of the common errors of reasoning present in your practice? What strategies do you use to minimize errors?

THREE FRAMEWORKS TO SITUATE CLINICAL REASONING IN PHYSIOTHERAPY

Clinical reasoning is increasingly acknowledged as important in clinically focussed publications, conference presentations and professional association practice competencies. However, outside of scholarly works that focus on clinical reasoning (e.g., Edwards et al., 2004a; Jensen et al., 2007, and this *Clinical Reasoning in the Health Professions* text), it is often referred to as a broad construct without reference to the scope of clinical judgements that should be considered or the dynamics of the reasoning process. Reference to clinical reasoning is usually focussed on pathoanatomical diagnosis and

management despite significant limitations in the associations between pathology, symptoms and disability. Three frameworks that can provide context and focus to the learning and practice of clinical reasoning in physiotherapy are the 'biopsychosocial' framework (Engel, 1977), 'clinical reasoning strategies' and 'hypothesis categories'.

Clinical Reasoning in a Biopsychosocial Framework

Physiotherapists must consider all factors potentially contributing to a person's health, whether working with patients having musculoskeletal/sports, neurological, oncological or cardiorespiratory problems from infants through to old age or when working in health promotion/injury prevention. Although physiotherapists are often perceived as having a focus on the 'physical', a contemporary biopsychosocial understanding of health and disability (Borrell-Carrió et al., 2004; Epstein and Borrell-Carrió, 2005; Imrie, 2004) requires full consideration of environmental and psychosocial factors that may influence physical health, within the scope and limits of the therapists' education. This requires a holistic philosophy of health and disability, assessment and management knowledge (including referral pathways) and skills to address any potential contributing factors. In addition, clinical reasoning proficiency is required to recognize whether these contributing factors are relevant to the individual patient to make appropriate clinical judgements that will contribute to the patient's optimal health care.

The biopsychosocial perspective recognizes that disability is the result of the cumulative effects of the biological health condition (disease, illness, pathology, disorder), external environmental influences (e.g., physical, social, economic, political) and internal personal influences (e.g., age, gender, education, beliefs, culture, coping style, self-efficacy). The World Health Organization (WHO) International Classification of Functioning, Disability and Health (ICF) model (Fig. 23.1) provides an excellent overarching biopsychosocial framework that illustrates the scope of knowledge that clinical reasoning physiotherapists need to be competent to holistically understand and manage their patients.

The boxes across the middle of the diagram depict the relationship between a patient's body function and impairments, his or her capabilities to do activities and

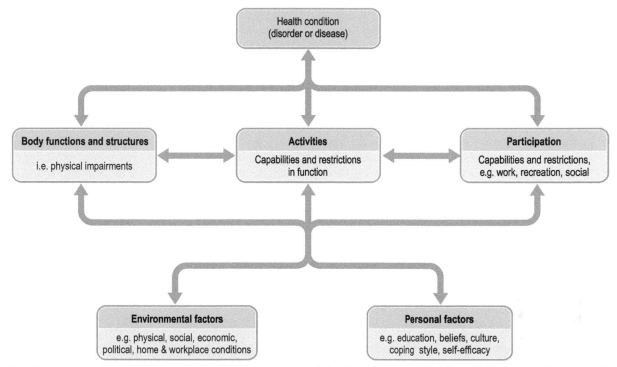

Fig. 23.1 ■ Adaptation of World Health Organization International Classification of Functioning, Disability and Health Framework. (From World Health Organization, 2001. International Classification of Functioning, Disability and Health. World Health Organization, Geneva, with permission.)

his or her participation in life situations (e.g., work, family, sport, leisure). Bidirectional arrows reflect the reciprocal relationships whereby different factors have the potential to influence each other (Borrell-Carrió et al., 2004; Duncan, 2000; Pincus, 2004). Formerly, functional restrictions, physical impairments and pain would have been conceptualized as the end result of a specific injury/pathology or syndrome, but the reciprocal arrows highlight that these also can be associated with, and even maintained by, environmental and personal influences. A holistic understanding of a patient's clinical presentation therefore necessitates attention and analysis of his or her physical health, environmental and personal factors. The ICF model provides an excellent contextualization of the scope of knowledge and clinical reasoning required in physiotherapy practice. A framework of 'clinical reasoning strategies' provides further assistance to understanding and learning clinical reasoning.

Focus of Our Clinical Reasoning: Clinical Reasoning Strategies

As previously mentioned, it is common for clinical reasoning presentations and discussions to focus on diagnosis alone, with diagnosis limited to categorizing the type of problem, injury or pathology. Pathology is important because red flags, signs and symptoms suggestive of undiagnosed, possibly sinister health problems, require further investigation. However, clinical reasoning that overfocusses on pathology at the expense of other factors, such as the psychosocial, physical impairment and environmental, is at risk of incomplete understanding of a patient's issues. Pathology can be asymptomatic, and symptoms can exist without detectable pathology. Symptomatic pathology will have a continuum of presentations, relating to stage and severity of pathology and interactions from other health comorbidities and psychosocial and environmental contributing factors. Reasoning about diagnosis/pathology represents only a portion of the reasoning that actually occurs in clinical practice. Physiotherapy diagnostic reasoning should, arguably, be broader than the categorization focus of our medical colleagues and include physiotherapy-specific features important to our subsequent management. Research and theory across a range of health professions (e.g., physiotherapy, medicine, nursing, occupational therapy) have identified a range of clinical reasoning foci (Edwards et al., 2004a). We suggest the following clinical reasoning strategies capture the scope of reasoning necessary to apply the ICF biopsychosocial model to physiotherapy practice (Box 23.2).

Expert physiotherapists have been shown to attend to these various reasoning strategies and also move dialectically in their reasoning between a biological and psychosocial focus in a fluid and seemingly effortless manner (Edwards et al., 2004a). For example, a diagnostic test may elicit a patient response that is more reflective of his or her fear of movement rather than any underlying pathology. Even though the diagnostic test may be associated with good sensitivity, specificity and likelihood ratios, the expert clinician will recognize the need to dialectically switch from biological to biopsychosocial thinking. Although the clinical reasoning strategies provide a framework to assist students and practicing physiotherapists, to recognize the different foci of reasoning required in biopsychosocial practice, it is also helpful to recognize that different categories

---

BOX 23.2

APPLYING THE INTERNATIONAL CLASSIFICATION OF FUNCTIONING, DISABILITY AND HEALTH BIOPSYCHOSOCIAL MODEL TO PHYSIOTHERAPY

Diagnostic reasoning: Reasoning underpinning the formation of a diagnosis related to functional limitation(s) and associated physical and movement impairments with consideration of pain type, potential sources of symptoms, pathology and the broad scope of potential contributing factors.

Narrative (or psychosocially focussed) reasoning: Reasoning associated with understanding patients' pain, illness and/or disability experiences. This incorporates their personal perspectives on their experiences including their understanding of their problem(s) and the meanings they hold, their expectations regarding management, associated cognitions and emotions, ability to cope and the effects these personal perspectives have on their clinical presentation, particularly whether they are facilitating or obstructing their recovery.

Reasoning about procedure: Reasoning underpinning the selection, implementation and progression of treatment procedures. Although clinical guidelines provide broad direction, typically focussing only on diagnostic categorization, practicing therapists need to adaptively reason how best to apply those guidelines to patients' individual presentations and goals. Progression of treatment is mostly then guided by judicious outcome reassessment that attends to both impairment and function/disability-related outcomes.

Interactive reasoning: Reasoning guiding the purposeful establishment and ongoing management of therapist–patient rapport.

Collaborative reasoning: The shared decision making between patient and therapist (and others) as a therapeutic alliance in the interpretation of examination findings, setting of goals and priorities and implementation and progression of treatment (see Edwards et al., 2004b, and Trede, Higgs, 2008, for further detail).

Reasoning about teaching: Reasoning associated with the planning, execution and evaluation of individualized and context-sensitive teaching of patients, including education for conceptual understanding (e.g., medical and physiotherapy diagnosis, pain, management options), education for physical performance (e.g., rehabilitative exercises) and education for behavioural change.

Predictive reasoning: Reasoning utilized in judgements regarding effects of specific interventions and overall prognosis. Although prognostic judgements regarding whether physiotherapy can help and expected time frames are not precise, thorough consideration of biological, environmental and personal factors that recognizes both facilitators and barriers (i.e., positives and negatives in a patient's presentation) and what is and is not modifiable will assist this reasoning strategy.

Ethical reasoning: Reasoning underpinning the recognition and resolution of ethical dilemmas that impinge upon the patient's ability to make decisions concerning his or her health and upon the conduct of treatment and its desired goals (see Chapter 16 for further detail).

of clinical judgements are required across these different reasoning strategies.

REFLECTION POINT 2

Do you explicitly assess patients' psychosocial status? If so, what do you assess, how do you assess it and how do you judge a psychosocial feature is contributing to a patient's presentation?

Categories of Clinical Judgements Required: Hypothesis Categories

One would hope that all physiotherapists know the purpose of every question they ask their patients and every physical assessment they perform. That is, what do you want to find out, and what clinical judgements will that information inform? It is not appropriate to stipulate a definitive list of clinical judgements all physiotherapists must consider as this has not been established and would only stifle the independent and creative thinking important to the evolution of our profession. However, active reflection on all, and any, information about a patient helps clinicians in a number of ways. Reflection can help clinicians understand the purpose of the questions they ask and the assessments they do. Reflection can encourage clinicians to think more broadly beyond the immediate diagnosis. Finally, reflection can encourage the creation of frameworks to organize clinical knowledge in ways that allow good decisions to be made. A minimum list of categories of judgements was initially proposed by Jones (1987). This has continued to evolve to its current format (Box 23.3).

There is now plentiful research evidence about the focus of clinical reasoning, including reasoning across and within these different categories (e.g., Barlow, 2012; Doody and McAteer, 2002; Edwards et al., 2004a; Jensen et al., 2007; Rivett and Higgs, 1997; Smart and Doody, 2006). This research, combined with reflective discourse from experienced clinicians and clinical educators, broadly supports the relevance and use of a hypothesis categories framework. Nevertheless, physiotherapists should not use these specific hypothesis categories uncritically. Whatever categories of judgements are adopted should continually be reviewed to ensure they reflect contemporary health care and clinical practice.

Clinicians' abilities to engage in ongoing self-assessment through reflection and self-monitoring are an essential lifelong skill (Schumacher et al., 2013).

As physiotherapists (or students) follow their structured examination (i.e., review of records, patient interview, physical assessment depending on work setting) appropriate for each area of practice (e.g., musculoskeletal, clinical neuroscience, cardiorespiratory, paediatrics), they should recognize patient cues that in turn should elicit hypotheses in one or more categories. That is, clinical reasoning across the different hypothesis categories occurs simultaneously and with varying emphasis depending on the context and nature of the clinical situation and problems encountered. There are many different types of clinical patterns, including patterns within all hypothesis categories (Box 23.4).

As specific hypotheses are considered, informed by knowledge of clinical patterns, tentative judgements should be 'tested' for the remaining features of the pattern through further patient inquiry, physical tests and ultimately with the physiotherapy intervention. Thinking of interpretations of patient information as hypotheses discourages premature conclusions and promotes synthesis of the full clinical story and physical assessment.

Patient information typically has implications for several different hypothesis categories. Consider the following case study (Case Study 23.1).

The reasoning regarding each of these hypothesis categories would then continue to evolve throughout the ongoing initial assessment and ongoing management. As proposed earlier in the chapter, we believe the biopsychosocial framework, clinical reasoning strategies and hypothesis categories framework collectively highlight core areas of knowledge essential to holistic clinical reasoning. Together, these ideas can assist students and practicing physiotherapists to better understand and improve their own reasoning.

Although cognitive processes such as cue perception, interpretation, planning and synthesis are integral to clinical reasoning, on their own they do not capture all that contributes to skilled reasoning. Additional factors, influencing proficiency in clinical reasoning, include critical thinking, higher-order metacognition, knowledge organization, data-collection skills and the therapeutic alliance between patient and therapist.

BOX 23.3
HYPOTHESIS CATEGORIES FRAMEWORK

- Activity and Participation capability and restriction
  - Activity: functional abilities and restrictions (e.g., walking, lifting, sitting) that are volunteered and further screened for. To gain a complete picture, it is important that the clinician identifies those activities the patient is capable of alongside those that are restricted.
  - Participation: abilities and restrictions to participate in life situations (e.g., work, recreation/sport, family), including modified participation (e.g., modified work duties).
- Patient's perspectives on his or her experiences (i.e., psychosocial status) incorporating, for example:
  - Understanding of his or her problem (including attributions about the cause, beliefs about diagnosis and pain and associated cognitions)
  - Response to stressors in his or her life and any relationship these have with his or her clinical presentation
  - Effects the problem and any stressors appear to have on his or her thoughts, feelings, coping, motivation and self-efficacy to participate in management
  - Goals and expectations for management
- In the 'Clinical Reasoning Strategies' framework presented earlier, hypotheses regarding patient perspectives fit within 'Narrative Reasoning' focussed on understanding patients' pain, illness and/or disability experiences.
- Pain type (i.e., 'mechanisms')
  - Nociceptive pain (with and without inflammation): Nociceptive pain is protective and represents the sensation associated with the detection of potentially tissue-damaging noxious stimuli. Nociceptive inflammatory pain occurs with tissue damage and/or immune cell activation in the case of systemic inflammation, facilitating repair by causing pain hypersensitivity until healing occurs (Wolf, 2010).
  - Neuropathic pain: pain arising as a direct consequence of a lesion or disease affecting the somatosensory system further differentiated into peripheral or central neuropathic pain depending on the anatomical location of the lesion (Jensen et al., 2011; Trede et al., 2008).
  - Maladaptive central nervous system (CNS) sensitization: dysfunctional pain operationally defined as 'an amplification of neural signalling within the central nervous system that elicits pain hypersensitivity' (Wolf, 2010, p. s5) (see also Nijs et al., 2014; Wolf, 2011).
- Sources of symptoms: specific tissues, structures, body regions and body systems hypothesized as responsible for the presenting symptoms without specific reference to pathology.
- Pathology: structural and functional changes in the body caused by disease or trauma hypothesized to be associated with presenting symptoms and/or disability.
- Impairments in body function or structure: any loss or abnormality of psychological, physiological or anatomical structure or function (World Health Organization, 2001).
- Contributing factors to the development and maintenance of the problem: predisposing or associated factors involved in the development or maintenance of the patient's problem(s). Both intrinsic and extrinsic factors should be considered, including environmental, psychosocial, behavioural, physical/biomechanical and hereditary.
- Precautions and contraindications to physical examination and treatment: medical (e.g., comorbidities), environmental, psychosocial, behavioural and physical factors and 'Red Flags' (signs and symptoms that may indicate the presence of more serious pathology and systemic or viscerogenic pathology/disease) identified that inform:
  - whether a physical examination should be carried out at all (versus immediate referral for further medical consultation/investigation) and, if so, the extent of examination that can be safely performed that will minimize the risk for aggravating the patient's symptoms/condition
  - whether specific safety tests are indicated (e.g., cervical arterial dysfunction testing, neurological examination, blood pressure/heart rate, balance assessment, instability tests)
  - whether any treatment should be undertaken (versus referral for further consultation/investigation)
  - the appropriate dose/strength of any physical interventions planned.
- Management/treatment selection and progression: 1) overall health management of the patient, including consultation and referral to other healthcare professionals, health promotion interventions (e.g., fitness assessment and management) and patient advocacy as required (e.g., with insurers or employers) and 2) specific therapeutic interventions (educational and physical) carried out during an appointment and the underlying reasoning required to determine which impairments to address, which to address first, the strategy/procedure and dosage to use, the outcome measures to reassess and the self-management appropriate for optimizing change (in understanding, impairment, activity and participation). Progression of treatment informed by outcome reassessment has the same considerations.
- Prognosis: the therapist's judgement regarding his or her ability to help the patient and an estimate of how long this will take. Broadly a patient's prognosis is determined by the nature and extent of the problem(s) and the patient's ability and willingness to make the necessary changes (e.g., lifestyle, psychosocial contributing factors, physical contributing factors) to facilitate recovery or improved quality of life. Clues will be available throughout the subjective and physical examination and the ongoing management.

BOX 23.4
DIFFERENT TYPES OF CLINICAL PATTERNS

- Epidemiology of different health conditions
- Diagnostic and clinical syndromes (physiological processes, activity and participation restrictions, associated sources of symptoms, associated symptomatic pathologies)
  - Patterns of 'processes' (e.g., degenerative, inflammatory, ischaemic, tissue strain)
  - Patterns of activity and participation restrictions, symptoms and physical impairments common to different diagnostic and clinical syndromes (e.g., spinal stenosis, functional instability, chronic obstructive pulmonary disease [COPD], different strokes)
  - Patterns of sources of symptoms (spinal posterior intervertebral joint, vascular, respiratory)
  - Patterns of symptomatic pathology (tendinopathy, pulmonary embolus, vascular aneurysm)
- Factors predisposing or contributing to patients' health conditions, physical impairments activity and participation restrictions

- Patterns of predisposing physical and environmental risk factors to musculoskeletal and sports-related problems (e.g., mobility, control/strength, sport training and equipment), cardiovascular disease (e.g., diet, weight, blood pressure, stress, smoking), chronic disability (e.g., socioeconomic status, inactivity, failure to return to work, beliefs about pain)
- Patterns of common environmental, social, cultural and personal contributing factors facilitating or restricting people's activity and participation
- Patterns of medical conditions, medications, symptoms and signs that signal the need for precautions to physical examination and treatment and/or referral for further medical consultation
- Patterns of management strategies for different diagnostic and clinical health conditions
- Patterns of factors suggesting poor to good prognosis (e.g., pathology/illness, impairments, environmental and personal factors)

CASE STUDY 23.1

Patient Information and Clinical Reasoning

A 72-year-old man is asked what aggravates his back and bilateral leg pains. His response is: 'Walking. I'm afraid to even try anymore. Even short walks make the back and legs worse, and then I have to sit down to ease it off. Sitting is good, but I can't sit all day! I can't even help out around the house anymore or get over to see the grandchildren. I'm really worried it might be something serious'. The following preliminary interpretations (hypotheses) can be made:

- Activity restriction: walking
- Activity capability: sitting
- Participation restrictions: helping around house and seeing grandchildren
- Patient perspectives: afraid to try walking, worried it may be serious

- Pain type: consistent mechanical pattern – nociceptive? neuropathic?
- Sources of symptoms: lumbar joints and neural (peripheral? central?) implicated
- Pathology/syndrome: vascular claudication, stenosis (neuropathic claudication)?
- Contributing factors: age
- Precautions: age, easily aggravated, bilateral leg pain, patient's fears/worry
- Prognosis: (negatives) age, extent of symptoms and disability, neuropathic features, potential for patient's perspectives to be a barrier; (positives) specific easing factor

---

REFLECTION POINT 3

Which of the different types of clinical patterns listed in Box 23.4 do you use in your clinical judgements? If there are some you agree are important but are not well developed in your working knowledge, you might consider building your knowledge of these through further study and peer discussions.

FACTORS INFLUENCING CLINICAL REASONING

Critical Thinking

Critical thinking involves analyzing and assessing information, issues, situations, problems, perspectives and thinking processes (Paul and Elder, 2007). It requires reflection and critique of assumptions embedded in current knowledge, reasoning and practice; openmindedness to other perspectives; critique of information regarding its accuracy, precision, completeness and relevance; and imagination to look beyond one's own perspective, including contemplation of possibilities beyond what is empirically known at the present time (Brookfield, 2008; Paul and Elder, 2007). Critical thinking underpins clinical reasoning and is a prerequisite to transformative learning where the assumptions of taken-for-granted perspectives are subjected to critical appraisal, leading to construction of new understandings and creation of new insights, knowledge and solutions (Mezirow, 2012).

Everyone has assumptions that underpin what he or she believes, feels, knows and does. These assumptions manifest in different forms, including professional beliefs, values and stereotypical views about human nature and social organization that underpin our attitudes and actions. Becoming aware of your own perspectives and habitual ways of thinking and acting in practice, along with the assumptions that form the basis for those perspectives and actions, is an essential element of critical thinking and skilled clinical reasoning. That is, transforming habits of thinking requires critical reflection of the premises or assumptions underpinning your thinking. The need for this is not always obvious as people often acquire their beliefs/perspectives, points of views and habits of thinking unconsciously through their professional and personal experiences. As such, there is a tendency to fall back on what is available and familiar rather than critically appraising what you 'know' or believe. An example of a reflection on assumptions in clinical practice could include reflection on the biopsychosocial practice you believe you follow. Although physiotherapists may claim to adopt the biopsychosocial framework, frank reflection may reveal incomplete understanding and superficial attention to psychosocial factors in assessment and management (Singla et al., 2015). Unjustified assumptions in clinical practice can

> **BOX 23.5**
> **SOME SAFEGUARDS AGAINST UNJUSTIFIED ASSUMPTIONS**
>
> - Qualifying patients' meanings
> - Screening to ensure information is not missed
> - Testing for competing hypotheses
> - Attending to 'negatives' or features of a presentation that do not fit favoured hypotheses and explanations
> - Verifying your assessment of the patient's story with the patient
> - Openly subjecting and comparing your own reasoning to others

be minimized through a range of safeguards, including those listed in Box 23.5.

Metacognition

In addition to physiotherapists' critical thinking and analytical skills, their metacognitive skills also influence their clinical reasoning proficiency. Metacognition is a form of reflective self-awareness that incorporates monitoring of yourself (e.g., your performance, your thinking, your knowledge) as though you are outside yourself observing and critiquing your practice. There is an integral link among cognition (i.e., perception, interpretation, synthesis, planning), metacognition and learning from clinical practice experience (Higgs et al., 2008). For example, following protocol assessments can require little cognition beyond remembering a routine. In contrast, questions and physical assessments can provide a more complete picture of the patient's presentation if the specific purpose is to test working hypotheses or recognize clinical patterns. Although, hopefully, all therapists think, not all therapists think about their thinking. It is this self-awareness and self-critique that prompt the metacognitive therapist to reconsider his or her hypotheses, plans and management.

This self-awareness is not limited to testing formal hypotheses and thinking about treatments. Metacognitive awareness of performance is also important. This, for example, underpins the experienced therapist's immediate recognition that a particular phrasing of a question or explanation is not clear to a patient. Similarly, metacognitive sensitivity enables immediate recognition that a procedure needs to be adjusted or perhaps should be abandoned. For example, cues such as an increase in muscle tone or the patient's expression can signal a procedure is not achieving its desired effect. Effective metacognition contributes to the responsibility (that the physiotherapist shares with the patient) for fully understanding the patient versus simply 'judging or labelling the patient' and consequently relieving the physiotherapist of responsibility for the outcomes of care.

Lastly, metacognition is important to recognizing limitations in knowledge and ability. The student or therapist who lacks this metacognitive awareness will learn less. Experts not only know a lot in their area of practice, but they also know what they do not know. That is, the expert is typically very quick to recognize a limitation in his or her knowledge (e.g., a patient's medication he or she is unfamiliar with, a medical condition, the distribution of a peripheral sensory or motor nerve) and act on this by consulting a colleague or appropriate resource. In short, metacognition and critical reflection are important means to continue professional career-long learning.

Data Collection and Procedural Skills

Clinical reasoning is only as good as the information on which it is based. Incomplete and inaccurate information obtained through the patient interview, physical examination and monitoring of outcomes (during and after treatments) can lead to inaccurate analyses that compromise specific treatment and overall management. Broadly, the patient interview (supplemented by review of available records) serves the purpose of obtaining information to understand the problem(s) and the person. It also provides the initial means for developing an effective patient–therapist therapeutic alliance, as discussed later in the chapter. Each area of physiotherapy practice will have its own core routine information sought within the patient interview. This core information needs to be complete and accurate and applies to all patients. The breadth of this information will then be complemented by the depth needed to understand individual patients in their uniqueness and clarify what is meaningful for them.

There are many situations in which patient responses require clarification to accurately understand their meaning. For example, patients' perceptions of their problems may be based on superficial accounts of what their doctors, or others, have told them. Our assessments need to find out what these perceptions actually mean to the patient with respect to the cause, management and the future. Clarifying relationships between beliefs, cognitions, emotions and behaviours with the history and behaviour of the patient's symptoms and disability helps identify the key factors contributing to a patient's pain/disability experience. Explicit 'Screening Questions' that assess beyond what the patient spontaneously offers, such as screening for other symptoms, aggravating or easing factors and screening general health, are examples of ways to establish this completeness.

As with the patient interview, the quality of information obtained from the physical examination is influenced by the physiotherapist's procedural skills. Errors in subjective assessments of physical tests (e.g., posture, range of active and passive movement, kinematics, judgements regarding stiffness, laxity/instability, motor performance and soft tissue) underpin the importance of using reliable objective measures and diagnostic procedures with the greatest validity, wherever possible. When objective measurement is not available, findings should be rechecked for consistency, related to other findings (e.g., passive accessory movement findings compared with physiological movement findings) and cautiously integrated with more objective findings to guide reasoning judgements.

Knowledge Organization

The importance of knowledge to physiotherapists' clinical reasoning is highlighted in Jensen's expertise research. Expert physiotherapists were seen to possess a broad, multidimensional knowledge base acquired through professional education and reflective practice where both patients and other health professionals were valued as sources for learning (Jensen et al., 2007). Well-structured knowledge is essential to domain competence. Research in cognitive psychology and artificial intelligence (e.g., Greeno and Simon, 1986), categorization (e.g., Hayes and Adams, 2000), expertise (e.g., Boshuizen and Schmidt, 2008; Jensen et al., 2007) and education (e.g., Pearsall et al., 1997) have collectively demonstrated the importance of well-developed knowledge to successful performance. Well-structured knowledge is not simply how much an individual knows but how that knowledge is organized. For knowledge to be accessible in practice, it needs to be linked to practice.

All forms of knowledge are important, including clinicians' broader worldviews, their philosophy of practice and their medical and profession specific knowledge. The ICF biopsychosocial model and the clinical reasoning strategies and hypothesis categories frameworks provide means for physiotherapy knowledge organization that directly link theory to practice. Physiotherapy theory continues to grow in unison with the growth in research across the sciences and health professions. Equally important, but generally with less research attention, is our professional craft knowledge (Higgs et al., 2008). Craft knowledge comprises professional knowledge such as procedural, communication and teaching knowledge and skills. It is underpinned by theory (e.g., anatomy, biomechanics, neurophysiology, psychology, sociology) that has been contextualized through clinical experience.

Although clinical trials, clinical guidelines, clinical prediction rules and theory extrapolated from basic science all provide helpful guides to management for different problems, as mentioned at the start, these should not be taken as prescriptions (Greenhalgh et al., 2014). Instead, physiotherapists must judge how their patient matches the population in the research reported and then tailor their management to the individual patient's unique lifestyle, goals, activity and participation restrictions, perspectives, pain type, potential pathology and physical impairments. Because research-supported management efficacy is still lacking for most clinical problems, advanced theoretical and craft knowledge, combined with skilled reasoning, is the physiotherapist's best tool to optimize management effectiveness for individual patients.

Therapeutic Alliance

Ferreira et al. (2013, p. 471) define the therapeutic alliance as 'the sense of collaboration, warmth, and support between the client and therapist'. The manner in which an examination and therapy are provided is important, especially with respect to patient rapport. If the physiotherapist shows interest, empathy and confidence, then patients are likely to respond positively. Patients are more willing to volunteer relevant information, more willing to participate in self-management, and more motivated to change (Ferreira et al., 2013; Hall et al., 2010). Although the patient interview and physical examination are largely about gaining information to understand the

patient and his or her problems, the nature and manner in which this is done are all important. The tone of voice, the nonverbal behaviours, the time allowed and the responses to patients all affect how a patient perceives the therapist. These factors are a strong influence on the confidence of the patient and the success of the therapeutic relationship (Ferreira et al., 2013; Hall et al., 2010).

The patient–therapist relationship is founded on the perceptions each has about the other and by how each person perceives and understands him or herself (and his or her roles) as a 'self'. Merleau-Ponty offered a concept of the 'self' as embodied (1962, p. 137), meaning that a person's sense of self (and his or her consciousness) is expressed in the physical and social world of that person via such things as his or her gestures, movements and actions. The idea of embodiment helps us understand that illness or disability 'is not simply a biological dysfunction of a body part but a pervasive disturbance of our being in the world' (Carel, 2012, p. 326). In other words, pain and disability can profoundly affect a person's sense of self and how he or she experiences his or her 'place' in the world. Our questions and responses (verbal and nonverbal) are interpreted by patients with pain and disability from this position of a changed sense of self (Greenfield and Jensen, 2010). If we forget this, then in our clinical reasoning conclusions, we can reduce the experiences of a person with pain and disability to a merely prescriptive label, such as 'pain behaviour', and we can then also reduce his or her capacity to act for change (Edwards et al., 2014; Ricoeur, 2006). Sensitivity to embodiment needs empathy.

Empathy in a clinical context refers to therapists' cognitive abilities to understand what their patients are experiencing and therapists' affective abilities to imaginatively project themselves into their patients' situations (Braude, 2012). Having and conveying empathy are probably personal skills acquired throughout life. When empathy is applied in practice, patients are more likely to feel they have been given a voice, have been heard and have been believed, all of which strengthen the therapeutic alliance. Many patients report negative experiences with medical and other healthcare professionals whom they felt did not listen or believe them (e.g., Edwards et al., 2014; Epstein et al., 2005; Johnson, 1993; Payton et al., 1998). Without good rapport and empathy, the patient is less likely to collaborate, potentially compromising clinical reasoning and jeopardizing the eventual outcome. The importance of empathic collaboration (as in the reasoning strategy collaborative reasoning), not simply cooperation, is underscored by the evidence that patients who have been given an opportunity to share in the decision making take greater responsibility for their own management, are more satisfied with their health care and have a greater likelihood of achieving better outcomes (Arnetz et al., 2004; Edwards et al., 2004b; Trede and Higgs, 2008).

CHAPTER SUMMARY

In this chapter, we have outlined:

- the critical need for physiotherapists to understand the components of clinical reasoning including common errors in human judgement, fast and slow reasoning processes and the critical role of adaptive expertise,
- how clinical reasoning fits within a biopsychosocial framework and is aligned with the ICF model,
- a framework of clinical reasoning strategies that provides assistance to understanding and learning clinical reasoning,
- a framework of hypothesis categories, or clinical judgements, required across the different clinical reasoning strategies and
- factors that influence clinical reasoning, including critical thinking, metacognition, knowledge organization and the therapeutic alliance.

REFLECTION POINT 4

How can you synthesize the ideas, frameworks and strategies presented in this chapter into a coherent model to guide your own clinical reasoning?

REFERENCES

Arnetz, J.E., Almin, I., Bergström, K., et al., 2004. Active patient involvement in the establishment of physical therapy goals: effects on treatment outcome and quality of care. Adv. Physiother. 6, 50–69.

Barlow, S.E., 2012. The barriers to implementation of evidence-based chronic pain management in rural and regional physiotherapy outpatients: realizing the potential, HETI Report, Rural Research Capacity Building Program. NSW Ministry of Health. Viewed 13 April 2017. Available from: www.aci.health.nsw.gov.au.

Borrell-Carrió, F., Suchman, A.L., Epstein, R.M., 2004. The biopsychosocial model 25 years later: principles, practice, and scientific inquiry. Ann. Fam. Med. 2, 576–582.

Boshuizen, H.P.A., Schmidt, H.G., 2008. The development of clinical reasoning expertise. In: Higgs, J., Jones, M.A., Loftus, S., et al. (Eds.), Clinical Reasoning in the Health Professions, third ed. Elsevier, Edinburgh, pp. 113–121.

Braude, H.D., 2012. Conciliating cognition and consciousness: the perceptual foundations of clinical reasoning. J. Eval. Clin. Pract. 18, 945–950.

Brookfield, S., 2008. Clinical reasoning and generic thinking skills. In: Higgs, J., Jones, M.A., Loftus, S., et al. (Eds.), Clinical Reasoning in the Health Professions, third ed. Elsevier, Edinburgh, pp. 65–75.

Carel, H., 2012. Nursing and medicine. In: Luft, S., Overgaard, S. (Eds.), The Routledge Companion to Phenomenology. Routledge, Taylor & Francis Group, London, UK, pp. 623–632.

Cooke, S., Lemay, F., 2017. Transforming medical assessment: integrating uncertainty into the evaluation of clinical reasoning in medical education. Acad. Med. 92, 746–751.

Cutrer, W.B., Miller, B., Pusic, M.V., et al., 2017. Fostering the development of master adaptive learners: a conceptual model to guide skill acquisition in medical education. Acad. Med. 92, 70–75.

de Bono, E., 2014. Lateral Thinking: An Introduction. Vermilion, New York, NY.

Doody, C., McAteer, M., 2002. Clinical reasoning of expert and novice physiotherapists in an outpatient orthopaedic setting. Physiotherapy 88, 258–268.

Duncan, G., 2000. Mind-body dualism and the biopsychosocial model of pain: what did Descartes really say? J. Med. Philos. 25, 485–513.

Edwards, I., Jones, M., 2013. Movement in our thinking and our practice. Man. Ther. 18, 93–95.

Edwards, I., Jones, M., Carr, J., et al., 2004a. Clinical reasoning strategies in physical therapy. Phys. Ther. 84, 312–335.

Edwards, I., Jones, M., Higgs, J., et al., 2004b. What is collaborative reasoning? Adv. Physiother. 6, 70–83.

Edwards, I., Jones, M., Thacker, M., et al., 2014. The moral experience of the patient with chronic pain: bridging the gap between first and third person ethics. Pain Med. 15, 364–378.

Engel, G.L., 1977. The need for a new medical model: a challenge for biomedicine. Science 196, 129–136.

Epstein, R.M., Borrell-Carrió, F., 2005. The biopsychosocial model: exploring six impossible things. Fam. Syst. Health. 23, 426–431.

Epstein, R.M., Franks, P., Fiscella, K., et al., 2005. Measuring patient-centred communication in patient-physician consultations: theoretical and practical issues. Soc. Sci. Med. 61, 1516–1528.

Ferreira, P.H., Ferreira, M.L., Maher, C.G., et al., 2013. The therapeutic alliance between clinicians and patients predicts outcomes in chronic low back pain. Phys. Ther. 93, 470–478.

Greenfield, B., Jensen, G., 2010. Understanding the lived experience of patients: the application of a phenomenological approach to ethics. Phys. Ther. 90, 1185–1197.

Greenhalgh, T., Howick, J., Maskrey, N., 2014. Evidence based medicine: a movement in crisis? BMJ 348, g3725.

Greeno, J.G., Simon, H.A., 1986. Problem solving and reasoning. In: Atkinson, R.C., Hersteing, R., Lindsey, G.L., et al. (Eds.), Steven's Handbook of Experimental Psychology, 2, Learning and Cognition, second ed. Lawrence Erlbaum Associates, Hillsdale, NJ, pp. 572–589.

Hall, A.M., Ferreira, P.H., Maher, C.G., et al., 2010. The influence of the therapist-patient relationship on treatment outcome in physical rehabilitation: a systematic review. Phys. Ther. 90, 1099–1110.

Hayes, B., Adams, R., 2000. Parallels between clinical reasoning and categorization. In: Higgs, J., Jones, M. (Eds.), Clinical Reasoning in the Health Professions, second ed. Butterworth-Heinemann, Oxford, pp. 45–53.

Higgs, J., Fish, D., Rothwell, R., 2008. Knowledge generation and clinical reasoning in practice. In: Higgs, J., Jones, M.A., Loftus, S., et al. (Eds.), Clinical Reasoning in the Health Professions, third ed. Elsevier, Edinburgh, pp. 163–172.

Higgs, J., Jones, M.A., Titchen, A., 2008. Knowledge, reasoning and evidence for practice. In: Higgs, J., Jones, M.A., Loftus, S., et al. (Eds.), Clinical Reasoning in the Health Professions, third ed. Elsevier, Edinburgh, pp. 151–161.

Hogarth, R.M., 2005. Deciding analytically or trusting your intuition? The advantages and disadvantages of analytic and intuitive thought. In: Betsch, T., Haberstroh, S. (Eds.), The Routines of Decision Making. Lawrence Erlbaum Associates, Mahwah, NJ, pp. 67–82.

Imrie, R., 2004. Demystifying disability: a review of the international classification of functioning, disability and health. Sociol. Health Illn. 26, 287–305.

Jensen, G.M., Gwyer, J., Hack, L., et al., 2007. Expertise in Physical Therapy Practice, second ed. Saunders-Elsevier, St. Louis, MO.

Jensen, T.S., Baron, R., Haanpää, M., et al., 2011. A new definition of neuropathic pain. Pain 152, 2204–2205.

Jones, M.A., 1987. The clinical reasoning process in manipulative therapy. In: Dalziel, B.A., Snowsill, J.C. (Eds.), Proceedings of the Fifth Biennial Conference of the Manipulative Therapists Association of Australia. Melbourne, VIC, pp. 62–69.

Jones, M., Grimmer, K.A., Edwards, I., et al., 2006. Challenges in applying best evidence to physiotherapy. Internet J. Allied Health Sci. Pract. 4. Viewed 13 April 2017. Available from: http://ijahsp.nova.edu/.

Johnson, R., 1993. Attitudes just don't hang in the air... disabled people's perceptions of physiotherapists. Physiotherapy 79, 619–626.

Jull, G., Moore, A., 2012. Hands on, hands off? The swings in musculoskeletal physiotherapy practice. Man. Ther. 17, 199–200.

Kahneman, D., 2011. Thinking, Fast and Slow. Allen Lane, London, UK.

Kahneman, D., Slovic, P., Tversky, A., 1982. Judgment Under Uncertainty: Heuristics and Biases. Cambridge University Press, New York, NY.

Kaufman, D.R., Yoskowitz, N.A., Patel, V.L., 2008. Clinical reasoning and biomedical knowledge: implications for teaching. In: Higgs, J., Jones, M.A., Loftus, S., et al. (Eds.), Clinical Reasoning in the Health Professions, third ed. Elsevier, Edinburgh, pp. 137–149.

Kerry, R., Madouasse, A., Arthur, A., et al., 2013. Analysis of scientific truth status in controlled rehabilitation trials. J. Eval. Clin. Pract. 19, 617–625.

Lehrer, J., 2009. How We Decide. Houghton Mifflin Harcourt, Boston, MA.

Merleau-Ponty, M., 1962. Phenomenology of Perception. Routledge, London, UK.

Mezirow, J., 2012. Learning to think like an adult: core concepts of transformative theory. In: Taylor, E.W., Cranton, P. (Eds.), The Handbook of Transformative Learning: Theory, Research and Practice. Jossey-Bass, San Francisco, CA, pp. 73–95.

Moseley, A.M., Elkins, M.R., Janer-Duncan, L., et al., 2014. The quality of reports of randomized controlled trials varies between subdisciplines of physiotherapy. Physiother. Can. 66, 36–43.

Nijs, J., Torres-Cueco, R., van Wilgen, C.P., et al., 2014. Applying modern pain neuroscience in clinical practice: criteria for the classification of central sensitization pain. Pain Physician 17, 447–457.

Paul, R., Elder, L., 2007. A Guide for Educators to Critical Thinking Competency Standards. Foundation for Critical Thinking, Dillon Beach, CA.

Payton, O.D., Nelson, C.E., Hobbs, M.S.C., 1998. Physical therapy patients' perceptions of their relationships with health care professionals. Physiother. Theory Pract. 14, 211–221.

Pearsall, N.R., Skipper, J.E.J., Mintzes, J.J., 1997. Knowledge restructuring in the life sciences: a longitudinal study of conceptual change in biology. Science Educ. 81, 193–215.

Pincus, T., 2004. The psychology of pain. In: French, S., Sim, K. (Eds.), Physiotherapy: A Psychosocial Approach. Elsevier, Edinburgh, pp. 95–115.

Ricoeur, P., 2006. Capabilities and rights. In: Nebel, M., Sagovsky, N. (Eds.), Transforming Unjust Structures: The Capability Approach. Springer, Dordrecht, The Netherlands, pp. 17–26.

Rivett, D.A., Higgs, J., 1997. Hypothesis generation in the clinical reasoning behavior of manual therapists. J. Phys. Ther. Educ. 11, 40–45.

Schumacher, D., Englander, R., Carraccio, C., 2013. Developing the master learner: applying learning theory to the learner, the teacher and the learning environment. Acad. Med. 88, 1635–1645.

Schwartz, A., Elstein, A.S., 2008. Clinical reasoning in medicine. In: Higgs, J., Jones, M.A., Loftus, S., et al. (Eds.), Clinical Reasoning in the Health Professions, third ed. Elsevier, Edinburgh, pp. 223–234.

Singla, M., Jones, M., Edwards, I., et al., 2015. Physiotherapists' assessment of patients' psychosocial status: are we standing on thin ice? A qualitative descriptive study. Man. Ther. 20, 328–334.

Smart, K., Doody, C., 2006. Mechanisms-based clinical reasoning of pain by experienced musculoskeletal physiotherapists. Physiotherapy 92, 171–178.

Trede, F., Higgs, J., 2008. Collaborative decision making. In: Higgs, J., Jones, M.A., Loftus, S., et al. (Eds.), Clinical Reasoning in the Health Professions, third ed. Elsevier, Edinburgh, pp. 31–41.

Treede, R.D., Jensen, T.S., Campbell, J.N., et al., 2008. Neuropathic pain: redefinition and a grading system for clinical and research purposes. Neurology 70, 1630–1635.

Villas Boas, P.J., Spagnuolo, R.S., Kamegasawa, A., et al., 2013. Systematic reviews showed insufficient evidence for clinical practice in 2004: what about in 2011? The next appeal for the evidence-based medicine age. J. Eval. Clin. Pract. 19, 633–637.

Wolf, C.J., 2010. What is this thing called pain? J. Clin. Invest. 120, 3742–3744.

Wolf, C.J., 2011. Central sensitization: implication for diagnosis and treatment of pain. Pain 152, s2–s15.

World Health Organization, 2001. International Classification of Functioning, Disability and Health. World Health Organization, Geneva.

24

CLINICAL REASONING IN DENTISTRY

SHIVA KHATAMI ■ MICHAEL MACENTEE ■ STEPHEN LOFTUS

CHAPTER AIMS

The aims of this chapter are to:

■ present a conceptual framework for clinical reasoning in dentistry,

■ identify the sources of uncertainty in clinical reasoning of dentists and

■ provide direction for future research and education of clinical reasoning.

KEY WORDS

Clinical reasoning

Uncertainty

Dental education

ABBREVIATIONS/ ACRONYMS

H-D Hypothetico-deductive

PBL Problem-based learning

WHO World Health Organization

EVOLUTION OF CLINICAL REASONING

Clinical reasoning is a core component of healthcare practice. It involves a process of thinking and interacting with 'problem spaces' within a multilayered context of the clinician, the patient and the clinical problem, surrounded by a larger social, cultural and global environment. Using this interactive and interpretive process, clinicians attempt to understand clinical situations, make diagnostic and therapeutic decisions and frame and solve clinical problems (Khatami et al., 2012).

Historically, healthcare professions have evolved their awareness of the scope and diversity of health-related problems. From the birth of scientific health care (Foucault, 1994), the biomedical model has dominated how the health professions conceptualized health and disease (Adams, 1999). More recently, other models, such as 'sick role theory' (Parsons, 1951), have challenged the biomedical model. Subsequent emphasis on the patient's role in health care led to development of the biopsychosocial model of health care (Engel, 1977). From this perspective, the concept of health has evolved to include a general feeling of physical, psychological and social well-being or, according to Svenaeus (2000), a sense of 'homelike being in the world' (p. 114).

Dentistry has seen a parallel evolution from treating disease to treating the whole person within a specific sociocultural context (Khatami and MacEntee, 2011) and beyond a predominantly surgical approach (e.g., extractions and fillings) to include a more medical and preventive model of care (Baelum and Lopez, 2004). A focus on prevention has highlighted the social and behavioural context of diseases together with a need for equitable access to oral healthcare services. The focus now on equity has broadened dental practice from private dental clinics to hospitals, schools, community-based clinics and long-term care facilities, along with an interdisciplinary approach to care (Field, 1995; Formicola et al., 2006). The advent of telemedicine and teledentistry will further expand the context of dental practice from physical to virtual interactions with patients and peers (Daniel and Kumar, 2014).

After the Institute of Medicine report was published (Field, 1995), dental educators were challenged to accommodate a broader awareness of environmental and psychosocial determinants of health in an already crowded professional curriculum focussed narrowly on science and psychomotor skills (Hendricson and Cohen, 2001; MacEntee, 2010). Alternative curricular models emerged promoting problem-solving skills, developing competencies and community-service learning (Khatami and MacEntee, 2011). However, the effectiveness of these curricular models is unclear in developing and evaluating the clinical reasoning of dentists, possibly due to limited understanding of the process of clinical reasoning. It is worth taking a short look at the history of how clinical reasoning has been understood in dentistry.

EXPLORING CLINICAL REASONING

Inconsistencies in diagnosis and treatment planning revealed by earlier psychometric studies resulted in repeated calls for sensitive and specific diagnostic tests, practice guidelines and decision-support systems for dentists (Kay et al., 1992; Kawahata and MacEntee, 2002). Decision analysis, preference-based measurement, rating scales, standard gamble techniques, time trade-offs, quality-adjusted life (tooth) years, game theory and Bayesian-based utility measures have all been applied as theoretical bases for exploring decision making in dentistry. These approaches collectively come under the banner of medical decision theory (Matthews et al., 1999).

Decision analysis applies a sequential process of developing and revising diagnostic and treatment decisions by constructing and proceeding along the trunk and branches of decision trees (Kawahata and MacEntee, 2002). Bayesian rules are applied to weigh all possible decisions by identifying the expected outcomes, estimating their probability, evaluating their risks and benefits and assigning a utility value to each. The probability and utility values are evaluated to reach the most 'rational' decision. However, Chambers et al. (2010) found that applications of Bayesian formulas to epidemiological data were not a typical part of how dental students or experienced dentists made decisions

about the presence or prognosis of disease. The uncertainty of available evidence frequently compromises confidence in diagnosis of pathologies (Pena and Andrade-Filho, 2009). Moreover, rational treatment decisions based on the rules of decision analysis can conflict with the patient's preference for treatment and the clinician's ethical principles (Patel et al., 2002). Decision trees require a certain degree of artistry; however, the creativity for constructing and interpreting them can contradict the conceptual framework of decision theory.

Bayes' theorem informed the development of earlier computer-based decision support systems for diagnosis and treatment planning in dentistry (e.g., Sims-Williams et al., 1987), followed by neural networks (e.g., Brickley and Shepherd, 1996) and fuzzy logic (e.g., Wang et al., 2016). There has also been an emphasis on language, symbols and semantics within the context of dentistry, even in the presence of uncertainty (Kawahata and MacEntee, 2002). Symbolic computations, such as fuzzy logic, for example, offer the possibility of managing uncertainty in rule-based clinical decisions (Zadeh, 2008). However, decision support systems such as those used in telemedicine and teledentistry apply essentially reductionist methods to solving problems and pose ethical and legal concerns when there is inadequate empirical evidence to support the decision recommended by the system (Goodman, 2007). Computerized systems cannot always manage the multilayered meanings within the clinical interactions between patient and dentist (Loftus, 2015). However, support systems offer educational opportunities for practicing diagnostic and treatment decisions on virtual patients (Cook et al., 2010).

The hypothetico-deductive (H-D) model has been the dominant theory explaining how experienced dentists move through 'forward reasoning' to search, identify and organize key points of information and generate a diagnosis (Crespo et al., 2004). Dental students and novice dentists usually start this diagnostic process by generating a list of hypotheses and working backwards to confirm or reject each hypotheses. Experts usually move more rapidly by acknowledging the influence of psychosocial issues on their decisions and relying on experience to recognize patterns or 'illness scripts' from previous clinical encounters (Charlin et al., 2000). From this viewpoint, for example, caries is recognized from a script describing the colour and size of demineralized dental lesions (Bader and Shugars, 1997). Dental students, in contrast, tend to use a more laborious 'dual processing' model with H-D reasoning and pattern recognition to the same end (Maupomé et al., 2010). However, the accuracy of diagnosis between one 'system' versus the other is unclear (Monteiro and Norman, 2013).

Alternatively, a narrative explanation posits that experienced dentists, unlike computers, are sensitive to the intricate beliefs and behaviours of their patients, which points to the need for more inductive and interpretive explorations of how dentists, like other clinicians, work towards making clinical decisions (Loftus, 2015). For example, encounters with anxious patients can be eased by allowing patients to tell stories that explain their clinical problems beyond the more typical biomedical narrative of disease.

Dentists can also benefit from developing phrónêsis or a practical disposition to act wisely when confronted by an unusual clinical situation (Kinsella and Pitman,

2012). Apparently, phrónêsis is acquired by practical encounters, especially when clinicians have opportunities to reflect on what they learned from each encounter (Schön, 1983). The development and sharing of such stories allow clinicians to acquire practical wisdom that they recall when confronted later by similar problems.

CONCEPTUAL FRAMEWORK

Fig. 24.1 portrays a conceptual model of clinical reasoning in dentistry developed from studies of dental students and specialists across different levels of expertise (Khatami, 2010). The multilayered context of clinical reasoning is shown as overlapping ovals integrating the personal frame of reference of the dentist, the frame of reference of the patient, the problem(s) and the larger healthcare environment. The following describes the components of the model and the similarities and differences in reasoning of dentists across different levels of expertise and problems.

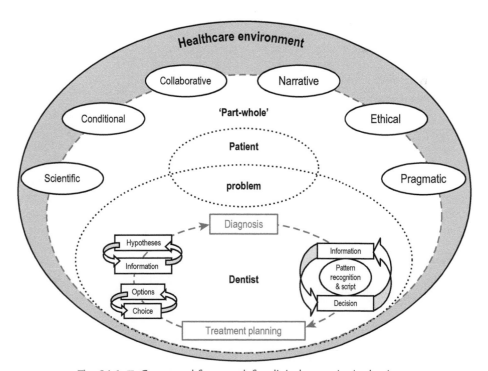

Fig. 24.1 ■ Conceptual framework for clinical reasoning in dentistry.

PROCESSES OF CLINICAL REASONING

Ritual

The notion of ritual is borrowed from the field of medical anthropology and plays a role in many aspects of health care (Helman, 2007). We use it here to emphasize that following a systematic and standardized approach is not new or exclusive to science or health care. Most dentists follow a systematic approach to acquire medical, dental and social histories and evaluate clinical data and diagnostic aids, such as radiographs and study models. Subsequently, they plan a sequence of treatment, usually starting with management of disease, followed by rehabilitation and maintenance of health. Being familiar with the routines and rituals of assessment means that one can concentrate on the goal of reaching a diagnosis without having to explicitly remember all the details that need to be included in the process. With practice, the routines and rituals become embodied and automatic. An expert can be sure that the relevant questions and procedures will be addressed. Beyond this, more experienced dentists seem to have individualized rituals and routines that allow them to reason rapidly and efficiently and collect only information pertinent to the case. This may be because experienced clinicians are keenly sensitive to what is salient in a particular setting (Benner et al., 2011).

Backward (Deductive) and Forward (Inductive) Reasoning

Although it is often said that experts tend to reason in a forward direction and novices in a backward direction, this is not always the case (Laufer and Glick, 1996). It is more likely that experienced dentists go backwards and forwards to diagnose clinical problems. Even in forward reasoning, experts will form several tentative diagnoses early in the process. Experts typically hold tentative diagnoses lightly and change their focus as information is gathered, whereas novices, often restricted to a backwards process of reasoning, tend to remain firmly attached to the initial diagnoses, as others have explained within the context of critical thinking (McKendry, 2015).

Pattern-Recognition Through Scripts

Visual and descriptive cues help dentists recognize the pattern of specific diseases, such as caries, periodontal disease and other abnormalities. These allow the dentist to bypass unconsciously the intricate processes of making and testing hypotheses.

Demineralized carious lesions on teeth present in a wide range of colours, appearances and textures from which a dentist can define a pattern recognized from previous experiences. However, assessing the aetiology and risk for caries and tooth loss requires a more elaborate exploration that extends from physical to psychosocial considerations (Baelum, 2010). The 'caries scripts' often consist of information about the composition of saliva and oral bacteria and details of a patient's diet, hygiene and socioeconomic status that leads to an assessment of 'caries risk' and therapeutic options. Similarly, visual cues about the normal versus abnormal appearance of gingiva and periodontium trigger the scripts for gingivitis and periodontal disease (Baelum and López, 2004). However, to classify the severity of each disease and appropriate treatment, additional clinical and possibly radiographic information is required.

Decision Analysis

Most dentists do not quantify the probability or utility value associated with Bayes' theorem. Instead they integrate their knowledge and experience practically to interpret the problem and select treatment options (Chambers et al., 2010; Khatami et al., 2012).

CLINICAL REASONING STRATEGIES

The following reasoning strategies help dentists interpret and address clinical problems.

Scientific Reasoning

The H-D process of reasoning, described earlier, follows a scientific method of systematically observing, measuring and collecting information, followed by the formation, testing and modification of hypotheses or tentative diagnoses (Khatami et al., 2012). However, as explained earlier, the experienced clinician usually brings professional experience and common sense to the reasoning process in ways that seem to increase directly with the extent of clinical uncertainty.

Conditional Reasoning

Predicting the prognosis of treatment needs biological, psychological and socioeconomic measurements tempered by clinical experiences and pattern recognition. Nonetheless, the uncertainty of treatment outcomes challenges most clinical decisions. Consequently, conditional reasoning helps anticipate and reduce future problems through a tentative or wait-and-see approach whereby the clinician defers definitive or irreversible decision until the uncertainty is reduced to a level agreeable to both the dentist and patient (Khatami, 2010).

Collaborative Reasoning

Communicating with patients and colleagues is an integral part of good clinical practice. It should aim to share the responsibility of making decisions and an understanding of the most desirable and feasible treatment outcome available, especially when treatment involves a change in the patient's beliefs and behaviour (Khatami et al., 2012).

Narrative Reasoning

This strategy manages the experience and multilayered meaning of disease and health from the perspective of patients and how they influence health-related behaviours and expected treatment outcomes. Reflecting on the assumptions that dentists bring to this interpretive process allows them to compare their own values and beliefs with those of a patient. This might include stories of previous encounters with similar problems that help to interpret the current situation and offer similar treatment options (Khatami, 2010).

Ethical Reasoning

Principle-based ethics have dominated the way many dentists resolve problems; however, virtue and narrative ethics provide greater scope for dealing with the difficulties of clinical uncertainty (Charon et al., 2016). Virtue ethics dwells more on developing the moral character of the dentist through personal reflection and allowance for personal strengths, weaknesses and motives rather than on ethical generalities that hallmark the principled approach to ethical practice (Oakley, 2016). Similarly, narrative ethics dwells directly but broadly on individual needs with all the nuances and contradictions that permeate the life of each patient (Geisler, 2006). It explores problems

and solutions through the unique experiences of each participant.

Pragmatic Reasoning

This strategy offers a pragmatic approach to the issues relating to the social, economic, or political environment of the healthcare system. Availability of resources, risks and benefits and cost-effectiveness of treatment modalities and abilities of the clinician to deliver the required care often influence the approach to care from idealistic or theoretical to realistic and practical (Schell, 2008).

Part-Whole Reasoning

Several reasoning strategies are used as clinicians focus in and out of different 'conceptual spaces'; refocus on different aspects of a clinical problem; move from one problem to another; and decide how all the parts relate to the patient as a whole (Fiorini et al., 2014; Khatami et al., 2012). Often, interpreting problems and evaluating options for treatment involve a combination of analytical and nonanalytical reasoning processes, integrating several reasoning strategies and moving from a specific problem to consider the larger context in which the problem occurs. Part-whole reasoning is also a significant part of hermeneutic reasoning (Svenaeus, 2000).

KEY FEATURES IN CLINICAL REASONING OF DENTISTS

A personal frame of reference is a major feature of how dentists interpret problems, assess treatment options and make clinical decisions (Khatami et al., 2012). They draw on past experiences to recognize the pattern of problems or diagnostic and management scripts. Novice dentists typically follow strict rules or rituals to collect information and plan treatment. Experienced dentists use more flexible routines in response to the familiar patterns of common problems, the expectations and motivations of their patients and their own personal context for prioritizing problems, and they plan interventions accordingly (Khatami, 2010).

REFLECTION POINT 1

How does your personal frame of reference influence your approach to Angela's care?

Considering Different Clinical Decisions – What's Your Opinion?

Angela is a 74-year-old retired teacher who presents to your practice with Wendy, her daughter. Angela does not speak English. She moved from China 4 years ago to live with Wendy and her family. Wendy tells you that you are the third dentist they have seen this week. They are frustrated with the high cost of treatment suggested by the previous dentists to replace missing teeth, and Angela does not have dental insurance.

Her medical status includes high blood pressure, which is currently under control, and Parkinson's disease. Angela is missing all posterior teeth and has a crowned upper-left central incisor that is sensitive to cold. She has abraded away about half of her lower incisors, but this does not concern her. Wendy asks if you could replace all of her mother's teeth with complete dentures to minimize the cost of treatment. How would you address this request?

UNCERTAINTIES IN CLINICAL REASONING

The uncertainty of clinical practice poses a significant challenge to all clinical practitioners, from students to mature clinicians. Fox (1980) observed that medical students struggle with three domains of uncertainty: 1) their own incomplete mastery of available knowledge; 2) the limitation of available knowledge; and 3) the distinction between their personal limitations and their emerging awareness of the limitations of the profession at large. In addition, they are readily confused by different approaches to analyzing and addressing clinical problems, especially when confronted by unpredictable responses from patients. Beresford (1991) explained the technical, personal and conceptual uncertainties of clinical practice. He identified technical uncertainty in the limitations of scientific evidence and personal uncertainty in the limitations of the clinician's knowledge and experience, compounded by the unpredictable response of patients. Finally there is conceptual uncertainty in the clinical application of incommensurable criteria to the concrete problems of patients. Han et al. (2011) define uncertainty as a subjective perception of ignorance constructed and managed 'through the interactions of patients and health professionals' (p. 834). They proposed an organized conceptual taxonomy or framework that is sufficiently broad to account for the full range of salient issues experienced by patients and clinicians yet narrow enough to be meaningful and practical. They believe that practically patients worry about uncertainty pertaining to the probability

of beneficial treatment, the ambiguity of accompanying advice and the complexity of the disorder itself, especially because these issues are frequently unquantifiable scientifically, practically or personally. Identifying the issues and sources of uncertainty in this manner, they contend, will enable the clinician to reduce them to the extent warranted by each patient. However, they stress, the therapeutic goal is not necessarily to eliminate uncertainty but rather to acknowledge it within the bounds of current knowledge and enable patients to make informed decisions.

More experienced clinicians are more likely to admit their uncertainties and develop a professional rhetoric of uncertainty when confronted by technical, personal or conceptual uncertainties (Lingard et al., 2003). Katz (1984) reminds us that physicians have a long history of therapeutic deception by hiding uncertainty from patients to enhance the placebo effect in the practice of medicine. Justification for masking uncertainty, he believes, depends on the 'kinds of faith, hope and reassurance' (p. 40) that a patient seeks from a doctor, and the patient must make this decision. This dilemma illustrates quite clearly the ongoing conflict between art and science in clinical decisions, a dilemma that also confronts dentists (MacEntee, 2007). Relationships between clinicians and their patients are strongly influenced by the professionalism and communication skills of the clinician. Denial of uncertainty can be a deceptive strategy to create an illusion of control leading to a dogmatic certainty that brings bias and error to clinical reasoning (Katz, 1984; MacEntee and Mathu-Muju, 2014).

REFLECTION POINT 2

Which of the technical, personal or conceptual uncertainties influence your clinical reasoning in everyday practice? How do you communicate uncertainty to your patients?

Light (1979) argued that the degree of technical uncertainty in each profession reflects the paradigm development underlying its practice and the paradigm strength explaining the phenomena it addresses. However, Knafl and Burkett (1975) referred to treatment philosophies in a context similar to paradigm development but concluded from an ethnographic study of residents in orthopaedic surgery that the 'fundamental importance attached to personal clinical experience in the exercise of judgement may lead physicians to reject established scientific opinion in favor of personal preferences' (p. 403).

The prognosis of dental treatment, as in all health care, is often difficult to predict. Uncertainties are exacerbated beyond the personal professional realms of patients and dentists by different philosophies of care and conflicting opinions within and across different specialties (Knafl and Burkett, 1975). The availability, validity and quality of evidence are inconsistent both within and across the specialties. Advances in biomaterials, computer-aided design/computer-aided manufacturing (CAD/CAM) and treatment modalities are rapid, challenging, uncertain and ongoing (Marinello, 2016). The validity and reliability of diagnostic indicators for caries, periodontal disease and other disorders of the mouth are all subject to interpretive challenges (Baelum, 2010; Baelum and López, 2004; Fuller, 2015).

The market trend and media may also influence the demand for specific dental treatments and approaches to care even if untested or lacking good supportive evidence (MacEntee, 2005; Newsome and Langley, 2014). Discrepancies in priorities and definitions of treatment objectives by clinicians, patients and third-party payers create conflict of opinions and interests and often lead to uncertainties and ethical dilemmas. The cost of treatment and coverage of the cost by dental insurances can influence patients and ultimately clinicians' choices for treatment (Vernazza et al., 2015). Sometimes treatment is postponed or rejected when a dental insurer does not cover the cost.

Inconsistencies and unclear definitions for standard of care lead to ethical dilemmas, fear of litigation and neglect of appropriate care (Bryant et al., 1995). Respecting a patient's autonomy can clash with the ethical principles of the clinician. Furthermore, a collaborative approach involving several clinicians in search of optimal care can be a double-edged sword. There is shared responsibility for managing uncertainty but also shared legal liability for the outcome. Indeed, this fear of litigation may sway many clinical decisions towards an overly conservative and possibly ineffective approach to treatment.

ASSESSMENT OF CLINICAL REASONING

The acquisition of skills to think critically and reason competently in clinical situations is a continuous and dynamic process, extends beyond predoctoral education and poses an assessment challenge for dental educators (Khatami and MacEntee, 2011). There is little evidence that dental educational methods based on problem-based learning (PBL) and the H-D model of problem solving can enhance the critical skills of dental students (Whitney et al., 2016). Moreover, uncertainty around the competency needed for dentistry in this dynamic environment tests the assessment methods currently used in dental education. Comparison of dental competency statements from Europe and the Americas reveals notable differences in format, detail and expected outcomes (American Dental Education Association, 2015; Plasschaert et al., 2005; Whitney et al., 2016). As in all healthcare disciplines, there is no common language or core of professional competencies. Consequently, dental educators struggle to define competencies appropriate to specific regions or modify existing competency statements from other regions (American Dental Education Association, 2015; Plasschaert et al., 2005).

REFLECTION POINT 3

How has your competency in clinical reasoning evolved in the course of your professional development?

Recent statements highlight the importance of professionalism, critical thinking, information management and decision-making for competent patient care (American Dental Education Association, 2015; Newsome and Langley, 2014). PBL and the H-D model of problem solving continue to dominate the learning environment and assessment methods in dental education despite questionable achievements in teaching clinical reasoning (Whitney et al., 2016). Nonetheless, despite the limitations of PBL, there remains the likelihood that clinical learning will be enhanced by Ericsson's (2004) concept of deliberate practice in which diagnosis and treatment planning in a classroom or virtual settings encourage the development of the knowledge networks required for clinical reasoning, through a process of repetition, reflection and feedback (Eva, 2005; Khatami et al., 2012).

Dental educators still rely heavily on multiple-choice questions and the objective structured clinical examination (OSCE) to assess professional competency, although with increasing concerns about their construct or predictive validity (Albino et al., 2008). There is now an awareness of the need to revise and probably replace these methods so that the public can be assured that a newly graduated dentist has 'at least minimal levels of competence on many different fronts' (Karimbux, 2013, p. 1555).

CHAPTER SUMMARY

It is through clinical reasoning that dentists, like other clinicians in health care, understand and solve clinical problems. Competent dentists make reasonable clinical decisions in a multilayered problem space that encompasses the social, cultural, political and economic environments in which they and their patients live. Their reasoning involves a nonlinear but typically recursive process of investigation and intervention involving both analytical and nonanalytical reasoning, dictated by the problem at hand and by previous experiences. The frame of reference guides the decision process along interpretive paths where problems are identified, assessed, prioritized and managed preferably through a shared understanding of the uncertainty by both the dentist and patient.

Competent dentists integrate a mix of reasoning strategies to form and implement effective treatments. In practice, they zoom in and out of problems from a local anatomical level to the wider psychosocial context in which their patients live. They are sensitive to uncertainties that arise from their limitation of knowledge and skills. They are aware also of the complexity of oral health–related problems and unpredictable outcomes of interventions. They acknowledge the limitations of diagnostic aids and multiple interpretations of clinical information, and they wrestle constantly with conflicts between ethical principles, fear of litigation and conflicting priorities of patients, colleagues and others involved in paying for health care.

REFLECTION POINT 4

How do the reasoning strategies introduced in this chapter help identify and address the uncertainties involved in your clinical reasoning?

REFERENCES

Adams, T., 1999. Dentistry and medical dominance. Soc. Sci. Med. 48, 407–420.

Albino, J.E., Young, S.K., Neumann, L.M., et al., 2008. Assessing dental students' competence: best practice recommendations in the performance assessment literature and investigation of current practices in predoctoral dental education. J. Dent. Educ. 72, 1405–1435.

American Dental Education Association, 2015. ADEA competencies for the new general dentist. J. Dent. Educ. 79, 813–816.

Bader, J.D., Shugars, D.A., 1997. What do we know about how dentists make caries-related treatment decisions? Community Dent. Oral Epidemiol. 25, 97–103.

Baelum, V., 2010. What is an appropriate caries diagnosis? Acta Odontol. Scand. 68, 65–79.

Baelum, V., López, R., 2004. Periodontal epidemiology: towards social science or molecular biology? Community Dent. Oral Epidemiol. 32, 239–249.

Benner, P.E., Hooper-Kyriakidis, P.L., Stannard, D., 2011. Clinical Wisdom and Interventions in Acute and Critical Care: A Thinking-in-Action Approach. Springer, New York, NY.

Beresford, E.B., 1991. Uncertainty and the shaping of medical decisions. Hastings Center Rep. 21, 6–11.

Brickley, M.R., Shepherd, J.P., 1996. Performance of a neural network trained to make third-molar treatment-planning decisions. Med. Decis. Making 16, 153–160.

Bryant, S.R., MacEntee, M.I., Browne, A., 1995. Ethical issues encountered by dentists in the care of institutionalized elders. Spec. Care Dentist. 15, 79–82.

Chambers, D.W., Mirchel, R., Lundergan, W., 2010. An investigation of dentists' and dental students' estimates of diagnostic probabilities. J. Am. Dent. Assoc. 141, 656–666.

Charlin, B., Tardif, J., Boshuizen, H.P., 2000. Scripts and medical diagnostic knowledge: theory and applications for clinical reasoning instruction and research. Acad. Med. 75, 182–190.

Charon, R., DasGupta, S., Hermann, N., et al., 2016. The Principles and Practice of Narrative Medicine. Oxford University Press, Oxford, UK.

Cook, D.A., Erwin, P.J., Triola, M.M., 2010. Computerized virtual patients in health professions education: a systematic review and meta-analysis. Acad. Med. 85, 1589–1602.

Crespo, K.E., Torres, J.E., Recio, M.E., 2004. Reasoning process characteristics in the diagnostic skills of beginner, competent, and expert dentists. J. Dent. Educ. 68, 1235–1244.

Daniel, S.J., Kumar, S., 2014. Teledentistry: a key component in access to care. J. Evid. Based Dental Pract. 14, 201–208.

Engel, G.L., 1977. The need for a new medical model: a challenge for biomedicine. Science 196, 129–136.

Ericsson, K.A., 2004. Deliberate practice and the acquisition and maintenance of expert performance in medicine and related domains. Acad. Med. 79, S70–S81.

Eva, K.W., 2005. What every teacher needs to know about clinical reasoning. Med. Educ. 39, 98–106.

Field, M.J. (Ed.), 1995. Dental Education at the Crossroads: Challenges and Change. National Academies Press, Washington, DC.

Fiorini, S.R., Gärdenfors, P., Abel, M., 2014. Representing part-whole relations in conceptual spaces. Cogn. Process. 15, 127–142.

Formicola, A.J., Myers, R., Hasler, J.F., et al., 2006. Evolution of dental school clinics as patient care delivery centers. J. Dent. Educ. 70, 1271–1288.

Foucault, M., 1994. The Birth of the Clinic: an Archaeology of Medical Perception. Pantheon Books, New York, NY.

Fox, R.C., 1980. The Evolution of Medical Uncertainty. Milbank Mem. Fund Q. Health and Soc. 1–49.

Fuller, C., Camilon, R., Nguyen, S., et al., 2015. Adjunctive diagnostic techniques for oral lesions of unknown malignant potential: systematic review with meta-analysis. Head Neck 37, 755–762.

Geisler, S.L., 2006. The value of narrative ethics to medicine. J. Phys. Assist. Educ. 17, 54–57.

Goodman, K.W., 2007. Ethical and legal issues in decision support. In: Berner, E.S. (Ed.), Clinical Decision Support Systems. Springer, New York, NY, pp. 126–139.

Han, P.K., Klein, W.M., Arora, N.K., 2011. Varieties of uncertainty in health care a conceptual taxonomy. Med. Decis. Making 31, 828–838.

Helman, C.G., 2007. Culture, Health and Illness. CRC Press, Boca Raton, FL.

Hendricson, W.D., Cohen, P.A., 2001. Oral health care in the 21st century: implications for dental and medical education. Acad. Med. 76, 1181–1206.

Karimbux, N.Y., 2013. Knowing where we're going in assessment. J. Dent. Educ. 77, 1555.

Katz, J., 1984. Why doctors don't disclose uncertainty. Hastings Center Rep. 14, 35–44.

Kawahata, N., MacEntee, M.I., 2002. A measure of agreement between clinicians and a computer-based decision support system for planning dental treatment. J. Dent. Educ. 66, 1031–1037.

Kay, E.J., Nuttall, N.M., Kniil-Jones, R., 1992. Restorative treatment thresholds and agreement in treatment decision-making. Community Dent. Oral Epidemiol. 20, 265–268.

Khatami, S., 2010. Clinical Reasoning in Dentistry. University of British Columbia, Vancouver, BC.

Khatami, S., MacEntee, M.I., 2011. Evolution of clinical reasoning in dental education. J. Dent. Educ. 75, 321–328.

Khatami, S., MacEntee, M.I., Pratt, D.D., et al., 2012. Clinical reasoning in dentistry: a conceptual framework for dental education. J. Dent. Educ. 76, 1116–1128.

Kinsella, E.A., Pitman, A. (Eds.), 2012. Phronesis As Professional Knowledge: Practical Wisdom in the Professions 1. Springer Science & Business Media, Germany.

Knafl, K., Burkett, G., 1975. Professional socialization in a surgical specialty: acquiring medical judgment. Soc. Sci. Med. 9, 397–404.

Laufer, E.A., Glick, J., 1996. Expert and novice differences in cognition and activity: a practical work activity. In: Engeström, Y., Middleton, D. (Eds.), Cognition and Communication at Work. Cambridge University Press, Cambridge, MA, pp. 177–198.

Light, D., Jr., 1979. Uncertainty and control in professional training. J. Health Soc. Behav. 310–322.

Lingard, L., Garwood, K., Schryer, C.F., et al., 2003. A certain art of uncertainty: case presentation and the development of professional identity. Soc. Sci. Med. 56, 603–616.

Loftus, S., 2015. Embodiment in the practice and education of health professionals. In: Green, B., Hopwood, N. (Eds.), Body/Practice: The Body in Professional Practice, Learning and Education. Springer, London, UK, pp. 139–156.

MacEntee, M., 2005. Prosthodontics: have we misjudged the cause and lost direction? The Int. J. Prosthodont. 18, 185–187.

MacEntee, M.I., 2007. Where science fails prosthodontics. Int. J. Prosthodont. 20, 377.

MacEntee, M.I., 2010. The educational challenge of dental geriatrics. J. Dent. Educ. 74, 13–19.

MacEntee, M.I., Mathu-Muju, K.R., 2014. Confronting dental uncertainty in old age. Gerodontology 31, 37–43.

Marinello, C., 2016. The digital revolution in prosthodontics: can it benefit older people? Gerodontology 33, 145–146.

Matthews, D.C., Gafni, A., Birch, S., 1999. Preference based measurements in dentistry: a review of the literature and recommendations for research. Community Dent. Health 16, 5–11.

Maupomé, G., Schrader, S., Mannan, S., et al., 2010. Diagnostic thinking and information used in clinical decision-making: a qualitative study of expert and student dental clinicians. BMC Oral Health 10, 1.

McKendry, S., 2015. Critical Thinking Skills for Healthcare. Routledge, London, UK.

Monteiro, S.M., Norman, G., 2013. Diagnostic reasoning: where we've been, where we're going. Teach. Learn. Med. 25 (Suppl. 1), S26–S32.

Newsome, P.R., Langley, P.P., 2014. Professionalism, then and now. Br. Dent. J. 216, 497–502.

Oakley, J., 2016. Virtue ethics and public policy: upholding medical virtue in therapeutic relationships as a case study. J. Val. Inq. 50, 769–779.

Parsons, T., 1951. The Social System. The Free Press, New York, NY.

Patel, V.L., Kaufman, D.R., Arocha, J.F., 2002. Emerging paradigms of cognition in medical decision-making. J. Biomed. Informat. 35, 52–75.

Pena, G.P., Andrade-Filho, J.S., 2009. How does a pathologist make a diagnosis? Arch. Pathol. Lab. Med. 133, 124–132.

Plasschaert, A.J.M., Holbrook, W.P., Delap, E., et al., 2005. Profile and competences for the European dentist. European J. Dent. Educ. 9, 98–107.

Schell, B.A.B., 2008. Pragmatic reasoning. In: Schell, B.A.B., Schell, J.W. (Eds.), Clinical and Professional Reasoning in Occupational Therapy. Lippincott Williams & Wilkins, Philadelphia, PA, pp. 169–187.

Schön, D.A., 1983. The Reflective Practitioner: How Professionals Think in Action. Basic Books, New York, NY.

Sims-Williams, J.H., Brown, I.D., Matthewman, A., et al., 1987. A computer-controlled expert system for orthodontic advice. Br. Dent. J. 163, 161–166.

Svenaeus, F., 2000. The Hermeneutics of Medicine and the Phenomenology of Health: Steps Towards a Philosophy of Medical Practice. Kluwer, Dordrecht, The Netherlands.

Vernazza, C.R., Rousseau, N., Steele, J.G., et al., 2015. Introducing high-cost health care to patients: dentists' accounts of offering dental implant treatment. Community Dent. Oral Epidemiol. 43, 75–85.

Wang, K.J., Chen, K.H., Huang, S.H., et al., 2016. A prognosis tool based on fuzzy anthropometric and questionnaire data for obstructive sleep apnea severity. J. Med. Systems 40, 1–12.

Whitney, E.M., Aleksejuniene, J., Walton, J.N., 2016. Critical thinking disposition and skills in dental students: development and relationship to academic outcomes. J. Dent. Educ. 80, 948–958.

Zadeh, L.A., 2008. Is there a need for fuzzy logic? Inf. Sci. 178, 2751–2779.

CLINICAL REASONING IN OCCUPATIONAL THERAPY

CHRISTINE CHAPPARO ■ JUDY RANKA

CHAPTER AIMS

The aims of this chapter are to examine clinical reasoning in occupational therapy from four perspectives, including:

■ a brief *history of clinical reasoning* in occupational therapy,

■ the *content of therapist thinking* that has been found to influence occupational therapy action,

■ the conceptual notions about the *thinking processes* that underpin clinical decision making in occupational therapy and

■ how occupational therapists may use *cognitive strategies* during the process of reasoning.

KEY WORDS

Diagnostic, procedural, conditional, pragmatic and ethical reasoning

Personal beliefs

Cognitive strategy use

ABBREVIATIONS/ ACRONYMS

OT Occupational therapy

OTs Occupational therapists

PRPP Perceive, Recall, Plan and Perform system of task analysis

INTRODUCTION

Answers to six questions lie at the heart of occupational therapy (OT) assessment and intervention, which is a complex, dynamic process based on observation of the interaction between people and their environments as they perform relevant and valued everyday activity.

1. What is the situation?
2. What is wanted/needed/possible in this situation?
3. What will I do?
4. How will I do it?
5. Why am I doing it?
6. Did it work?

People access OT when they, family and community members or other professionals perceive that they are not adequately performing their daily occupations or activities. Disruptions to occupational performance are inherently complex, severe and enduring, affecting all ages and sociocultural backgrounds. OT can be applied in many situations such as medical, community and educational. Both social services and private practices may use OT. The professional practice of all therapists is affected by a configuration of demographic, social, cultural, political, technological or epidemiological sources, contributing to the complexity of therapy. Under conditions of such complexity, uncertainty and change, occupational therapists aim to develop and implement therapy programs that support clients and their families to participate in desired life skills and ensure their quality of life. 'Thinking like a therapist' is critical to selecting the 'right' therapeutic intervention for a particular setting and implementing it in the interest of each client. For over three decades, therapist thinking in OT has been termed *clinical reasoning* (Mattingly and Fleming, 1994). It is a nonlinear, recursive style of thinking that involves gathering and analyzing client information and deciding on therapeutic actions specific to a client's circumstances and wishes. It combines cognitive and metacognitive strategies such as analysis, problem solving and evaluation together with precognitive intuition. Finally information is synthesized with visualization of the client's future needs in his or her unique physical, social and cultural context (Durning et al., 2011).

Although the importance of reasoning in OT has been clearly established (Mattingly and Fleming, 1994), it remains a hypothetical construct, the understanding of which has continued to evolve (Unsworth, 2011). Several questions remain unanswered about the thinking processes used in clinical reasoning. What personal and contextual elements are involved in the reasoning process? How do therapists combine science, practical knowledge and their personal commitments to make decisions about their actions? Why do therapists make decisions the way they do?

CLINICAL REASONING IN OCCUPATIONAL THERAPY: HISTORICAL PERSPECTIVE

Throughout the development of OT, clinical reasoning has been referred to as treatment planning (Day, 1973), the evaluative process (Hemphill, 1982), clinical thinking (Line, 1969), a subset of the OT process (Christiansen et al., 2005) and problem solving (Hopkins and Tiffany, 1988). The clinical reasoning process has been described as a largely tacit, highly imagistic and deeply phenomenological mode of thinking, 'thinking about thinking' (Schell and Schell, 2008). More recently, there has been a move away from use of the term 'clinical reasoning' in preference to 'professional reasoning' (Turpin and Iwama, 2011, p. 33) and 'occupational reasoning' (Rogers, 2010, p. 57). This is because many therapists are employed outside clinical settings and provide interventions for 'clients' and 'people' rather than 'patients'. Current understandings of clinical reasoning have been influenced by the diverse nature and goals of OT practice, the philosophical development

of the profession itself and the various epistemologies of individual researchers.

OT was founded on humanistic values (Meyer, 1922). The view of occupation that was accepted by the profession early in its development centred on the relationship between health and the ability to organize the temporal, physical and social elements of daily living (Keilhofner and Burke, 1983). Therapy depended on an analysis to understand the unique significance and meaning of activity in a person's everyday life. Today's practice continues this, using the notion of *health and ability for all* and with a social awareness that locates disability, illness and the need for therapy in exclusionary social, economic and cultural barriers to human occupational performance (Townsend and Polatajko, 2007). OT thinking is increasingly seen in nontraditional public health roles such as aid agencies (Kronenberg et al., 2011). Public policy has become an everyday working arena for occupational therapists, requiring the use of reasoning skills to determine how occupational performance fits with social need (Braveman and Suarez-Balcazar, 2009).

The development of medical and rehabilitation paradigms in the middle of the 20th century influenced how OT clinical reasoning was conceptualized. Therapists sought kinesiological, neurophysiological and psychodynamic explanations of human function and dysfunction (Molineux, 2011). Clinical decision making focussed on improving isolated units of function, such as particular physical or psychological attributes. Systems approaches were used to explain and teach clinical reasoning (Box 25.1).

The last two decades have seen a resurgent demand for scientific reasoning prompted by evidence-based practice that assumes a systematic approach to

---

BOX 25.1
SYSTEMS APPROACH TO CLINICAL REASONING

Day (1973) created a unidirectional model of decision making comprising problem identification, cause identification, treatment principle or assumption selection, activity selection and goal identification. Central to this model was a procedural reasoning style that continues to be recognized as one element of therapist thinking.

therapist thinking (Taylor, 2000). Derived from medicine, evidence-based decisions were, originally, to be made by integrating knowledge of individual client characteristics and preferences, together with the therapist's clinical experience and evidence from clinical research in the formulation of clinical decisions (Sackett et al., 1996). An evidence-based approach to clinical reasoning emphasizes knowledge generated by randomized controlled trials and statistical measurement (National Health and Medical Research Council, 2009). It can be argued that assumptions that underpin this view of evidence include:

- health is a simple construct that can be measured the same way for all people and
- ill health and disability can be reduced to small units of measurement that accurately reflect a larger problem.

The influence upon OT thinking is clear. Contemporary writers frequently prefer clinical reasoning based on evidence established by certain kinds of research only. The client's input and the therapist's expertise tend to be downplayed. In these instances, clinical reasoning has been described as not aligned with the social rights to health (Di Constanzo, 2012) and therefore distant from the original focus of OT.

In summary, OT practice in the 21st century continues to be characterized by theoretical conflict, as the profession reexamines its direction and focus (Molineux, 2011; Turner and Knight, 2015). A number of theories, models and frames of reference have emerged to explain the concept of occupation, the purpose of OT and to guide practice, each with an associated reasoning pathway. The original belief in clients' rights to choice and autonomy is reflected in the phenomenological and hermeneutic approaches that have largely been used to study OT clinical reasoning, and the influence of medicine on clinical reasoning is illustrated by the analytic EBM (Evidence-based medicine) approach.

REFLECTION POINT 1

OT clinical reasoning processes will continue to form a basis for OT identity. Their importance was summed up by Pedretti (1982, p. 12), who stated, 'perhaps our real identity and uniqueness lies not as much in what we do, but in how we think'.

KNOWLEDGE AND CLINICAL REASONING IN OCCUPATIONAL THERAPY

There are both internal and external influences on OT clinical reasoning. These include the therapy context, the client situation, theory, the identity of the therapist, attitudes about therapy and expectancies of OT outcomes. These influences affect decision making and address the question '*what* do therapists think *about*' when they reason.

The Therapy Context

The context of therapy contains powerful factors that establish knowledge about the conditions (e.g., organizational, cultural and societal values) and constraints (e.g., human and financial resources, policies) that affect therapy (Kristensen et al., 2012). Therapy experiences are remembered by therapists as total contextual patterns of what is possible and include people, actions, contexts and objects, rather than as decontextualized elements or general rules (Schell and Schell, 2008). Contextual patterns contribute to therapists' perceptions of the amount of control they have over their ability to carry out planned actions. These perceptions have a direct effect on their feelings of efficacy, self-confidence and autonomy (Sharafaroodi et al., 2014). Therapists reason according to both personal values and professional perspectives. If the therapy context does not permit these values and perspectives, then therapists face a dilemma. There is a conflict between what *therapists perceive should be done,* what the *client wants done* and what the *system will allow*. These constraints can impose major restrictions on clinical reasoning.

Clients and Their Life Contexts

Sensitivity to clients and their life situation is fundamental to the clinical reasoning process. A core ethical tenet of OT is that interventions should be in concert with clients' needs, goals, lifestyles and personal and cultural values (Chapparo et al., 2017a). To this end, Mattingly and Fleming (1994) originally described one of the primary goals of clinical reasoning as determining the meaning of occupational need from the client's perspective. Understanding of the client's perspective becomes a source of knowledge that is used during assessment and intervention and is constantly updated to build a conceptual model of the client situation (Mattingly and Fleming, 1994; Schell and Schell, 2008) (Box 25.2).

Theory and Science

Therapists' knowledge about disease, human function and human occupation, gleaned largely from scientific theory and evidence gives direction for thinking, information about alternatives and predictions of function. Termed 'professional knowledge', it is conceptualized as applied theory when used in a process of 'naming' and 'framing' the problem (Kielhofner, 2009). This process requires classifying findings in terms of abstract constructs (such as function, depression, sensory processing, motor control, occupational role, cognitive ability or social justice). The identified construct becomes a cognitive mechanism that facilitates the selection of strategies for assessment and treatment (Schell and Schell, 2008). However, OT has a theory base that is incomplete and is characterized by philosophical conflict. Additionally, therapists are required to make decisions in situations of uncertainty that stem from multiple sources or for which there is little evidence. Under these conditions, therapists may have to use their own personal beliefs and experience as a basis for decision making.

Personal Beliefs of the Therapist

The fourth type of knowledge that guides reasoning is personal knowledge incorporating the beliefs and values of the therapist. These are the fundamental beliefs and assumptions about *what we know 'to be true'* about ourselves, others and OT. Therapists use themselves as referents when creating a model of the client situation (Chapparo, 1999), ascribing meaning to the client's individual situation according to his or her own reality. Therapists probably develop an internal model of what they believe is the client's perspective and work from that belief model. Such beliefs and values are used to define the limits of acceptable behaviour in any given therapy situation (Chapparo, 1999).

Attitude-Behaviour Expectancy

Scheffer and Rubenfeld (2000) suggest that attitude, philosophical perspective and beliefs set up a thinking 'disposition' that influences the clinical reasoning process. Attitude-behaviour theory has been used to demonstrate the effect of attitude on OT reasoning (Chapparo, 1999). This model proposes therapy is mediated through intention (what therapists choose to do) and expectancies (the perceived expectations of self and others). Attitude (seen here as what therapists imagine as positive or negative outcomes of therapy possibilities) develops from sets of beliefs derived from the personal, theoretical and contextual knowledge outlined earlier in the chapter. This conceptual model of reasoning is an explanation of the effects of attitude on clinical reasoning. Attitudes of therapists about their therapy can be triggered by specific and changing events in therapy and contribute to the development of an internal frame of reference about the processes they choose to use during therapy.

Personal Internal Frame of Reference

The existence of a personal paradigm (Creek and Lawson-Porter, 2007) is believed to underlie all decisions made in professional practice. Clearly, clinical reasoning in OT balances a number of personal, client-related, theoretical and organizational sets of knowledge. How therapists determine which type of knowledge receives precedence in reasoning for each individual therapy situation is not yet clear. One emerging hypothesis is that all sources of knowledge used for clinical reasoning are housed within a complex internal framework structure that has precognitive and cognitive elements that represent the therapist's personally constructed view of any therapy event (Chapparo, 1999) and affect clinical reasoning (Fig. 25.1).

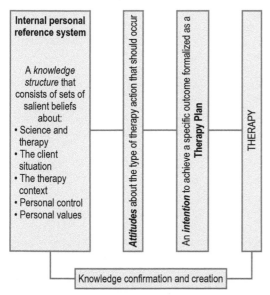

Fig. 25.1 ■ **The therapist internal personal reference system.** A personal knowledge structure that is shaped by beliefs, attitudes and expectations. Therapy (action) is preceded by an *intention* to act in a particular way (therapy plan). Intentions are shaped by *attitudes* towards the salient therapy situation. Attitudes are shaped by a *constellation of beliefs* about aspects of the therapy situation.

Lines of Reasoning

In the third section of this chapter, we explore the ways in which therapists use different lines of thinking to form pictures of client problems, client potential, therapy action and outcome. We address the question "how do therapists use their knowledge during clinical reasoning?" The majority of this information has been derived from what has been considered the keystone study into clinical reasoning in OT (Mattingly and Fleming, 1994). Although a relatively small, culturally and geographically localized study with inherent biases, it exerts disproportional influence on how clinical reasoning in OT is described and taught today.

Scientific Reasoning: "What Is the Presenting Problem?"

Two forms of scientific reasoning identified by early OT researchers are diagnostic reasoning and procedural reasoning (Mattingly and Fleming, 1994). These processes involve a progression from problem sensing to problem definition and problem resolution. This line

of reasoning is the "how to" of the therapeutic process. The focus is on the problem, and therapists draw on their knowledge of occupations, therapy procedures, diseases and conditions to address it. Problem identification, goal setting and intervention planning are part of these diagnostic and procedural reasoning modes. Therapists generate two to four hypotheses about the cause and nature of functional problems and several more concerning possible directions for treatment (Mattingly and Fleming, 1994) (see Case Study 25.1). Hypotheses are then subjected to a process of critical reflection and consideration of evidence. Newer therapists tend to generate fewer hypotheses (Unsworth, 2011). The danger for experienced therapists is placing exclusive dependence on past experiences that have not been subjected to critical analysis through evidentiary inquiry.

Narrative and Interactive Reasoning: "What Does It Mean to the Person?"

Implementing a therapy program that will potentially change life roles and functions for the client requires understanding the *meaning* of a client situation. Two dimensions of meaning making are involved and have been referred to as narrative and interactive reasoning. *Meaning perspectives* are the assumptions and beliefs within which new experiences are interpreted. For example, OTs make interpretations about client situations based on perceived client satisfaction with occupational roles and tasks, interpretation of client past life experiences and future desires.

Therapists construct perspectives of the client experience into a *personal narrative* or a *story* of the situation in a way that parallels the hermeneutic process (Chapparo, 2016). The therapist's views of the situation become gradually 'fused' with the client's until the client's experience, rather than the problem per se, becomes paramount (Mattingly and Fleming, 1994). This interpretive process prompts decisions about therapy action (or nonaction) (see Case Study 25.1).

Ethical Reasoning: "What Should Happen?"

As outlined previously, personal values substantially affect clinical reasoning processes in OT. A therapist–client interaction becomes an ethical *dilemma* when it seems that an OT treatment decision will violate the therapist's values. In the process of choosing a

CASE STUDY 25.1

Brief Example of How Some Narrative and Scientific Lines of Reasoning Contribute to Generating Hypotheses About the Nature and Cause of the Occupational Problem

Danny is 4 years of age and was referred to OT early-intervention services. Julia is his therapist and is experienced in early-intervention service delivery. Julia observes that Danny notices toys and picks them up now and then. During mealtime he uses his left hand to pick up his food to eat but seems more interested in the touch and feel of it, often throwing it on the floor. Although he is aware of his family, his social responses are inconsistent. He often appears 'distant' and 'anxious' when family members leave the room.

SCIENTIFIC REASONING

Julia further constructs a picture of the problem from evidence about Danny's diagnosis and her knowledge of typical and atypical childhood social and occupational performance.

Medical: Danny has reduced motor control on his right body side in comparison with the left and was given a diagnosis of cerebral palsy (unilateral) and developmental delay. Social/Occupational: Delayed ability to interact with other children, reduced potential to play with toys and others and reduced independence in eating and drinking often result from these conditions.

NARRATIVE REASONING

Julia further constructs a picture of Danny's occupational life by talking to his family to obtain their perspective of the problem and what they expect from therapy services.

As a result of an abusive early childhood for the first 3 years of life, Danny was placed with foster parents who have two other children younger than 5 years of age. He has received no previous intervention. He attends a day-care facility 3 days a week for 7 to 8 hours each day with his foster siblings. There are positive reports about the day-care providers. Danny has made progress since being fostered. The family would like Danny to:

- use a cup and feed himself without throwing food,
- develop more play skills and engage in social interaction,
- use his right hand and arm and
- have a regular sleep/wake schedule.

Hypotheses About Danny's Situation Generated From Scientific and Narrative Reasoning

Julia uses this information to generate the following hypotheses:

The underlying causes of the child and family's identified needs, concerns or problems are as follows:

- Danny's problems are linked to his early developmental experiences.
- Danny has not had the physical, social and sensory opportunities that prompt early skill development and will need to spend time experiencing these.
- He has experienced less social attachment and interactions than needed to develop play and social-emotional skills, and foster parents may need some support in the best ways to develop these.
- Danny may not have had parent-supported routines and schedules to develop sleep patterns, social interactions and eating routines in early infancy and needs to learn these.
- Danny may have needed early intervention services to address the effect of reduced developmental opportunities and did not receive these.

---

therapeutic action, occupational therapists are often forced to balance one value against another. Although this process is typically unconscious, it can drive decision making at any point in the therapist–client interaction (Jordens and Little, 2004) (Box 25.3).

Conditional Reasoning: "What Will Be the Outcome?"

Mattingly and Fleming (1994) described a line of reasoning termed 'conditional reasoning', which involves projecting an imagined future for the client. They used the term 'conditional' in three different ways. First, problems are interpreted and solutions are realized in relation to people within their particular context. Second, therapists imagine how the present situation could be changed. Third, success is determined by the level of client participation and satisfaction. It is a line of thinking used to reconcile the actual (therapy) and the possible (intention) in terms of therapy outcome. This involves *reflection,* when the therapist's action turns in on itself, *conflict,* when therapists seek to reconcile choices made, and *judgement,* when therapists weigh soundness of decisions.

Pragmatic Reasoning: "What Can Be Done?"

Pragmatic reasoning addresses what is achievable in the contexts in which therapy occurs (Schell and Schell, 2008). As outlined earlier in the chapter, this includes organizational constraints, values and resources, practice trends, reimbursement issues and therapist skills. Evans (2010), for example, highlights the place of social influence and conformity to the expectations of colleagues. Curtin and Jaramazovi (2001) demonstrated how, despite a positive disposition towards evidence-based practice, therapists cite lack of skills and resources as barriers to inclusion of evidence in their reasoning.

Famously, Mattingly and Fleming (1994) created an image of an occupational therapist with a 'three-track mind' (p. 119). Tracks are lines of thinking that are related to thought content rather than describing how thinking happens. All lines of reasoning may be used in one therapy session. The procedural track is used when therapists reason about the client's diagnosis. The interactive-narrative track occurs when therapists focus on the client as a person. The conditional track creates an image of the client that is provisional, holistic and conditional on the client's participation. The line of thinking used at any time during therapy is related to the salient goal of therapy (e.g., determining occupational diagnosis, exploring alternatives with clients, setting short-term goals, evaluating intervention, discharge planning).

REFLECTION POINT 2

It is unclear whether therapists use exclusive forms of thinking or whether the different styles of reasoning that have been identified in each piece of research were constructed through the research process of attempting to describe in words a largely internal, tacit phenomenon (Robertson, 2012). Therapists may seem more rational in their decision making when interviewed after the fact because of the coherence that comes with reflection and the rules of narration. Descriptions of the different clinical reasoning processes that exist may reflect the epistemology of various researchers at the time (Robertson, 2012), such as anthropology (Mattingly and Fleming, 1994), medicine, cognitive psychology (Chapparo and Ranka, 2016) and social psychology (Chapparo, 1999; Unsworth, 2011).

INFORMATION PROCESSING, COGNITIVE STRATEGY USE AND CLINICAL REASONING

It has been argued that conceptualizations of clinical reasoning within the profession have not kept pace with cognitive research about thinking and reasoning (Robertson, 2012). Here we address the question "how do therapists think?"

Kahneman (2011) proposes two distinct cognitive systems underpinning reasoning. System 1 operates automatically and quickly, with little or no effort or control, and is sensory dependent. For example, as we talk to a client, we automatically alert to their facial expression of pain, or reposition equipment, without conscious thought. System 2 comprises complex effortful deliberate thinking. How this type of cognition is applied in OT reasoning is just beginning to be explored (Pelaccia et al., 2011). Next, we briefly describe a recent model of cognitive strategy use that incorporates this dual-process paradigm.

Clinical reasoning in OT requires therapists to extend their thinking beyond what they know and beyond the context in which they do therapy (Carr and Shotwell, 2007). In many instances, OT requires therapists to 'know the unknown'. At the same time, therapists must access and use some knowledge so automatically that they can 'do without thinking', for example, be able to think ahead to the next sequence of a therapy session while automatically positioning a client or themselves safely for a wheelchair transfer. Of particular relevance is how therapists might use a range of cognitive strategies during everyday reasoning to achieve the best outcome for clients.

Cognition has been defined many ways. In this chapter, it is defined as an interaction of processes that involve *all forms of awareness and knowing* such as sensing, remembering, questioning, judging, problem solving and decision making (VandenBos, 2015) and subsumes metacognition (thinking about one's own thinking). *Cognitive strategies* are mental thinking tactics, or how we use our cognition. They are used when we are faced with the need to identify important, unfamiliar or difficult information; understand and retain information; retrieve information from memory stores; manipulate and apply information; plan and modify responses using information; and simultaneously cope with internal and external distractions during task performance (Ramsden, 2013).

Cognitive strategy use is dependent on information processing. This processing system is controlled by an executive system that monitors thinking processes and engages in corrective strategies when processing is not going smoothly (Huitt, 2003). Central to applying notions of cognitive strategy use to clinical reasoning is the assumption that successful reasoning requires both automatic (System 1) and deliberate use of information (System 2) processed through application of a set of cognitive strategies that suit each situation. During clinical reasoning, therapists gather information from people, things and events in their environment (using sensory gathering strategies). They organize this information in their minds and code it in ways that keep it usable and easily understood (memory storing strategies). They match the sensory information with what they have learned and experienced, noticing similarities and differences and store the information for future use (recall strategies). As these representations

of therapy become deeper and more powerful with repetition over time, therapists' understanding of client problems, worldviews and therapy outcomes becomes more precise, and they are able to apply their knowledge using a range of cognitive strategies across a wide range of clients and therapeutic tasks (generalizing, planning, decision making and self-evaluating strategies). They become *strategic thinkers,* using internally generated cognitive strategies.

Cognitive strategies can be classified as *general* (generic thinking strategies that are applied to any task) or more *specific* (strategies that relate to a particular task, such as a specific way to use particular equipment) (Chapparo, 2017). Each therapy session demands *particular client information* to be chosen, constructed, processed, stored, recalled, organized and used for a *particular therapy purpose.* Cognitive strategy use implies salience or use of a general set of cognitive strategies in a particular moment. Chapparo et al. (2017b) hypothesize that people do not use 'different' lines of thinking for clinical reasoning but rather learn to *apply* a generic set of thinking strategies that they already use in daily life to a specific situation. Although therapists develop particular and specialized *knowledge structures* about occupation, disability and therapy, they learn to *apply* or *manipulate* this knowledge to problems of occupation in their role as a therapist using an already existing generic set of thinking strategies. Perhaps this is what is meant by learning to 'think like a therapist'.

Chapparo et al. (2017b) constructed a conceptual model of how people use cognitive strategies during task performance. Termed the Perceive, Recall, Plan and Perform (PRPP) system (Fig. 25.2), it is centred on four processing 'quadrants' connected by multidirectional arrows that mirror the four-staged flow of information in theoretical models of information processing. These quadrants include attention and sensory perception (Perceive), memory (Recall), response planning and evaluation (Plan) and performance monitoring (Perform). Built on earlier notions from instructional psychology (Romiszowski, 1984) and applied cognitive task analysis (Schraagen et al., 2000), it has been used to explain people's ability to use cognitive strategies to effectively think through routine and complex work tasks (Bootes and Chapparo, 2010; Lewis et al., 2016). Here, we apply this model to therapist thinking.

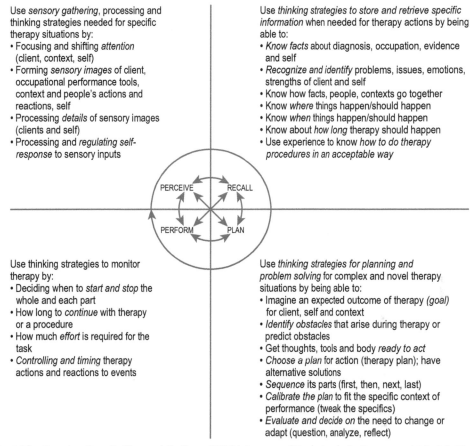

Use *sensory gathering*, processing and thinking strategies needed for specific therapy situations by:
• Focusing and shifting *attention* (client, context, self)
• Forming *sensory images* of client, occupational performance tools, context and people's actions and reactions, self
• Processing *details* of sensory images (clients and self)
• Processing and *regulating self-response* to sensory inputs

Use *thinking strategies to store and retrieve specific information* when needed for therapy actions by being able to:
• *Know facts* about diagnosis, occupation, evidence and self
• *Recognize and identify* problems, issues, emotions, strengths of client and self
• Know how facts, people, contexts go together
• Know *where* things happen/should happen
• Know *when* things happen/should happen
• Know about *how long* therapy should happen
• Use experience to know *how to do therapy procedures in an acceptable way*

PERCEIVE   RECALL

PERFORM   PLAN

Use thinking strategies to monitor therapy by:
• Deciding when to *start and stop* the whole and each part
• How long to *continue* with therapy or a procedure
• How much *effort* is required for the task
• *Controlling and timing* therapy actions and reactions to events

Use *thinking strategies for planning and problem solving* for complex and novel therapy situations by being able to:
• Imagine an expected outcome of therapy *(goal)* for client, self and context
• *Identify obstacles* that arise during therapy or predict obstacles
• Get thoughts, tools and body *ready to act*
• *Choose a plan* for action (therapy plan); have alternative solutions
• *Sequence* its parts (first, then, next, last)
• *Calibrate the plan* to fit the specific context of performance (tweak the specifics)
• *Evaluate and decide on* the need to change or adapt (question, analyze, reflect)

Fig. 25.2 ■ The Perceive, Recall, Plan and Perform (PRPP) System of Task Analysis Conceptual Model: Hypothesized Cognitive Strategies Used in Clinical Reasoning During Every Therapy Situation.

Perceive Strategies: Attention and Sensory Perception Strategies (Strategies for Attending to and Sensing Information)

Once sensory input from a client or therapy context captures our attention, and we focus on it, details of the information are registered. Initial interpretation of sensory data is thought to precede conscious thinking, suggesting that client and contextual information is always interpreted preconsciously in the first instance (Hogarth, 2005), mirroring the System 1 concept outlined earlier in the chapter. The more attention we pay to a given bit of sensory information (e.g., a painful wrist joint or listening to a client narrative), the more

elaborately the information will be learned and retained. The top-left quadrant (Perceive) in Fig. 25.2 outlines some specific cognitive strategies from the PRPP system associated with this first stage of information processing. These strategies are observable behaviours that signal whether therapists are attending to and dealing with sensory input that is needed for therapy (Chapparo and Ranka, 2016).

Recall Strategies (Strategies to 'Know' and Use What Is Known)

Sensory images of people, things and contexts are transferred to a working memory, which is what we are thinking about at any given time. Memories of our personal, client and therapy experiences are then configured into long-term memory structures called 'schemas.' Schemas serve as filters for ongoing experience, allowing us to come to conclusions about what we see, hear or do automatically (Hattie and Yates, 2014) without having to 'think too hard' and is often referred to as 'automaticity' (Chapparo, 2017). This line of thinking is depicted by arrows from Perceive to Recall to Perform in the central part of Fig. 25.2. During clinical reasoning, this enables us to interpret the present based on experience from the past and answer the question *"Do I know…?"* (Chapparo and Ranka, 2016).

Three broad categories of information are stored and retrieved for use during clinical reasoning. These are explained in the following sections.

Factual Knowledge (Facts) – 'Do I Know WHAT…?'

The storing and recalling of facts enable therapists to recognize sensory data from clients and situations and the meaning that is attached to them. It makes a major contribution to *practical knowledge* and is the basis for diagnostic and procedural reasoning. Sensory images are assigned technical labels that assist with efficient storage and retrieval. Labels such as pain, depression and stroke become fused with our own personal understanding of these terms and are used to assign meaning to client and therapy events. This builds the 'internal frame of reference' outlined previously and becomes the sum total of *what we know about ourselves and others* and is probably used during what has been termed 'narrative' or 'interactive' reasoning.

Schematic Knowledge (Schemes) – 'Do I Know WHERE…?'; 'Do I Know WHEN…?'; 'Do I Know HOW LONG…?'

Schematic memory represents what we have learned about where, when and how long something happens. This type of memory is based on particular experiences that are located in *personal* time and space and may contribute to pragmatic reasoning. Schematic information provides us with a personally constructed 'map' or model for when and where to act as a therapist.

Procedural Knowledge – 'Do I Know HOW…?'

Procedural memory enables us to perform therapeutic techniques 'automatically' based on past experience.

Procedural memory has been shown to be the most resistant to forgetting and foremost in the natural inclination for therapists to 'do what they know' in the first instance. Experienced therapists often seem to 'do therapy' without thinking because they have highly developed procedural knowledge. Therapists moving from one specialized practice to another will have to develop new procedural knowledge.

The top-right quadrant (Recall) in Fig. 25.2 outlines some specific cognitive strategies from the PRPP system associated with this second stage of information processing.

Plan Strategies (Strategies to Map Out, Program and Evaluate Future Action)

Organization, problem solving, decision making and insight are all part of the third stage of information processing and can be thought of as the 'rules of operation' that we apply to problem solving and analyzing information in any situation that is novel or complex. Planning strategies are not linked to any particular type of sensory information or ability but are executive functions that are applied to all information that has to be organized for use in a particular way or when *what we know is not enough*. When reasoning through complex therapy events, we process information with reference to a particular goal, an idea or an understanding of an outcome *(what will happen?)*. With an outcome in mind, effective thinkers use cognitive strategies that enable them to put a therapy plan into action. Although knowledge is used as a platform for this aspect of reasoning (arrow from Recall to Plan, see Fig. 25.2), planning strategies are different from the recall strategies described earlier and involve 'figuring out' extensions to habitual responses that may be demanded by the client situation. This can involve rapid searches for additional information to solve a problem (arrow from Plan to Perceive, see Fig. 25.2).

Effective clinical reasoning happens when therapists reflect on their own plans and performance and make considered decisions (Kieran and Christoff, 2014). Some of the cognitive strategies involved in the planning aspect of information processing during clinical reasoning are listed in the lower-right quadrant in Fig. 25.2 (Plan).

REFLECTION POINT 3

Problem solving is paramount when planning around complexity or novelty and is stimulated by the following self-generated questions:

- What obstacles might/did get in the way?
- How can I get myself and the client ready for therapy?
- What is the best choice of therapy approach, place and tool to use for this specific therapy task?
- How do I have to sequence therapy?
- What do I have to do to make my responses fit the client expectation/therapy context/my abilities?
- What personal reactions to client and therapy events do I have to consciously inhibit?

Perform Strategies (Strategies Used to Time, Control and Monitor Therapy)

After planning, the last stage of information processing focusses on using thinking strategies to 'do' therapy (arrow from Plan to Perform, see Fig. 25.2). New information requires therapists to dynamically respond 'in the moment'. Therapists' own actions are fed back into the system as sensory input and result in not only remembering what has been done and how (arrows from Perform to Perceive, Perform to Recall, see Fig. 25.2) but also the thinking that preceded it (arrow from Perform to Plan, see Fig. 25.2). For this attending, sensing, knowing, thinking, doing system to be effective, therapists must have a firm outcome (goal) in mind and be able to bring the goal back into focus for review as they *do therapy*.

CHAPTER SUMMARY

Clinical reasoning in OT is based on the complex interaction between people and their environments as they perform relevant and valued everyday activity. As contemporary therapy becomes increasingly aligned with community service delivery systems in public health, social welfare and education, there are suggestions for 'clinical' reasoning to be termed 'professional' reasoning. There is general agreement that:

- There are multiple lines of reasoning in OT, providing a multifaceted view of clients' problems, capacities, futures and therapy outcomes. Ethics

and pragmatics further frame our views of clinical reasoning.

- Each therapist constructs a personal internal frame of reference, in which information about clients and the client situation are thought to be 'fused' with the therapist's personal beliefs about such things as perceived level of skill, ethics and perceived level of control. Such images serve to make clinical reasoning an intensely personal process.
- From a cognitive perspective, clinical reasoning is thought to be served by a dual-process system that is part automatic use of professional and personal knowledge and part deliberate thinking. Reasoning is carried out through application of multiple cognitive strategies that are applied in the moment to suit the goal of therapy.

REFLECTION POINT 4

Current explanations of clinical reasoning in OT are continually evolving. It is a highly individualistic mode of social interaction that is informed by scientific knowledge and method, creative imagination, intuition and interpersonal skill and that uses an attending, sensing, knowing, thinking, doing cognitive system that operates strategically within the frame of the OT profession.

REFERENCES

Bootes, K., Chapparo, C., 2010. Difficulties with multitasking on return to work after TBI: a critical case study. Work 36, 207–216.

Braveman, B., Suarez-Balcazar, Y., 2009. Social justice and resource utilization in a community-based organization: a case illustration of the role of the occupational therapist. Am. J. Occup. Ther. 63, 13–23.

Carr, M., Shotwell, M., 2007. Information processing theory and professional reasoning. In: Schell, B.A., Schell, J.W. (Eds.), Clinical and Professional Reasoning in Occupational Therapy. The Netherlands, Wolters Kluwer, pp. 36–68.

Chapparo, C., 1999. Working out: working with Angelica—interpreting practice. In: Ryan, S.E., McKay, E.A. (Eds.), Thinking and Reasoning in Therapy: Narratives from Practice. Stanley Thomes, Cheltenham, UK, pp. 31–50.

Chapparo, C., 2016. Hermeneutik. In: Ritschl, V., Weigl, R., Stamm, T. (Eds.), Weissenschaftliches Arbeiten und Schribein: Verstehen, Anwenden, Nutzen für die Praxis. Springer, Berlin, Germany, pp. 98–112.

Chapparo, C., 2017. Perceive, Recall, Plan and Perform (PRPP): occupation-centred task analysis and intervention system. In: Rodger, S. (Ed.), Occupation Centred Practice with Children: A

Practical Guide for Occupational Therapists, second ed. Wiley-Blackwell, Hoboken, NJ, pp. 189–208.

Chapparo, C., Ranka, J., 2016. The Perceive, Recall, Plan and Perform system of task analysis assessment and research manual. Discipline of Occupational Therapy, Faculty of Health Sciences. University of Sydney, Sydney, NSW.

Chapparo, C., Ranka, J.L., Nott, M., 2017a. Occupational Performance Model (Australia): a description of constructs, structure and propositions. In: Curtin, M., Egan, M., Adams, J. (Eds.), Occupational Therapy for People Experiencing Illness, Injury or Impairment: Promoting Occupation and Participation, seventh ed. Elsevier, London, UK, pp. 134–147.

Chapparo, C., Ranka, J.L., Nott, M., 2017b. Perceive, Recall, Plan and Perform (PRPP) system of task analysis and intervention. In: Curtin, M., Egan, M., Adams, J. (Eds.), Occupational Therapy for People Experiencing Illness, Injury or Impairment: Promoting Occupation and Participation, seventh ed. Elsevier, London, UK, pp. 243–257.

Christiansen, C.H., Baum, C.M., Bass-Haugen, J. (Eds.), 2005. Occupational Therapy: Performance, Participation, and Well-Being, third ed. SLACK Incorporated, Thorofare, NJ.

Creek, J., Lawson-Porter, A., 2007. Contemporary Issues in Occupational Therapy: Reasoning and Reflection. John Wiley & Sons, West Sussex, UK.

Curtin, M., Jaramazovic, E., 2001. Occupational therapists' views and perceptions of evidence based practice. Br. J. Occup. Ther. 64, 212–222.

Day, D.J., 1973. A systems diagram for teaching treatment planning. Am. J. Occup. Ther. 27, 239–243.

Di Constanzo, C., 2012. Science and rights: the 'clinical reasoning' within health needs assessment. GSTF Int. J. Law Soc. Sci 1, 84–89.

Durning, S.J., Artino, A.R., Pangaro, L.N., et al., 2011. Context and clinical reasoning. Adv. Health Sci. Educ. 45, 927–938.

Evans, J., 2010. Thinking Twice: Two Minds in One Brain. Oxford University Press, Oxford, UK.

Hattie, J.A.C., Yates, G.C.R., 2014. Using feedback to promote learning. In: Benassi, V.A., Overson, C.E., Hakala, C.M. (Eds.), Applying Science of Learning in Education: Infusing Psychological Science into the Curriculum. American Psychological Association, Washington, DC, pp. 45–58.

Hemphill, B.J., 1982. The evaluative process. In: Hemphill, B.J. (Ed.), The Evaluative Process in Psychiatric Occupational Therapy. Charles Slack, Thorofare, NJ, pp. 17–26.

Hogarth, R.M., 2005. Deciding analytically or trusting your intuition? The advantages and disadvantages of analytic and intuitive thought. In: Betsch, T., Haberstroh, S. (Eds.), Routines of Decision Making. Erlbaum, Mahwah, NJ, pp. 67–82.

Hopkins, H.L., Tiffany, E.G., 1988. Occupational therapy: a problem-solving process. In: Hopkins, H.L., Smith, H.D. (Eds.), Willard and Spackman's Occupational Therapy, seventh ed. Lippincott, Philadelphia, PA, pp. 102–111.

Huitt, W., 2003. The information processing approach to cognition, Educational psychology interactive. Viewed 5 May 2017. Available from: http://chiron.valdosta.edu/whuitt/col/cogsys/infoproc.html.

Jordens, C.F.C., Little, M., 2004. In this scenario I do this, for these reasons: narrative, genre and ethical reasoning in the clinic. Soc. Sci. Med. 58, 1635–1645.

Kahneman, D., 2011. Thinking, Fast and Slow. Penguin, London, UK.

Kielhofner, G., 2009. Conceptual Foundations of Occupational Therapy Practice, fourth ed. FA Davis, Philadelphia, PA.

Keilhofner, G., Burke, J., 1983. The evolution of knowledge in occupational therapy: past, present and future. In: Keilhofner, G. (Ed.), Health Through Occupation. FA Davis, Philadelphia, PA, pp. 149–162.

Kieran, C.R.F., Christoff, K., 2014. Metacognitive facilitation of spontaneous thought processes: when metacognition helps the wandering mind find its way. In: Fleming, S.M., Frith, C.D. (Eds.), The Cognitive Neuroscience of Metacognition. Springer-Verlag, Berlin, pp. 293–319.

Kristensen, H., Borg, T., Hounsgaard, L., 2012. Aspects affecting occupational therapists' reasoning when implementing research-based evidence in stroke rehabilitation. Scand. J. Occup. Ther. 19, 118–131.

Kronenberg, F., Pollard, N., Sakellariou, D. (Eds.), 2011. Occupational Therapy Without Borders: Towards an Ecology of Occupation Based Practices, vol. 2. Churchill Livingstone Elsevier, Edinburgh, UK.

Lewis, J., Chapparo, C., Mackenzie, L., et al., 2016. Work after breast cancer: identification of cognitive difficulties using the Perceive, Recall, Plan, and Perform (PRPP) system of task analysis. Br. J. Occup. Ther. 79, 323–332.

Line, J., 1969. Case method as a scientific form of clinical thinking. Am. J. Occup. Ther. 23, 308–313.

Mattingly, C., Fleming, M.H., 1994. Clinical Reasoning: Forms of Inquiry in a Therapeutic Practice. FA Davis, Philadelphia, PA.

Meyer, A., 1922. The philosophy of occupational therapy. Arch. Occup. Ther. 1, 1–10.

Molineux, M., 2011. Standing firm on shifting sands. N. Z. J. Occup. Ther. 58, 21–28.

National Health and Medical Research Council, 2009. NHMRC levels of evidence and grades for recommendations for developers of guidelines, NHMRC, Canberra, ACT, viewed 5 May 2017. Available from: http://citeseerx.ist.psu.edu/viewdoc/download;jsessionid=A EFFDA62A5245D6D07F060B56789ED5A?doi=10.1.1.177.4984&r ep=rep1&type=pdf.

Pedretti, L.W., 1982. The compatibility of current treatment methods in physical disabilities with the philosophical case of occupational therapy, PhD thesis. San Jose University, San Jose, CA.

Pelaccia, T., Tardif, J., Triby, E., et al., 2011. An analysis of clinical reasoning through a recent and comprehensive approach: the dual-process theory. Medical Education Online 16, 1–9.

Ramsden, P., 2013. Applications of the concepts of strategy and style. In: Schmeck, R.A. (Ed.), Learning Strategies and Learning Style: Perspectives on Individual Differences. Springer Science, New York, NY, pp. 159–185.

Robertson, D.M., 2012. Critical thinking and clinical reasoning in new graduate occupational therapists: a phenomenological study, PhD thesis. Robert Gordon University, Aberdeen, UK.

Rogers, J., 2010. Occupational reasoning. In: Curtin, M., Molineux, M., Supyk-Mellson, J. (Eds.), Occupational Therapy and Physical Dysfunction: Enabling Occupation. Churchill Livingstone Elsevier, Edinburgh, UK, pp. 57–66.

Romiszowski, A., 1984. Designing Instructional Systems. Hogan Page, London, UK.

Sackett, D.L., Rosenberg, W.M., Gray, J.A., et al., 1996. Evidence based medicine: what it is and what it isn't (editorial). BMJ 312, 71–72.

Sharafaroodi, N., Kamali, M., Parvizy, S., et al., 2014. Factors affecting clinical reasoning of occupational therapists: a qualitative study. Med. J. Islam. Repub. Iran 28, 8.

Scheffer, B.K., Rubenfeld, M.G., 2000. A consensus statement on critical thinking. J. Nurs. Educ. 39, 352–359.

Schell, B.A., Schell, J.W., 2008. Clinical and Professional Reasoning in Occupational Therapy. Lippincott & Wilkins, Philadelphia, PA.

Schraagen, J.M., Chipman, S.F., Shalin, V., 2000. Cognitive Task Analysis. Lawrence Erlbaum Associates, Mahwah, NJ.

Taylor, M.C., 2000. Evidence-Based Practice for Occupational Therapists. Blackwell Science, Oxford, UK.

Townsend, E.A., Polatajko, H.J., 2007. Enabling Occupation II: Advancing an Occupational Therapy Vision for Health, Well-Being, & Justice Through Occupation. CAOT ACE, Ottawa, ON.

Turner, A., Knight, J., 2015. A debate on the professional identity of occupational therapy. Br. J. Occup. Ther. 78, 664–673.

Turpin, M., Iwama, M., 2011. Using Occupational Therapy Models in Practice: A Field Guide. Churchill Livingstone Elsevier, Edinburgh, UK.

Unsworth, C.A., 2011. The evolving theory of clinical reasoning. In: Duncan, E. (Ed.), Foundations for Practice in Occupational Therapy. Churchill Livingstone Elsevier, Edinburgh, UK.

VandenBos, G.R., 2015. APA dictionary of psychology, second ed. American Psychological Association, Washington, DC.

CLINICAL DECISION MAKING IN EMERGENCY MEDICINE

PAT CROSKERRY

CHAPTER AIMS

The aims of this chapter are to:

- review the recent emergence of clinical decision making in the context of patient safety,
- emphasize the critical role of rationality in clinical decision making,
- review the main facilitators of rationality,
- examine the components of dysrationalia and
- outline some of the special characteristics of clinical decision making in emergency medicine.

KEY WORDS

Patient safety

Dual-process theory

Emergency medicine

Mindware

Cognitive bias

ABBREVIATIONS/ ACRONYMS

CDM Clinical decision making

IOM Institute of Medicine

ED Emergency department

EP Emergency physician

INTRODUCTION

Several decades ago, it could have been reasonably said that the average emergency physician (EP) did not give a lot of thought to his or her decision making. For most, clinical decision making (CDM) was largely a reactive process. Patients came to the emergency department (ED) with various symptoms and signs, were diagnosed, treated and either admitted or discharged. Clinical reasoning and decision making were embedded somewhere in the process, but it was rarely if ever thought about in any depth and certainly did not merit much discussion in the literature. David Eddy, one of the pioneers of evidence-based medicine, noted that in the 1970s: 'Medical decision making as a field worthy of study did not exist' (Eddy, 2005, pp. 9–17).

However, since the turn of the century, two major developments have taken place that have significantly affected the way we look at decision making in emergency medicine: the development of the patient safety movement and the incorporation of the cognitive science approach to decision making into mainstream medicine and emergency medicine.

REFLECTION POINT 1

The current emphasis on clinical decision making can be seen as a confluence of developments in patient safety and cognitive science.

The patient safety movement gathered momentum through the last part of the 20th century but was galvanized by the US Institute of Medicine (IOM) report *To Err Is Human* (Kohn et al., 1999). Described as 'the shot heard around the world', the report became the tipping point for a whole new approach to patient safety. Following general overviews of the topic (Aspden et al., 2004; Vincent, 2006), several disciplines produced their own specialized treatments, including emergency medicine (Croskerry et al., 2009), in which CDM received considerable attention. It was clear that CDM was an important, if not dominant, aspect of patient safety, although this had not been fully appreciated in the IOM report. Wachter (2010) noted that whereas medication error was mentioned 70 times, diagnostic error (often the outcome of poor CDM) was mentioned only twice (p. 1605). This omission was corrected in 2015, when the former IOM (now the National Academies of Sciences, Engineering, and Medicine) published *Improving Diagnosis in Health Care* (Balogh et al., 2015). An important chapter in the book was devoted to the diagnostic process, which included a review of clinical reasoning and decision making. From a relatively obscure position, CDM was now catapulted to the forefront.

The second major development was the cognitive revolution in psychology and the emergence of the 'heuristics and biases' literature. This began in the 1970s with the publication of several papers that were the harbinger of hundreds of others to follow over the next 40 years (e.g., Kahneman, 2013). Collectively, they demonstrated that human reasoning and decision making, at times, are significantly compromised. Systemic irregularities in human cognition were widespread. The ultimate focus of this failure was on the rationality of the decision maker, a characteristic that is extremely important in the makeup of the emergency physician.

EMERGENCE OF DUAL-PROCESS THEORY IN CLINICAL DECISION MAKING

Before discussing rationality, it would be helpful to look at how the brain actually makes decisions. The dominant model has been dual-process theory, which has been widely incorporated into decision making in multiple fields of human activity, including medical decision making (Croskerry 2009). Fig. 26.1 shows a schematic adapted from that paper. It is now widely taught and forms the basis of a recently published educational module on cognitive error and debiasing in emergency

medicine (Daniel et al., 2017). Dual-process theory proposes two ways in which we make decisions. These have been termed System 1 or Type 1 processing (intuitive), which is typically automatic, autonomous, fast, nonverbal and often driven by pattern recognition, and System 2 or Type 2 processing (analytical), which is slow, deliberate, verbal and generally less prone to error (Croskerry, 2009). In Fig. 26.1, the two dotted-line boxes leading into each system contain proposed determinants, respectively, of the two systems.

REFLECTION POINT 2

Dual-process theory is the dominant model for characterizing the two systems of decision making: intuitive (System 1) and analytical (System 2) processing.

The model runs from left to right. The patient presents with symptoms or signs that may form a pattern that is immediately recognized (e.g., the rash of shingles), and the diagnosis can be made in fractions of a second. The four major channels of Type 1 processing, not elaborated upon here, are described in more detail elsewhere (Croskerry et al., 2013). Most biases reside in System 1. If the pattern is not recognized, Type 2 processing is required and is enacted deliberately through a single channel, which, typically, may take considerably longer. Repetitive Type 2 processing can lead to Type 1 processing, in the acquisition of a skill such as intubation. System 2 may exert executive override of the output from System 1 – this decoupling is at the basis of reflection, metacognition and mindfulness and provides the means for cognitive bias mitigation. System 1 can also override System 2, such that despite knowing the most rational thing to do, intuitive responses can preponderate. This is referred to as dysrationalia. In the model, T represents a toggle function, the ability to move back and forth between the two systems. Overall, there is a tendency to default to System 1, where less cognitive effort is required – referred to as cognitive miserliness. We spend most of our time in System 1.

RATIONALITY IN CLINICAL DECISION MAKING

Normative decision making is characterized as the best possible decision by ideal decision makers who are able

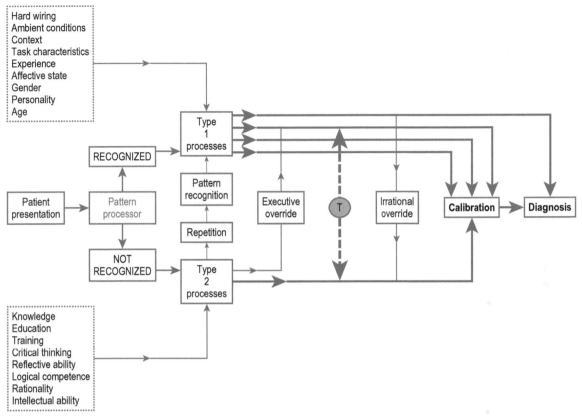

Fig. 26.1 ▪ Dual-process model of clinical decision making. (Adapted from Croskerry, P., 2009. A universal model of diagnostic reasoning. Acad. Med. 84, 1022–1028, with permission.)

to compute with high degrees of accuracy and rationality with sufficient resources at their disposal. It is clear, however, that this normative ideal is often not reached. Over the past 40 years, cognitive science has unequivocally established the general vulnerability of human decision making. Extensive nonnormative decision failures have been described. There are significant individual differences that affect decision making (Croskerry, 2017a) and, therefore, substantial variation. Thus just like intelligence, human rationality is normatively distributed. Generally, it is optimal when the decision maker is knowledgeable about the topic, has the intellectual capacity to think at the level of complexity the task demands, demonstrates critical thinking skills and has favourable individual characteristics (e.g., mindfulness, metacognitive awareness, actively open-minded thinking and others) as illustrated in Fig. 26.2 (Croskerry, 2017b).

REFLECTION POINT 3

Rationality is the quintessential characteristic of a good decision maker in emergency medicine.

FACILITATORS OF RATIONALITY

For optimal rationality, there need to be sufficient facilitators (Fig. 26.3) and minimal inhibitors (see Fig. 26.4). Facilitators are cognitive components that support and promote rationality. The dual-process model provides a good conceptual scaffold for thinking about decision making. In particular, it illustrates the important capability of decoupling from System 1 and using System 2 to modulate decision making. This is accomplished, for example, through the basic processes of metacognition, reflection and mindfulness. An awareness of cognitive biases and logical fallacies, and how they work, is also important. Having identified bias in one's decision making, the capacity to apply cognitive bias mitigation techniques (mindware) may be necessary to deal with them. Being able to reflect upon one's reasoning and decision making is important because it allows a second look at what has been done or is about to be done. Similarly, mindfulness is the ability to apply attitudinal

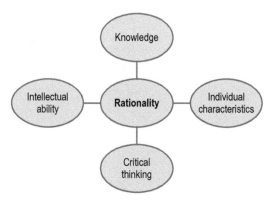

Fig. 26.2 ■ Major components of rationality. (Croskerry, P. 2017b. The rational diagnostician. In: Croskerry, P., Cosby, K.C., Graber, M.L., Singh, H. (Eds.), Diagnosis: Interpreting the Shadows. CRC Press, Boca Raton, FL, forthcoming, with permission.)

qualities that may improve thinking, such as patience, beginner's mind, trust, nonjudging, nonstriving, acceptance and letting go, originally described by Kabat-Zinn (1990). These qualities of mind can be used to mitigate some well-known cognitive biases (Sibinga and Wu, 2010). Further, although a number of individual faculties are associated with optimal decision making (Croskerry, 2017a), chief among them are those that support Actively Open-Minded Thinking (AOT), a personality trait that correlates highly with rationality (Baron, 1993; Stanovich et al., 2016). Other cognitive faculties that avoid cognitive miserliness, such as perseverance, effortful thinking and conscientiousness, also support rationality.

DYSRATIONALIA

Inhibitors of rationality lead to *dysrationalia*, defined as 'the inability to think and behave rationally despite having adequate intelligence' (Stanovich, 2009a, p. 35). These can be divided into process and content problems (Fig. 26.4) (Stanovich, 2009b). An important processing problem is cognitive miserliness. Although we do not have a deliberate strategy not to use our brains, we are inclined to engage thinking that is fast and

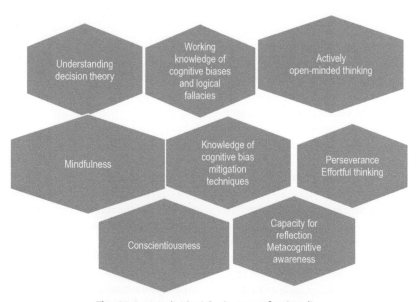

Fig. 26.3 ■ Individual facilitators of rationality.

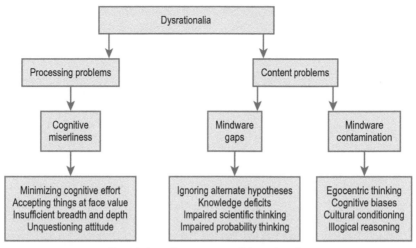

Fig. 26.4 ▪ Components of dysrationalia.

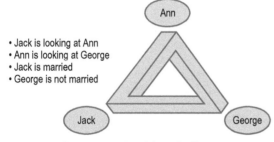

• Jack is looking at Ann
• Ann is looking at George
• Jack is married
• George is not married

Fig. 26.5 ▪ Cognitive miserliness.

computationally inexpensive. Such cognitive miserliness is often the best strategy in emergency medicine – we often rely on not overthinking issues that can be reliably dealt with quickly. Thus cognitive thriftiness often serves us well, but occasionally it may result in missing the correct solution.

Fig. 26.5 illustrates a problem originally attributed to Bob Moore (Levesque 1986, p. 85). In Fig. 26.5, we are given four true statements and asked the question: Is a married person looking at an unmarried person? About 80% of people will say the answer cannot be determined (Stanovich, 2009b). Because Ann's marital status is unknown, they choose not to pursue the search for a solution and leave it there. The problem appears insoluble, and no further effort is made. However, with

a little perseverance some people realize that because Ann has only two states, married and unmarried, they can compute the correct answer by considering each separately. If Ann is married, the answer is yes because she is looking at George who is unmarried. If Ann is unmarried, then the answer is still yes because Jack is looking at her. Whether she is married or not, the answer is yes. Thus the correct solution is available with a little extra cognitive effort, involving disjunctive reasoning.

Consider now the clinical example in Case Study 26.1. There are several biases that contribute to the correct diagnosis not being made in a timely fashion at the first visit. The patient is well known for being a frequent visitor to the ED. Physicians who see her experience a sense of futility that they will ever find a diagnosis to explain her symptoms given she has been seen by numerous specialists in the past. This is an example of the Yin-Yang Out bias – the patient has been 'worked up the Yin-Yang' with no firm diagnosis, therefore, further efforts are probably futile. Unfortunately, she has acquired the pejorative label of 'frequent flyer', which means she is perceived as inappropriately using the ED. Also, she has the psychiatric diagnosis of somatic symptom disorder, which may manifest in several ways; in this case, it appears to be illness anxiety disorder. One of the Psych-Out biases is to ascribe somatic symptoms to a psychiatric condition rather than evaluate them objectively. The EP is also fatigued, and the department is very busy, and he fails to muster sufficient reserve to complete a more thorough evaluation. This is an example of cognitive miserliness associated with significant contributory factors (decision fatigue, general fatigue, possible dysphoria from fatigue and/or the pressures from overcrowding and likelihood of minimal yield for cognitive effort).

REFLECTION POINT 4

Cognitive miserliness allows EPs to deal with many routine decisions in the ED using minimal effort, but occasionally miserliness may lead to significant difficulties.

The other major factors that contribute to dysrationalia are content problems (see Fig. 26.4). These are divided into *mindware gaps* and *mindware contamination*. Simple knowledge deficits, such as not knowing that knee pain may be a manifestation of a hip problem

in children or that hypoglycaemia may mimic almost any neurological condition, or indeed medical knowledge generally, may certainly cause problems for clinical reasoning, but such medical knowledge deficits can be distinguished from mindware gaps, which are specific deficiencies in *knowledge about reasoning*. Stanovich and West cite numerous studies demonstrating such failings:

> *people's responses sometimes deviate from the performance considered normative on many reasoning tasks. For example, people assess probabilities incorrectly, they test hypotheses inefficiently, they violate the axioms of utility theory, they do not properly calibrate degrees of belief, their choices are affected by irrelevant context, they ignore the alternative hypothesis when evaluating data, and they display numerous other information processing biases (2000, p. 645).*

CASE STUDY 26.1

Stacey (a Frequent Visitor to the Emergency Department)

Stacey is a 28-year-old patient who presents to the emergency department (ED) with lower abdominal pain. She has had numerous visits to the ED over the past few years with similar complaints and is known to have visited all four EDs in the city in the same evening. She is described as a 'frequent flyer'. She has been extensively investigated by gynaecology, urology, gastroenterology and psychiatry. Despite numerous investigations including ultrasound, abdominal CT and hysterosalpingogram, no somatic cause has been found for her discomfort.

The ED is extremely busy with 30 people in the waiting room. The EP who assesses her has seen her several times in the past. Her abdominal discomfort is mostly on the left side. Her vital signs are stable. She has a soft abdomen with good bowel sounds and vague tenderness in the left lower quadrant. Her urinalysis is normal.

The EP reassures her that she doesn't have a urinary tract infection and does not appear to have any serious condition. He comments on the extensive workups she has had in the past for similar symptoms. She

tells him that she feels different this time, but he reminds her that she has said that numerous times before. She responds well to further reassurance, and he discharges her from the ED.

The next afternoon, she is brought back to the same ED having collapsed at the local mall. She is pale and hypotensive. Bloodwork shows a haemoglobin of 6 and a positive pregnancy test. Pelvic ultrasound revealed a complex adnexal mass on the left side with a large amount of free fluid. She is diagnosed with a ruptured ectopic pregnancy and taken immediately to the operating room.

Comment. The EP was aware of the patient's label as a 'frequent flyer' and her diagnosis of somatoform disorder and well aware of the perils of making assumptions about such patients. However, he saw her in the closing hours of an 8-hour shift in a very busy ED and was fatigued. Had he simply allowed the patient the benefit of the doubt and performed a pregnancy test on the first visit, he may well have made the correct diagnosis.

Common examples of mindware gaps are poor probabilistic reasoning, fallacies in logical reasoning and impaired scientific reasoning. Much of this mindware content knowledge is taught in medical undergraduate courses on clinical epidemiology and biostatistics and is well covered in textbooks (Weingart and Wyer, 2006; Rao, 2007). Students are taught about test specificity, sensitivity, likelihood ratios, Bayesian reasoning, number needed to treat and other bio-statistical tests that will enable them to critically evaluate tests and studies published in the literature. Most EPs will have had the benefits of such training. However, this knowledge and the skills necessary to apply it will fade unless it becomes a routine of practice, so there is an imperative to reinforce it in practicing EPs. In emergency medicine, excellent coverage of potential mindware gaps together with a strong dose of critical thinking and evidence-based medicine is provided in a book by Weingart and Wyer (2006). Many of the clinical examples given by Gigerenzer in a chapter on physicians' decision making titled 'What doctors need to know' are mindware gaps of this type (2014, pp. 159–186).

Problems with probability reasoning are illustrated in Case Study 26.2. The nurse first recognizes the pattern of leg pain and chest pain, which are consistent with pulmonary embolus (PE) and, especially in view of her recent experience with two cases of PE (availability bias), orders a D-dimer test. The test is sensitive but has very low specificity, which means that it is good for ruling out deep venous clots and PE but not good at ruling them in. In this case, given the very low pretest probability that the patient has this diagnosis, the test should not have been ordered. Elevated levels may be caused by recent surgery, trauma, infection and some other conditions. Minor elevations above the cutoff value are not uncommon. Once the test has been done, however, and yields a positive result, there is an onus on the physician to explain it. The physician failed to stick with the original judgement and agreed to an unnecessary test thus exposing the patient to unnecessary radiation.

The second area in which mindware fails is when it is contaminated (see Fig. 26.3). In contrast to mindware gaps where essential knowledge about reasoning is

CASE STUDY 26.2

Brad (Worried About His Heart)

Brad, a 32-year-old male patient, comes to the ED with pleuritic chest pain and feeling slightly short of breath. He is very anxious. He is concerned he may be having a heart attack. His brother-in-law had similar symptoms 1 week ago and is currently in the cardiac care unit (CCU). His vital signs are stable at triage other than a slightly elevated respiratory rate (22) and tachycardia (110). He is triaged to the cardiac room. The ED is busy. Routine bloodwork is done, including cardiac enzymes, and a cardiogram and chest x-ray are ordered.

He is assessed by the EP after about 20 minutes. Brad's wife is with him and appears anxious. His cardiogram is first reviewed. It shows normal sinus rhythm with a rate of 86 bpm. He relates that the pain started the day before and seems to be a little worse on inspiration. He has been pain-free since being placed in the cardiac room.

He has no risk factors for heart disease and no prior chest pain or respiratory problems. He has no significant medical history or history of anxiety disorder. He appears to be in good physical shape and runs regularly. He feels he may have strained a calf muscle running a few days ago. On examination, his cardiovascular and respiratory examinations are normal. His heart rate and respiratory rate are now both normal at 78 and 18, respectively. He has some localizing pain at the insertion of his left Achilles tendon, but the calf is supple with no pain on deep palpation.

The EP reads his chest x-ray as normal. He reassures Brad that all seems fine and if his troponin is normal he can probably go home. Brad's wife is concerned about an elevated test result that was mentioned to her by the nurse. The EP tells her he will check the bloodwork and return shortly. He finds the nurse as soon as he leaves the room. She immediately asks

Continued on following page

CASE STUDY 26.2

Brad (Worried About His Heart) *(Continued)*

him if he has seen the D-dimer result. She added the test to the bloodwork because she had a strong intuition this might be a PE. She had seen two cases of PE the previous week. The D-dimer was 350 (in this laboratory, threshold is 200 for a positive test), and the patient's troponin level was <14 (normal). The nurse asked the physician if she should order a chest CT.

The physician pointed out that he had not ordered the D-dimer test and did not believe the patient had a PE. The nurse was uncomfortable with this decision,

given her recent experiences with PEs. She states that for one of the cases 'no-one believed he had a PE either'. She is also concerned with the patient's wife, who now knows her husband has a 'positive' test result. The EP acquiesces and orders a chest CT, which is normal. The patient is reassured that everything appears fine and that the episode was likely caused by anxiety over his brother-in-law's recent CCU admission. He is discharged home with a diagnosis of chest pain NYD (not yet diagnosed) to return to the ED if his symptoms recur.

missing, in this case the decision maker has mindware, but it is flawed. When it is applied to the decision-making process, it has a negative effect on the quality of rationality. Systematic deviations from normative decision making are called biases, and there are many of them, enough in fact, that bias may be considered a normal operating characteristic of the brain (Croskerry, 2014a, pp. 23–27). Wikipedia lists over 100 and a number of social and memory biases.[i] Every discipline in medicine has now acknowledged their relevance to decision making (Croskerry, 2014a). Importantly, Stanovich specifically defines irrationality as the vulnerability to cognitive bias: 'Degrees of rationality can be assessed in terms of the number and severity of such cognitive biases that individuals display. Conversely, failure to display a cognitive bias becomes a measure of rational thought' (Stanovich, 2011, pp. 343–365). Thus biases are a major source, but not the only source, of mindware contamination.

In Case Study 26.3, the first cognitive failure is actually a logical fallacy perpetrated by the patient herself. The fallacy is *cum hoc, ergo propter hoc* (with this, therefore because of this) and is committed when the patient infers causation between twisting her shoulder and the onset of shoulder pain (whereas it appears to be referred pain from her heart associated with physical effort). Prompted by the patient's

assumption and framing of the problem, the triage nurse perpetrates the fallacy by sending the patient to the Minors' area (triage cueing). The EP believes he is dealing with a benign problem (ascertainment bias). On the shoulder x-ray, he sees changes of osteoarthritis, which confirm his belief that the problem is not serious (confirmation bias). The outcome of this sequence of cognitive errors and biases is that a potentially life-threatening condition is missed.

HOW DOES CDM IN EMERGENCY MEDICINE DIFFER FROM THAT IN OTHER SETTINGS?

The basic approach towards decision making is universal. Wherever decision makers are, and whatever decisions are being made, all decision making follows similar patterns, and the general properties described by cognitive science apply. Within medicine, there will be predictable differences depending on specialty and on ambient and other conditions. In the visual specialties (dermatology, radiology and anatomical pathology), pattern recognition is high, and the signal is often less ambiguous and well defined. This is reflected in a fairly low rate of diagnostic failure in the order of 1% to 2% (Berner and Graber 2008, pp. 2–23). In some specialties, such as orthopaedics, plastics, urology and others, by the time the patient arrives in clinic, much of the uncertainty has been removed, and the diagnosis is often unambiguous. In contrast, emergency medicine ranks

---

[i]List of cognitive biases. Viewed 10 Feb 2017. Available from: <https://en.wikipedia.org/wiki/List_of_cognitive_biases>

Geography Is Destiny

A sprightly 68-year-old female presents at an ED, complaining of shoulder pain. When mowing her lawn today, the mower got stuck in an awkward spot and she had to twist and push hard to release it. She feels she may have strained her shoulder in the process (framing bias).

At triage, she is noted to have shoulder sprain brought on by mowing (triage cueing). Her vital signs are all stable, and she is triaged to the Minors' (fast-track) area, where after a brief wait she is seen by an emergency physician. It was the practice in this department that emergency physicians would work the first 6 hours of their shift on the main floor and then go to the Minors' area for the last 2 hours. The implicit assumption made by those working in the Minors' area is that they will not be dealing with complex cases (ascertainment bias), also a manifestation of the Geography is Destiny bias.

The EP takes a brief history and examines the patient. Her shoulder is slightly limited in range of motion but appears otherwise normal. He orders an x-ray, which shows no acute injury, but notes some osteoarthritic changes (confirmation bias). He orders a sling for the patient and advises her to take anti-inflammatories and rest it for the next few days. His discharge diagnosis is 'Osteoarthritis'.

Several hours later, the patient returns to the same ED having experienced a 'weak spell' associated with some nausea and vomiting. She is pale, diaphoretic and hypotensive. An ECG at triage reveals an acute inferior myocardial infarct.

---

alongside family practice and internal medicine in having the highest levels of diagnostic failure at 10% to 15%, reflecting more challenging clinical decision making (Croskerry and Sinclair, 2001). Patients may present with headache, for example, which has approximately 300 aetiologies, or chest pain, which has at least about 25. More possibilities on the differential diagnosis mean higher levels of uncertainty and an increased use of heuristics. Further, there is a growing awareness of how individual and ambient factors, especially in such environments as the ED (decision fatigue, general fatigue, sleep deprivation, cognitive overload, stress, dysphoria and others) may contribute to compromises in decision making (Croskerry, 2014b; Croskerry, 2017a).

The requirements for good decision making in EM are rigorous and demanding. Although certain individual characteristics will facilitate rationality, EPs need to be able to toggle effectively between the fast pattern recognition of Type 1 processing and the slower more deliberate decision making of Type 2, with the thoughtful application of appropriate mindware when needed, and ever mindful of mindware gaps and contamination. Through it all, they need to be aware of the effect of ambient conditions on their decision making in what is seen to be the most chaotic of medical environments.

CHAPTER SUMMARY

In this chapter, we have outlined:

- antecedents of the recent emphasis on CDM in emergency medicine,
- the appropriateness of dual-process theory as a platform for clinical decision making,
- the central role of rationality in all decision making,
- sources of dysrationalia in clinical decision making and
- the special features of CDM in emergency medicine.

REFLECTION POINT 5

Cognitive biases are a major contributor to mindware contamination. The number and severity of biases that EPs display reflect their level of rationality.

REFERENCES

Aspden, P., Corrigan, J.M., Wolcott, J., et al. (Eds.), 2004. Patient Safety: A New Standard for Care. Institute of Medicine of the National Academies, Quality Chasm Series. National Academies Press, Washington, DC.

Balogh, E.P., Miller, B.T., Ball, J.R. (Eds.), 2015. Improving Diagnosis in Health Care. The National Academies of Sciences, Engineering and Medicine. National Academies Press, Washington, DC.

Baron, J., 1993. Why teach thinking? an essay. Appl. Psychol. 42, 191–214.

Berner, E.S., Graber, M.L., 2008. Overconfidence as a cause of diagnostic error in medicine. Am. J. Med. 121 (Suppl. 5), S2–S23.

Croskerry, P., 2009. A universal model of diagnostic reasoning. Acad. Med. 84, 1022–1028.

Croskerry, P., 2014a. Bias: a normal operating characteristic of the diagnosing brain. Diagnosis 1, 23–27.

Croskerry, P., 2014b. ED Cognition: any decision by anyone at any time, ED administration series. Can. J. Emerg. Med. 16, 13–19.

Croskerry, P., 2017a. Individual variability in clinical decision making and diagnosis. In: Croskerry, P., Cosby, K.C., Graber, M.L., et al. (Eds.), Diagnosis: Interpreting the Shadows. CRC Press, Boca Raton, FL.

Croskerry, P., 2017b. The rational diagnostician. In: Croskerry, P., Cosby, K.C., Graber, M.L., et al. (Eds.), Diagnosis: Interpreting the Shadows. CRC Press, Boca Raton, FL. (forthcoming).

Croskerry, P., Cosby, K.S., Schenkel, S.M., et al. (Eds.), 2009. Patient Safety in Emergency Medicine. Lippincott Williams & Wilkins, Philadelphia, PA.

Croskerry, P., Sinclair, D., 2001. Emergency medicine: a practice prone to error? Canadian J. Emerg. Med. 3, 271–276.

Croskerry, P., Singhal, G., Mamede, S., 2013. Cognitive debiasing 1: origins of bias and theory of debiasing. BMJ Qual. Saf. 22 (Suppl. 2), ii58–ii64.

Daniel, M., Khandelwal, S., Santen, S., et al., 2017. Cognitive debiasing strategies for the emergency department. Acad. Emerg. Med. Educ. Train. 1, 41–42.

Eddy, D.M., 2005. Evidence-based medicine: a unified approach. Health Aff. (Millwood) 24, 9–17.

Gigerenzer, G., 2014. What doctors need to know. In: Gigerenzer, G. (Ed.), Risk Savvy: How to Make Good Decisions. Allen Lane, London, UK, pp. 159–186.

Kabat-Zinn, J., 1990. Full Catastrophe Living: Using the Wisdom of Your Body and Mind to Face Stress, Pain, and Illness. Delta, New York, NY.

Kahneman, D., 2013. Thinking, Fast and Slow. Farrar, Strauss and Giroux, New York, NY.

Kohn, L.T., Corrigan, J.M., Donaldson, M.S. (Eds.), 1999. To Err Is Human: Building a Safer Health Care System, Report of the Institute of Medicine of the National Academies. National Academies Press, Washington, DC.

Levesque, H.J., 1986. Making believers out of computers. Artif. Intell. 30, 81–108.

Rao, G., 2007. Rational Medical Decision Making: A Case-Based Approach. McGraw-Hill, New York, NY.

Sibinga, E.M., Wu, A.W., 2010. Clinician mindfulness and patient safety. JAMA 304, 2532–2533.

Stanovich, K.E., 2009a. Rational and irrational thought: the thinking that IQ tests miss. Sci. Am. Mind 20, 34–39.

Stanovich, K.E., 2009b. What Intelligence Tests Miss: The Psychology of Rational Thought. Yale University Press, New Haven, CT.

Stanovich, K.E., 2011. On the distinction between rationality and intelligence: implications for understanding individual differences in reasoning. In: Holyoak, K.J., Morrison, R.G. (Eds.), The Oxford Handbook of Thinking and Reasoning. Oxford University Press, Oxford, UK, pp. 343–365.

Stanovich, K.E., West, R.F., 2000. Individual differences in reasoning: implications for the rationality debate? Behav. Brain Sci. 23, 645–726.

Stanovich, K.E., West, R.F., Toplak, M.E., 2016. The Rationality Quotient: Toward a Test of Rational Thinking. MIT Press, Cambridge, MA.

Vincent, C., 2006. Patient Safety. Churchill Livingstone, London, UK.

Wachter, R.M., 2010. Why diagnostic errors don't get any respect—and what can be done about them. Health Aff. (Millwood) 29, 1605–1610.

Weingart, S., Wyer, P., 2006. Emergency Medicine Decision Making: Critical Choices in Chaotic Environments. McGraw-Hill, New York, NY.

CLINICAL DECISION MAKING IN PARAMEDICINE

BILL LORD ■ PAUL SIMPSON

CHAPTER AIMS

The aims of this chapter are to:

- describe the nature of contemporary paramedic practice,
- outline the context of clinical reasoning within paramedicine,
- explain models of clinical reasoning relevant to paramedic practice,
- discuss the effect of cognitive bias on the quality of clinical reasoning and
- provide strategies for cognitive de-biasing using metacognition and reflective practice.

KEY WORDS

Paramedic

Reflection

Metacognition

Cognitive bias

Cognitive disposition to respond

Dual processing

ABBREVIATIONS/ ACRONYMS

BVM Bag-valve-mask

CDR Cognitive disposition to respond

EtCO₂ End-tidal carbon dioxide

ICP Intensive care paramedic

SGA Supraglottic airway

SpO₂ Peripheral capillary oxygen saturation

INTRODUCTION

Paramedic practice throughout the world has undergone a remarkable transformation over the past two decades as the role of the paramedic has responded to changing population health demands. In this chapter we use our experience of these changes in Australia to show how the clinical reasoning required has been affected. The changing population health demands reflect the increasing prevalence of chronic health problems associated with increasing length of life and initiatives that aim to expand community-based health care as a substitute for in-hospital care (Caplan et al., 2012).

Paramedics' professional identity has traditionally centred on management of acute health emergencies including major trauma and cardiac arrest. However, the incidence of these cases in Australia is falling (Boyle et al., 2008; Dyson et al., 2015), largely a result of public health interventions and legislation to change behaviour that is associated with risk for injury or illness. In contrast, paramedics are increasingly caring for older people (Lowthian et al., 2011) with complex healthcare needs, and a call to the emergency number is now likely to involve exacerbation of a chronic health condition or injury sustained after a fall.

The changing nature of the cases managed by ambulance services is reshaping the paramedic role. Although paramedics have traditionally functioned in an 'assess, treat, stabilize and transport' paradigm, contemporary models of care now entail advanced patient examination and treatment with a view to determining a clinically appropriate disposition that is as likely to involve referral of the patient to an integrated community-based care pathway as it is transport to an emergency department. Paramedics now also actively engage in health promotion by way of opportunistic counselling for issues relating to management of chronic disease and illness and contribute to injury prevention strategies such as prevention of falls in the elderly by conducting evidence-based risk assessment and screening.

Scope of practice has substantially increased at each end of the spectrum of acuity. In lower acuity contexts, paramedics may perform suturing, wound care, indwelling urinary catheterization and administration of antibiotics. At the higher end, paramedic-initiated thrombolysis for STEMI (ST-segment elevation myocardial infarction) and sedation and paralysis for airway management, surgical airways and management of cardiac dysrhythmias have become standards of care in many practice settings.

The ability to provide safe and effective health care in an increasingly complex and autonomous environment justifies an examination of the nature of clinical reasoning in paramedicine. Given the important influence that clinical decision making has on the delivery of safe and effective care, this chapter describes models of clinical reasoning identified in the health professions literature, the relevance of these models to paramedic practice and the potential effects of cognitive errors and affective bias on clinical decisions and patient outcomes.

THE NATURE OF PARAMEDIC PRACTICE

Paramedics provide unscheduled health care to individuals in the community. A call for an emergency ambulance results in a response based on the outcome of the telephone triage process. From that initial call, information about patient age and gender and a brief description of the nature of the problem are available for paramedics to review while travelling to the case.

The initial patient encounter is commonly associated with inaccessible or incomplete health records, limited access to diagnostic tests and competing priorities that include organizational requirements to minimize time spent 'on scene' to maximize operational responsiveness. Initial attempts to gather a history and examine a patient are frequently impeded by scene management and situational logistics.

Paramedics must gather data of varying reliability and integrity from several sources to formulate a clinical impression and subsequent treatment plan. Data sources include the patient and others present, which may include friends, relatives and other healthcare professionals. Contextual sources of information include the patient's social environment that may provide evidence of ability to live independently, verification of mechanism of injury or suspicion of illness. Paramedics are required to interpret salient features of the environment in which the clinical encounter takes place to build an impression of the factors that may be associated with the patient's current health status. Finally, the patient's subjective narrative and the paramedic's objective clinical observations complete the data-collection process.

Research has described the complexity of paramedic decisions and the multiple levels of system influences that may be associated with increased risk (O'Hara et al., 2015). Decision making by paramedics is characteristically performed in a state of high 'cognitive load', increasing propensity for error (Burgess, 2009). Clinical reasoning demands compete against multiple priorities that may include maintenance of situational awareness, assessment of safety, counselling and reassurance of bystanders, friends or family and communication with and coordination of other emergency service or healthcare professionals in what is generally a task-heavy, human resource-poor environment.

REFLECTION POINT 1

Paramedics operate most commonly in a dual-crew capacity. Consider the multiple concurrent tasks and functions that must be managed in the initial 10 minutes of a medium-acuity case involving an older person who has fallen and sustained a fractured hip. What strategies could be implemented or adopted at the point of care to reduce cognitive load in this scenario?

Well-developed clinical reasoning skills, including the ability to self-monitor for factors that may compromise the resulting clinical judgements, are central to the delivery of safe and effective care.

CLINICAL REASONING IN PARAMEDICINE PRACTICE

There is scant research evidence investigating clinical reasoning specific to paramedic practice, with existing studies focussing on decision outcomes rather than the cognitive processes involved in arriving at these decisions.

Shaban et al. described theories of decision making in paramedic practice, in a practice environment described as a state of 'constant uncertainty' (Shaban et al., 2004). Earlier research from the United States has identified the importance of critical thinking and diagnostic reasoning skills, with the authors advocating for more emphasis on the development of these skills in entry-to-practice paramedic education (Dalton, 1996; Janing, 1994). This research describes the use of inductive and deductive reasoning with an emphasis on the influence that personal beliefs and values can have on the quality of clinical judgements and decisions. Despite arguments for the integration of clinical reasoning and de-biasing strategies within paramedic curricula, there has been little evidence of educational design that aims to enable these skills.

A 2016 survey of Canadian paramedics identified a dominant perception by respondents that they use a rational (conscious) style of thinking over an experiential (intuitive) approach to thinking and problem solving (Jensen et al., 2016). The authors suggest that these styles of thinking correlate with the Dual-Process theory systems of reasoning (Evans, 2003; see later in the chapter for more detail). Research has proposed that a mix of approaches are used and that these include rule-out-worst-scenario, algorithmic thinking and exhaustive thinking, with each of these associated with System 2 thinking (Jensen, 2010).

This absence of substantial research exploring clinical reasoning in the context of paramedicine has led to the extrapolation of theory from other clinical disciplines, most notably emergency medicine. In a generic sense, clinical reasoning involves context-dependant thinking that leads to a clinical judgement, diagnosis, intervention or other action. Clinical reasoning is an essential component of professional competence, which is dependent on technical skills, communication, knowledge and reflection on practice (Epstein and Hundert, 2002).

Core skills involved in safe and effective decision making include the use of appropriate domain-specific knowledge – both propositional knowledge derived from theory and research and nonpropositional knowledge derived from professional and personal experience – and reasoning skills and an ability to reflect on the quality of the individual's cognitive processes and the influence of bias, including affective bias (Croskerry et al., 2010).

The demands occurring during the patient encounter include the complexity of the task, experience and ability of the individual and the delegated responsibility for the task. Decisions associated with a significant level of risk demand a high level of reasoning and problem solving. Reasoning may also be influenced by cultural beliefs and values, risk factors, interpersonal interactions with others on scene and personal beliefs, values and attitudes (Brandling et al., 2016). Overlaying these variables are personal factors such as fatigue. Given the possible consequences of flawed or inadequate thinking and reasoning processes in the prehospital environment, sound clinical reasoning is required to provide safe and effective care for patients.

COGNITIVE STRATEGIES INVOLVED IN CLINICAL REASONING

Although few published studies have described processes of paramedic reasoning and decision making, clinical reasoning strategies described in medicine (Elstein and Schwarz, 2002) and the specialty of emergency medicine will be used as a reference because of similarities in dealing with incomplete information in often hectic and time-poor environments. This literature describes hypothesis testing, inductive reasoning, pattern recognition and the use of heuristics or 'illness scripts' that are based on known descriptions of disease or common features of a particular disease (Kovacs and Croskerry, 1999). These models of reasoning are detailed elsewhere in this book.

One model of reasoning and decision making is known as Dual-Process theory (DPT), or System 1 and System 2 models of reasoning (Sloman, 1996) System 1 has been described as intuitive decision making, where rapid decisions arise from comparing a familiar pattern of cues with prior examples derived from prior experience (Croskerry, 2009a). This style of thinking enables efficient processing of information to form an impression while reducing cognitive load and fits neatly within the context of paramedic decision making. With experience, thinking becomes automatic, and a more conscious and analytical form of thinking (System 2) is only engaged when complex, novel or atypical situations are encountered. System 1 has been described as a form of universal cognition (Evans, 2003).

Clinical reasoning in medicine has been shown to involve a System 1 process of reasoning where the clinical features are recognized, resulting in a rapid generation of a hypothesis or definition of the problem. In the emergency medicine setting, a 'recognition primed' model of decision making has been described (Weingart, 2009), which corresponds to the System 1 model of pattern recognition. When the clinical features associated with a patient presentation fail to activate prior recognition because of unusual or atypical clinical findings, a more analytical pathway of clinical decision making System 2 is likely to be employed.

The use of pattern recognition by expert paramedics, and the way this differs from novice reasoning, can be identified by observing personal (expert versus novice) differences in the approach to the interpretation and classification of a cardiac electrocardiogram (ECG). Given an ECG showing atrial fibrillation, experts can quickly classify the dysrhythmia without the need for extensive analysis. This is largely a function of exposure to many prior examples so that the distinctive pattern of irregular R-R intervals and lack of regular P-wave activity are recognized automatically. In contrast, novices with knowledge of cardiac electrophysiology but lacking exposure to repeated examples of this dysrhythmia and confirmation of the correct classification may rely on a more analytical and time-consuming dissection of waveform morphology to form a decision regarding the type of dysrhythmia.

ERRORS IN CLINICAL REASONING

Reasoning that underpins the formulation of a diagnosis and subsequent case management plans must be logically sound, defensible and appropriate. This requirement spans all clinical decisions, from the management of minor injury to decisions to withhold or withdraw resuscitation in cases of sudden cardiac arrest. Errors in the field of paramedicine that compromise patient safety or that lead to poor patient outcomes are difficult to find because of limitations of existing reporting practice. A surrogate measure is the incidence of medical indemnity claims in Australia, with paramedics involved in 1.2% of all claims in 2012 to 2013 in Australia (Australian Institute of Health and Welfare, 2014).

A case involving a 50-year-old male reporting a sudden onset of substernal pain that radiates to his left shoulder may initiate a System 1 approach, particularly where the paramedic sees a familiar pattern of clinical signs that may include nonverbal cues. In contrast, a case involving a 22-year-old male reporting a recent onset of chest pain may initiate a System 2 or hypothetico-deductive approach if there is no overt external cause of the pain or when the patient's presentation – including his or her behaviour – is inconsistent with prior examples of nontraumatic chest pain in this age group. The lack of a defining clinical pattern may prompt a more analytical approach to assessment. However, when the pattern of the patient's presentation does not conform to the paramedic's expectations or beliefs about behaviour normally associated with severe pain, judgements about the veracity of the patient's complaint may influence decisions to offer analgesia or refer for further treatment. This may be more likely if the paramedic has developed a model of pain-related behaviour associated with a history of malingering and drug abuse that has similarities with the current case. Hence, if the patient does not conform to prior exemplars of a 'normal' presentation of acute pain, the diagnosis and management may be compromised by cognitive errors such as 'premature closure' (Croskerry, 2003b), particularly when the diagnosis is influenced by judgements regarding the patient's motives for reporting pain.

Cognitive failures associated with decision making have been collectively referred to as cognitive bias or, more recently, 'cognitive dispositions to respond' (CDR) (Croskerry, 2003b). In addition, the influence of emotions on decision making has been classified as 'affective dispositions to respond' (ADR) (Croskerry, 2009b). The ED has been described as a perfect environment for the study of CDR because of the often imperfect information and time limitations that physicians have to work with, but it could be argued that the setting in which paramedics operate is equally challenging.

CDR that are not recognized and result in an adverse outcome can be considered a cognitive error. Upwards of 30 types of CDR have been described in the literature relating to medical decision making (Croskerry, 2002). Although research investigating CDR in paramedic practice has not been reported, they are highly likely to be relevant and present in paramedic clinical reasoning. For an extensive description of CDR, the reader is referred to the work of Croskerry (2009b). Several common CDR factors likely to affect clinical decision making are illustrated in Case Study 27.1.

EDUCATIONAL STRATEGIES TO IMPROVE CLINICAL REASONING

Despite continuing debate about whether it is possible to teach diagnostic reasoning skills (Graber, 2009), there is support for educational design that aims to reduce clinical errors arising from flawed diagnostic reasoning processes (Croskerry et al., 2013). One strategy used to help individuals learn how to monitor their thinking strategies involves the development of self-diagnosis of thinking to enable identification and remediation of thinking errors. Reflection on thinking refers to the conscious assessment of the individual's thinking process,

---

CASE STUDY 27.1

Factors Influencing CDM

Paramedics attend a private residence in the inner city where they encounter a 19-year-old male who is unconscious. The dispatch information provided en route states a 'suspected drug overdose'. The paramedics recognize the address and the patient from a previous incident involving a heroin overdose. The front door to the residence is unlocked. The interior of the residence is untidy, and evidence of what appears to be illicit drug paraphernalia, including syringes, is noted on the kitchen bench. A brief examination involving an attempt to rouse the patient and measurement of his pulse is performed. Profuse diaphoresis is noted. The paramedics form a clinical impression of a narcotic overdose and administer naloxone intramuscularly with no response. Two further doses of naloxone result in no improvement. The paramedics decide to load the patient and transport him to a nearby emergency department (ED). During handover, the triage nurse asks for the blood glucose level (BGL) taken on scene, to which the paramedics report that it was not taken due the diagnosis of narcotic overdose. A BGL is quickly taken revealing a measurement of 1.1 mmol/L. After administration of glucose intravenously, the patient's level of consciousness begins to improve.

UNPACKING THE CASE

This incident is rich in flawed clinical reasoning, underpinned by the presence of several CDR and a failed heuristic decision-making process. 'Anchoring', 'premature diagnostic closure' and 'confirmation bias' are all present to some degree. 'Anchoring' is the common tendency to lock onto early features of a case and not consider or look for other information that might point to another diagnosis. In this example, the call data provided en route and prior knowledge of the address and the patient contributed to the anchoring bias. 'Premature diagnostic closure' is the tendency to terminate the formation of other differential diagnoses as a result of committing to an early diagnosis but without fully confirming it. 'Confirmation bias' results in the clinician neglecting to search for signs or symptoms that might disprove an early clinical impression, tending rather to search for those that will confirm their early impression. This case also illustrates the contextual nature of paramedic clinical reasoning through the powerful influence of the immediate environment and context in which the patient was found. This is a distinct feature of paramedic reasoning, which can be extremely informative and useful on the one hand but cognitively biasing on the other and capable of overshadowing the clinical presentation itself.

or rather it represents thinking about thinking, which is also known as metacognition. Reflection offers the novice the opportunity to be aware of his or her thinking processes, to understand the effect that cognition has on clinical judgements and to support the transition from novice to expert. Metacognition allows the clinician to think about his or her thinking while he or she is thinking, providing self-monitoring in real time at the point where cognitive biases may be actually at play.

When developing the abilities of metacognition and reflective practice, the value of these skills must be evident to the individual, particularly in paramedic practice where technical skills are highly valued by both novices and experts. Students can be taught about metacognition, but its value must be manifest and explicit before students and novice practitioners are likely to accept this skill. Cosby (2011) argues that reflection must be guided by an experienced facilitator or mentor to identify and avoid incorrect conclusions.

REFLECTION POINT 2

Reflect on the context in which paramedics conduct clinical reasoning. What clinical, cultural, environmental or situational barriers may exist that would affect the translation of metacognitive education into the ability to be metacognitive in real time when clinical reasoning is occurring?

The development of metacognitive skills can help clinicians to develop strategies for minimizing or avoiding cognitive error, thus 'inoculating' the clinician against error. Prerequisites for effective inoculation are:

- an understanding of error theory, common clinical errors and cognitive de-biasing techniques involving metacognition;
- development of a 'forcing strategy' to prevent common cognitive errors such as anchoring or early diagnostic closure through the use of scenarios or case studies where this error is likely to occur and
- demonstration of a cognitive forcing strategy that is appropriate to the context to avoid error (Croskerry, 2003a).

The use of case-based learning or simulation can be used to develop these skills in the paramedic education setting. Consideration needs to be given to designing learning activities that contain cognitive error traps or that include information about the patient's environment, history and initial presentation that are likely to trigger bias.

As an example, a case contains information about a call to a suburban home to a 25-year-old male with a recent onset of abdominal pain. Stock photographs of the fictional location can be used to create a vignette to illustrate low socioeconomic circumstances. Additional stock photographs can be used to illustrate the patient presentation. Alternatively, actors or standardized patients can be used to play the role of the patient. History may include a 3-hour history of severe (8/10) hypogastric abdominal pain and nausea. The patient volunteers a history of opioid dependence, and current medications include methadone. Students should complete the case and then a case debrief with an experienced facilitator, where reasons for actions or decisions can be explored. For example, if the student elects to withhold analgesia, the reasons for the decision should be explored. This process may reveal concerns about the patient's motives for reporting pain. A forcing strategy that may be used in this case is to 'consider the opposite' (Croskerry et al., 2013), where the student is asked to use evidence to rule out the possibility of pain.

Although there is limited evidence of the effectiveness of cognitive de-biasing strategies, the development of strategies that help the clinician to evaluate his or her thinking to consider alternative explanations for the patient's presentation and to check for the potential influence of emotions or bias on decision making has the potential to reduce clinical errors. In the previous example, the inability to objectively validate and quantify pain in others may lead to errors in reasoning, including errors in judging the patient's motives for reporting pain that has no obvious pathological basis. As such, strategies that support personal development of cognitive strategies that reduce the risk for error may reduce the risk for poor clinical judgements and improve the quality of patient care.

CHAPTER SUMMARY

In this chapter we have:

- described contemporary models of paramedic practice,

- discussed the context in which clinical reasoning occurs in the discipline of paramedicine,
- explored the evidence describing clinical reasoning in paramedicine,
- discussed theories of clinical reasoning relevant to paramedicine,
- discussed cognitive error in the context of clinical reasoning performed by paramedics,
- illustrated the effect of CDR on clinical reasoning and
- proposed strategies for enhancing the quality of clinical reasoning through development of meta-cognition in paramedics.

REFLECTION POINT 3

What are the challenges faced by paramedic educators who need to teach clinical reasoning skills to novices? Consider both field education and education in the classroom.

REFERENCES

Australian Institute of Health and Welfare, 2014. Australia's medical indemnity claims 2012–13: safety and quality of healthcare 15, cat. no. HSE 149. AIHW, Canberra, Australia.

Boyle, M.J., Smith, E.C., Archer, F.L., 2008. Trauma incidents attended by emergency medical services in Victoria, Australia. Prehosp. Disaster Med. 23, 20–28.

Brandling, J., Kirby, K., Black, S., et al., 2016. Paramedic resuscitation decision-making in out of hospital cardiac arrest: an exploratory study. Emerg. Med. J. 33, e11–e12.

Burgess, D.J., 2009. Are providers more likely to contribute to healthcare disparities under high levels of cognitive load? How features of the healthcare setting may lead to biases in medical decision making. Med. Decis. Making 30, 246–257.

Caplan, G.A., Sulaiman, N.S., Mangin, D.A., et al., 2012. A meta-analysis of 'hospital in the home'. Med. J. Aust. 197, 512–519.

Cosby, K., 2011. The role of certainty, confidence, and critical thinking in the diagnostic process: good luck or good thinking? Acad. Emerg. Med. 18, 212–214.

Croskerry, P., 2002. Achieving quality in clinical decision making: cognitive strategies and detection of bias. Acad. Emerg. Med. 9, 1184–1204.

Croskerry, P., 2003a. Cognitive forcing strategies in clinical decision-making. Ann. Emerg. Med. 41, 110–120.

Croskerry, P., 2003b. The importance of cognitive errors in diagnosis and strategies to minimize them. Acad. Med. 78, 775–780.

Croskerry, P., 2009a. A universal model of diagnostic reasoning. Acad. Med. 84, 1022–1028.

Croskerry, P., 2009b. Cognitive and effective dispositions to respond. In: Croskerry, P., Cosby, K., Schenkel, S., et al. (Eds.), Patient Safety in Emergency Medicine. Lippincott Williams & Wilkins, Philadelphia, PA, pp. 219–227.

Croskerry, P., Abbass, A., Wu, A.W., 2010. Emotional influences in patient safety. J. Patient Saf. 6, 199–205.

Croskerry, P., Singhal, G., Mamede, S., 2013. Cognitive debiasing 2: impediments to and strategies for change. BMJ Qual. Saf. 22, ii65–ii72.

Dalton, A.L., 1996. Enhancing critical thinking in paramedic continuing education. Prehosp. Disaster Med. 11, 246–253.

Dyson, K., Bray, J., Smith, K., et al., 2015. Paramedic exposure to out-of-hospital cardiac arrest is rare and declining in Victoria, Australia. Resuscitation 89, 93–98.

Elstein, A.S., Schwarz, A., 2002. Clinical problem solving and diagnostic decision making: selective review of the cognitive literature. BMJ 324, 729–732.

Epstein, R.M., Hundert, E.M., 2002. Defining and assessing professional competence. JAMA 287, 226–235.

Evans, J.S.B., 2003. In two minds: dual-process accounts of reasoning. Trends Cogn. Sci. 7, 454–459.

Graber, M.L., 2009. Educational strategies to reduce diagnostic error: can you teach this stuff? Adv. Health Sci. Educ. Theory Pract. 14, 63–69.

Janing, J., 1994. Critical thinking: incorporation into the paramedic curriculum. Prehosp. Disaster Med. 9, 238–242.

Jensen, J.L., 2010. Paramedic clinical decision making, Master of Applied Health Services research thesis. Dalhousie University, Halifax, Nova Scotia.

Jensen, J.L., Bienkowski, A., Travers, A.H., et al., 2016. A survey to determine decision-making styles of working paramedics and student paramedics. CJEM 18, 213–222.

Kovacs, G., Croskerry, P., 1999. Clinical decision making: an emergency medicine perspective. Acad. Emerg. Med. 6, 947–952.

Lowthian, J.A., Jolley, D.J., Curtis, A.J., et al., 2011. The challenges of population ageing: accelerating demand for emergency ambulance services by older patients. 1995–2015. Med. J. Aust. 194, 574–578.

O'Hara, R., Johnson, M., Siriwardena, A.N., et al., 2015. A qualitative study of systemic influences on paramedic decision making: care transitions and patient safety. J. Health Serv. Res. Policy 20 (1 Suppl.), 45–53.

Shaban, R., Wyatt-Smith, C., Cumming, J., 2004. Uncertainty, error and risk in human clinical judgment: introductory theoretical frameworks in paramedic practice. J. Emerg. Primary Health Care 2, 1–12.

Sloman, S.A., 1996. The empirical case for two systems of reasoning. Psychol. Bull. 119, 3.

Weingart, S., 2009. Critical decision making in chaotic environments. In: Croskerry, P., Cosby, K., Schenkel, S., et al. (Eds.), Patient Safety in Emergency Medicine. Lippincott Williams & Wilkins, Philadelphia, PA, pp. 209–212.

28

CLINICAL DECISION MAKING IN OPTOMETRY

CATHERINE SUTTLE ■ CAROLINE FAUCHER

OPTOMETRY AND ITS SCOPE OF PRACTICE

According to the World Council of Optometry, 'Optometry is a healthcare profession that is autonomous, educated, and regulated (licensed/registered) and optometrists are the primary healthcare practitioners of the eye and visual system who provide comprehensive eye and vision care, which includes refraction and dispensing, detection/diagnosis and management of disease in the eye and the rehabilitation of conditions of the visual system'.[i]

Optometry's scope of practice varies around the world and even within provinces or states of the same country. This variation results, in part, from the fact that in some geographical locations (e.g., Australia and the United Kingdom) scope of practice has increased considerably over time to a level at which the optometrist's role includes the prescription of therapeutic drugs to treat eye disease (Cooper, 2012; Harper et al., 2016; Kiely and Slater, 2015), and in others scope of practice is limited to the provision of spectacles (European Council of Optometry and Optics, 2015). Comprehensive routine eye and vision examinations remain the main reason to visit an optometrist (American Optometric Association, 2015; Boadi-Kusi et al., 2015; Thite et al., 2015). Although the optometrist's role varies globally, a comprehensive eye and vision examination includes evaluation of the functional status of the eyes and visual system, assessment of ocular health conditions, establishment of diagnoses, formulation of a treatment and a management plan and counselling and education of the patient regarding his or her visual and ocular healthcare status (American Optometric Association, 2015). The nature of the eye and vision system is such that many conditions have similar symptoms. Moreover, in asymptomatic patients, comprehensive

---

[i]http://www.worldoptometry.org/en/about-wco/who-is-an-optometrist/index.cfm

routine optometric examinations can lead to the detection of a significant number of new eye conditions (including a change in spectacle prescription and new critical diagnosis) and/or result in management changes (Dobbelsteyn et al., 2015; Irving et al., 2016). Therefore an eye and vision examination can rarely be driven only by the patient's symptoms (problem-oriented examination). It is rather a thorough investigation of many aspects of vision and eye health (systems examination), embedded in a routine but flexible protocol.

Fig. 28.1 shows two formats that an optometric examination can take, according to the main reason for the encounter. Optometrists have their habitual routine of examination in which they review the oculovisual systems: visual function, refraction, binocular vision and ocular health (Elliott, 2014). Of course, history taking is vital, as many patients presenting for a routine eye examination without initially reporting any complaints finally declare some vision or eye-related symptoms when questioned specifically by their optometrist (Webb et al., 2013). When patients present complex clinical features, optometrists deviate from their routine according to each clinical situation. They are planning, on an ongoing basis, what they will be doing later during the encounter (Faucher et al., 2012). Because a routine optometric examination often leads to incidental findings that were not indicated by the initial reason for the visit, optometrists have to balance the importance of the examination's incidental findings and the patient's

expectations or concerns. For example, a patient comes to change her spectacles, but the optometrist uncovers an unsuspected eye disease needing an urgent referral to a specialist. This is a potential site of tension between the patient's and optometrist's respective agendas (Varpio et al., 2007).

This routine aspect of the optometric profession has aspects in common with some health professions, such as dentistry. Traditional medical textbooks describe very detailed and systematic physical examination of each organ system. Mostly used by students, the value of such a systematic database examination is questioned by some authors, who state that it divorces data collection from clinical reasoning (Benbassat et al., 2005) and that it may be impractical in clinical settings where time is of the essence (Elliott, 2014; Ramani, 2008). Thus most published papers or books specifically dedicated to clinical reasoning focus on managing ill patients or patients presenting with problems/complaints.

Despite several decades of research on decision making and clinical reasoning in many healthcare professions, optometry remains underrepresented, and the clinical decision making literature in optometry is largely focussed on evidence-based practice and the effect of training and guidelines (Myint et al., 2014). Only a few articles have specifically focussed on optometrists' or optometry students' clinical reasoning (Corliss, 1995; Faucher et al., 2012; Faucher et al., 2016; Kurtz, 1990; Werner, 1989). This chapter provides an

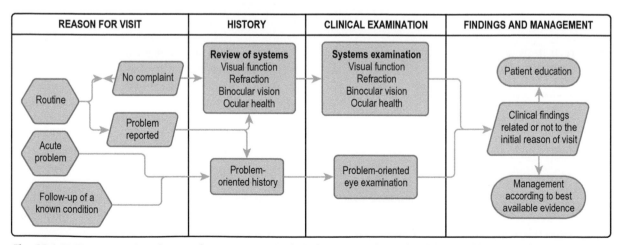

Fig. 28.1 ■ Two categories of reason for an optometric clinical encounter (a routine visit or a visit to investigate an acute or ongoing condition) and the type of investigation related to each.

overview of decision making and clinical reasoning in optometry.

EVIDENCE-BASED DECISION MAKING IN OPTOMETRY

Clinical reasoning requires critical thinking, and the two concepts are related but distinct. Critical thinking is a way of thinking that is free from bias, suspends judgement and considers different perspectives. It requires not only skills but also an attitude, such that the critical thinker approaches ideas and concepts without bias (da Silva Bastos Cerullo and de Almeida Lopes Monteiro da Cruz, 2010). Clinical reasoning requires this approach in addition to clinical knowledge and information from a wide range of sources. The patient's signs, symptoms, preferences and circumstances are used in addition to knowledge and information from education, colleagues, research and other sources to make a clinical decision with the patient. The use of experience and information from a range of sources is captured by the concept of evidence-based practice (EBP), which combines three key factors used in clinical decision making: the practitioner's experience, the patient's circumstances and preferences and the best available evidence from research (Dawes et al., 2005; Sackett et al., 1996). The clinical decision is made in the environmental context of the practice (Satterfield et al., 2009), so the process may be affected by factors such as Internet access, practice policy and attitudes of colleagues within the practice. Fig. 28.2 illustrates this model, with three key factors contributing to decision making.

Viewed from this perspective, it is clear that the quality of clinical decision making depends on the quality of any evidence used. For some clinical questions, research evidence may not be available at all, and in such cases the clinical decision is not informed by research. For those clinical questions with relevant research evidence, the optometrist must be aware of its validity or strength, including its relevance and clinical significance for the patient concerned. The model shown in Fig. 28.2 includes the patient's preferences and circumstances, indicating that these should be taken into account in decision making and that the reliability and clinical significance of any evidence should be discussed with the patient so that the patient and practitioner

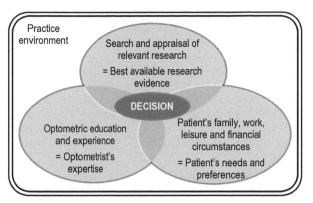

Fig. 28.2 ■ The connection between three key factors in evidence-based clinical decision making: the practitioner's expertise, the patient's preferences and the best available evidence. The decision is made in the clinical environment, which may limit or facilitate the extent to which best evidence is used. (Based on Satterfield, J.M., Spring, B., Brownson, R.C., Mullen, E.J., Newhouse, R.P., Walker, B.B., et al., 2009. Toward a transdisciplinary model of evidence-based practice. Milbank Q. 87, 368–390. Fig. 5, with permission.)

make an informed clinical decision in the context of that patient's situation.

Evidence and Its Quality

Hierarchies of evidence present 'levels' of evidence, showing nonresearch sources such as advice from colleagues as low level, with case studies just higher than this and with randomized controlled trials and systematic reviews of evidence at higher levels, as illustrated in Table 28.1. This hierarchy reflects the fact that sources such as case studies present us with evidence based on only one or a small number of patients and with results that may be unlikely to apply to our patient. In addition, intervention studies in which the researcher and/or patient is aware of the intervention and expected outcome are subject to bias, and randomized controlled trials are important to account for this and to provide more reliable evidence of the efficacy of interventions.

In addition to the level of evidence, the quality of evidence should be rated by critical appraisal, looking for indicators of bias. This can be achieved using critical appraisal tools (CATs) such as those made freely available by the Critical Appraisal Skills Programme (CASP, no date). Critical appraisal of this kind is important because a high-level (e.g., randomized controlled) study may

| | TABLE 28.1 | |
| | **Levels of Evidence** | |
Level	Form of Evidence	Description and Examples
High ↑	Systematic review of evidence with or without meta-analysis; Evidence-based synopsis of research	Review of research using a wide literature search and a set of criteria to judge research quality. A meta-analysis combines research findings to find a pooled estimate of effect from a large sample.
	Treatment trial with randomization and control	Research in which patients have been randomly allocated to treatment and control groups.
↓	Treatment trial without control group or with historical control; Case-control study; Cohort study	Research in which the sample size may be adequate but the control is not, or research in which control is not included as part of the study design (e.g., a cohort study).
Low	Individual case study or small case series	A report of clinical findings in one or a small number of patients.
	Recommendation from expert	Advice from a respected colleague, a seminar speaker or author of a CET article.

CASE STUDY 28.1

Evidence for CDM

Mark is an adult with amblyopia who has found a possible treatment on a website. He tells you that the treatment is a special pair of glasses with flickering coloured lights presented to either eye. The website suggests a high likelihood of successful treatment of amblyopia, and Mark would like to know whether this is worth trying. Your search for research evidence using PubMed and Google Scholar using appropriate key words finds no relevant research. You then access the website Mark was talking about and find no references to research on this method. How do you manage this situation?

be in some cases of poor quality, perhaps caused by inadequate control or a lack of masking. Studies described in scientific journals have generally been through a process of peer review, in which a number of experts (usually two) in the area have read the article and provided feedback before publication. It might be supposed that the articles passing this process are providing good quality evidence, but it is important to realize that this is not a safe assumption (Henderson, 2010; Smith, 2006). Quality and reliability should be gauged by the practitioner's own critical appraisal and to some extent on the basis of the level and type of evidence. For example, a systematic review has been generated by a process designed to minimize bias and is likely to provide more reliable evidence than a traditional literature review (though as outlined earlier in the chapter, the method followed in a particular review may be flawed, and this would be determined by critical appraisal).

As outlined earlier in the chapter, for some clinical questions, there may be no research evidence at all, or the research evidence may be of poor quality. To illustrate these situations and their implications for clinical decision making, Case Studies 28.1 and 28.2 show hypothetical clinical scenarios in which the practitioner finds no evidence (Case Study 28.1) or high-level evidence (Case Study 28.2). The resulting recommendation to the patient is discussed briefly in the following section.

In Case Study 28.1, because there is no research evidence, the practitioner must base clinical decision making on information from other sources, experience and existing knowledge, in addition to the patient's preferences. The practitioner advises the patient that although there is no evidence that the method will be harmful, there is also no reliable evidence that this treatment will be effective. In Case Study 28.2, research evidence indicates that dietary supplementation with omega 3 fatty acids has no effect on progression of the disease. The evidence is high level, and quality is likely to be high because it has been generated using a method that minimizes bias. Thus the patient can be

Basing CDM and Client Advice on Evidence

Karen is a 75-year-old patient with mild age-related macular degeneration. She has heard that progression can be slowed by increasing dietary intake of omega 3 fatty acids and asks whether this is correct. A search of the PubMed database and the Cochrane Database of Systematic Reviews finds that high-level evidence (a Cochrane systematic review) is available on this particular clinical topic. It indicates that dietary supplementation with omega 3 fatty acids has no effect on progression of the disease. What advice do you offer Karen?

---

advised that this evidence is likely to be reliable and that the supplementation is unlikely to affect disease progression.

Basis of Optometrists' Clinical Decision Making

Optometrists, as with all other healthcare practitioners, have access to a plethora of information on which clinical decisions could potentially be based. Some of this information is presented to them in the form of continuing education lectures or articles or marketing information on the use of certain diagnostic or therapeutic tools or interventions. Other information is not presented but is available for the practitioner to obtain, such as advice from colleagues, research-based information in peer-reviewed journals and information in books or other journals. Sources such as CET lectures, articles and books are likely to be research based, at least in part, but are unlikely to present full research details and are therefore not readily open to appraisal by the optometrist.

The sources of information used by nurses and other healthcare practitioners have been identified in a number of research studies. These have demonstrated that nurses tend to consult colleagues, particularly those who they perceive to be experts who are credible and trustworthy (Marshall et al., 2013), rather than directly accessing and appraising research (e.g., Clarke et al., 2013). In optometry, the basis of decision making has been explored by a small number of studies. In a questionnaire-based study, Suttle et al. (2012) asked 3589 registered optometrists in Australia and New Zealand about the sources of information they use as a basis for clinical decision making. 279 (8%) responded (note that a low response rate reduces the quality of this evidence, but because there is little available on this issue it is part of the best available evidence base). Respondents were presented with 11 potential sources of information and were asked to rank these in order of importance as a basis for clinical decision making. More than three-quarters ranked undergraduate education highly, as the first, second or third most important of these sources, and almost four-fifths ranked postgraduate/continuing education at one of these levels, indicating that this sample relies heavily on information gained from undergraduate or postgraduate/continuing education. The questionnaire also asked whether respondents had modified their clinical practice within the past 2 years in the light of new information and, if so, to state the source of the information. 85% of respondents had modified their practice, and more than one-half of these did so based on information from a continuing education seminar. These findings demonstrate that, at least in this Australasian sample, optometrists rely on information provided to them by presenters of continuing, postgraduate or undergraduate education. This information is provided through the filter of the educator and may not be critically appraised. The practitioner receiving and using this information may assume that it is of high quality, but this may not be the case.

In a United Kingdom–based study, Lawrenson and Evans (2013) invited 8735 optometrists to complete a questionnaire on dietary and lifestyle advice for patients with or at risk of age-related macular degeneration, and 1414 responses were received (16% response rate). The questionnaire asked about the sources of evidence used as a basis for advice to patients about nutritional supplements, and there were 1196 responses to this question. Optometrists frequently cited professional magazines (with non–peer-reviewed articles) as sources of evidence. These findings further demonstrate that optometrists tend to depend on sources other than peer-reviewed published research.

The fact that a high proportion of optometrists, at least in these samples, say that they are using information from undergraduate, postgraduate, continuing education and professional magazines as a basis for their clinical decision making suggests that this is not seen as problematic by those practitioners. However, as outlined earlier in the chapter, that information is provided through the filter of the educator or writer, and the practitioner cannot easily determine whether it is up to date or reliable. Peer-reviewed, published research is preferable as a source of evidence because the practitioner can appraise it and gauge its quality before applying it as part of decision making. Intuitively, it seems that the use of more reliable evidence would lead to better patient outcomes, because flawed evidence (e.g., wrongly suggesting high efficacy of a treatment method) would be identified as low quality and treated as such by the practitioner. Surprisingly, to date there is little high-level evidence on the relationship between evidence-based practice and patient outcomes. A number of studies, however, have demonstrated lower patient mortality with evidence-based practice (involving the use of best available evidence) than with standard practice (e.g., Emparanza et al., 2015). There is not yet, to our knowledge, any such evidence on the effectiveness of evidence-based practice in eye care, but the evidence in medicine cited earlier in the chapter does suggest that the practice has a positive effect on health outcomes, and optometry seems unlikely to be an exception.

Finding and appraising evidence may not be feasible within a clinical encounter, and indeed a lack of time is a major barrier to evidence-based practice in optometry (Alnahedh et al., 2015). Resources that may help to reduce this barrier include systematic reviews focussed on clinical questions, such as those available from the Cochrane Eyes and Vision Group (eyes.cochrane.org) and the Translating Research into Practice (TRIP) database, which provides an indication of the level of research evidence relevant to given key words (www.tripdatabase.com). Databases providing free access to preappraised evidence are available for some health disciplines (e.g., speechbite.com for speech pathology) but not yet for optometry. Evidence-based clinical guidelines such as those provided by the College of

Optometrists[ii] provide advice based on the best available evidence relevant to certain eye conditions but do not address a wide range of clinical scenarios. The National Institute for Health and Care Excellence (NICE)[iii] in the UK provides evidence-based guidance relevant to the investigation and management of a range of conditions, but many optometric clinical encounters would have no relevant guidelines or guidance. Given this situation, in which the practitioner is faced with a number of barriers to finding and appraising evidence within the clinical encounter, evidence-based practice requires search and appraisal that occurs to some extent outside of the clinic. The practitioner should, for example, use critical thinking skills to consider the evidence presented in CET seminars or articles, where full details are not usually provided but the recipient of this evidence can find and appraise evidence based on the topic and any clinical claims. In addition, it may be possible in some cases to anticipate clinical questions, such as asking whether a new intervention is effective or whether a new diagnostic method has high sensitivity. Thus barriers such as time do limit the extent to which the optometrist can apply EBP, but resources may help and strategies can be adopted to ensure that the practitioner is aware of the best evidence relevant to at least some clinical encounters.

FROM DECISION MAKING TO CLINICAL REASONING

The decision-making theory was originally a model of idealized rationality (Elstein, 2000), which could be seen as a prescriptive approach telling practitioners how they should make decisions based on probabilities and statistics. As outlined earlier in the chapter, decisions in the clinical situation need to call on knowledge of the best available evidence, and this may need to be sourced and appraised in anticipation, caused by time limitations in the clinic. It is important to note that patients rarely come with classic textbook characteristics. For example, it may be difficult to identify the cause of vision loss, particularly if a patient is seen for the first time: is the loss caused by amblyopia, worsening

[ii]http://www.college-optometrists.org/en/professional-standards/clinical_management_guidelines/index.cfm

[iii]https://www.nice.org.uk/

TABLE 28.2		
Uncertainty in Optometric Clinical Decision Making		
Source of Uncertainty	**Examples or Explanations**	**Strategies for Addressing It**
Limited availability of clinical information	Special populations (limited patient's ability to respond to testing) Invasive procedures (if risks outweigh benefits)	Be familiar with special testing procedures Consider alternative strategies
Limited quality of information	Unreliable responses from patients	Ensure the patient understands Repeat or clarify the directions Use alternative tests
Limited ability to gather definitive information	It is physically impossible to inspect directly every part of the body (e.g., optic chiasm)	Stay up to date Acquire specialized equipment if possible Consider patient referral for certain types of testing
Ambiguity in interpreting clinical data	Reliable data may be subject to interpretation	Consider closer follow-ups Combine multiple tests
Uncertainty in patients' responses to treatment	Efficacy of treatment varies among patients and for the same patient on a different period of time	Monitor patients' response to treatment over time Educate patient about side effects
Examiners' uncertainty	Optometrist's own confidence in generating hypotheses, gathering and analyzing data, making diagnoses and choosing treatment plans	Monitor successful cases Reinforce knowledge by additional training, reading and continual education Solicit feedback from clinical experts

of a retinal disease or a developing cataract? A combination of multiple conditions may complicate the diagnosis. The frequent need for subjective responses from patients also influences clinical results and may render data harder to interpret. Ettinger (1997) has identified six sources of uncertainty in optometry. They are provided in Table 28.2 with examples and strategies for addressing them.

It becomes obvious that, to address those multiple sources of uncertainty in clinical practice, optometrists will have to mobilize several resources (including their own knowledge) and exercise judicious and efficient clinical reasoning.

Scripts Formation and Activation

It is often claimed that the structure of knowledge in memory plays a central role in clinical reasoning. Originating from cognitive psychology, the script theory of reasoning provides a theoretical framework to illustrate how knowledge can be structured for clinical problem solving (Charlin et al., 2000). Scripts are cognitive structures stored in the memory. They contain a complex network of meaningful links among clinical features

(e.g., enabling conditions, causes and consequences of specific diseases or anomalies) that allow a healthcare practitioner to resolve clinical problems, via diagnosis, investigation or treatment. Scripts develop progressively by applying knowledge through regular practice with patients. To take an example: students in optometry with no clinical experience with glaucomatous patients do possess theoretical (pathophysiological) knowledge about concepts such as physiology of the aqueous humour; intraocular pressure; ocular anatomy; vascularization of the eye; and perception, perimetry and pharmacology. Once in clinical settings, students gradually reorganize what they know about glaucoma into a series of scripts. Meaningful links are created between various bits of information, particularly with regard to diagnosis and treatment. Students' growing experience with diverse cases of glaucoma (various presentations, degrees of severity, rates of progression and responses to treatment) helps them internalize many examples of glaucoma, which enrich any glaucoma script they have already stored. Later, when experienced optometrists recognize cases of glaucoma (script activation), the knowledge required for appropriate case management comes to mind: they will have no need to retrieve pathophysiological details from their long-term memory (Faucher et al., 2016). Keeping up to date with evolving research evidence can also contribute to underpin optometrists' scripts.

Dual-Process Reasoning

Given the multifaceted, complex context of practice, and the constantly evolving field of practice, how do optometrists actually reason during an optometric encounter? Unfortunately, only a few investigators have studied clinical reasoning in optometry. Some authors have adapted medical models to the optometry profession (Corliss, 1995; Ettinger and Rouse, 1997; Kurtz, 1990; Werner, 1989) without conducting any research involving practicing optometrists. Part of the answer may be found in work by Faucher et al. (2012). They have conducted a qualitative study aiming to make explicit the clinical reasoning processes of optometrists from two contrasting levels of professional development and to highlight the characteristics of clinical reasoning expertise in optometry. Their results are consistent with the script theory of reasoning on several points. They show that optometrists quickly construct a mental representation of the patient's clinical situation (activation of relevant scripts). Through hypothetico-deductive reasoning, optometrists also anticipate clinical findings throughout the encounter and constantly readjust their initial mental representation of the clinical situation based on any additional clinical findings. According to the script theory of reasoning, this corresponds to the assessment of a fit between activated scripts and the clinical situation (Charlin et al., 2000). Finally, optometrists formulate their management and treatment plan throughout the encounter, not just at the end of it.

These findings show that clinical reasoning in optometry is also consistent with the dual-process theory of reasoning, originating from the cognitive psychology literature (Wason and Evans, 1975) and more recently proposed to describe clinical reasoning processes (Marcum, 2012; Pelaccia et al., 2011). According to the dual-process theory, clinical reasoning is a multidimensional and complex process involving both nonanalytic and analytic cognitive processes. Nonanalytic processes include tacit or intuitive knowledge, relying on a clinician's previous experience. They are used in an unconscious manner: the clinician automatically recognizes a configuration of signs and symptoms. For example,

an optometrist can suspect hyperopia and esotropia as soon as a patient walks in simply by noticing that the patient's spectacles have a magnifying effect on his or her eyes. Analytic processes represent critical thinking and objective analysis that are deliberate and reflective. In the same example, analytic processes will be necessary to put together the clinical findings (patient's history, visual function, refraction, binocular vision, ocular health) to confirm – or not – the presence of hyperopia and esotropia and to make decisions based on the patient's conditions and needs. Analytic and nonanalytic processes are actually intertwined in clinical practice, working in synergy to rapidly understand a clinical situation, investigate further and make the appropriate decisions for a given patient.

CONCLUSION

Optometrists are primary providers of comprehensive eye and vision care. They usually follow a routine but flexible sequence of examination. Any clinical finding – within normal limits or not – triggers the activation of clinical reasoning processes and leads to the understanding of the clinical situation as a whole. Because of time constraints, finding and appraising evidence often have to occur outside of the clinical encounter. Clinical reasoning then helps practitioners to make judgements about the relevance of particular research and clinical evidence for a specific clinical situation (Higgs et al., 2001). Clinical knowledge, which is essential to clinical reasoning, is constantly enriched by every clinical situation and updated by applying evolving research evidence. Studies suggest, however, that optometrists mostly base their clinical decisions on information from undergraduate, postgraduate and continuing education, rather than on peer-reviewed published research. Further research is needed to assess the effectiveness of evidence-based practice in optometry and to better understand the clinical reasoning processes, which are essential to optometrists' actions.

CHAPTER SUMMARY

In this chapter, we have outlined that:

- optometrists are comprehensive eye and vision care providers who have seen their scope of practice expand considerably over time,

- clinical decision-making literature in optometry is largely focussed on evidence-based practice, guidelines and the effect of training,
- optometrists do not base their decisions on peer-reviewed published research as much as they could do,
- optometrists' clinical reasoning is consistent with both the dual-process and the script theories of reasoning and
- evidence-based practice, decision making and clinical reasoning need to be investigated further specifically for the optometry profession.

REFLECTION POINT 1

As the scope of practice in optometry increases and optometrists take on more responsibility, there is an urgent need to ensure that the clinical reasoning involved in practice and education is as rigorous as it can be.

REFERENCES

Alnahedh, T., Suttle, C.M., Alabdelmoneam, M., et al., 2015. Optometrists show rudimentary understanding of evidence-based practice but are ready to embrace it: can barriers be overcome? Clin. Exp. Optom. 98, 263–272.

American Optometric Association, 2015. Evidence-Based Clinical Practice Guideline: Comprehensive Adult Eye and Vision Examination. American Optometric Association, St. Louis, MO.

Benbassat, J., Baumal, R., Heyman, S.N., et al., 2005. Viewpoint: suggestions for a shift in teaching clinical skills to medical students: the reflective clinical examination. Acad. Med. 80, 1121–1126.

Boadi-Kusi, S.B., Ntodie, M., Mashige, K.P., et al., 2015. A cross-sectional survey of optometrists and optometric practices in Ghana. Clin. Exp. Optom. 98, 473–477.

Charlin, B., Tardif, J., Boshuizen, H.P., 2000. Scripts and medical diagnostic knowledge: theory and applications for clinical reasoning instruction and research. Acad. Med. 75, 182–190.

Clarke, M.A., Belden, J.L., Koopman, R.J., et al., 2013. Information needs and information-seeking behaviour analysis of primary care physicians and nurses: a literature review. Health Info. Libr. J. 30, 178–190.

Cooper, S.L., 2012. 1971–2011: forty year history of scope expansion into medical eye care. Optometry 83, 64–73.

Corliss, D.A., 1995. A comprehensive model of clinical decision making. J. Am. Optom. Assoc. 66, 362–371.

Critical Appraisal Skills Programme (CASP), n.d. Viewed 25 January 2017. Available from: www.casp-uk.net.

da Silva Bastos Cerullo, J.A., de Almeida Lopes Monteiro da Cruz, D., 2010. Clinical reasoning and critical thinking. Rev. Lat. Am. de Enfermagem 18, 124–129.

Dawes, M., Summerskill, W., Glasziou, P., et al., 2005. Sicily statement on evidence-based practice. BMC Med. Educ. 5, 1.

Dobbelsteyn, D., McKee, K., Bearnes, R.D., et al., 2015. What percentage of patients presenting for routine eye examinations require referral for secondary care? a study of referrals from optometrists to ophthalmologists. Clin. Exp. Optom. 98, 214–217.

Elliott, D.B., 2014. Evidence-based eye examinations. In: Elliott, D.B. (Ed.), Clinical Procedures in Primary Eye Care. Elsevier Saunders, Philadelphia, PA, pp. 1–12.

Elstein, A.S., 2000. Clinical problem solving and decision psychology: comment on 'the epistemology of clinical reasoning'. Acad. Med. 75 (10 Suppl.), S134–S136.

Emparanza, J.I., Cabello, J.B., Burls, A.J., 2015. Does evidence-based practice improve patient outcomes? an analysis of a natural experiment in a Spanish hospital. J. Eval. Clin. Pract. 21, 1059–1065.

Ettinger, E.R., 1997. Dealing with clinical uncertainty. In: Ettinger, E.R., Rouse, M.W. (Eds.), Clinical Decision Making in Optometry. Butterworth-Heinemann, Boston, MA, pp. 39–64.

Ettinger, E.R., Rouse, M.W. (Eds.), 1997. Clinical Decision Making in Optometry. Butterworth-Heinemann, Boston, MA.

European Council of Optometry and Optics (ECOO), 2015. ECOO blue book, ECOO, Brussels, Belgium. Viewed 1 June 2017. Available from: http://www.ecoo.info/about-optics-and-optometry/.

Faucher, C., Dufour-Guindon, M.P., Lapointe, G., et al., 2016. Assessing clinical reasoning in optometry using the Script Concordance Test. Clin. Exp. Optom. 99, 280–286.

Faucher, C., Tardif, J., Chamberland, M., 2012. Optometrists' clinical reasoning made explicit: a qualitative study. Optom. Vis. Sci. 89, 1774–1784.

Harper, R., Creer, R., Jackson, J., et al., 2016. Scope of practice of optometrists working in the UK Hospital Eye Service: a national survey. Ophthalmic Physiol. Opt. 36, 197–206.

Henderson, M., 2010. Problems with peer review. BMJ 340, 1409.

Higgs, J., Burn, A., Jones, M., 2001. Integrating clinical reasoning and evidence-based practice. AACN Clin. Issues 12, 482–490.

Irving, E.L., Harris, J.D., Machan, C.M., et al., 2016. Value of routine eye examinations in asymptomatic patients. Optom. Vis. Sci. 93, 660–666.

Kiely, P.M., Slater, J., 2015. Optometry Australia entry-level competency standards for optometry 2014. Clin. Exp. Optom. 98, 65–89.

Kurtz, D., 1990. Teaching clinical reasoning. J. Optom. Educ. 15, 119–122.

Lawrenson, J.G., Evans, J.R., 2013. Advice about diet and smoking for people with or at risk of age-related macular degeneration: a cross-sectional survey of eye care professionals in the UK. BMC Public Health 13, 564.

Marcum, J.A., 2012. An integrated model of clinical reasoning: dual-process theory of cognition and metacognition. J. Eval. Clin. Pract. 18, 954–961.

Marshall, A.P., West, S.H., Aitken, L.M., 2013. Clinical credibility and trustworthiness are key characteristics used to identify colleagues from whom to seek information. J. Clin. Nurs. 22, 1424–1433.

Myint, J., Edgar, D.F., Murdoch, I.E., et al., 2014. The impact of postgraduate training on UK optometrists: clinical decision-making in glaucoma. Ophthalmic Physiol. Opt. 34, 376–384.

Pelaccia, T., Tardif, J., Triby, E., et al., 2011. An analysis of clinical reasoning through a recent and comprehensive approach: the dual-process theory. Medical Education Online 16, 5890.

Ramani, S., 2008. Twelve tips for excellent physical examination teaching. Med. Teach. 30, 851–856.

Sackett, D.L., Rosenberg, W.M., Gray, J.A., et al., 1996. Evidence based medicine: what it is and what it isn't. BMJ 312, 71–72.

Satterfield, J.M., Spring, B., Brownson, R.C., et al., 2009. Toward a transdisciplinary model of evidence-based practice. Milbank Q. 87, 368–390.

Smith, R., 2006. Peer review: a flawed process at the heart of science and journals. J. R. Soc. Med. 99, 178–182.

Suttle, C., Jalbert, I., Alnahedh, T., 2012. Examining the evidence base used by optometrists in Australia and New Zealand. Clin. Exp. Optom. 95, 28–36.

Thite, N., Jaggernath, J., Chinanayi, F., et al., 2015. Pattern of optometry practice and range of services in India. Optom. Vis. Sci. 92, 615–622.

Varpio, L., Spafford, M.M., Schryer, C.F., et al., 2007. Seeing and listening: a visual and social analysis of optometric record-keeping practices. J. Bus. Tech. Commun 21, 343–375.

Wason, P.C., Evans, J.S.B.T., 1975. Dual processes in reasoning. Cognition 3, 141–154.

Webb, H., vom Lehn, D., Heath, C., et al., 2013. The problem with 'problems': the case of openings in optometry consultations. Res. Lang. Soc. Interact 46, 65–83.

Werner, D.L., 1989. Teaching clinical thinking. Optom. Vis. Sci. 66, 788–792.

29

CLINICAL REASONING IN DIETETICS

RUTH VO ■ MEGAN SMITH ■ NARELLE PATTON

CHAPTER AIMS

The aims of this chapter are to:

■ describe what is known of clinical reasoning within dietetics as portrayed in contemporary literature and

■ illuminate the sociocultural and physical context of dietetics reasoning through descriptions of the dietetic profession including practice models and roles and physical practice settings.

KEY WORDS

Clinical reasoning

Collaborative decision making

Critical thinking

Dietetics

ABBREVIATIONS/ ACRONYMS

DAA Dietitians Association of Australia

NCPM Nutrition Care Process model

CDM Collaborative decision making

INTRODUCTION

A dietitian is a qualified healthcare professional who 'applies the science of nutrition to the feeding and education of individuals or groups in health and disease' (International Confederation of Dietetic Associations, 2004, p. 3). This application of the science of nutrition in clinical situations is underpinned by dietitians' clinical reasoning capabilities. Clinical reasoning is considered to be an essential component of dietetic clinical practice (Gates, 1992). Clinical reasoning has been described as the way a practitioner thinks in a particular context, including the use of knowledge, reasoning and meta-cognition at micro, macro and meta levels and may be undertaken individually or collaboratively (Higgs and Jones, 2008). Shared or collaborative decision making between practitioners and patients has been described as providing an additional dimension to this clinical reasoning framework (Higgs and Jones, 2008; Trede and Higgs, 2003). Interestingly, this highlights an important need to distinguish between *clinical reasoning* and *clinical decision making*. In the literature, these two terms are often used interchangeably, which can cause misunderstanding. Therefore in this chapter we have chosen to distinguish between these terms and identify clinical decision making as the process by which decisions are made. Clinical reasoning is the broader phenomenon that involves decision making but includes contextual factors such as the affordances and restrictions of the clinical environment, the patients' values and desires and what the clinicians themselves can bring to these settings.

Effective clinical reasoning capability enables dietitians to make appropriate decisions regarding patients' overall nutritional status and nutritional management plans and being able to monitor and review patient progress effectively. Thus clinical reasoning is key to achieving optimum outcomes for patients. Currently, dietitian-specific literature around clinical reasoning is limited. Therefore this chapter draws heavily upon clinical reasoning literature from related health professions and translates this knowledge to dietetic practice.

THE CONTEXT OF DIETETICS

Dietetics is a relatively young and evolving profession (Calabro et al., 2001). The past 50 years has seen dietetics move away from its roots in home economics. As a consequence, this move has led to a clear diversification of the dietitian's role (Erickson-Weerts, 1999). Dietitians' roles have come to include practice areas such as:

- clinical dietetics – inpatient and outpatient,
- clinical nutrition – long-term care,
- food and nutrition management,
- community and public health management,
- private consultation and business and
- education and research (Hooker et al., 2012).

To work as a dietitian in most countries requires tertiary undergraduate and/or postgraduate education in nutrition and dietetics that has been recognized by a national authority (International Confederation of Dietetic Associations, 2004). In some countries this involves professional registration with a governing body, for example in New Zealand or the United Kingdom. However, even in some industrialized countries, such as Australia, the profession is yet to be fully recognized as an allied health profession as it has not been included in the recently constituted Australian Health Practitioner Regulation Agency. Instead, the Dietitians Association of Australia oversees dietitian education, with strict credentialing processes for university programs, completion of which certifies graduates as an Accredited Practising Dietitian. In some countries, like Australia, there is a distinction between dietitians and other occupations in the nutrition and food science field, including that of a nutritionist (Dietitians Association of Australia, 2017). Unlike a dietitian, a nutritionist does not have an industry-specific assessing authority of his or her qualifications and is not qualified to provide diet therapy to individuals or groups (Dietitians Association of Australia, 2017).

Dietitians' clinical reasoning is significantly shaped by the practice contexts in which they work. These practice contexts embrace both clinical (in hospitals and community) and public health settings (with a focus on preventive strategies). The different domains of nutrition service delivery in the Australian context have been defined, including clinical and community dietetics, community nutrition and public health nutrition (Hughes and Somerset, 1997). Hughes and Somerset defined clinical dietetics as 'the application of dietetics in hospital or health care institutional settings' and community dietetics as 'the application of dietetics in community settings, including continuity of care for discharged patient populations' (p. 41). Traditional understandings of clinical reasoning practices, involving interactions with individual clients, align well with the context of clinical and community dietetics. In these settings, dietitians have a role in making decisions about the nutritional concerns of patients and determining appropriate therapeutic protocols. This differs from community and public health nutrition service types, where the focus is on primary prevention strategies, such as influencing nutrition-related public policy, food supply, communities and populations (Hughes and Somerset, 1997).

Clinical dietetics is the largest practice area and includes assessing the nutritional needs of individual patients and planning appropriate nutrition therapy and education of patients and their families, mostly in the setting of a hospital or aged care facility. Dietitians in this area can work in either a specialized clinical area or maintain a broad scope of practice (O'Sullivan-Maillet, 2009). Clinical dietetics has evolved into a healthcare professional practice whose role now extends beyond diet prescription, advice and counselling for behaviour change to include provision of medical nutrition therapy. Medical nutrition therapy refers to the implementation of specific nutrition services to treat an illness, injury, or condition and involves assessment and treatment phases (American Dietetic Association, 1994).

Much of clinical dietetic practice occurs in hospitals, and these institutions provide an important physical and sociocultural context for the practice of clinical dietetics. Within these spaces, dietitians work with other dietitians, nurses, doctors, other allied healthcare practitioners, administrative support staff, patients, their families and carers. This means that the clinical reasoning of dietitians is complex and can involve interactions with all these people. This puts limits on the autonomy that dietitians can exercise in decision making. As an example, there are decisions that dietitians routinely make such as if, and what type of, oral nutrition support is provided. However, for interventions such as artificial nutrition, dietitians need to engage with, and often seek permission from, the treating medical team. This is in direct contrast to other allied healthcare professionals such as physiotherapists, speech pathologists and occupational therapists, who routinely use clinical reasoning to determine the most appropriate therapy interventions and then implement them autonomously, often without the need to gain permission. Many of the outcomes of dietitians' clinical reasoning, such as what interventions should be provided, are not independently enacted. For example, if a dietitian decides that a patient needs parenteral nutrition (intravenous nutrition), then a prescribing doctor, pharmacist, specialist nurse, ward nurse, treating team doctor and the patient are all involved in the process of making this happen. This example also reiterates the fact that much clinical reasoning in dietetics is collaborative with other healthcare professionals being involved.

REFLECTION POINT 1

Clinical reasoning in dietetics is largely influenced by physical and sociocultural contextual factors. Think about your most recent patient assessment, and identify how your clinical reasoning was influenced by contextual factors such as:
- degree of autonomy,
- who else was involved,
- available resources and
- how the patient made you feel.

How might these factors change your practice in the future?

CLINICAL REASONING IN CLINICAL DIETETICS

Clinical reasoning is core to the practice of clinical dietetics and underpins decision-making processes that allow identification and treatment of the nutritional concerns of patients. Building on Higgs and Jones (2008), we now explore three key dimensions involved in the clinical reasoning process in clinical dietetics. These are

the knowledge, cognition and metacognition required for clinical reasoning. There is currently no single encompassing framework for how dietitians integrate these components, so they are explored here individually in relation to dietetic practice as we understand it today.

Knowledge

Clinical decisions made in clinical dietetics rely upon strong nutrition and dietetic-specific knowledge. The knowledge categorization framework that includes propositional, professional craft and personal knowledge (Higgs and Titchen, 1995; Titchen and Ersser, 2001) provides a useful framework for understanding the forms of knowledge that inform the clinical decisions made by dietitians. Propositional knowledge used in dietetics includes a large volume of biomedical and technical information such as caloric value of nutrients, vitamin and mineral needs, digestion and metabolic processes and the nutrient composition of foods (Hwalla and Koleilat, 2004). Professional craft knowledge in dietetics is that knowledge gained from direct practice experience in and around patient care. For example, a dietitian can, through repeated exposure to patients who are experiencing certain gastrointestinal problems, develop the practical knowledge that high-fibre foods are generally less well tolerated than low-fibre foods in this particular patient group. Knowing and adapting to the common postoperative feeding practices of the gastrointestinal surgeon a dietitian may be working with is another example of professional craft knowledge. In dietetics, this personal knowledge, derived from direct experience with particular conditions, may have to be integrated with the customs and dietary trends of certain cultures. This integration can profoundly shape dietitians' clinical reasoning. This integration will also include evidence-based practice.

The emergence and dominance of evidence-based practice in many health professions highlight the privileged position of propositional knowledge in clinical reasoning. Evidence-based practice emerged initially in medicine in the 1980s and quickly evolved into a clinical reasoning model and focus for medicine (Sackett et al., 1996) and other health professions, including dietetics. This is perhaps unsurprising as evidence-based practice was viewed as a way to ensure the provision of safe and high-quality health care.

Evidence-based practice in dietetics reflects the integration of a broad range of information sources (usually scientific in nature) mediated by practitioner qualities. The International Confederation of Dietetic Associations put out a consensus statement acknowledging the key contribution of knowledge and evidence to clinical reasoning but also recognizing the importance of an individual dietitian's expertise and a client's unique values and circumstances:

> *'evidence-based practice is about asking questions, systematically finding research evidence, and assessing the validity, applicability and importance of that evidence. This evidence-based information is then combined with the dietitian's expertise and judgement and the client's or community's unique values and circumstances to guide decision-making in dietetics'*
>
> **(Maclellan and Thirsk, 2010, p. 2).**

The integration of propositional knowledge (the best available evidence) with the personal expertise of the clinician and the desires and values of the patient was put forward early in the move to evidence-based practice (Sackett et al., 1996). It can be argued that although other health professions seem to have forgotten the need for this integration, dietitians see it as important and a key aspect of clinical reasoning.

Cognition

For dietitians, cognition includes critical thinking skills such as analysis, synthesis and evaluation of data about a patient (Higgs and Jones, 2008). Critical thinking is integral to clinical reasoning that results in good patient care. The Nutrition and Dietetic Process (British Dietitians Association, 2016) highlights the central position of critical thinking to dietetic practice in its outline of the steps involved in the provision of nutrition intervention to patients: 1) assessment, 2) identification of nutrition and dietetic diagnosis, 3) plan nutrition and dietetic intervention, 4) implement nutrition and dietetic intervention, 5) monitor and review and 6) evaluation (Fig. 29.1). Within each of these steps, required critical thinking elements are described to carry out the step. For example, to complete an 'assessment', the dietitian needs to determine appropriate data to collect and how to collect it, validate the data, compare patient data with nutritional, biochemical and anthropometric standards

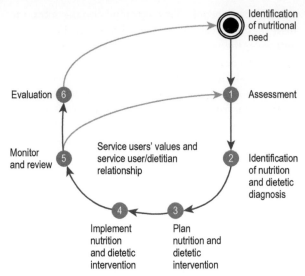

Fig. 29.1 ■ Process for nutrition and dietetic process. (From British Dietitians Association, 2016. Model and process for nutrition and dietetic practice. Viewed 16 February 2017. Available from: <https://www.bda.uk.com/publications/professional/model_and_process_for_nutrition_and_dietetic_practice_>, p. 6, with permission.)

and identify other healthcare professionals that may need to be consulted regarding the patient's nutritional problems (British Dietitians Association, 2016). Each step of the process requires critical thinking to effectively facilitate the nutritional care the patient requires. Although the Nutrition and Dietetic Process neatly lists the procedural components in clinical decision making, it does not explore how this integrates broader elements of clinical reasoning.

Critical thinking is an abstract concept that is difficult to quantify. However, one tool that has been used in dietetics that attempts to measure critical thinking is the California Critical Thinking Disposition Inventory (CCTDI) (Facione and Facione, 2001). This inventory describes seven different qualities that are associated with a critical thinking disposition (Facione and Facione, 2001):

- open-mindedness,
- inquisitiveness,
- truth seeking,
- analyticity,
- systematicity,
- confidence and
- cognitive maturity.

This tool highlights the importance of these qualities, and if we see clinical reasoning as a form of critical thinking, then they matter to all clinicians, not just dietitians.

There have been attempts to quantify the degree to which a group of student dietitians demonstrate critical thinking dispositions upon completing their clinical placement using the CCTDI (Schumacher, 2014). Answers for each quality were simply identified in three categories as weak, neither weak nor strong or strong. Only a few participants in this study demonstrated a strong critical thinking disposition. This study unfortunately did not offer any insights into what using critical thinking as clinical decision making actually looks like in a novice dietitian. There is clearly a need for further research focussing on critical thinking as an important component of a dietitian's clinical reasoning. For this, an acceptable model of clinical reasoning in dietetics would help.

In dietetic practice, recent development of the Nutrition Care Process Model (NCPM) has largely standardized the process and language of clinical reasoning (Bueche et al., 2008). The NCPM describes the steps a dietitian should take to identify and solve the nutritional problems of patients, regardless of context or setting, based on evidence-based practice. The four steps in this process involve:

- nutrition assessment,
- nutritional diagnosis,
- nutrition intervention and
- nutrition monitoring and evaluation or reevaluation (p. 1113).

The NCPM also includes contextual elements that influence the clinical reasoning process, including healthcare system, practice settings, social systems and economic systems. Central to the model is the relationship the dietitian has with the patient or client. This model introduces the language of medical practice when describing the step of determining a nutritional diagnosis and its aetiology together with measurable evidence or symptoms. Dietitians who do not use the NCPM still identify the key nutritional issues, but these are often labelled as their concluding 'assessment' or 'issue' rather than diagnosis. The NCPM aims to provide a means by which outcomes related to nutritional therapy can be monitored, measured and reported to either highlight or justify dietetic services. The NCPM recognizes some of the elements shown to be involved in clinical reasoning in other health professions such as critical thinking, evaluation, interpreting data, knowledge, skills, collaboration and ethics (Bueche et al., 2008). A critique of the NCPM is that it is similar to the Nutrition and Dietetics Process (British Dietitians Association, 2016) and provides limited insight into the complexity and dynamic nature of clinical reasoning in different contexts. Recognizing the importance of context can be seen as a part of metacognition and reflexivity.

Metacognition

This core dimension of clinical reasoning refers to the practitioner's reflective self-awareness, essentially his or her ability to critique his or her own thinking (Higgs and Jones, 2008). In the context of dietetics, this can relate to the dietitian knowing his or her professional and personal limitations with respect to knowledge and/or skills and then developing a strategy to rectify this. It is a cognitive capability that allows for ongoing evaluation of his or her own practice with a view to continue to improve his or her care for patients. The scarce evidence that exists about reflection and self-critique as part of dietetic practice is found mostly in the advanced practice literature and is seen as an attribute of an advanced practitioner (Bradley et al., 1993; Brody et al., 2012; Skipper and Lewis, 2007; Wildish and Evers, 2010). Advanced practitioners recognize the importance of collaborating closely with patients.

REFLECTION POINT 2

Practitioner reflexivity alongside other qualities and dispositions is core to developing expertise in clinical reasoning.

When you are working with patients do you:
- critique your own thinking, e.g., look for flaws in your logic or biases and assumptions;
- examine the influence you are having on your critical thinking, e.g., are you tired or distracted or lacking motivation;
- examine the degree of trust established with your patient and the consequent quality of the information being provided;
- identify environmental influences on your thinking, e.g., time constraints and high workloads leading to rushed assessment and treatment and

- identify sociocultural influences, e.g., how is your thinking shaped by expectations or needs of other staff members such as doctors or nurses?

COLLABORATIVE DECISION MAKING IN DIETETICS

Collaborative decision making (CDM) is sometimes referred to as shared decision making. This is a model of clinical reasoning that includes the patient in a two-way discussion leading to a decision made through mutual deliberation (Charles et al., 1999; Trede and Higgs, 2003). The CDM model has various elements in common with the NCPM such as the patient–clinician relationship being central to the process and the emphasis on collaboration and communication (Bueche et al., 2008). The focus of the available research on

communication in dietetics, such as Bueche et al. (2008), is on collaboration with patients.

One good example of research into collaboration and the clinical reasoning capabilities of dietitians is that of Olsen (2013). Her focus was on novice dietitians in rural Australia. She used hermeneutic phenomenology as the research framework. Olsen's results illuminated the core capabilities and conditions required for collaborative decision making (Fig. 29.2) and how these novice dietitians may have acquired these capabilities. Core capabilities that were shown to facilitate CDM were:

- developing self-awareness,
- building caring and trusting relationships,
- establishing and maintaining open and transparent dialogues,
- responding to the given situation,

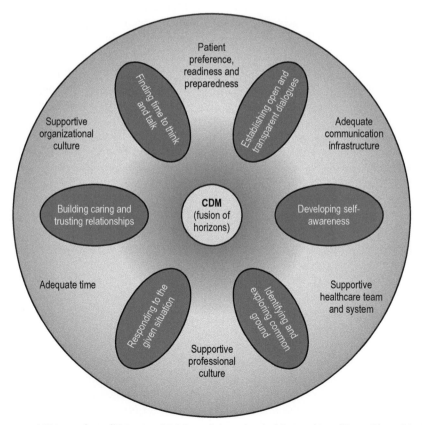

Fig. 29.2 ■ The core capabilities and conditions required for collaborative decision making. (From Olsen, M., 2013. Collaborative decision making in early career dietetic practice, PhD thesis. Charles Sturt University, NSW 3, p. 220, with permission.)

- identifying and exploring common ground and
- finding time to think and talk.

This research adds to our understanding of how CDM contributes to dietetic practice in settings such as generalist practice in rural Australia. In these rural settings, practitioners are often working as solo dietitians with limited support. Olsen's work could be used to refine the development of these capabilities for practitioners who must work in these settings.

However, little is known about the use of CDM in different practice settings such as hospitals or with different patient groups. The identification of core capabilities for CDM highlights the metaskills needed to effectively undertake patient-centred decision making. A limitation of the CDM model in dietetics is that it was developed from a specific context, specifically the decision making of novice dietitians in mostly outpatient settings in rural Australia. As noted earlier in the chapter, context significantly influences the requirements of the clinician's clinical reasoning. There is a need to extend this kind of research into the clinical reasoning of dietitians in other contexts.

CLINICAL REASONING IN ADVANCED DIETETIC PRACTICE

Clinical reasoning research in dietetics has had a strong focus on advanced practice with a particular aim of describing the qualities and skills associated with the advanced practitioner (Bradley et al., 1993; Brody et al., 2012; Skipper and Lewis, 2007; Wildish and Evers, 2010). If we can articulate the qualities and skills that characterize advanced practitioners, then this would provide us with a model that teachers could use to help novices develop their own expertise. Similar work has been done to develop models of advanced practice in nursing (Benner et al., 2011; Bobbs, 1990; Rew, 1990). These models also pay attention to the aspects of knowledge, cognition and metacognition (Higgs and Jones, 2008). Advanced-level clinical dietetics involves using expert clinical reasoning and the skilful integration of information from various sources to streamline activities, increasing productivity and effectiveness (Skipper and Lewis, 2006).

Advanced practice in clinical dietetics has been researched in broad terms (Brody et al., 2012) and more specifically in the practice of providing medical nutrition therapy such as in the hospital setting (Skipper and Lewis, 2006). The ability to integrate and synthesize disparate details into organized systems using general principles has been identified as a key ability of advanced dietetic practitioners (Bradley et al., 1993). Brody et al. (2012) showed that an ability to communicate complex scientific concepts to patients by using plain language is also characteristic of advanced dietitians. This ability is closely related to expert abilities in interviewing and counselling. The experts are also able to demonstrate mastery of evidence-based practice and integrate information from the biomedical sciences that underpins dietetics, such as pathophysiology, pharmacology and metabolism. The experts also demonstrated high-level practical skills such as a physical assessment that is part of the Nutrition Care Process (Brody et al., 2012; Bueche et al., 2008; Skipper and Lewis, 2006). Case Study 29.1 demonstrates how a dietitian may apply the elements of knowledge, cognition and metacognition through the different domains of a nutrition assessment. The case study highlights the advanced critical thinking skills needed and the ability to integrate multiple sources of information and to evaluate their relevance.

Finally, one last ability that is considered necessary for advanced clinical reasoning is a high tolerance for ambiguity and uncertainty (Bradley et al., 1993). Specialist knowledge and experience alone were not considered sufficient for expertise in the Bradley model. Later studies have confirmed high tolerance for ambiguity to be a very common characteristic of advanced-level practice (Brody et al., 2012; Skipper and Lewis, 2006; Wildish and Evers, 2010). These studies showed that, although being comprehensive in their assessments, advanced practitioners were still able to deal with complexity and ambiguity. This may be a result of their ability to simplify problems into manageable parts while maintaining a 'big-picture' perspective at the same time.

Approaches to patient care in advanced practice dietitians also appear to involve initiative, creativity, intuition and a high degree of adaptability (Bradley et al., 1993; Brody et al., 2012; Skipper and Lewis, 2006; Wildish and Evers, 2010). Little further is known, however, of the cognitive processes that may be facilitating this advanced-level practice in advanced dietitians in different contexts. We know these practitioners can make complex decisions, but we are not certain exactly

Questions an Advanced-Practice Dietitian May Ask in Each Domain of the Nutrition Assessment Illustrating Critical Thinking

A 31-year-old woman is admitted to a hospital ward with severe acute pancreatitis and develops a splenic infarct caused by a portal vein thrombus in her liver. She has a history of repeated presentations of acute on chronic pancreatitis caused by familial hypertriglyceridemia. She also has type 2 diabetes treated with insulin. During her admission, she develops a gastric outlet obstruction, multiple liver abscesses, ongoing sepsis, chylous ascites and diarrhoea. She has an extended admission with gradual decline in her body weight going from 88 kg to 45 kg in 6 months and is now considered malnourished.

Domain	Critical Thinking Questions
Anthropometry	How are fluid and energy balance affected by acute pancreatitis? What is the effect of sepsis, diarrhoea and chylous ascites on weight, fluid balance and other anthropometric measures such as lean body mass changes? What factors may cause and worsen chylous ascites?
Biochemical data, medical tests and procedures	What biochemical alterations are likely with extended periods of sepsis? What effect does acute and chronic pancreatitis have on biochemical nutrition markers such as fat-soluble vitamin levels? What effect do pancreatitis and sepsis have on blood sugar control, and what is the role of diet in optimizing these levels? What interventions can be made for overcoming the gastric outlet obstruction to achieve enteral nutrition? What measures can be used to support suspected pancreatic exocrine insufficiency?
Clinical history	How do the gastric outlet obstruction and inflammation from the pancreatitis affect gastrointestinal function and other nutrient requirements? How does chronic pancreatitis affect nutrient utilization? Is the diarrhoea exclusively caused by pancreatic exocrine insufficiency, or what other factors could be contributing to this? Through what means of administration does the patient have access to effective pancreatic enzyme replacement therapy? What available modes of nutrition support are appropriate given the ascites, gastric outlet obstruction and diarrhoea?
Diet/nutrition-related history	How do the sepsis and the pancreatitis affect appetite? When and under what conditions will nonoral feeding need to be considered? What means should be used to determine tolerance of route and macronutrient absorption of feeding? What effect is the long admission having on interest in hospital menu items and therefore calorie and protein intake? Is there a risk for micronutrient deficiency considering the gastrointestinal function? How can the different nutrition support routes help slow down the worsening and then try to reverse the malnutrition when there are ongoing sepsis- and pancreatitis-related complications? What nutrition support options are available in the community to facilitate ongoing improvement in nutritional status upon discharge?

how they do it. It seems that, just as in other health professions, 'competence is context-dependent' (Epstein and Hundert, 2002). Based on the characteristics identified, it is likely that advanced clinical dietitians use clinical reasoning approaches similar to those found in medicine and physiotherapy such as diagnostic reasoning (Bowen, 2006; Edwards et al., 2004) and intuitive reasoning (Barrows and Feltovich, 1987).

What is needed from further studies? Key questions are as follows:

- What is the nature of dietitians' clinical reasoning in different settings?
- How is professional judgement relevant to their clinical reasoning?
- How is clinical reasoning related to expertise in dietetics?
- What factors are associated with optimal reasoning?
- Is there a relationship between dietitians' clinical reasoning and patient outcomes?

CHAPTER SUMMARY

In this chapter, we have:

- contextualized current understanding of clinical reasoning in the discipline of clinical dietetics,
- explored three key domains of thinking that underpin clinical reasoning: knowledge (propositional, professional-craft and personal), cognition and metacognition and
- discussed strengths and limitations of two practice models in dietetics.

REFLECTION POINT 3

Clinical reasoning in dietetics is considered a complex and dynamic process that incorporates key dimensions of knowledge, cognition and metacognition occurring in specific contexts. Clinical reasoning approaches have been explored in early career dietitians in rural settings, and we have some insights into the skills and qualities of advanced practice dietetics. There is need for deeper understanding of the nature of clinical reasoning in dietitians in different contexts. How could exploration of your own clinical reasoning practices contribute to the current gap in understanding this phenomenon in dietetics?

REFERENCES

American Dietetic Association, 1994. Identifying patients at risk: ADA's definitions for nutrition screening and nutrition assessment. J. Am. Diet. Assoc. 94, 838–839.

Barrows, H.S., Feltovich, P.J., 1987. The clinical reasoning process. Med. Educ. 21, 86–91.

Benner, P., Hooper-Kyriakidis, P., Stannard, D., 2011. Clinical Wisdom and Interventions in Acute and Critical Care: A Thinking-in-Action Approach, second ed. Springer, New York, NY.

Bobbs, J.K., 1990. Critical care voices: intuition in nursing practice. Dimens. Crit. Care Nurs. 9, 38.

Bowen, J.L., 2006. Educational strategies to promote clinical diagnostic reasoning. N. Engl. J. Med. 355, 2217–2225.

Bradley, R.T., Young, W.Y., Ebbs, P., et al., 1993. Characteristics of advanced-level dietetics practice: a model and empirical results. J. Am. Diet. Assoc. 93, 196–202.

British Dietitians Association, 2016. Model and process for nutrition and dietetic practice. Viewed 16 February 2017. Available from: https://www.bda.uk.com/publications/professional/model_and_process_for_nutrition_and_dietetic_practice_.

Brody, R.A., Byham-Gray, L., Touger-Decker, R., et al., 2012. Identifying components of advanced-level clinical nutrition practice: a Delphi study. J. Acad. Nutr. Diet. 112, 859–869.

Bueche, J., Charney, P., Pavlinac, J., et al., 2008. Nutrition care process and model part I: the 2008 update. J. Am. Diet. Assoc. 108, 1113–1117.

Calabro, K.S., Bright, K.A., Bahl, S., 2001. International perspectives: the profession of dietetics. Nutrition 17, 594–599.

Charles, C., Gafni, A., Whelan, T., 1999. Decision-making in the physician–patient encounter: revisiting the shared treatment decision-making model. Soc. Sci. Med. 49, 651–661.

Dietitians Association of Australia, 2017. Dietitian or nutritionist? Viewed 2 February 2017. Available from: https://daa.asn.au/what-dietitans-do/dietitian-or-nutritionist/.

Edwards, I., Jones, M., Carr, J., et al., 2004. Clinical reasoning strategies in physical therapy. Phys. Ther. 84, 312–330, discussion 331–335.

Epstein, R.M., Hundert, E.M., 2002. Defining and assessing professional competence. JAMA 287, 226–235.

Erickson-Weerts, S., 1999. Past, present, and future perspectives of dietetics practice. J. Am. Diet. Assoc. 99, 291–293.

Facione, P.A., Facione, N.C., 2001. California Critical Thinking Disposition Inventory Test Manual. California Academic Press, Millbrae, CA.

Gates, G., 1992. Clinical reasoning: an essential component of dietetic practice. Top. Clin. Nutr. 7, 74–80.

Higgs, J., Jones, M.A., 2008. Clinical decision making and multiple problem spaces. In: Higgs, J., Jones, M.A., Loftus, S., et al. (Eds.), Clinical Reasoning in the Health Professions, third ed. Elsevier, Edinburgh, pp. 1–18.

Higgs, J., Titchen, A., 1995. Propositional, professional and personal knowledge in clinical reasoning. In: Higgs, J., Jones, M. (Eds.), Clinical Reasoning in the Health Professions, second ed. Butterworth-Heinemann, Oxford, pp. 129–146.

Hooker, R.S., Williams, J.H., Papneja, J., et al., 2012. Dietetics supply and demand: 2010-2020. J. Acad. Nutr. Diet. 112, S75–S91.

Hughes, R., Somerset, S., 1997. Definitions and conceptual frameworks for public health and community nutrition: a discussion paper. Austr. J. Nutr. Diet. 54, 40–45.

Hwalla, N., Koleilat, M., 2004. Dietetic practice: the past, present and future. East. Mediterr. Health J. 10, 716–730.

International Confederation of Dietetic Associations, 2004. The education and work of dietitians. Viewed 6 December 2016. Available from: http://www.internationaldietetics.org/Downloads/Education-and-Work-of-Diettiians-2004.aspx.

MacLellan, D., Thirsk, J., 2010. Final Report of the International Confederation of Dietetic Associations (ICDA) Evidence-Based Practice Working Group. International Confederation of Dietetics Associations, Toronto, Ontario.

Olsen, M., 2013. Collaborative decision making in early career dietetic practice, PhD thesis. Charles Sturt University, NSW.

O'Sullivan-Maillet, J., 2009. A historical perspective on specialty and advanced-level practice in dietetics. Top. Clin. Nutr. 24, 236–242.

Rew, L., 1990. Intuition in critical care nursing practice. Dimens. Crit. Care Nurs. 9, 30–37.

Sackett, D.L., Rosenberg, W.M.C., Gray, J.A.M., et al., 1996. Evidence based medicine: what it is and what it isn't. BMJ 312, 71–72.

Schumacher, J., 2014. Critical-thinking dispositions among dietetic interns at the completion of their internship. J. Fam. Consum. Sci. 106, 55–57.

Skipper, A., Lewis, N., 2007. Advanced medical nutrition therapy practice: what are the future needs? Nutr. Today 42, 200–205.

Skipper, A., Lewis, N.M., 2006. Using initiative to achieve autonomy: a model for advanced practice in medical nutrition therapy. J. Am. Diet. Assoc. 106, 1219–1225.

Titchen, A., Ersser, S.J., 2001. The nature of professional craft knowledge. In: Higgs, J., Titchen, A. (Eds.), Practice Knowledge and Expertise in the Health Professions. Butterworth-Heinemann, Oxford, pp. 35–41.

Trede, F., Higgs, J., 2003. Re-framing the clinician's role in collaborative clinical decision making: re-thinking practice knowledge and the notion of clinician-patient relationships. Learn. Health Soc. Care 2, 66–73.

Wildish, D.E., Evers, S., 2010. A definition, description, and framework for advanced practice in dietetics. Can. J. Diet. Pract. Res. 71, e4–e11.

30

CLINICAL REASONING IN PHARMACY

W. CARY MOBLEY ■ ROBIN MOORMAN-LI

CHAPTER AIMS

The aims of this chapter are to:

■ discuss the roles of a systematic patient care process and clinical reasoning in assessing and resolving medication-related problems as part of a collaborative effort to provide patient-centred care,

■ provide the reader with a case study example illustrating medication-related problem solving in the Pharmacists' Patient Care Process and

■ discuss common sources of error in clinical reasoning.

KEY WORDS

Clinical reasoning

Clinical problem solving

Collaborative health care

Medication-related problems

Pharmacists' Patient Care Process

Explanations and arguments

Cognitive biases

INTRODUCTION

In a broad sense, clinical reasoning is the reasoning employed in clinical problem solving that is 'the process of forming conclusions, judgements, or inferences for facts or premises' (Dictionary.com Unabridged no date) in clinical problem solving. In clinical reasoning, the facts or premises from which decisions are made include signs and symptoms, treatment facts, principles of disease and care and the practitioner's understanding of how the patient views his or her health and quality of life. For a pharmacist, clinical reasoning is centred on solving problems related to medications, which generally involve questions related to the appropriateness, effectiveness and safety of the medications, as well as compliance to the medication regimen. Within these broad categories, specific types of medication-related problems that pharmacists typically encounter are listed in Box 30.1 (Cipolle et al., 2012). Though clinical problems can vary in different ways (e.g., simple vs complex, or acute vs chronic, urgent vs preventive), an important common goal for problem resolution will be an individualized recommendation in accordance with the patient's 'needs, goals, lifestyle, and personal and cultural values' (Rogers, 1983, p. 36).

With this goal in mind, for the resolution of many clinical problems, it may be best that the pharmacist adopts a holistic mindset that visualizes an individual's health in the context of his or her physical, mental and social well-being (Huber et al. 2011; Jayasinghe, 2012). In this context, a patient's health can be viewed as a function of multiple interacting and dynamic systems including the biochemical, cellular, physiological systems that are at the physiological source of ill health, along with the psychological, social and value systems that shape an individual's attitudes and lifestyle (Jayasinghe, 2012; Wilson et al., 2001). The patient's attitudes and lifestyle can be influential in the development or course of many acute and chronic health problems. For example, an individual's stress or sedentary lifestyle can be important factors in the development and course of various cardiovascular, inflammatory and psychiatric conditions (Booth et al., 2012; Schneiderman et al., 2005; Slavich, 2016). Viewing an individual's health problem(s) as part of a complete system favours a holistic, integrated approach to clinical reasoning, whereby ideas from different disciplines are associated to connect different health factors (or determinants) to an individual's health problems. These factors are considered in the creation of a complete plan for maintenance or reestablishment of the patient's health.

THE PHARMACIST AS PART OF A COLLABORATIVE TEAM

The pharmacist contributes his or her unique expertise in medication management as part of a collaborative interdisciplinary effort to maintain or reestablish a patient's health. In this team approach to health care, the knowledge, experience and judgement of different practitioners are integrated to make patient-centred healthcare decisions. Given that the assessment and resolution of the patient's health problems will involve understanding the perspectives of patients and of fellow

practitioners, it is incumbent on the pharmacist to develop an interdisciplinary mindset. The pharmacist should possess enough insight from other healthcare disciplines to be able to understand and evaluate the reasoning of his or her fellow practitioners to evaluate potential conflict or synergy between their treatment approaches and that of the pharmacist. All this means that the pharmacist has to work effectively as a member of a team dedicated to creating a unified, synergistic and comprehensive plan for achieving health goals for the patient.

CLINICAL PROBLEM SOLVING FOR THE PHARMACIST

There are different models for problem-solving processes related to a patient's medication-related needs, but as with other healthcare professions, the models tend to follow a certain order (American College of Clinical Pharmacology, 2014; Gambrill, 2012; Martin et al., 2016; Rogers, 1983; Steiner et al., 2002; Tietze, 2012). The clinical problem-solving process begins with the gathering and evaluation of information, going as deeply and broadly as the situation warrants, with a goal of developing an understanding of the patient's current clinical status. On the basis of this understanding, the process continues with the generation and selection of strategies to resolve or ameliorate the patient's health problems. The selected strategy is then implemented and monitored for its effectiveness. For this chapter, the Pharmacists' Patient Care Process is the model used to provide a framework to describe clinical reasoning for pharmacists. The process includes the following five sequential steps: Collect, Assess, Plan, Implement, and Follow up (see Bennett et al., 2015, for details). The following case study will be used to exemplify the results of each stage of this clinical problem-solving process.

BOX 30.1
SEVEN BASIC CATEGORIES OF DRUG THERAPY PROBLEMS

- Unnecessary drug therapy
- Need for additional drug therapy
- Ineffective drug therapy
- Dosage too low
- Dosage too high
- Adverse drug reaction
- Noncompliance with drug regimen

CASE STUDY 30.1

Introduction

Cally is a 68-year-old female who presents to her primary care physician's office with a chief complaint of excessive daytime sedation and continued burning sensations in her feet. Her primary care physician

has referred her to clinical pharmacy services for evaluation of her medications and a recommendation for management of her painful diabetic neuropathy.

The Collection and Assessment of Patient Information

The collection and assessment of patient information are a quest for understanding and explicating the patient's health status. In this phase, information about the patient is collected, interpreted, and evaluated based on the knowledge, experience and reasoned judgement of the practitioner. The goal is to create a clear, accurate and comprehensive assessment that will serve as the basis for rational medication-related decisions.

Collection

The collection of information may proceed in different ways depending on the nature of the practice and of the clinical encounter. For example, it may begin with a visual cue (e.g., a worried look, a cough or skin discoloration), a verbal description of symptoms by the patient or caregiver, an examination of prescription vials and refill histories, a computer alert during prescription processing, a routine examination of a medical record or (as in the case mentioned earlier) a referral from a physician. Further information may also be gathered in different ways, including direct communication with the patient, communication with caregivers, surrogates and fellow clinicians and/or continued examination of a medical record.

During the collection phase, the pharmacist will systematically and thoroughly gather and record subjective and objective information in a manner dictated by the clinical issues and the practice of the pharmacist. Subjective data are commonly described as data provided by the patient. Objective data are commonly described as information that is reported, observed or documented by a healthcare provider, can be reproduced and are fact based. Medication-related information that may be routinely gathered includes a current medication list and medication use history. Other pertinent information includes age, gender, ethnicity, allergies, laboratory and other test results, vital signs, physical assessment data and the patient's healthcare goals (Bennett et al., 2015). The pharmacist will also seek to gain the patient's perspectives by ascertaining understandings, beliefs, attitudes and behaviours related to medication therapy (Cipolle et al., 2012) as well as factors that may present barriers, such as issues of health literacy, distrust or economics (Bennett et al., 2015).

The collection phase may also have a significant diagnostic element as the pharmacist will be on a quest to discover and evaluate potential medication-related problems (such as those listed in Box 30.1), along with their contributing factors. This pharmaceutical diagnosis will typically proceed in a hypothetico-deductive manner, whereby the acquisition of cues leads to a hypothesis of a medication-related problem, which will be tested with a deductive investigation for confirmatory and disconfirmatory information. This information may come from many sources, including how the patient uses the medications; changes in disease status or functional parameters (such as liver or kidney function); symptom onset, severity, aggravating and remitting factors; prescribing or dispensing issues; and social or economic issues. This process may also include judging when a referral or further testing (e.g., laboratory) is warranted.

It is important to note that when eliciting information directly from patients, proper communication skills are imperative, and include effective wording of the questions, using open-ended questions, using active listening skills and developing a good rapport with the patient.

Assessment

During the assessment, all collected information is meticulously analyzed, interpreted and evaluated with a goal of creating a clear, comprehensive and accurate assessment of the patient's medication-related needs. The subjective and objective information is grouped and evaluated for possible relationships to hypothesize potential medication-related problems, which will be confirmed or disconfirmed based on other patient information (Tietze, 2012).

Aside from focussing on the medications, the pharmacist evaluates the patient's function, perceptions of quality of life, current healthcare goals and overall understanding and agreement with the current healthcare plan. Additionally, it is important for the pharmacist to evaluate preventive healthcare issues such as diet concerns, substance use and immunization status to ensure all aspects of medication-related needs have been thoroughly evaluated.

When multiple medication-related problems are identified and characterized, they must be prioritized to capture the most urgent issues that could lead to the most immediate negative effect on the patient and thus should receive priority.

CASE STUDY 30.2

Collect

Cally is a 68-year-old female who presents to the Pharmacotherapy clinic today at the request of Dr. Jones for evaluation of her current medication regimen and recommendations for her painful diabetic neuropathy. Cally reports a burning sensation in her feet that has become unbearable over the past month. Upon further discussion, her description of this pain includes burning pain, with numbness and tingling in both feet. The pain seems to be greater at night, rating the pain a 10/10 and averaging about 8/10 during the day. She has decreased her daily activities because of her pain. Her sleep quality has progressively worsened despite the addition of amitriptyline, which she has been taking for about 1 month. She reports that amitriptyline is causing daytime sedation, dry mouth and eyes, increased constipation and periodic episodes of confusion. She is concerned about the constipation, because before amitriptyline she was having a bowel movement once a day with no straining, and now she is having a bowel movement every other day, and it is painful to pass. She is hoping these side effects will start to resolve now that she has been taking this medication for 1 month. She is hoping there are some treatment options that could at least decrease her pain to a 6/10 on average so she can enjoy her daily activities, begin exercising again and improve her overall sleep quality.

(Information that was collected about Cally included: current medications [including over-the-counter medications, herbals and dietary supplements], adherence evaluation, past medications and reason for discontinuation, medication allergies, social history [including smoking, alcohol, substance abuse], past medical history, current immunizations, lifestyle habits [including exercise, diet and psychosocial functioning], personal healthcare goals, vital signs and laboratory results.)

CASE STUDY 30.3

Assess

1. Uncontrolled Painful Diabetic Neuropathy: leading to decreased function, quality of sleep and quality of life. Patient is also experiencing adverse reactions to amitriptyline: daytime sedation, dry mouth and eyes, increased constipation and intermittent confusion. Additionally, amitriptyline is on the Beer's list of drugs to avoid in older adults, and its use in the elderly is not recommended because of adverse drug reactions.

2. Constipation: Adverse drug reaction secondary to anticholinergic effects of amitriptyline. Decreased physical activity caused by increased pain from diabetic peripheral neuropathy could also be contributing to symptoms.

3. Poorly Controlled Type 2 Diabetes: Haemoglobin A1C is currently 9.1% and is contributing to painful diabetic peripheral neuropathy. Based on patient's current age and health status, her haemoglobin A1c goal is <7.5%, which translates into fasting and preprandial glucose levels averaging between 140 and 150 mg/dL.

4. Controlled Hypertension and Dyslipidaemia: Patient is currently reaching treatment goals. Hypertension: goal <140/90. Lipid levels are acceptable. No adverse drug reactions reported.

Reasoning in the Collection-Assessment Phase

An assessment is an evaluative process, where diagnostic reasoning is applied to collected information to determine the existence and nature of clinical problems, with a particular emphasis on elucidating their aetiology.

With this emphasis of determining the causes and contributing factors of medication-related problems, from a reasoning perspective, the assessment phase is largely an explanation-creating phase. To create an explanation, the practitioner infers a working hypothesis (e.g., patient is noncompliant) to explain a set of collected information (e.g., unmet clinical outcomes). The pharmacist then seeks to deductively test the hypothesis by ascertaining further information (e.g., refill history) (Kelley, 1998). With new information, a working hypothesis may be confirmed, or disconfirmed and discarded, and new hypotheses may be inferred and tested. To validate a particular explanation as the best explanation and to avoid premature closure on a hypothesis, the pharmacist must purposefully create, test and rule out alternate explanations for the collected information.

The collection-assessment process does not typically continue indefinitely to achieve absolute certainty. Rather, it continues until explanations emerge that can be used to define the patient's clinical status and clinical problems with sufficient adequacy and accuracy that maximize understanding while minimizing the risk for any remaining uncertainty. Thus the decision on when to stop the assessment is in part an ethical decision for the practitioner (Rogers, 1983).

Care Plan Development, Implementation and Follow-up: the Therapeutic Phase

With assessment of the patient's medication-related needs complete, the pharmacist is now able to rationally create an individualized care plan in collaboration with the patient and other healthcare practitioners.

Planning

Care planning begins by establishing goals of therapy that are defined in terms of measurable outcomes that will be used to measure the effectiveness and safety of recommended interventions (Bennett et al., 2015; Tietze, 2012). Potential medication-related goals include curing or preventing a disease, slowing or halting disease progression, reducing or eliminating signs or symptoms, normalizing laboratory values or providing palliative care (Cipolle et al., 2012). The goals are structured to include observable, measurable and realistic clinical parameters for goal achievement, the desired value or observable change for those parameters and the expected time frame for their achievement (Cipolle et al., 2012).

With goals of therapy established, the pharmacist proceeds to develop strategies to achieve them. A list of drug and nondrug strategies is generated and evaluated. Some are eliminated and others are selected, with

the best strategy selected and alternatives identified (Tietze, 2012). Selection of patient-specific medication interventions involves the weighing of the comparative effectiveness and safety of the options. Multiple patient-specific factors that can influence the chosen therapy and its outcomes are considered in this decision-making process. These factors include comorbid conditions; other therapeutic interventions; patient attitudes, beliefs, healthcare goals and healthcare access; affordability; and the capacity and willingness to comply with the recommendation. Because the patient is at the centre, he or she is encouraged to be an active participant in this care-planning process and to take responsibility for his or her own health care.

The recommended plan must be acceptable to all parties involved and developed with a collaborative mindset. When the pharmacist is making treatment recommendations, the plan should be evidence based, focussed on clinical goals and should have sound reasoning. As the plan is documented, all clinical goals should be matched to the treatment recommendations, and the monitoring parameters that measure the effectiveness of the treatment plan should be clearly indicated. The plan should be clearly written so every healthcare provider involved in the patient's care can follow the pharmacist's thought pattern. It should include the specific drug, dose, route and duration, and the type and frequency of monitoring, any necessary referrals and follow-up instructions to ensure proper monitoring of the patient and achievement of the healthcare goals.

Implementation

Once the developed plan is accepted by the healthcare team, it is imperative to implement it fully. The most important part of this phase is proper communication to all stakeholders and effective patient education. Thus the pharmacist will need to possess the cognitive flexibility and empathy to be able to tailor the communication to different individuals involved in plan implementation, including the specific patient, surrogate and/or caregiver to assure optimal understanding and compliance with the plan.

For the patient, the pharmacist will need to employ a communication strategy that will enable the assessment of the patient's understanding of his or her illness and medication plan as well the level of motivation and commitment. The pharmacist will need to take the

CASE STUDY 30.4

Plan

1. Uncontrolled painful diabetic neuropathy
   - Goals: Goals include improving pain symptoms and reaching patient-set pain goal of 6/10 within 4 to 6 weeks and improving function, quality of life and sleep within next month as treatment regimen is titrated appropriately based on patient's response. Minimize adverse drug reactions with treatment options.
   - Discontinue amitriptyline.
   - Refer to primary care provider to evaluate diabetes medication to achieve better blood glucose control (A1c Goal <7.5% within next year to help prevent worsening of diabetic peripheral neuropathy). Consider referral to diabetic education class for improvement of self-management skills.
   - Start slow titration of gabapentin 300 mg by mouth at bedtime for 1 week, then may increase to 300 mg by mouth two times daily for 1 week, then increase again to 300 mg by mouth three times daily. Titration to continue with goal dosing of gabapentin 600 mg by mouth three times daily to achieve optimal efficacy and tolerability. Monitor for signs of daytime sedation, confusion or peripheral oedema. Evaluate pain levels associated with diabetic peripheral neuropathy.
   - Encourage proper foot care: Daily examination of each foot to identify cracking, dryness or signs of infection. Stress importance of proper shoe selection.

2. Constipation: Adverse drug reaction secondary to amitriptyline
   - Goal: Improve symptoms with Bristol stool score of 4 (i.e., like a sausage or snake, smooth and soft), and achieve a daily regular bowel movement within the next 1 to 4 days without straining.
   - Initiate polyethylene glycol 3350: Mix 17 grams in 8 ounces of beverage, and drink once daily for 3 days; then use as needed when Bristol is less than 3 or other symptoms of constipation occur. Hold dose for loose stools. Provide education on Bristol stool chart. Encourage proper hydration and adequate dietary fibre via fruits and vegetables and stress the importance of doing as much exercise as can be tolerated.

3. Poorly controlled type 2 diabetes
   - Goal: Achieve haemoglobin A1c goal <7.5% within next year to prevent worsening of diabetic peripheral neuropathy.
   - Referral to diabetic education class for improvement of self-management skills.
   - Primary care provider (PCP) to evaluate diabetes medication for adjustment of oral medications to dual therapy to achieve better blood glucose control.

4. Controlled hypertension and dyslipidaemia: Continue current regimen.

proper amount of time to explain the treatment plan to the patient, including not only what the patient will be asked to do but also why this particular plan is deemed the best plan for the particular situation. It is imperative the patient not only understands the entire plan but also agrees to it. Pharmacists should be keenly aware of communication tips and well educated on adult education to ensure all information is provided in an effective manner and the patient is not overwhelmed or confused by the information.

Follow-up: Monitoring and Evaluation

The follow-up phase includes the ongoing monitoring and evaluation of the treatment plan. Focussing on the medications, the pharmacist will monitor to ensure treatment efficacy, possible side effects and the patient's overall response and satisfaction with the treatment. During this time, it is also important to continually align clinical outcomes with healthcare goals to ensure progress is being made towards achieving these goals. These goals must be continually evaluated to ensure they remain appropriate and achievable because a patient's health can change frequently.

When considering healthcare outcomes to measure, the pharmacist must not only focus on the clinical measures but must also evaluate the humanistic measures such as patient functioning, ability to participate in self-management and understanding of current medication therapy. Additionally, economic-related measures are important to evaluate including, for example, frequency and reasons for emergency department visits and hospitalizations and overall medication costs.

Reasoning in the Therapeutic Phase

In the therapeutic phase, the practitioner uses the collected information and assessment as the basis, or the premises, to create goals for improvement of the patient's health. In turn, the assessment and goals provide the basis for the generation and selection of therapeutic and monitoring strategies. Thus therapeutic reasoning in each of these steps involves the generation and substantiation of arguments for what should be done to maintain or improve the patient's health (Kelley, 1998). In the process of therapeutic selection, the pharmacist will employ dialectical reasoning, as he or she will argue one therapeutic option against another or in some cases against an argument for no treatment.

As with other arguments, the proposed strategy must satisfy the basic criteria for valid arguments, namely that its premises (e.g., the assessment and goals) are true and that the conclusion of what to do logically follows (Kelley, 1998). Additionally, the argument for a recommended strategy must be communicated in a way that it can be readily understood and evaluated by each stakeholder. The pharmacist should be able to articulate the evidence on which the recommendation is based and should be able to logically explain how the proposed intervention will affect the underlying pathophysiological processes to achieve the outcomes stipulated in the therapeutic goals and how it may lead to adverse effects (Hawkins et al., 2010).

Ethical reasoning will also be an essential component of therapeutic reasoning, as choices are made in the best interest of and with the consent of the patient whose valued goals must be considered, whose active participation in care planning and implementation is desired and who is the ultimate change agent for his or her own health (Hawkins et al., 2010; Rogers, 1983).

Common Sources of Reasoning Errors

Reasoning is our best guide to the truth, and therefore the more effective at reasoning we are, the closer to the truth and the more valid our assertions, conclusions and arguments relating to caring for a patient can be. However, we are fallible, and there are many controllable factors that contribute to our fallibility, which we are obligated to recognize and remediate to achieve optimal

---

CASE STUDY 30.5

Monitor and Evaluate

1. Uncontrolled painful diabetic neuropathy
   - Improved symptoms based on pain levels, improved function and quality of life, improved sleep quality.
   - Signs and symptoms of side effects upon initiation and slow titration of gabapentin: daytime sedation, confusion.
   - Improved haemoglobin A1C every 3 months following adjustments after follow-up with PCP for diabetes mellitus (DM) management, attendance of diabetes self-management skills class.

2. Constipation
   - Bristol stool chart and signs and symptoms of constipation (signs of straining, incomplete evacuation).
   - Frequency of use of polyethylene glycol 3350 to determine whether this should be scheduled.

3. Hypertension/dyslipidaemia
   - Continued control with current regimen, no reports of adverse drug reaction (ADRs).

care for our patients. Among these factors are inadequate knowledge and cognitive biases that undermine our reasoning and are at the source of many of our clinical reasoning errors.

Inadequate Knowledge

Reasoning and all of its elements rely on our understanding of what it is we are reasoning about to make accurate interpretations, evaluations, inferences and arguments. This requirement places an onus on the pharmacist to continuously develop a deep, broad, accurate and integrated knowledge base that includes a wide range of concepts, principles and facts. It includes knowledge about diseases and their mechanisms, psychosocial determinants, manifestations, diagnostic elements and morbidity. It includes knowledge about drug and nondrug therapeutic remedies, their mechanisms, risks, benefits, costs and evidentiary support. It also includes knowledge about the practices and perspectives of other healthcare practitioners who join in a collective pursuit of helping the patient to achieve his or her healthcare goals. This knowledge about what underlies a patient's health and health care is integrated with knowledge about the patient (e.g., signs and symptoms) to develop a clear and comprehensive clinical picture and therapeutic plan.

Cognitive Biases

In the process of becoming a competent reasoning clinician, the pharmacist must strive to develop a mindset that excludes the cognitive biases that are destructive to the reasoning process and, consequently, are often found at the root of many clinical errors. These biases, along with inadequate knowledge, can also lead to suboptimal problem assessment and resolution. There are over 100 potential biases that can affect our reasoning (Croskerry et al., 2013a). See Box 30.2 for some of the more common examples for pharmacists to be aware of (Croskerry, 2003; Croskerry et al., 2013a; Croskerry et al., 2013b; Scott, 2009).

When considering this short list of biases, it is not difficult to envision how a pharmacist can fall victim to them. For example, when evaluating the patient who is experiencing dry mouth and dry eyes, intuitively the pharmacist may focus on the drugs listed on the patient's medication list that have anticholinergic effects rather than evaluating the patient in a more holistic systematic

---

BOX 30.2
COMMON EXAMPLES OF POTENTIAL BIASES THAT CAN AFFECT REASONING

Aggregate bias: Believing that the aggregate data used in documents, such as clinical guidelines, do not apply to the current patient's situation.

Anchoring: Prematurely settling on a single diagnosis or drug-related problem based on the initial data and initial presentation and failing to adjust the hypothesis as further data are collected.

Ascertainment bias: Prior experiences are used to shape current thinking, leading to seeing what you expect to see.

Availability: While diagnosing a patient or working to identify the reasons associated with a possible drug-related concern, only considering disease states or drug-related issues most frequently seen in current practice, not considering less-common disease states or drug reactions.

Confirmation bias: Focussing on the signs and symptoms that can confirm a leading diagnostic hypothesis and discounting any data that would counter or refute them.

Fundamental attribution error: Overweighting of a patient's personality when considering causes of the particular reported problem or possible drug-related problem.

Order effects: Focussing on information gathered at the beginning and end of the interview and failing to adequately take into account the information gathered in between.

Premature closure: Forming a hypothesis before gathering sufficient information and exploring alternatives.

Representativeness restraint: Judging a situation based on the typical prototype and matching up the current situation to this prototype, leading to a risk for missing an atypical presentation.

---

manner to develop a more complete hypothesis list before assuming the reported side effects are drug related. It is imperative that all healthcare providers, including pharmacists, are keenly aware of these common errors that can negatively affect clinical reasoning and lead to possible negative outcomes for the patient. It is vital to take a step back and look at the entire picture and actively engage in the problem-solving process to allow for appropriate arguments to be developed and evaluated, leading to the best treatment options for the patient.

CHAPTER SUMMARY

In this chapter, we have outlined:

- how pharmacists apply their medication-management expertise and clinical reasoning in clinical problem solving as part of a collaborative effort to achieve effective patient-centred care,
- how pharmacists employ clinical reasoning and a systematic patient care process to assess and resolve medication-related problems and
- the contributions of inadequate knowledge and cognitive biases to clinical reasoning errors.

REFLECTION POINT 1

Pharmacists have in-depth knowledge of medications and their interactions. This knowledge gives their clinical reasoning a valuable role in contributing to the interprofessional care that is needed by many patients who have complex needs and require multiple medications.

REFERENCES

American College of Clinical Pharmacology, 2014. Standards of practice for clinical pharmacists. Pharmacotherapy 34, 794–797.

Bennett, M., Kliethermes, M.A., American Pharmacists Association, 2015. How to implement the pharmacists' patient care process: a systematic approach. American Pharmacists Association, Washington, DC.

Booth, F.W., Roberts, C.K., Laye, M.J., 2012. Lack of exercise is a major cause of chronic diseases. Compr. Physiol. 2, 1143–1211.

Cipolle, R.J., Strand, L.M., Morley, P.C., 2012. Pharmaceutical Care Practice: The Patient-Centered Approach to Medication Management Services, third ed. McGraw-Hill Medical, New York, NY.

Croskerry, P., 2003. The importance of cognitive errors in diagnosis and strategies to minimize them. Acad. Med. 78, 775–780.

Croskerry, P., Singhal, G., Mamede, S., 2013a. Cognitive debiasing 1: origins of bias and theory of debiasing. BMJ Qual. Saf. 22 (Suppl. 2), ii58–ii64.

Croskerry, P., Singhal, G., Mamede, S., 2013b. Cognitive debiasing 2: impediments to and strategies for change. BMJ Qual. Saf. 22 (Suppl. 2), ii65–ii72.

Dictionary.com. Unabridged n.d. Viewed. 30 November 2016. Available from: http://www.dictionary.com/browse/reasoning.

Gambrill, E.D., 2012. Critical Thinking in Clinical Practice: Improving the Quality of Judgments and Decisions, third ed. Wiley, Hoboken, NJ.

Hawkins, D.R., Paul, R., Elder, L., 2010. The Thinker's Guide to Clinical Reasoning. Foundation for Critical Thinking, Dillon, CA.

Huber, M., Knottnerus, J.A., Green, L., et al., 2011. How should we define health? BMJ 343, d4163.

Jayasinghe, S., 2012. Complexity science to conceptualize health and disease: is it relevant to clinical medicine? Mayo Clin. Proc. 87, 314–319.

Kelley, D., 1998. The Art of Reasoning, third ed. WW Norton, New York, NY.

Martin, L.C., Donohoe, K.L., Holdford, D.A., 2016. Decision-making and problem-solving approaches in pharmacy education. Am. J. Pharm. Educ. 80, 52.

Rogers, J.C., 1983. Eleanor Clarke Slagle Lectureship—1983: clinical reasoning: the ethics, science, and art. Am. J. Occup. Ther. 37, 601–616.

Schneiderman, N., Ironson, G., Siegel, S.D., 2005. Stress and health: psychological, behavioral, and biological determinants. Annu. Rev. Clin. Psychol. 1, 607–628.

Scott, I.A., 2009. Errors in clinical reasoning: causes and remedial strategies. BMJ 338, b1860.

Slavich, G.M., 2016. Life stress and health: a review of conceptual issues and recent findings. Teach. Psychol. 43, 346–355.

Steiner, W.A., Ryser, L., Huber, E., et al., 2002. Use of the ICF model as a clinical problem-solving tool in physical therapy and rehabilitation medicine. Phys. Ther. 82, 1098.

Tietze, K.J., 2012. Clinical Skills for Pharmacists, third ed. Mosby, St. Louis, MO.

Wilson, T., Holt, T., Greenhalgh, T., 2001. Complexity and clinical care. BMJ 323, 685.

Section 5 TEACHING CLINICAL REASONING

31

PEDAGOGIES FOR TEACHING AND LEARNING CLINICAL REASONING

NARELLE PATTON ■ NICOLE CHRISTENSEN

CHAPTER AIMS

The aims of this chapter are to explore:

■ the complex nature of clinical reasoning,

■ pedagogies for teaching clinical reasoning,

■ how clinical reasoning is currently taught in academic and workplace settings and

■ future directions for teaching and learning clinical reasoning.

KEY WORDS

Clinical reasoning

Theory

Practice

Capability

Dispositions

Reification

WHAT IS CLINICAL REASONING?

Clinical reasoning is a very complex and multifaceted phenomenon, a vast and complex construct that is described and used in different ways by different people (Gruppen, 2017). Because of this inherent complexity and range of understandings and usages, clinical reasoning is in danger of becoming a catchall phrase for an ill-defined process. Clarity around the nature and shared understanding of clinical reasoning provides a firm foundation for the development of pedagogies for

successfully teaching clinical reasoning to healthcare students and facilitation of clinical reasoning capabilities in healthcare practitioners.

This chapter is based on the premise that clinical reasoning is a complex, fluid, situated and embodied journey towards expertise that sits at the heart of ethical professional practice. This understanding of clinical reasoning acknowledges both the cognitive, problem-solving and decision-making capabilities at the heart of effective clinical reasoning and the influence of a broader range of practitioner qualities and contextual dimensions. It also moves beyond consideration of clinical reasoning as a process and views it as an unremitting journey, as practitioners seek to develop their capability to achieve the best outcomes for those with whom they work (Higgs and Jones, 2008).

Clinical reasoning extends well into conscious and nonconscious processes with a great deal of research on clinical reasoning addressing the various cognitive processes involved, for example, problem solving, analytic skills, knowledge synthesis and metacognitive skills. However, increasingly recent explorations of clinical reasoning also acknowledge a broader range of individual dispositional (such as emotion and motivation) dimensions (Durning et al., 2015) and social and contextual dimensions of clinical reasoning (Ratcliffe and Durning, 2015).

Acknowledgement of the influence of contextual factors on clinicians' clinical reasoning processes highlights the importance of consideration of how the inherent dynamic characteristics of clinical workplaces contribute to the fluid nature and quality of clinicians' clinical reasoning. In clinical environments, time constraints result from heavy workloads, staff shortages and the fast pace of clinical environments themselves (Courtney-Pratt et al., 2012). These time constraints in combination with other contextual factors such as resource provision and equipment availability can significantly shape the character of clinicians' clinical reasoning. The fluid nature of clinical reasoning is further captured in the evolution of descriptions of clinical reasoning over time, reflecting both the dynamic and transformative nature of clinical reasoning and our deepening understanding of the concept itself. The contribution of practitioner qualities and capabilities, contextual factors such as patients, other clinicians and clinic arrangements and social relationships to the ongoing development of clinical reasoning is captured in Fig. 31.1.

Multiple perspectives and theories that frame our thinking about clinical reasoning are needed to develop a full and deep understanding of this complex construct (Gruppen, 2017) and the pedagogies underpinning successful clinical reasoning teaching and learning practices. Therefore development of a comprehensive perspective of clinical reasoning must involve a multi-dimensional exploration of the application of theories and practice of clinical reasoning and how it is taught. Acknowledging the complexity of clinical reasoning and the influence of this complexity on clinical reasoning teaching practices, the following sections explore two key dimensions of clinical reasoning that are its embodied

and situated nature and theoretical and practical approaches to understanding and teaching clinical reasoning.

REFLECTION POINT 1

As you embark on the exploration of clinical reasoning offered in this chapter, take a moment to think about your own journey of clinical reasoning capability development. 'Clinical reasoning capability' is a term used here to represent the cognitive abilities, technical skills and personal qualities (such as integrity, empathy, respect and work ethic) that are enacted through the practitioner's clinical reasoning.

> How does the description of clinical reasoning as a journey resonate with your experience of developing your own clinical reasoning capability?
> How can conceptualizing clinical reasoning as a journey enhance ongoing development of your own clinical reasoning capabilities and shape how you might better teach clinical reasoning in the future?

EMBODIED NATURE OF CLINICAL REASONING

Clinical reasoning has long been considered as an embodied action, at its simplest as a cognitive process undertaken by individuals and at its more complex as encompassing clinicians' motivations, emotions and values. Simply put, clinical reasoning is the sum of the thinking and decision-making processes associated with clinical practice (Higgs and Jones, 2008). Many defini-tions converge on these cognitive, predominantly problem-solving dimensions of clinical reasoning including a broad range of cognitive processes such as observation, collection and analysis of information leading to decision making and action that takes into account a patient's specific circumstances and preferences (Ratcliffe and Durning, 2015). More recent explorations of clinical reasoning also encompass how clinical reason-ing is shaped by clinicians' motivations and emotional states (Durning et al., 2015).

Clinical reasoning has been described as a process including dimensions of knowledge, cognition, meta-cognition and mutual decision making (Higgs and

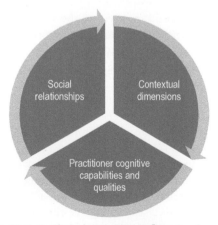

Fig. 31.1 ▪ Clinical reasoning: Influencing factors.

Jones, 2008). In this process, a strong discipline-specific knowledge base, cognitive thinking skills (such as collection, analysis and synthesis of data) and metacognition or reflective self-awareness and ability to undertake mutual decision making with clients are all required (Higgs and Jones, 2008). In these definitions of clinical reasoning, although there is a focus on individuals' knowledge acquisition and organization, interpersonal skills required for mutual decision making are also highlighted. These definitions underline the embodied nature of clinical reasoning, as individual capabilities including cognitive abilities and interpersonal skills lie at its heart.

As an embodied phenomenon, clinical reasoning necessarily encompasses clinicians' cognitive capabilities and their motivations and emotional states (Durning et al., 2015). The idea that reasoning is influenced by an individual's motivation is not new. John Dewey (1916) identified motivational components of reasoning in his description of the criticality of a willingness in the individual to undergo the effort of seeking a solution to the problem at hand to the quality of the reasoning process. Dewey clearly linked individuals' dispositional qualities such as motivation, habits and predictable behaviours to the character of reasoning that is undertaken. More recently, Ratcliffe and Dunning (2015) further emphasized the important contribution of individuals' dispositions and qualities to clinical reasoning in their description of the particular significance of motivational beliefs and self-efficacy to the quality of clinical reasoning. This understanding of the contribution of individual dispositions to the quality of clinical reasoning has particular resonance for healthcare students and practitioners who undertake professional practice experiences and consequently clinical reasoning in often busy healthcare contexts and across a range of settings and practice fields in which their interests, priorities and confidence may vary.

SITUATED NATURE OF CLINICAL REASONING

In addition to its cognitive and dispositional domains, clinical reasoning is increasingly viewed as a situated and social construct (Ratcliffe and Durning, 2015), further highlighting both its fluid nature and complexity.

The centrality of context to clinical reasoning has been underlined in descriptions of excellence in clinical reasoning as a state rather than a trait, with clinical reasoning abilities being situation specific, for example residing with a particular patient in a specific setting with specific resources and interactions with both patients and environment (Durning et al., 2015). This description, although acknowledging an important contribution of resources, also draws attention to the intrinsically human and relational nature of clinical reasoning in its acknowledgement of the significant contribution of patients and their circumstances to the quality of clinicians' clinical reasoning capabilities and outcomes.

This emphasis on social and contextual dimensions of clinical reasoning opens possibilities for consideration of clinical reasoning as a reciprocal process between clinicians and a broad range of people with whom they work including patients, clients, carers and colleagues. This view of the reciprocal nature of clinical reasoning is supported by situated cognition theories that transform the traditional view of cognitively isolated clinicians into clinicians whose interactions with other healthcare providers, patients and environments profoundly affect their diagnostic or clinical reasoning ability (Ratcliffe and Dunning, 2015). Situated cognition argues that cognition or thinking is situated in the specifics of a given encounter, for example, the patient, the physician and other healthcare team members and the environment or system (Ratcliffe and Dunning, 2015). Contemporary patient-centred models of health care emphasize the importance of centring clinical reasoning on the patient, who as a powerful source of clinical knowledge, makes a significant contribution to clinical reasoning processes. This view of clinical reasoning as being strongly shaped by other people aligns with Brookfield's (1995) and Barnett's (1997) emphasis on the social construction of critical thinking and their recognition that critical thinking is sustained by interactions with colleagues around collective standards. Although critical thinking is only one of the cognitive abilities employed in good clinical reasoning, it does play a significant role in the questioning of assumptions that must be ongoing during excellent clinical reasoning. In this way, clinical reasoning can be viewed as being critically constructed by interactions between clinicians, patients and colleagues around professional standards and evidence-based practices.

As further evidence of the influence of social and contextual factors on the quality of clinical reasoning, Smith et al. (2010) identified that the evolving nature of clinical reasoning was in part underpinned by ongoing critical appraisal of knowledge and practice and relationships with work colleagues. These authors also found that clinical reasoning developed along a continuum from novice to expert with more experienced or expert practitioners withholding judgement or the judging of patients, which allowed them to fully engage with the patient as a moral agent. Additionally, expert practitioners adopted approaches to clinical reasoning that empowered patients to be active participants in their own therapy, demonstrated greater capability in the management of social relationships with their patients and colleagues and were more specific, creative and refined towards individual needs of patients and the contexts in which they worked.

PEDAGOGIES FOR TEACHING CLINICAL REASONING

Clinical reasoning is central to effective healthcare practice and as such is often the focus of specific courses and forms a key goal of almost any course, clinical subject or clinical placement, often with considerable resource allocation to ensure its success. Recent innovations for the teaching of various aspects of clinical reasoning, including the use of carefully designed and selected cases, mnemonics for gathering information, identification of critical information and appropriate methods for managing uncertainty, although useful, neglect critical contextual and dispositional influences on clinical reasoning (Gruppen, 2017). Therefore the following exploration of pedagogies for teaching clinical reasoning embraces a broad range of pedagogies including those directed towards illuminating the invisible aspects of clinical reasoning, enhancing cognitive process and those that acknowledge the inherently situational and dispositional nature of clinical reasoning. This broad range of pedagogies underpinning successful teaching of clinical reasoning is captured in Fig. 31.2.

There is a deep compatibility between pedagogical approaches to teaching and learning clinical reasoning grounded in a sociocultural theoretical framework, especially when clinical reasoning is viewed as a complex, ongoing professional development journey for the learner. In particular, educational theory concerned with the interdependence of professional socialization and identity development and learning for participation in communities of practice (Wenger, 1998) provides guidance when developing clinical reasoning learning experiences.

Professional formation implies the creation of an identity as a healthcare professional, an adoption of the spirit and ethos of that profession (Colby and Sullivan, 2008). Participation in and becoming a member of a professional community of practice therefore affect not only what the practitioner knows how to do, but it transforms that person's identity (Wenger, 1998). Therefore professional formation directly influences and is influenced by personal beliefs and shapes the ways learners embody their professional and moral role in relationship with their patients and others in the healthcare context. Through this journey of becoming, individuals learn to focus their professional 'lens' to frame and interpret situations, identify problems and clinically reason through to enacted solutions (Christensen and Nordstrom, 2013). Contextualizing the teaching and learning of clinical reasoning by situating it within simulated participation experiences (e.g., in academic settings) or within authentic practice experiences helps entrench the learning of how to 'do' practice activities within the larger context of learning to think or clinically reason like a member of one's professional community. This would address, to some extent, Colby and Sullivan's concern that although professionals are about knowing, doing and being, too little of our current educational focus is on the being dimension of professional practice.

Wenger (1998) also describes *reification*, the utilization of a process by which the community gives form to concepts and experiences central to practice to facilitate the shaping of experiences. Reification is complementary and intrinsic to participation when learning in a community of practice. Giving form to complex and abstract aspects of practice results in 'focusing our attention in a particular way and enabling new kinds of understanding' (Wenger 1998, p. 60). Clinical reasoning, although complex and abstract in nature, can be reified or given form to make it more visible to learners (Christensen et al., 2008). Explicit

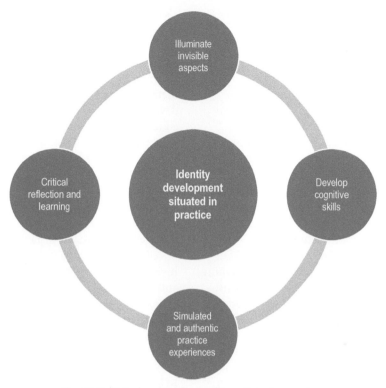

Fig. 31.2 ■ Pedagogies for teaching clinical reasoning.

exploration of definitions, descriptions and theoretical and research-derived models of clinical reasoning can all help to make clinical reasoning explicit and visible to the learner and can provide a language and a structure around which teachers and learners can expose, explore and critically reflect on individual contributions, contextual factors and relationships and interdependencies at work in any given practice scenario. This type of explicit conceptualization of clinical reasoning allows educators to 'create points of focus around which the negotiation of meaning becomes organized' (Wenger, 1998, p. 58).

Educators can best facilitate the learning of a complex phenomenon like clinical reasoning by making visible and fostering learners' awareness of all participants and related components involved in a particular clinical reasoning encounter (e.g., patients, carers, psychological and sociocultural factors, relevant structural health disparities, clinical context, health systems context) and most importantly by exploring the interdependent relationships between the individuals and components at play in any given situation. Explicit exploration of the ways in which clinical reasoning is enacted in various contexts can allow educators to 'create points of focus around which the negotiation of meaning becomes organized' (Wenger, 1998, p. 58). The use of a common language, derived from the descriptions, definitions and models used, provides a critical channel through which learners and teachers can describe, reflect on and learn from reasoning experiences (their own or those of others).

REFLECTION POINT 2

In your specific context (academic or workplace), how can you reify clinical reasoning to make it more visible to students?

How do you use theoretical models of clinical reasoning to enhance your own clinical reasoning practice and in your teaching of clinical reasoning?

How can you assist students to identify the influence of all participants (including themselves) and contextual factors inherent in a particular clinical reasoning encounter?

TEACHING CLINICAL REASONING IN CLASSROOMS

As a complex, abstract practice phenomenon, the teaching and facilitation of learning of clinical reasoning are challenging in both the classroom and workplace settings. Aided by the adoption of a model and language of clinical reasoning as a curricular framework, educators in a classroom setting can situate the teaching and learning of profession-specific technical skills within a larger curricular context of clinical reasoning (Christensen and Nordstrom, 2013). Clinical reasoning therefore becomes the background context or scaffold to which profession-specific technical knowledge is added. This scaffold is an existing visible 'structure' that provides clinical context and relevance to new knowledge and skills. This type of curricular framework encourages deep learning and discourages learning of discrete pieces of knowledge disconnected from the bigger practice context.

Essential to the development of curricula aiming to facilitate the learning of and from clinical reasoning is an explicit focus on development of related thinking and experiential learning skills. Transformative learning theory (Cranton, 2006; Mezirow, 2009), a branch of reconstructivist learning theory, provides a pedagogical foundation for educational strategies. Transformative learning is a process of using a prior understanding to construct a new or revised interpretation to guide future action. This learning transforms the learner by expanding his or her understanding, resulting in knowledge that is more 'inclusive, discriminating, reflective, open and emotionally able to change' (Mezirow, 2009, p. 22). Transformative learning is particularly relevant to using critical reflection on clinical reasoning experiences as the stimulus for learning from those experiences. Mezirow (2009) describes an outcome of transformative learning as when 'adults learn to reason for themselves—to advance and reassess reasons for making a judgement—rather than act on the assimilated beliefs, values, feelings and judgements of others' (p. 23).

In the classroom setting, today's educators have many options to bring simulated or authentic patient encounters to life – for example, having their students engage in clinical reasoning through the use of standardized patients or interaction with volunteer community members with real impairments. To facilitate the development of students' clinical reasoning skills, educators can engage learners with strategic questions to stimulate constructive dialogue rather than 'teaching' or 'telling' learners what they 'need to know'. In this way, students get practice in reasoning through a situation but also in explicit facilitation aimed at constructing new understandings based on their own reasoning experiences and those of their peers. This guided, experiential approach to facilitating the development of clinical reasoning capabilities illuminates often invisible aspects of clinical reasoning and scaffolding students' clinical reasoning capability development through a gradual trajectory from protected, authentic experiences towards clinical reasoning proficiency in real clinical situations with real patients, real timeframes and real consequences.

Expertise in clinical practice can be viewed as a result of excellence in learning from clinical experiences. The facilitation of critical self-reflection on clinical reasoning creates opportunities for challenging clinical knowledge and any potentially unsubstantiated assumptions underlying that knowledge. This type of challenge allows for growth and transformation of existing frames of reference, including theoretical or research-derived and experience-derived knowledge that, through application and testing with a recent clinical experience, may be revealed to have been inadequate. Facilitation of critical self-reflection on clinical reasoning experiences involves dialogue and questioning so that learners can figure things out for themselves, as they are facilitated in thinking about and making explicit to an external audience their own thinking (Cranton, 2006). Critical self-reflection, when facilitated by questioning and dialogue, can help to solidify the learner's understanding about his or her areas of strength, areas needing improvement and potentially any knowledge gaps or blind spots that were surfaced during a simulated or authentic clinical practice encounter. This in turn serves to further facilitate the building of skill in a process of active, systematic self-reflection and promotes self-directed learning.

TEACHING CLINICAL REASONING IN WORKPLACES

Professional practices are largely enacted and richly learned in workplace contexts. This juxtaposition of practice and learning in workplaces adds further complexity to the development of professional practice capabilities, such as clinical reasoning, in workplaces. When student education is located in workplace contexts, there is potential for conflict between achievement of organizational goals and students' educational goals. Health and educational institutions have their own domains and missions; one is primarily concerned with health provision and patient care and the other with student education (Jaye and Egan, 2006). In clinical workplaces, clinicians have an ethical obligation to prioritize quality patient care and a contractual obligation to meet organizational targets; therefore, student education can take a secondary role to patient care and organizational goals. Clinical teachers are required to undertake dual reasoning; they simultaneously reason about the patient they are treating and the student they are supervising, with an obligation to do their best for both. In situations in which time is short or productivity is a barrier to the time it takes to facilitate students' learning, in the end, the care of the patient will 'win' (Irby, 2014). This privileging of institutional goals over educational goals may result in student education being compromised and highlights an important need to better understand how professional practice capabilities such as clinical reasoning are best developed in clinical workplaces.

Clinical workplaces represent unique, complex, contested and dynamic contexts where clinical reasoning capabilities are developed. Learning in clinical workplaces is a multifaceted phenomenon that involves complex webs of power, acceptance into a community of practice and transformation of both learners and practice communities (Patton et al., 2013). Workplace learning theories provide a solid foundation for clinical educators or supervisors to construct wise clinical education practices including strategies to enhance development of clinical reasoning capabilities in complex workplace contexts. Many contemporary theories of workplace learning, built upon Lave and Wenger's (1991) situated learning theory, foreground contribution of social dimensions of workplaces to workplace learning in descriptions of learning as predominantly occurring through participation and interaction with colleagues. This emphasis of learning occurring through participation and interaction aligns well with the experiential and social dimensions of clinical reasoning described earlier in this chapter. Clinicians responsible for student education are therefore encouraged to look beyond the teaching practices they employ and explicitly consider their individual clinical environments and identify potential pervasive influences of those environments on students' clinical reasoning development. For example, clinicians could examine the level of independent clinical reasoning students undertake in their workplace, evidenced in undertaking independent patient assessment and treatment activities. Students can learn a great deal about clinical reasoning through working with patients and experiencing real outcomes from their treatment protocols and critically reflecting on those experiences. As another example, clinicians could examine student access to role models or contextual guides in the form of more experienced colleagues who are able to articulate their clinical reasoning processes and reveal some of the invisible aspects of clinical reasoning for students.

Workplace learning theories also offer a great deal in the consideration of how individual dispositional factors including emotion and general levels of well-being can influence and shape clinical reasoning and the development of clinical reasoning capabilities in clinical workplaces. These theories draw attention to how students' general state of well-being influences their engagement with learning experiences including the development of clinical reasoning capabilities. Learners themselves ultimately determine how they participate in and learn from what is afforded them, premised on their values, goals and experiences (Billett, 2010). Moreover, individuals' dispositions, interests and brute facts of energy, strength, state of fatigue and emotion also shape how individuals engage with and learn from workplace practices (Billett, 2009). An example of the wide continuum of student dispositions that can influence student engagement during clinical placements is provided in Case Study 31.1.

These composite student profiles of two physiotherapy students, Imogen and Ivy, are drawn from Narelle's doctoral research (Patton, 2014). In this case study, Imogen is well placed to develop her clinical reasoning capabilities during the current placement. She arrives

Two Physiotherapy Students

Imogen is very excited to be undertaking her first block placement in her hometown, as she will be able to live at home for the duration of her placement. Imogen's home is a 10-minute walk from the health service where she is undertaking her placement. Imogen is feeling confident about this placement as she has previously worked as an Allied Health Assistant with the health service and is therefore familiar with the hospital layout and the particular ward in which she is undertaking placement. After work each day, Imogen has established a routine of going for a bike ride, which gives her an opportunity to reflect on the activities of the day. After her bike ride, Imogen joins her mother in meal preparations and enjoys her evening meal with her family. Imogen debriefs with her family during meal times. As Imogen's father is a general practitioner, she finds his viewpoints particularly useful. After the evening meal, Imogen uses the Internet to source information required for the next day, including evidence-based treatment protocols. Being at home allows Imogen to organize social gatherings with other students staying at the hospital accommodation, providing further opportunities to discuss clinical experiences.

Ivy is undertaking her first placement away from home and has recently experienced the breakdown of a long-term relationship with her boyfriend. Ivy is anxious about this placement, as she has no previous experience of acute care hospital settings. Ivy is staying with friends who live 40 minutes from the hospital. Ivy is also recovering from an ankle injury that is giving her considerable discomfort during the day and prevents her from undertaking any physical activity outside of work hours. After work, Ivy stays up late into the evening socializing with her friends. She has no access to the Internet and has limited time to undertake preparation for her placement outside of work hours. As a consequence, Ivy is feeling stressed and fatigued and is starting to develop a sore throat.

each day refreshed and ready to engage, she is familiar with the hospital environment and she is able to ensure she has the requisite knowledge for each day and has multiple opportunities to collaboratively construct her clinical reasoning capabilities. Conversely, Ivy is not so well placed, she is somewhat isolated from her peers, she arrives each day fatigued, she has distractions that take her thoughts away from the placement, she is experiencing physical pain that also decreases her ability to concentrate and she is unable to ensure that she has the requisite knowledge on which to build her clinical reasoning capabilities. Teachers in both academic and workplace learning environments are therefore encouraged to consider students' general state of well-being and motivation to engage when constructing learning experiences aimed at the development of clinical reasoning capabilities.

Clinical educators responsible for the development of students' clinical reasoning capabilities during clinical placements should remain aware of how students engage with workplace opportunities to practice their reasoning skills and individual student characteristics that may further shape their learning. The significant influence of relationships and quality of guidance that students receive from more experienced colleagues is also salient to the development of clinical reasoning capabilities. Finally, to further enhance the quality of clinical learning experiences, clinical educators are encouraged to facilitate active and independent student participation in real patient activities because of the inherently experiential nature of clinical reasoning and professional practice. It is anticipated that grounding clinical reasoning teaching practices in sound and appropriate learning theories will enhance students' clinical reasoning capabilities and contribute to the development of health practitioners able to practice wisely in a rapidly changing healthcare system.

FUTURE DIRECTIONS

Currently, although there is no clear best practice framework to guide the teaching of clinical reasoning

(Ledford and Nixon, 2015), we recommend a holistic approach that acknowledges the complex, situated and embodied nature of clinical reasoning to achieve optimum development of clinical reasoning capabilities. The reduction of clinical reasoning to its cognitive, problem solving and de-contextualized dimensions risks limiting capability development and inadequately preparing students for the complex and fluid nature of professional practice and complexity of contemporary healthcare environments. Context is integral to clinical reasoning performance and includes psychological variables such as fatigue or stress or immediately preceding patient experiences, social variables, such as team relationships and support, and institutional or environmental factors, such as inpatient/outpatient setting (Gruppen, 2017). This centrality of context to the development of clinical reasoning capabilities highlights the importance of authentic practice experiences in academic contexts and workplace learning during clinical placements to students' developing clinical reasoning capabilities.

Recent developments in medical education and workplace learning have centred on development of core competencies, milestones and in particular on the emerging development of entrustable professional activities (EPAs) schemas (Chen et al., 2015). These workplace-centred approaches are providing new insights into methods of facilitating and assessing the learning of complex capabilities such as clinical reasoning in authentic and meaningful ways, beyond checklists of observable behaviours (Ten Cate and Billett, 2014). Although there is some variability in how these emerging constructs are being implemented across medical education systems (e.g., the Netherlands and the United States), the underlying conceptual framework of assessment as being oriented around achievement of effective independent performance of various practice activities is extremely applicable to situated, contextually driven phenomena like clinical reasoning. Key concepts relevant to the assessment of clinical reasoning from within this type of assessment approach are the development of descriptions of learners' clinical reasoning abilities linked along a developmental continuum of developmental milestones indicating progressive levels of achievement over time and related to decreased levels of supervision required to perform adequately (Englander and Carraccio, 2014). EPAs provide a way of inferring competency in the authentic workplace context rather than measuring it, as learners are deemed ready to transition to unsupervised practice when they can be fully entrusted to effectively perform various aspects of clinical practice without supervision (Englander and Carraccio, 2014). The assessment of a learner as worthy of entrustment to perform in an unsupervised manner relies on demonstration of both accurate self-assessment of the learner's own gaps or deficits in knowledge and abilities and trustworthiness, in that the learner can be relied upon to seek help when appropriate and necessary (Association of American Medical Colleges, 2014).

Contemporary and future academic landscapes that are increasingly transitioning healthcare education to online or distance modes incorporating flipped classrooms for part or all of the academic component emphasize the importance of implementation of pedagogical strategies that allow learners to learn through and from clinical reasoning before entering supervised workplace educational settings to build clinical reasoning awareness and related metaskills ahead of time. Larger class sizes in professional education programs as universities seek to maximize student load will increasingly challenge educators to engage with and 'diagnose' learning gaps in clinical reasoning knowledge/skills/metaskills and place preparation for optimal clinical learning at risk. These challenges highlight the importance of ongoing professional development around clinical reasoning for academics and workplace learning supervisors responsible for the development of students' clinical reasoning capabilities. Academics and workplace learning supervisors are encouraged to reflexively interrogate and advance their own clinical reasoning capabilities as they develop students' capabilities.

CHAPTER SUMMARY

In this chapter, we have outlined:

■ the complex, fluid, situated and experiential nature of clinical reasoning through our description of clinical reasoning as a holistic, experiential journey towards expertise,

■ pedagogies underpinning the teaching of clinical reasoning in academic and workplace contexts,

- the centrality of context to clinical reasoning and consequent criticality of student engagement in authentic practice experiences to the development of clinical reasoning capabilities and
- the need for ongoing exploration of assessment and teaching methods that capture the complexity of clinical reasoning and foster the development of clinical reasoning capabilities in students, clinicians and academics.

REFLECTION POINT 3

How can you embed more authentic experiential clinical encounters in your subject or course curriculum?

What opportunities currently exist in your subject or course to scaffold the development of students' critical reflective capabilities?

REFERENCES

Association of American Medical Colleges, 2014. Core entrustable professional activities for entering residency: curriculum developers' guide. Association of American Medical Colleges, Washington, DC. Viewed 1 June 2017. Available from: https://members.aamc.org/eweb/upload/Core%20EPA%20Curriculum%20Dev%20Guide.pdf.

Barnett, R., 1997. Higher Education: A Critical Business. The Society for Research into Higher Education & Open University Press, Buckingham, UK.

Billett, S., 2009. Conceptualizing learning experiences: contributions and mediations of the social, personal and brute. Mind Culture Activity 16, 32–47.

Billett, S., 2010. Lifelong learning and self: work, subjectivity and learning. Stud. Contin. Educ. 32, 1–16.

Brookfield, S., 1995. Becoming a Critically Reflective Teacher. Jossey-Bass, San Francisco, CA.

Chen, H.C., van den Broek, W.E.S., Ten Cate, O., 2015. The case for use of entrustable professional activities in undergraduate medical education. Acad. Med. 90, 431–436.

Christensen, N., Jones, M., Edwards, I., et al., 2008. Helping physiotherapy students develop clinical reasoning capability. In: Higgs, J., Jones, M., Loftus, S., et al. (Eds.), Clinical Reasoning in the Health Professions, third ed. Elsevier, Edinburgh, pp. 389–396.

Christensen, N., Nordstrom, T., 2013. Facilitating the teaching and learning of clinical reasoning. In: Jensen, G.M., Mostrom, E. (Eds.), Handbook of Teaching and Learning for Physical Therapists, third ed. Butterworth-Heinemann Elsevier, St. Louis, MO, pp. 183–199.

Colby, A., Sullivan, W., 2008. Formation of professionalism and purpose: perspectives from the Preparation for the Professions Program, University of St. Thomas. Law J. 5, 404–427.

Courtney-Pratt, H., Fitzgerald, M., Ford, K., et al., 2012. Quality clinical placements for undergraduate nursing students: a cross sectional survey of undergraduates and supervising nurses. J. Adv. Nurs. 68, 1380–1390.

Cranton, P., 2006. Understanding and Promoting Transformative Learning: A Guide for Educators of Adults, second ed. Jossey-Bass Wiley, San Francisco, CA.

Dewey, J., 1916. Democracy and Education: An Introduction to the Philosophy of Education. McMillan, New York, NY.

Durning, S., Ranic, J., Trowbridge, R., et al., 2015. Afterward teaching clinical reasoning—where do we go from here? In: Trowbridge, R.L., Rencic, J.J., Durning, S.J. (Eds.), Teaching Clinical Reasoning. Versa Press, East Peoria, IL, pp. 13–29.

Irby, D.M., 2014. Excellence in clinical teaching: knowledge transformation and development required. Med. Educ. 48, 776–784.

Englander, R., Carraccio, C., 2014. From theory to practice: making entrustable professional activities come to life in the context of milestones. Acad. Med. 89, 1321–1323.

Gruppen, L., 2017. Clinical reasoning: defining it, teaching it, assessing it, studying it. West. J. Emerg. Med. 18, 4–7.

Higgs, J., Jones, M., 2008. Clinical decision making and multiple problem spaces. In: Higgs, J., Jones, M., Loftus, S., et al. (Eds.), Clinical Reasoning in the Health Professions, third ed. Elsevier, Edinburgh, pp. 3–18.

Jaye, C., Egan, T., 2006. Communities of clinical practice: implications for health professional education. Focus on Health Professional Education 8, 1–10.

Lave, J., Wenger, E., 1991. Situated Learning: Legitimate Peripheral Participation. Cambridge University Press, Cambridge, UK.

Ledford, C.H., Nixon, L.J., 2015. General teaching techniques. In: Trowbridge, R.L., Rencic, J.J., Durning, S.J. (Eds.), Teaching Clinical Reasoning. Versa Press, East Peoria, IL, pp. 77–116.

Mezirow, J., 2009. Transformative learning theory. In: Mezirow, J., Taylor, E.W., Associates (Eds.), Transformative Learning in Practice: Insights From Community, Workplace, and Higher Education. Jossey-Bass, San Francisco, CA, pp. 3–33.

Patton, N., 2014. Clinical learning spaces: crucibles for the development of professional practice capabilities, PhD thesis. Charles Sturt University, Albury, NSW.

Patton, N., Higgs, J., Smith, M., 2013. Using theories of learning in workplaces to enhance physiotherapy clinical education. Physiother. Theory Pract. 29, 493–503.

Ratcliffe, T., Durning, S., 2015. Theoretical concepts to consider in providing clinical reasoning instruction. In: Trowbridge, R.L., Rencic, J.J., Durning, S.J. (Eds.), Teaching Clinical Reasoning. Versa Press, East Peoria, IL, pp. 13–29.

Smith, M., Higgs, J., Ellis, E., 2010. Effect of experience on clinical decision making by cardiorespiratory physiotherapists in acute care settings. Physiother. Theory Pract. 26, 89–99.

Ten Cate, O., Billett, S., 2014. Competency-based medical education: origins, perspectives, and potentialities. Med. Educ. 48, 325–332.

Wenger, E., 1998. Communities of Practice: Learning, Meaning, and Identity. Cambridge University Press, Cambridge, UK.

32

TEACHING CLINICAL REASONING IN MEDICAL EDUCATION COURSES

DENISE M. CONNOR ■ GURPREET DHALIWAL ■ JUDITH L. BOWEN

CHAPTER AIMS

The aims of this chapter are to:

- describe the key elements, learning goals and teaching strategies for an integrated clinical reasoning curriculum for medical students and
- emphasize an approach for aligning a clinical reasoning curriculum with the developmental stage of learners, building in complexity and authenticity as students near immersive clinical training.

KEY WORDS

Clinical reasoning

Problem representation

Illness scripts

Metacognition

Curriculum design

ABBREVIATIONS/ ACRONYMS

A&P Assessment and plan

H&P History and physical

HPI History of present illness

SP Standardized patient

INTRODUCTION

Most medical schools do not explicitly teach students how doctors reason through patients' clinical problems. Instead, schools impart medical knowledge and then offer opportunities for students to apply that knowledge in examinations, simulations and patient care. This traditional approach to medical education creates adequate reasoners, but it is unlikely to cultivate exceptional ones. The persistent problem of diagnostic error in medicine (estimated to occur in 10% to 15% of patient encounters) demands a new approach to teaching clinical reasoning (National Academies of Sciences, Engineering, and Medicine [NASEM], 2016).

Clinical reasoning is a procedure akin to tying a surgical knot, listening to a heart or leading a family meeting. For students to reach their full potential as reasoners, they require longitudinal instruction, practice, coaching and formative feedback. In this chapter, we outline a curriculum for clinical reasoning for undergraduate medical education that accomplishes the following goals:

1. Introduces the science of reasoning, fosters use of the vocabulary of reasoning and provides a map of the reasoning process (Understanding Reasoning section).
2. Integrates reasoning practice with both medical knowledge acquisition and clinical skill building (Integration section).

345

3. Introduces the concepts of clinical uncertainty and diagnostic error (Introduction to Uncertainty and Diagnostic Error section).

Each of the following sections contains a description of key concepts paired with related learning goals and teaching strategies.

UNDERSTANDING REASONING

Clinical reasoning curricula should offer students a window into how experts solve clinical problems (the science of reasoning). This context prepares students to engage in learning the process of reasoning through defined, discrete steps (using a map of reasoning) that can be described (using the vocabulary of reasoning), practiced and intentionally improved upon over time.

Science of Reasoning

Introducing the science of reasoning gives students a rationale for engaging with the curriculum and the motivation to think about their own thinking. Cognitive psychology proposes two closely related reasoning modes: intuitive and analytic (Eva, 2005). Intuitive reasoning, also known as 'pattern recognition', describes a subconscious, rapid process. Analytic reasoning describes a deliberate, slower process. These processes represent two ends of a continuum. Clinicians do not consciously choose when to use intuitive or analytic reasoning. Instead, the relative contribution of each mode is determined by the task and by how the relevant knowledge is structured in memory.

Teachers should avoid setting up a false hierarchy between these strategies, as either mode can result in diagnostic success or error. Combined reasoning can be introduced as a strategy to mitigate error (e.g., performing a diagnostic time-out to mentally check a diagnosis arrived at using intuition with an analytic question like 'what else could this be?') (Ark et al., 2004; Lambe et al., 2016; Norman et al., 1999).

Learning Goals

After this introduction, students should be able to: compare and contrast intuitive versus analytic reasoning and describe the benefits of combined reasoning.

Teaching Strategies

Students' familiarity with reasoning modes can be developed through sessions that:

- Solicit examples of intuitive versus analytic problem solving from everyday life (e.g., automatically navigating the route home versus identifying the problem when a car will not start) and draw comparisons with clinical problem solving.
- Showcase a clinician thinking aloud while analyzing a case. After the expert discusses a segment of clinical data, a teacher offers a metacognitive commentary, describing the cognitive processes underlying the expert's reasoning. The *Journal of General Internal Medicine's Exercises in Clinical Reasoning Series* provides a useful illustration of this approach (Henderson et al., 2010).

Vocabulary of Reasoning

In all complex fields, students and teachers require a shared vocabulary to communicate effectively. Pathophysiology and ethics are examples of domains in which defined terminology (e.g., impaired diastolic relaxation) and frameworks (e.g., benevolence and autonomy) are necessary to learn and scrutinize complicated problems. Similarly, reasoning terms provide a shared language for examining how students think about, speak about and learn from clinical problems (Dhaliwal and Ilgen, 2016).

By learning how to transform patients' stories into medical terminology, students can begin to communicate their reasoning to other clinicians. Further, semantic qualifiers enable students to translate patients' stories into refined clinical problems that can be more easily solved (Fig. 32.1).

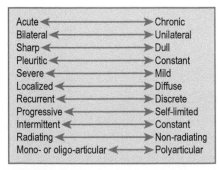

Fig. 32.1 ■ Examples of opposing semantic qualifiers.

Orientation to the language of reasoning should include the concepts elaborated in Table 32.1. Of note, the concept of problem representation has evolved over time, particularly within clinical teaching contexts. In the foundational reasoning literature, the problem representation connotes an early abstraction of the core problem-type being solved (e.g., acute monoarticular arthritis in an otherwise healthy man). As more data are gathered in the clinical encounter, the problem representation is refined and contextualized to form an assessment that comprehensively and specifically describes the patient's problem (e.g., 48-year-old man recently started on hydrochlorothiazide with acute right ankle arthritis, leukocytosis and elevated, C-reactive protein (CRP)). The meaning of problem representation has been extended in the clinical teaching literature to capture both the early abstraction of the core problem-type and the summative assessment. However, because early problem representation serves a different role in the reasoning process than the later summative assessment, we find it helpful to separate these concepts.

Learning Goals

After exposure to reasoning vocabulary, students should be able to:

■ Demonstrate accurate transformation of the components of patients' stories into medical terminology (e.g., 'shortness of breath with walking' becomes 'dyspnoea on exertion').

TABLE 32.1
Reasoning Vocabulary

Reasoning Concept	Definition	Purpose	Example
Semantic Transformation	Translation of specific characteristics of the patient's history into abstract terms using vocabulary with opposed concepts (e.g., acute vs chronic)	■ Acculturation ('talk like a doctor') ■ Recognizes the centrality of compare/contrast in defining a problem type	■ 'It started suddenly last night' becomes 'acute' ■ 'All of the joints in my arms and legs are aching' becomes 'symmetrical polyarthralgia'
Problem Representation	Abstracted core of a patient's clinical issue using medical terms and semantic qualifiers. Iteratively refined throughout H&P	■ Activates knowledge (triggers potential illness scripts), which continuously informs additional data acquisition (e.g., what data must be collected to retain/discard candidate scripts) ■ Developed and refined iteratively as new data is gathered (e.g., acute dyspnoea becomes acute dyspnoea in immunosuppressed patient)	■ Young man with acute, painless monocular blindness ■ Elderly smoker with chronic, episodic gross haematuria
Assessment (Summative Problem Representation)	Summary statement or 'one-liner'. Opens the A&P. Contextualizes key elements of a patient's abstracted problem. May include: predisposing conditions (epidemiology/risk factors), clinical consequences (time course/tempo, symptoms/signs); similar categories found in illness scripts	■ Enables justification of a prioritized differential diagnosis by comparing/contrasting candidate illness scripts with a summary of the patient's problem ■ Highlights features of a patient's H&P that justify a 'most likely' diagnosis	■ 48-year-old immunosuppressed woman with chronic productive cough, fevers, and progressive dyspnoea on exertion with left upper lobe rhonchi and egophany

Continued on following page

TABLE 32.1			
Reasoning Vocabulary *(Continued)*			
Reasoning Concept	Definition	Purpose	Example
Illness Script	Mental model of disease featuring: predisposing conditions (epidemiology/risk factors); clinical consequences (time course/tempo, signs/symptoms); pathophysiological fault (NB: Experts have elaborated scripts with additional data such as prognosis, treatment options)	■ Organizes medical knowledge about a diagnosis around the most relevant features and key categories ■ Emphasizes features that differentiate one diagnosis from related illnesses	■ An early script for vasovagal syncope may include: often in young, healthy patients; hyperacute, short duration; premonitory symptoms of nausea, pallor, diaphoresis with trigger (e.g., blood draw); transient hypotension caused by bradycardia and/or peripheral vasodilation from inappropriate neural input
Prioritized Differential Diagnosis	Organizes potential diagnoses as most likely, can't miss, less likely and least likely and provides a rationale for this ranking	■ Shares justification for prioritized diagnostic thinking by compare/contrast with patient's assessment ('think aloud')	■ The most likely diagnosis is migraine based on the subacute onset, unilateral and pulsatile qualities, with photophobia and vomiting ■ A less likely but 'can't miss' diagnosis is a subarachnoid haemorrhage (SAH). However, SAH is usually sudden onset with accompanying neurological deficits. ■ Finally, bacterial meningitis is very unlikely given the lack of fever, leukocytosis or meningismus.
Diagnostic Schema	A systematic approach or framework for thinking through a clinical problem	■ Links mechanistic thinking and pathophysiology with common clinical syndromes ■ Offers analytic approaches to developing differential diagnoses for complex problems	■ Acute kidney injury can be broken down into prerenal, intrinsic, or postrenal causes.

■ Demonstrate transformation of the HPI into abstract terms using semantic qualifiers (e.g., 'it's getting worse' becomes 'progressive').

■ Explain the role of problem representations, summative assessments, illness scripts, prioritized differential diagnoses and schema in the diagnostic process.

Teaching Strategies

■ Ask students to identify active problems from written, live, or videotaped histories and use medical terms and semantic qualifiers to describe each problem. Peer and facilitator feedback can clarify questions and generate discussion about the importance of abstraction and the value of identifying the crux of a problem.

■ During clinical exposure, encourage students to notice when clinicians use medical terminology versus plain language. Students can reflect on how technical language influences problem solving, while also considering the importance of plain language for patient communication.

Map of the Reasoning Process

Understanding the discrete steps of reasoning helps teachers and students to identify where students are succeeding or struggling and to target areas needing additional practice (Fig. 32.2). The ability to describe

MAP OF REASONING PROCESS   **TEACHING EMPHASIS**

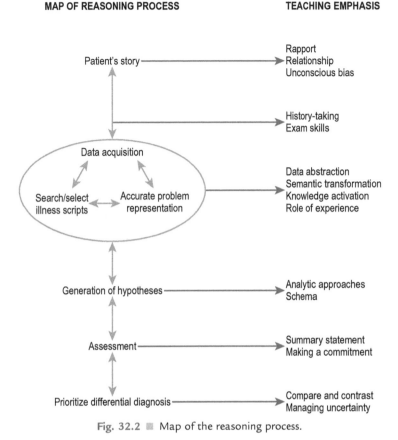

Fig. 32.2 ◼ Map of the reasoning process.

these steps using reasoning terms provides students with language for seeking specific feedback from clinical supervisors and a framework for analyzing their successes and errors in reasoning.

Because illness scripts serve as foundational knowledge structures in long-term memory, early scripts should emphasize typical features of classic presentations and aspects that differentiate related diagnoses. Armed with insight into the reasoning framework, students can begin to compare/contrast candidate illness scripts and develop hypothesis-driven approaches to patient encounters.

REFLECTION POINT 1

For the map of the reasoning process to have the greatest effect, teachers in both the preclinical and clinical domains must use a shared language to describe their own thinking process and to critique students' work. Consider how you would develop and implement a faculty development program at your institution with the aim of spreading the language of reasoning beyond isolated reasoning-focussed didactics.

How would such a faculty development campaign look at your institution?

Learning Goals

Learning goals should align with students' development. At the foundational level, students should be able to:

◼ abstract the key attributes of patients' chief complaints, including onset, site, chronology and severity and use them to create succinct problem representations;

- identify relevant data pertaining to the chief complaint (e.g., history of diabetes is relevant to a foot infection);
- identify relevant contextual information that pertains to the problem representation (e.g., recent international travel) and
- identify matches and mismatches between a patient's presentation and the typical features of candidate illness scripts.

At the clerkship preparation level, students should be able to:

- identify the most likely, can't miss and less likely diagnoses when analyzing clinical cases,
- defend selection of the most likely diagnosis based on the clinical data set,
- explain why other diagnoses are less likely based on the clinical data set,
- describe how the likelihood of a diagnosis is affected by pretest probability, base rate and incremental data, leading to a posttest probability and
- develop diagnostic approaches to commonly encountered clinical problems (e.g., chronic cough in the office setting).

Teaching Strategies

Case-based sessions engage students and prepare them for the clinical setting. Cases enable students to link history and examination findings with diagnostic considerations and pathophysiology while they develop diagnostic approaches to clinical problems. However, early learners are at risk for overwhelming their working memory with novel data and tasks during case-based learning. When this capacity is overextended, the ability to learn new concepts declines. Offering increasing complexity and cognitive demands over time can maximize learning by optimizing cognitive load (Schmidt and Mamede, 2015). Thus teaching strategies should follow a developmental trajectory:

- Cases in the preclinical curriculum should focus on simple, common presentations and diseases, not rare ones (e.g., the approach to dyspnoea should be developed through the juxtaposition of pneumonia and heart failure, not granulomatosis with polyangiitis and sarcoidosis). When

students reach the clinical environment, atypical presentations and rare diagnoses can be introduced and anchored to students' foundation of classic clinical presentations (Kassirer, 2010).

- Cases should progress from simple paper cases in which a complete data set is provided, to serial cue cases in which students must request necessary data, to SP cases in which students must gather data (Schmidt and Mamede, 2015). Initially, after eliciting students' ideas for possible diagnoses, teachers should fill in gaps in the differential diagnosis and provide examples of key content in the illness scripts under consideration.
- Sessions should include opportunities for students to practice defending their diagnostic considerations. Practicing the skill of 'thinking on your feet' prepares students for clerkships and facilitates their transition to clinical training.
- Cases presented near the end of preclerkship education should include opportunities to apply Bayesian reasoning. This form of analytic reasoning helps students think critically about the properties of diagnostic tests and the importance of assigning pretest probability before testing. Scenarios can include potential diagnoses with accessible data about pretest probability and well-defined test characteristics such as streptococcal pharyngitis (Centor criteria, throat swab test characteristics), pulmonary embolism (Wells score, D-dimer test characteristics) and coronary artery disease (Framingham risk score, stress test characteristics). Teachers should acknowledge the limits of applying quantitative approaches in real-world settings.

Students should consolidate application of clinical reasoning concepts by:

- Writing evolving problem representations at several steps of a paper case (e.g., after the HPI, after the medical history, after the examination). Facilitators should discuss students' choices at each step and point out how the evolving problem representation influences further data gathering and narrows the plausible differential diagnosis.
- Working with peers to create a flowchart delineating the categories of disease (e.g., cardiac, pulmonary or musculoskeletal) that may explain a clinical problem (e.g., acute chest pain), further

developing those categories with a facilitator (e.g., specifying subcategories and considering historical/examination features that differentiate between or within categories) and using this schema to guide the differential diagnosis.

- Practicing committing to a most likely diagnosis and describing why that diagnosis is more likely than competing possibilities.
- Committing to a pretest probability, gathering interval data with associated likelihood ratios and calculating posttest probability at several junctures (e.g., after history, after examination, after laboratories/radiology). Subgroups of students can be given different examination, laboratory, or imaging data that lead to differing posttest probabilities, stimulating discussion of the effect of pretest probability and testing on diagnosis. Teachers can emphasize that understanding these concepts in a quantitative way will prepare students for grasping the more qualitative Bayesian thinking that clinicians utilize in the real-world (e.g., assigning 'low', 'intermediate' or 'high' pretest probability) (Medow and Lucey, 2011).

REFLECTION POINT 2

A 'good teaching case' in the clinical setting is often shorthand for patients with rare diagnoses or atypical presentations. However, simple, typical, straightforward cases are the highest yield for early learners. Consider clinical cases in your specialty that would maximize learning for students who are just beginning to build their illness scripts for common diagnoses. What clinical syndromes (e.g., acute headache) are fundamental for students to understand, and which diagnoses causing those syndromes would you choose to highlight?

INTEGRATION

Integrating reasoning principles with medical knowledge acquisition, clinical skill building and communication training enables students to put the reasoning framework into practice, to create a pragmatic scaffold for early knowledge organization and to develop links between the cognitive and behavioural skills needed to solve clinical problems.

Integration With Medical Knowledge Acquisition

Preclinical students' early knowledge structures and learning habits may affect their ability to develop differential diagnoses in clinical encounters. Organizing knowledge in a fashion that mirrors how information will be accessed when faced with undifferentiated patients who present with symptoms – not assigned diagnoses – will prepare learners for their future problem-solving tasks (Stern et al., 2014). Emphasizing compare/contrast thinking helps students select which information to encode in their early illness scripts. For instance, as students think through the problem of acute chest pain and appreciate the need to differentiate pulmonary embolism (PE) from angina, they may recognize the value of exacerbating features of the pain (e.g., pleuritic in PE versus exertional in angina) in their diagnostic thinking and emphasize these distinguishing features as they develop and refine the relevant illness scripts.

Further, viewing disease processes through clinical reasoning and basic science lenses can help contextualize learning, reinforce key points and strengthen students' grasp of complex topics (Lisk et al., 2016a, 2016b; Woods, 2007).

Learning Goals

Students engaged in an integrated reasoning curriculum should be able to:

- outline illness scripts for common diagnoses organized around the categories of predisposing factors (epidemiology/risk factors), clinical consequences (time course/tempo, signs/symptoms) and pathophysiology (Custers, 2015);
- identify differentiating features for closely linked diagnoses (e.g., gout versus osteoarthritis);
- describe the defining (must be present) and differentiating (discriminate between related diagnoses) features of two to three scripts relevant to a problem representation (Bowen, 2006) (e.g., gout and osteoarthritis both cause knee pain, but only gout would have a synovial white blood cell count greater than 25,000 WBC/μL) and
- provide an example of how pathophysiology may be used to develop diagnostic schema for approaching a clinical problem (e.g., separate acute kidney injury into prerenal, intrinsic and postrenal causes).

TABLE 32.2
Compare/Contrast Illness Script Grid for the Clinical Syndrome of Transient Loss of Consciousness

Diagnosis	Vasovagal Syncope	Seizure	Syncope Caused by an Arrhythmia
Predisposing Conditions (Risk Factors, Epidemiology)	Frequently in young, healthy patients May present atypically in older patients Most common cause of syncope	Variable, depends on cause of seizure Many causes: e.g., metabolic abnormalities (electrolyte disturbances, renal failure); brain lesions (cancer, stroke)	Variable, depends on cause of arrhythmia, e.g., congenital long QT often presents at young age, may have family history of sudden death
Time Course, Pattern	Hyperacute Short duration	Hyperacute *Can* be prolonged duration	Hyperacute Short duration
Clinical Consequences (Symptoms (Sx), Signs)	Premonitory sx (increased vagal tone) common = nausea, diaphoresis, pallor Occurs when sitting/standing, recover when supine (increased blood flow to brain) Triggers: strong emotions, stress (e.g., pain, blood draws)	Premonitory sx common (may have aura) (e.g., déjà vu) or nonspecific sx (e.g., dizziness, paraesthesia) Prolonged recovery (postictal state) with confusion, abnormal level of consciousness	Minimal premonitory sx (may have palpitations) Injury common (sudden, without bracing for a fall) Triggers vary, e.g., congenital long QT syncope triggered by exertion, strong emotions Quick recovery, no prolonged confusion
Pathophysiology	Neural reflex → hypotension from bradycardia +/− peripheral vasodilation from faulty neural input	Abnormal neuronal firing (hyperexcitability, hypersynchrony)	Abnormal cardiac rhythm → poor forward flow/ hypotension → poor perfusion of brain

Teaching Strategies

To achieve these learning outcomes, we suggest several strategies (Table 32.2):

- Focus on compare/contrast learning (Lucey, 2015).
  - Instead of assigning reading or selecting didactic content that focusses on a single diagnosis, use a compare/contrast learning strategy that requires students to simultaneously consider two or three overlapping, competing diagnoses for a given clinical syndrome (e.g., oligoarticular arthritis) with an emphasis on differentiating characteristics (e.g., how to distinguish rheumatoid arthritis from osteoarthritis) (Stern et al., 2014).
  - Present two cases of dyspnoea (e.g., chronic obstructive pulmonary disease and asthma) within a single session, and require students to identify defining/differentiating features in the original data set.
  - Ask students to construct compare/contrast tables to crystallize learning (Table 32.3).

TABLE 32.3
Traditional Versus Compare/Contrast Approach to Clinical Learning

Traditional Approach	Compare/Contrast Approach
Disease (e.g., migraine)	Clinical syndrome (e.g., headache)
1 patient case = exemplar	2–3 related patient cases
Reinforce, contextualize medical knowledge about a *diagnosis*	Identify features that differentiate causes of a *syndrome*
Knowledge expertise	Knowledge application expertise
Diagnosis-facing	Patient-facing

Based on Stern et al., 2014

- Link medical knowledge content covered in reasoning sessions with the basic science curriculum.
- Although students are learning the pathophysiology of cerebral ischaemia, reasoning sessions should develop students' abilities to form problem representations for related clinical syndromes such as acute focal weakness and to develop illness scripts

for diagnoses that link the pathophysiology of ischaemia with the clinical presentation. Similarly, basic science sessions should make connections between pathophysiology and clinical presentations, focussing on mechanisms of disease that explain symptoms and signs.

Integration With Hypothesis-Driven Data Collection

Linking reasoning practice with clinical skill development builds students' appreciation of interview questions and examination manoeuvres as options on a menu of diagnostic tools to be actively selected while gathering relevant data. Integration of clinical skill building with reasoning means that the 'thorough H&P' becomes secondary to the hypothesis-driven H&P. In the former, students check off a long list of manoeuvres unrelated to a patient's problem. In the latter, students engage their diagnostic reasoning and make intentional decisions about how to focus their data gathering (e.g., focussing on data with defining and discriminating power) (Allen et al., 2016).

Learning Goals

Students should be able to:

- provide examples of how divergent findings on physical examination affect diagnostic thinking for a clinical syndrome (e.g., presence/absence of hypervolaemia in a dyspnoeic patient);
- demonstrate use of historical questions and examination manoeuvres that differentiate among candidate diagnoses during information gathering with an SP (e.g., ask about time to peak intensity of acute headache; assess for presence/absence of cervical lymphadenopathy with sore throat) and
- perform hypothesis-driven H&Ps with SPs with common symptoms.

Teaching Strategies

We suggest the following:

- Utilize clinical vignettes to contextualize physical examination skill development.
  - After students practice the cardiac examination, ask them to consider how differing abnormalities of the cardiovascular examination would modify the differential diagnosis for a dyspnoeic

patient, e.g., elevated jugular venous pulsation (JVP) and lower-extremity oedema versus a normal JVP and no oedema. In this way, the examination becomes a meaningful extension of students' diagnostic thinking.
- Integrate reasoning concepts into data-gathering sessions (e.g., during HPIs with SPs, take time-outs to ask students to articulate their working problem representation and reflect on how the problem representation activates diagnostic considerations and informs additional data gathering to distinguish among possible diagnoses).
- Feature H&Ps performed by experts who provide a parallel clinical reasoning narration – the expert reasons aloud as he or she learns new information in the history and then plans, executes and interprets results of examination manoeuvres.

Integration With Patient-Centred and Interprofessional Communication

Integrating reasoning concepts with data-collection skill building creates an opportunity to demonstrate that sensitive and skilful communication with both patients and the interprofessional team is essential for diagnostic success (e.g., a patient-centred approach enables providers to gather a full history and perform an appropriate examination).

Learning Goals

Students should:

- demonstrate use of open-ended questions and empathic and summarizing statements (e.g., 'to make sure I'm understanding correctly, I'd like to summarize what you've told me so far') while eliciting an SP's HPI;
- describe the value of rapport to the diagnostic process and
- describe how interprofessional and intraprofessional communication affects the diagnostic process.

Teaching Strategies

Authentic stories are powerful means to link communication with diagnosis. Sessions can do the following:

- feature panels in which patients highlight occasions when they did not share details of their clinical story with providers because of negative feelings (e.g., discomfort, shame) versus encounters when they revealed information because of positive rapport (Aper et al., 2015);

- bring together students across health professions for case-based, simulated role-play of interprofessional communication (e.g., nursing, medical student and pharmacy students practice solving a case together after their own independent analysis). Include time for discussion of how communication facilitated or hampered patient care within the context of a simulated case and
- include SP feedback after simulated encounters focussed on how the patient–provider interaction either facilitated or impaired disclosure of historical details. To achieve this sophisticated feedback, SPs require additional training to modify how they disclose information based on the quality of the rapport built by the student.

REFLECTION POINT 3

Effective integration of reasoning into existing curricula requires collaboration among many stakeholders. Who are the stakeholders at your institution within both the basic and clinical sciences? How would you engage these educational leaders to intentionally create clear linkages between traditional content and new reasoning-focussed content?

INTRODUCTION TO UNCERTAINTY AND DIAGNOSTIC ERROR

Once students understand the elements of diagnostic success, they can be introduced to the concepts of diagnostic uncertainty and error. Acknowledging the entire spectrum of diagnostic performance requires nurturing students' nascent self-efficacy while simultaneously instilling humility and a commitment to continuous self-improvement (Simpkin and Schwartzstein, 2016; Sommers and Launer, 2014). Diagnostic error should be introduced as a quality and safety issue with both cognitive and systems origins (NASEM, 2016).

Normalizing Uncertainty

Openly discussing uncertainty early in medical education and demonstrating that experts grapple with

this issue allow students to reflect on uncertainty throughout their training and professional lives. Diagnostic uncertainty is best explored after students have developed a solid foundation with the reasoning framework but before entering immersive clinical training. Students should begin to recognize uncertainty within clinical cases and communicate it with patients and colleagues. Familiarizing students with the language of probability and base rates can be a useful adjunct to discussions about uncertainty (Maserejian et al., 2009).

Learning Goals

Students should be able to:

- describe sources of uncertainty in diagnosis (e.g., patients with atypical presentations),
- convey diagnostic uncertainty surrounding a simulated case to a colleague in written and oral formats,
- engage an SP in a discussion about diagnostic uncertainty,
- involve an SP in shared decision making about next steps in the face of diagnostic uncertainty (e.g., the role of a therapeutic trial) and
- identify the utility of base rates when facing diagnostic uncertainty and provide an example of how consideration of base rates can influence the diagnostic process.

Teaching Strategies

- Hold panel presentations with providers from many practice settings discussing their experiences with uncertainty.
- Offer insight into the effect of uncertainty on patients (e.g., patients whose diagnoses remained elusive for an extended time are invited to discuss the effect of uncertainty on their quality of life).
- Present authentic cases in which a definitive diagnosis is not identified – with the help of facilitators, students can develop strategies to resolve uncertainty or to move forward after acknowledging unresolved uncertainty.
  - Students can then role-play how to convey their uncertainty to colleagues.
- Role-play shared decision making with SPs when a clear diagnosis is lacking.

Analyzing Error

Students should develop the capacity to recognize circumstances and thought processes that may contribute to diagnostic errors. To acquire this skill, students need practice in retrospectively analyzing diagnostic errors using a systematic approach for classifying the underlying causes of missed or delayed diagnoses. External circumstances such as patient handoffs and internal states such as fatigue that may increase the risk for error can be explored. Introducing a few common forms of cognitive error in a case-based fashion can bring this topic to life. Finally, students can explore the effect of unconscious social bias on clinical decision making.

Learning Goals

Students should be able to:

- describe a framework for the causes of diagnostic errors (e.g., systems, cognitive, no fault) (Graber et al., 2005),
- describe situations that may increase the risk for diagnostic error (e.g., multitasking, emotionally charged encounters, fatigue) (Johns et al., 2009; NASEM, 2016; Schmidt et al., 2017),
- describe three common cognitive tendencies (e.g., premature closure, anchoring, availability bias) and recognize examples in clinical vignettes and
- describe sources of unconscious social bias in clinical decision making (e.g., related to race or gender).

Teaching Strategies

During discussions of errors, care must be taken to create a safe learning environment and to set a positive, rather than a blaming, hypercritical tone. Options include:

- patient panels or videotaped testimonials discussing the effect of diagnostic error,
- facilitated discussions using written, live or video patient vignettes to explore common causes of cognitive error, situations at high risk for error and the effect of unconscious social bias (MedU, n.d.; Reilly et al., 2013) and
- sessions in which students discuss diagnostic errors they have witnessed (or experienced) to enable

an analysis of underlying cognitive, social and systems factors.

Strategies to Reduce Risk for Error

Introducing uncertainty and error without sharing strategies to deal with these issues can be counterproductive and may negatively affect students' self-efficacy. Offering insight into how clinicians manage these issues establishes a problem-solving mindset that can carry students forward into their professional lives.

Deliberate individuation of patients (e.g., learning about what makes a patient unique, counteracting the tendency to categorize patients within a particular social group) and the conscious cultivation of empathy can be introduced as tools to combat the unintended effect of unconscious social bias (Boscardin, 2015).

Discussion of the potentially negative effect of cognitive biases should be balanced with acknowledgement that heuristics, or mental shortcuts, are valuable problem-solving tools (Dhaliwal, 2017). Rather than leaving students with the impression that heuristics should be avoided, teachers can emphasize the importance of engaging in circumspection, recognizing when a heuristic is being used and using reflective practice to check a diagnosis arrived at quickly, particularly when faced with complex cases (Mamede et al., 2008). Teachers should also point out that excessively analytic approaches can lead to overweighting of features that distract clinicians during the reasoning process.

Learning Goals

Students should be able to:

- recognize common cognitive biases in simulated clinical cases,
- demonstrate the use of combined intuitive and analytic reasoning strategies in a simulated case (Ark et al., 2004; Eva et al., 2007),
- describe mechanisms for reducing the risk for error in high-risk situations (e.g., fatigue, handoffs) (Johns et al., 2009; NASEM, 2016; Starmer et al., 2014),
- describe how more elaborated illness scripts or schemas can lead to improved diagnostic performance and
- reflect on unconscious social bias and describe tools for deliberately individuating patients.

Teaching Strategies

- Case-based sessions can facilitate students' abilities to identify and define common forms of cognitive error; teachers should encourage students to critically review recent debates on the subject of mitigating cognitive errors (Graber et al., 2012).
- A panel of providers can discuss their experiences with system factors that increase the risk for error, such as a confusing interface for data entry into the electronic health record and describe their practices for reflection after diagnostic errors.
- Case presentations in which a diagnostic error is made because of inadequate knowledge (e.g., all asthma exacerbations present with wheezing) can open discussion into how clinicians learn from these experiences and revise their illness scripts accordingly.
- Videos demonstrating the effect of body language and differential responses to patient questions can be provocative tools for generating discussion about the effect of unconscious social bias on patient–provider communication.
- Students can take several versions of the Implicit Association Test (e.g., related to gender, race) followed by reflective writing or discussion to process the results (Greenwald et al., n.d.).

REFLECTION POINT 4

Explicit discussion of uncertainty and error in the preclinical domain should be followed by ongoing openness to these discussions in the patient care domain. Otherwise, the 'hidden curriculum' will quickly reverse students' perceptions of what topics are acceptable for discussion. Consider whether your institution currently has a climate that encourages or discourages dialogue about uncertainty and error. If these subjects are met with resistance, how might you embark on institutional culture change? If your institutional culture only accepts these discussions when focussed on 'systems errors,' reflect on what might be the first steps to expand that culture to include individual clinicians' experiences with uncertainty and cognitive error.

CONCLUSION

Just as we have historically used 'see one, do one, teach one' when instructing students on bedside procedures, we should similarly offer students opportunities to see the diagnostic reasoning process before expecting them to do this intricate procedure independently. Instruction should start at the beginning of medical school and be integrated throughout the curriculum, with increasing complexity and uncertainty introduced along the way.

Expert reasoning is often intuitive and therefore invisible to students. Classroom-based instruction can demystify this process. With an explicit reasoning map, students can analyze their own reasoning attempts, mark their progress and set goals for self-improvement. As students move from the preclinical domain to immersive patient care, it is important to prevent discourse around reasoning to fade into the background. Faculty development is essential to continuing this thread during clinical training. Clinical faculty should be armed with the same reasoning vocabulary and framework imparted to students and should have opportunities to practice giving feedback on the reasoning process.

A reasoning curriculum has the potential to empower students to see diagnostic thinking not as a black box but rather as a process that can be consciously improved upon over time. Patients will benefit from being cared for by thoughtful physicians who embrace the importance of reflection and self-improvement in the diagnostic process, who are aware of the risk for error and who can identify and manage uncertainty in a patient-centred manner. Developing an integrated reasoning curriculum is a challenging but rewarding process for educators who believe that clinical reasoning is one of the most important procedures in medicine.

CHAPTER SUMMARY

In this chapter, we have outlined:

- content for medical student education focussed on understanding reasoning, integrating reasoning practice with medical knowledge acquisition and strategies for approaching uncertainty and diagnostic error and

■ a teaching and learning approach for integration of a developmentally and intentionally aligned reasoning curriculum with other elements of students' education.

REFLECTION POINT 5

We have suggested a comprehensive and integrated reasoning curriculum. However, initiating curriculum redesign in a stepwise fashion is often what is most feasible. If stepwise curriculum development is more appropriate for your institution, consider which learning goals you would want to target first and which learning strategies might fit your institutional culture. How would you adapt these learning strategies to your educational context? What would be your elevator pitch to key stakeholders to gather support for launching a curricular innovation focussed on reasoning at your institution?

REFERENCES

Allen, S., Olson, A., Menk, J., et al., 2016. Hypothesis-driven physical examination curriculum. Clin. Teach. 14, 417–422.

Aper, L., Veldhuijzen, W., Dornan, T., et al., 2015. 'Should I prioritize medical problem solving or attentive listening?': the dilemmas and challenges that medical students experience when learning to conduct consultations. Patient Educ. Couns. 98, 77–84.

Ark, T.K., Brooks, L.R., Eva, K.W., 2004. November, The best of both worlds: Adoption of a combined (analytic and non-analytic) reasoning strategy improves diagnostic accuracy relative to either strategy in isolation. Annual Meeting at the Association of American Medical Colleges.

Boscardin, C.K., 2015. Reducing implicit bias through curricular interventions. J. Gen. Intern. Med. 30, 1726–1728.

Bowen, J.L., 2006. Educational strategies to promote clinical diagnostic reasoning. N. Engl. J. Med. 355, 2217–2225.

Custers, E.J., 2015. Thirty years of illness scripts: theoretical origins and practical applications. Med. Teach. 37, 457–462.

Dhaliwal, G., 2017. Premature closure? not so fast. BMJ Qual. Saf. 26, 87–89.

Dhaliwal, G., Ilgen, J., 2016. Clinical reasoning: talk the talk or just walk the walk? J. Grad. Med. Educ. 8, 274–276.

Eva, K.W., 2005. What every teacher needs to know about clinical reasoning. Med. Educ. 39, 98–106.

Eva, K.W., Hatala, R.M., LeBlanc, V.R., et al., 2007. Teaching from the clinical reasoning literature: combined reasoning strategies help novice diagnosticians overcome misleading information. Med. Educ. 41, 1152–1158.

Graber, M.L., Franklin, N., Gordon, R., 2005. Diagnostic error in internal medicine. Arch. Intern. Med. 165, 1493–1499.

Graber, M.L., Kissam, S., Payne, V.L., et al., 2012. Cognitive interventions to reduce diagnostic error: a narrative review. BMJ Qual. Saf. 21, 535–557.

Greenwald, T., Banaji, M., Nosek, B., et al., n.d. Project implicit. Viewed 10 March 2017. Available from https://implicit.harvard.edu/implicit/takeatest.html.

Henderson, M., Keenan, C., Kohlwes, J., et al., 2010. Introducing exercises in clinical reasoning. J. Gen. Intern. Med. 25, 9.

Johns, M.M., Wolman, D.M., Ulmer, C., 2009. Resident Duty Hours: Enhancing Sleep, Supervision, and Safety. National Academies Press, Washington, DC.

Kassirer, J.P., 2010. Teaching clinical reasoning: case-based and coached. Acad. Med. 85, 1118–1124.

Lambe, K.A., O'Reilly, G., Kelly, B.D., et al., 2016. Dual-process cognitive interventions to enhance diagnostic reasoning: a systematic review. BMJ Qual. Saf. 25, 808–820.

Lisk, K., Agur, A.M., Woods, N.N., 2016a. Examining the effect of self-explanation on cognitive integration of basic and clinical sciences in novices. Adv. Health. Sci. Educ. Theory Pract. 1–13.

Lisk, K., Agur, A.M., Woods, N.N., 2016b. Exploring cognitive integration of basic science and its effect on diagnostic reasoning in novices. Perspect. Med. Educ. 5, 147–153.

Lucey, C.R., 2015. Clinical problem solving: Dr Lucey, UCSF public online course content, University of California, San Francisco. Viewed 25 March 2017. Available from: https://vimeo.com/album/2358328.

Mamede, S., Schmidt, H.G., Penaforte, J.C., 2008. Effects of reflective practice on the accuracy of medical diagnoses. Med. Educ. 42, 468–475.

Maserejian, N.N., Lutfey, K.E., McKinlay, J.B., 2009. Do physicians attend to base rates? Prevalence data and statistical discrimination in the diagnosis of coronary heart disease. Health Serv. Res. 44, 1933–1949.

Medow, M.A., Lucey, C.R., 2011. A qualitative approach to Bayes' Theorem. Evid. Based Med. 16, 163–167.

MedU, n.d. DX: Diagnostic Excellence, MedU, Hanover, NH. Viewed 10 March 2017. Available from: http://www.med-u.org/diagnostic-excellence.

National Academies of Sciences, Engineering, and Medicine [NASEM], 2016. Improving Diagnosis in Health Care. National Academies Press, Washington, DC.

Norman, G.R., Brooks, L.R., Colle, C.L., et al., 1999. The benefit of diagnostic hypotheses in clinical reasoning: experimental study of an instructional intervention for forward and backward reasoning. Cogn. Instr. 17, 433–448.

Reilly, J.B., Ogdie, A.R., Von Feldt, J.M., et al., 2013. Teaching about how doctors think: a longitudinal curriculum in cognitive bias and diagnostic error for residents. BMJ Qual. Saf. 22, 1044–1050.

Schmidt, H.G., Mamede, S., 2015. How to improve the teaching of clinical reasoning: a narrative review and a proposal. Med. Educ. 49, 961–973.

Schmidt, H.G., van Gog, T., Schuit, S.C., et al., 2017. Do patients' disruptive behaviours influence the accuracy of a doctor's diagnosis? A randomised experiment. BMJ Qual. Saf. 26, 19–23.

Simpkin, A.L., Schwartzstein, R.M., 2016. Tolerating uncertainty: the next medical revolution? N. Engl. J. Med. 375, 1713–1715.

Sommers, L.S., Launer, J., 2014. Clinical Uncertainty in Primary Care. Springer, New York, NY.

Starmer, A.J., Spector, N.D., Srivastava, R., et al., 2014. Changes in medical errors after implementation of a handoff program. N. Engl. J. Med. 371, 1803–1812.

Stern, S., Cifu, A., Altkorn, D., 2014. Symptom to Diagnosis: An Evidence-Based Guide. McGraw Hill Professional.

Woods, N.N., 2007. Science is fundamental: the role of biomedical knowledge in clinical reasoning. Med. Educ. 41, 1173–1177.

33

TEACHING CLINICAL REASONING IN NURSING EDUCATION

TRACY LEVETT-JONES ■ JACQUELINE PICH ■ NICOLE BLAKEY

CHAPTER AIMS

The aims of this chapter are to:

■ present a suite of strategies that can be used by clinical educators[i] to facilitate the development of nursing students' clinical reasoning skills and

■ highlight the relationship between clinical reasoning and patient outcomes.

KEY WORDS

Clinical reasoning

Cognitive bias

Deliberate practice

Patient outcomes

Reflection

Think aloud

ABBREVIATIONS/ ACRONYMS

DP Deliberate practice

RN Registered nurse

TA Think aloud

---

[i]In this chapter, the term 'educator' refers to anyone who provides clinical teaching to nursing students, including those who are formally appointed (e.g., university-employed facilitators) and those who are informally allocated (e.g., preceptors or mentors).

INTRODUCTION

The importance of clinical reasoning in health care cannot be overstated, and a body of research attests to the relationship between clinical reasoning skills and patient outcomes (Rajkomar and Dhaliwal, 2011). Although nursing students generally learn the purpose and process of clinical reasoning in on-campus activities, clinical placements provide authentic, rich and dynamic opportunities for engagement in activities that can enhance this cognitive skill set. This chapter provides a suite of diverse teaching and learning strategies that can be used by educators to facilitate the development of nursing students' clinical reasoning skills. The activities are interlinked and progress in complexity, but each has a focus on patient safety.

PROVIDING OPPORTUNITIES FOR AUTONOMOUS PRACTICE

Beginning students, and sometimes even those who are more senior, often depend on their educator or mentor to identify patient problems, plan care and delegate tasks. This approach does not allow students to independently engage in higher-order thinking about their practice. An effective teaching strategy to enhance students' capacity for autonomous clinical reasoning is to ask them to imagine that they are the registered nurse (RN) who is fully responsible for the patient's care. This approach challenges students to make sense of clinical data to develop a nursing diagnosis and to grapple with challenging decisions rather than immediately deferring to their educator or mentor. Students can be asked to explain which cues they collect and why, how they make sense of the data they collect, the thinking that underpins their decision making and their rationales for care.

When students are lacking in confidence or unwilling to offer a nursing diagnosis or related nursing actions, educators can encourage them to simply 'take a guess', even if they are wrong. Similarly, when caring for patients with complex comorbidities and multiple management goals, students can be challenged to prioritize their nursing actions. For example, the educator could ask the student to identify and justify his or her immediate nursing priorities for the care of a person with a pain score of 7 out of 10 on a numerical rating scale, an oxygen saturation level of 88% and a blood glucose level of 3.0 mmol/L. Additionally, asking students to predict 'what might happen if no action were taken in this situation' prompts them to 'think ahead' and anticipate potential outcomes, depending on a particular course of action. These active learning strategies encourage learners to 'step up' when caring for patients and can enhance their clinical reasoning skills (Rencic, 2011).

REFLECTION POINT 1

What are some of the main challenges that you have encountered in clinical settings when attempting to teach nursing students to become competent and confident in clinical reasoning?

What strategies have you used to overcome these challenges?

FOCUSSING ON DELIBERATE PRACTICE

Deliberate practice (DP) is critical to the development of clinical reasoning skills. Although expertise is sometimes assumed to be an outcome of exposure, experience and knowledge, research demonstrates only a weak relationship between these factors and actual performance (McGaghie, 2008). For example, once an elite sportsperson reaches a level of expertise, more experience will not, by itself, result in further improvement. However, if a sports coach provides opportunities for DP by ensuring that every practice session has a specific purpose, improvement in targeted areas is more likely.

Similarly, individualized opportunities for purposeful, repetitive and systematic practice can be designed to improve nursing students' performance in specific aspects of clinical reasoning.

DP is most effective when educators provide:

■ well-defined learning goals related to discrete aspects of clinical reasoning,
■ immediate feedback that is clear and specific,
■ adequate time for problem solving and
■ opportunities for repeated practice to gradually refine specific aspects of clinical reasoning performance (Ericsson et al., 1993).

Educators frequently report that although nursing students typically manage the initial stages of clinical reasoning confidently, they often struggle with higher-order thinking skills. For example, although students may be able to accurately assess a person's vital signs, fluid balance and oxygen saturation level, they often find synthesizing and making sense of this information to be more challenging. By designing opportunities for DP, educators can focus on more challenging skills such as cue clustering, forming a nursing diagnosis and planning appropriate nursing actions, ultimately enhancing each learner's overall clinical reasoning ability.

USING HIGHER-ORDER QUESTIONING

The use of higher-order questions is key to the development of the critical thinking and clinical reasoning skills that are integral to nursing practice (Phillips and Duke, 2001). However, a number of studies have reported that in their interactions with students educators predominantly use low-level questions, centred on knowledge and comprehension (Phillips et al., 2017; Profetto-McGrath et al., 2004). Knowledge-based questions, according to Bloom's Taxonomy, represent the lowest category in the cognitive domain and require only simple recall of information. Although these types of lower-level questions are important to learning, the use of higher-order questions that require analysis, synthesis and evaluation are crucial to clinical reasoning (Profetto-McGrath et al., 2004).

Low-level questions can be answered by simple recall of previously learned information and often are framed using terms like 'what', 'when', 'who', 'which', 'define', 'describe', 'identify', 'list' and 'recall' (Profetto-McGrath et al., 2004). Other characteristics include the use of closed questions that will elicit a yes or no response, questions that elicit recall of factual information and leading questions that provide clues as to the answer required in their wording. By comparison, higher-order questions probe students' understanding and reasoning by asking them to critique or analyze their actions and to break down an idea into its component parts (Profetto-McGrath et al., 2004). See Box 33.1.

BOX 33.1
LEVELS OF QUESTIONS –
AN EXEMPLAR

EXAMPLES OF QUESTIONS RELATED TO
HAND HYGIENE

The clinical facilitator has concerns about a student's compliance with hand hygiene requirements and wants to test her understanding.

Low-level question: 'What are the five moments of hand hygiene?'

This leads the student to the answer by jogging her memory about the five moments required. The student is likely to frame the answer with the information given in the question; however, there is no way of knowing if the student understands the importance the five moments before being asked the question. In this way, the student can hide her lack of understanding.

Midlevel question: 'Can you tell me about the policy that relates to hand hygiene?'

This question is better in that it is not leading in nature; however, it is designed to elicit an answer based on the student's memory or recall of the policy rather than her application of the policy in practice.

High-level question: 'Can you critique your hand hygiene practice with reference to the relevant policy?'

This question also requires the student to recall her knowledge of the hand hygiene policy. However, by asking her to critique her practice, the student must evaluate her hand hygiene performance to determine whether or not she has complied with the policy.

Higher-level question: 'Whilst wearing gloves and attending your patient, you collected clean linen from the linen trolley. Critique your actions and the implications'.

This question takes a moment of practice that is related to a lapse in hand hygiene; however, there is no mention of hand hygiene. The student must critique her actions to firstly make the link to hand hygiene, then critique her practice with respect to the relevant policy/guidelines, and lastly consider the implications of her actions for patient safety.

EMPHASIZING THE IMPORTANCE OF EVIDENCE-BASED PRACTICE

A sound evidence base is critical to clinical reasoning. Without evidence to inform practice, nursing diagnoses and decisions may be based on little more than hunches and anecdotes. Although best practice guidelines and articles should inform students' decision making, role modelling by educators is essential if students are to value evidence-based literature. When asking students to provide an evidence-based rationale for their decisions, educators can encourage them to access contemporary literature by undertaking a quick but highly focussed Internet-based search (e.g., using a smartphone or tablet). When educators encourage students to use this approach to address specific and complex patient problems, it demonstrates that accessing evidence-based literature is both feasible and valuable (Rencic, 2011). Additionally, educators can ask students to discriminate among different levels of evidence, emphasize the importance and value of different sources of evidence (e.g., empirical studies, clinical expertise, patient's values and preferences) and help students develop an understanding of terms such as 'rigor', 'validity', 'reliability' and 'feasibility'. Most important, when educators role-model or facilitate the use of evidence-based resources, they are teaching students that clinical reasoning is a scientific and rigorous process that requires intelligence, integrity and a commitment to lifelong learning.

LEARNING TO THINK ALOUD

The think-aloud (TA) approach is both a teaching and a research strategy (Banning, 2008). In nursing education, TA can be used to engage students in the process of clinical reasoning by encouraging them to verbalize their thinking while attempting to analyze and solve clinical problems (Lundgrén-Laine and Salanterä, 2010). The aim of TA is to gain access to students' thought processes, including their train of thought, ability to make connections and identify relationships and application of prior learning to problem solving. TA also provides a diagnostic opportunity to gain insights into any difficulties being encountered by learners in regards to clinical reasoning (Banning, 2008).

When facilitating, TA educators can prompt students to verbalize their thoughts and the rationales underpinning their actions as they engage in critical thinking and problem solving (Banning, 2008). This enables errors in the student's clinical reasoning to be identified and rectified and 'faulty' clinical reasoning patterns to be remediated (Lee and Ryan-Wenger, 1997). The specific information that is gained from the TA process is highly useful as too often educators can identify *when* a student is not thinking critically, but without deep insights into his or her thinking processes, it is difficult to understand *why*. Thus the insights generated from TA can lead to the provision of structured and targeted learning support (e.g., using deliberate practice) designed to improve clinical reasoning skills (Linn et al., 2012).

The TA strategy can be employed in a classroom setting and in simulation, but it is equally suited for use in the clinical environment. When facilitating, TA educators may need to remind the student to keep talking aloud and prompt him or her to explain his or her thinking where required. The use of words like 'describe' can help orient the student, and subtle prompts such as 'what are you thinking now?', 'why are you are doing that?' and 'can you talk me though that process?' can be used as occasional reminders if students stop verbalizing their thoughts. However, although these prompts can be useful, they should not be confused with instruction and the provision of formative feedback (Todhunter, 2015). It is also valuable for educators to role-model TA when demonstrating patient care activities. This clarifies what is expected of students but also gives them insights into the thinking processes of expert clinicians. Although the TA approach can be time-consuming, it can lead to a significant improvement in students' clinical reasoning skills and confidence (Todhunter, 2015).

In a professional environment with real-time demands, it is maybe necessary to wait until the end of an activity before reviewing the thinking processes and outcomes. Retrospective TA can also be a useful strategy for improving clinical reasoning. Questioning after retrospective TA should aim to elicit students' thinking and to ensure that they understood the rationale behind their actions. Therefore closed questions that require a yes or no response should be avoided as should questions that are leading in nature. For example, asking the student 'At what blood pressure reading would you withhold metoprolol?' would be considered leading as this question provides the link between the medication and its indication for use and helps orient the student in his or her thinking. A better question would be 'Can you carefully describe your thinking as you administered Mr Smith's medications?' Educators should be aware that when engaging in retrospective TA, periods of silence are appropriate, as they allow students the opportunity to gather their thoughts if needed (Todhunter, 2015). See Case Study 33.1.

DECONSTRUCTING CRITICAL EVENTS

Deconstructing critical events during debriefing fosters critical thinking and informs clinical reasoning (Dreifuerst, 2012). This teaching strategy involves students working in groups to deconstruct a critical event using the clinical reasoning cycle as the organizing framework.

CASE STUDY 33.1

Example of the Use of the Think-Aloud Strategy

Betty Dobson is a 75-year-old patient who was admitted with a fractured wrist after an unwitnessed fall at home 2 days ago. She is complaining of feeling a bit lightheaded and dizzy and tells the nursing student caring for her that she was too tired to get out of bed today. The nursing student moves to collect a sphygmomanometer. The educator prompts the student to think aloud and to explain her reasoning. The student explains that the patient's symptoms may be caused by hypotension, so she wants to take the patient's blood pressure to confirm this. The student takes the blood pressure and obtains a reading of 98/60. She asks the patient how much she has been drinking, explaining to her educator that dehydration can be a cause of hypotension. The educator might then prompt the student to explain the link between hypotension and dehydration and to consider other clinical issues that can cause dehydration.

Students work systematically through the cycle using a table or a mind map to help them record and organize the patient information. In a similar approach to the TA method, students need to articulate their thoughts and the rationales behind their decision making. The complexity of the clinical exemplars used can increase as the students' progress in their nursing programs so that students can continually extend their clinical reasoning skills.

Mind maps provide students with a strategy for integrating critical thinking and problem-solving skills (Mangena and Chabeli, 2005). The advantages of mind mapping include its free-form and unconstrained structure, the generation of unlimited ideas and links, promotion of creativity and encouragement of brainstorming (Davies, 2010). In order for meaningful learning to occur, students must link new information with their existing knowledge. The multisensory nature of mind maps, which can incorporate colour and pictures, also facilitates the transfer of information from short- to long-term memory (D'Antoni et al., 2010). See Case Study 33.2.

REFLECTING ON COGNITIVE BIASES

Retrospective analyses of critical incident reports have identified that cognitive errors rather than a lack of knowledge are the major cause of errors in health care (Rajkomar and Dhaliwal, 2011). Decision making is a complex process, and generally an intuitive or an analytical approach is used (this is sometimes referred to as dual-process theory) (Croskerry, 2003). Intuitive decision making is used repetitively in our everyday lives and when at work. It is a largely unconscious thought-processing system that is fast, mostly effective but also more prone to failure (Kahneman, 2011). Intuitive

thinking is typically 'hardwired' to save time and mental effort, especially when we are familiar (or overly familiar) with a task, when there are time constraints and when there is a real or perceived need to take shortcuts (Croskerry et al., 2013). It is sometimes characterized by an 'I've got this … I've seen it a hundred times' attitude. By contrast, analytical decision making is a conscious process that is generally reliable, safe and effective, but it is also slow and deliberate (Croskerry, 2003).

Clinical educators have a responsibility to help nursing students become aware of cognitive factors that affect their clinical reasoning, for example:

■ the hardwired tendency for intuitive thinking,
■ the risk for cognitive overload – studies have shown that an average of only seven units of information can be held in the working memory (Miller, 1956) – and
■ the tendency to make errors when thinking is affected by fatigue, stress, prejudice and preconceptions (Croskerry et al., 2013).

REFLECTION POINT 2

Can you recall any personal or professional experiences in which your cognitive biases impeded your capacity for clinical reasoning? What did you learn from this experience? How could you use your learning to inform or improve your teaching?

One way of raising learners' awareness is through the provision of opportunities for reflection on and in practice. This allows for metacognition, or thinking about thinking, by stepping away from the immediate problem to examine and reflect on one's thinking or to reexamine a clinical situation after it has passed.

CASE STUDY 33.2

Example of a Mind-Mapping Activity

Jacob Chikuhwa is a 75-year-old patient who is 1 day postop after major surgery for oesophageal cancer. He has an IV running at 80 mL per hour and a patient-controlled analgesia (PCA) of morphine. At 0700 hours, his vital signs were T 37°C, pulse rate 110 beats per minute (weak and thready), respiratory rate

20 breaths per minute and blood pressure 110/55 mm Hg. His urine output is averaging 10 to 15 mL per hour. In groups, create a mind map that illustrates the pathophysiology related to Mr. Chikuhwa's current situation and the related thinking processes. See Fig. 33.1.

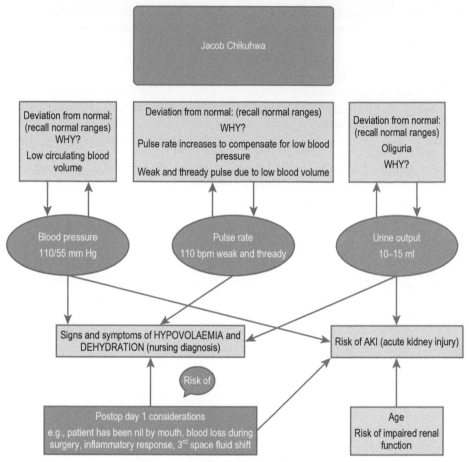

Fig. 33.1 ■ Mind map of a clinical case.

Both intuitive and analytical thinking, irrespective of level of nursing experience, can be influenced by cognitive biases. These types of thinking errors are one of the major causes of inaccurate clinical reasoning and consequently adverse patient outcomes. Educators must help students to become familiar with various types of cognitive biases (Table 33.1) and to consider how their clinical reasoning can be clouded by negative stereotypes, preconceptions and prejudices.

Educators should be alert to situations when students demonstrate thinking errors that are influenced by cognitive biases – for example, comments such as 'He is drug seeking, he doesn't really have pain' (fundamental attribution error), 'She is 85 … so confusion is not at all surprising' (ascertainment bias); and 'I'm sure it's just indigestion … I've seen it a hundred times'

(overconfidence bias). These thinking errors interfere with effective clinical reasoning and are therefore a risk to patient safety. Educators should question (and even challenge) students when they are concerned about their cognitive biases and use these opportunities for 'just in time teaching'. These situations can also be used to prompt students to reflect on and consider the basis to their flawed perceptions and thinking processes.

REFLECTION POINT 3

With reference to Table 33.1 and Case Study 33.3, how could you facilitate students' reflection on practice in a way that encourages and enables them to identify their own cognitive biases?

TABLE 33.1	
Examples of Cognitive Biases That Affect Clinical Reasoning	
Cognitive Bias	**Definition**
Anchoring	The tendency to lock onto salient features in the patient's presentation too early in the clinical reasoning process and failing to adjust this initial impression in the light of later information. Compounded by confirmation bias.
Ascertainment bias	When a nurse's thinking is shaped by prior assumptions and preconceptions, for example, ageism, stigmatism and stereotyping.
Confirmation bias	The tendency to look for confirming evidence to support a nursing diagnosis rather than look for disconfirming evidence to refute it, despite the latter often being more persuasive and definitive.
Diagnostic momentum	Once labels are attached to patients, they tend to become stickier and stickier. What starts as a possibility gathers increasing momentum until it becomes definite and other possibilities are excluded.
Fundamental attribution error	The tendency to be judgemental and blame patients for their illnesses (dispositional causes) rather than examine the circumstances (situational factors) that may have been responsible. Psychiatric patients, those from minority groups and other marginalized groups tend to be at risk for this error.
Overconfidence bias	A tendency to believe we know more than we do. Overconfidence reflects a tendency to act on incomplete information, intuition or hunches. Too much faith is placed on opinion instead of carefully collected cues. This error may be augmented by anchoring.
Premature closure	The tendency to apply premature closure to the decision-making process, accepting a diagnosis before it has been fully verified. This error accounts for a high proportion of missed diagnosis.

Adapted from Croskerry, 2003.

CASE STUDY 33.3

A Reflection About Cognitive Biases by a Third-Year Nursing Student

A 52-year-old male patient, John (pseudonym), was brought into the emergency department by the police and the local mental health team. John was in breach of his community treatment order. On presentation, John had slurred speech, was unable to stand or walk unassisted and was very aggressive. A code black was called after the triage nurse was punched and the attending nurse was bitten whilst obtaining a blood pressure. The emergency medical officer and two security personal responded, with John being restrained and sedation administered.

I had been asked to obtain a patient history. However, upon presentation I had already labelled John as an alcoholic who was homeless and suffering from some sort of mental illness. I didn't see the purpose of taking a full patient history and thought that we just needed to sober him up and then release him back to the mental health team. The clinical reasoning errors that influenced my attitude and thinking included fundamental attribution error – I believed the patient's illness and situation were self-inflicted as a result of his decision to drink; overconfidence bias and unpacking principle – I did not believe this patient had any real medical issues because of my labelling him as an alcoholic. As a result of my assumptions, I did not collect a thorough history or assessment of this patient and disregarded the real medical and social problems that he was presenting with.

John was homeless and had been for the past 6 years, since his wife, daughter and two grandchildren had been killed in a car accident; he was simply unable to function anymore. Three years ago, John had come to the attention of the mental health team, and he was diagnosed with an anxiety disorder, delusions, paranoia and panic attacks; he was also misusing alcohol and drugs; however, he had been clean and sober for the past 18 months. It was later established that John had a blood alcohol reading of zero. He was diagnosed with severe dehydration and a mild cerebrovascular haemorrhage.

Continued on following page

CASE STUDY 33.3

A Reflection About Cognitive Biases by a Third-Year Nursing Student (Continued)

I was fortunate to have been supervised throughout this experience so my personal judgements did not endanger this patient. However, this has been an invaluable experience for me as I have learnt that you need to treat every patient individually without judgement, and a thorough history is essential to understand what may be affecting the patient's health status. I will endeavour to remember this in the future and not allow my biases to cloud my thinking.

Source: Levett-Jones et al. (2010)

CHAPTER SUMMARY

In this chapter, we have explored seven creative strategies for facilitating the development of nursing students' clinical reasoning skills:

- providing opportunities for autonomous practice,
- focussing on deliberate practice,
- using higher-order questioning,
- emphasizing the importance of evidence-based practice,
- learning to think aloud,
- deconstructing critical events and
- reflecting on cognitive biases

Each of these strategies can be used to address students' specific learning needs in relation to clinical reasoning and to foster lifelong critical thinking habits.

REFLECTION POINT 4

Can you think of any upcoming opportunities to apply some of the suggestions in this chapter to your clinical teaching? What actions would you need to take to prepare for this teaching and to optimize effectiveness of the selected activity?

REFERENCES

Banning, M., 2008. The think aloud approach as an educational tool to develop and assess clinical reasoning in undergraduate students. Nurse Educ. Today 28, 8–14.

Croskerry, P., 2003. The importance of cognitive errors in diagnosis and strategies to minimize them. Acad. Med. 78, 775–780.

Croskerry, P., Singhal, G., Mamede, S., 2013. Cognitive debiasing 1: origins of bias and theory of debiasing. BMJ Qual. Saf. 22, ii58–ii64.

D'Antoni, A.V., Pinto Zipp, G., Olson, V.G., et al., 2010. Does the mind map learning strategy facilitate information retrieval and critical thinking in medical students? BMC Med. Educ. 10, 61.

Davies, M., 2010. Concept mapping, mind mapping and argument mapping: what are the differences and do they matter? Higher Ed. 62, 279–301.

Dreifuerst, K.T., 2012. Using debriefing for meaningful learning to foster development of clinical reasoning in simulation. J. Nurs. Educ. 51, 326–333.

Ericsson, K., Krampe, R., Tesch-Römer, C., 1993. The role of deliberate practice in the acquisition of expert performance. Psychol. Rev. 100, 363–406.

Kahneman, D., 2011. Thinking, Fast and Slow. Doubleday, Canada.

Lee, J.E., Ryan-Wenger, N., 1997. The 'Think Aloud' seminar for teaching clinical reasoning: a case study of a child with pharyngitis. J. Pediatr. Health Care 11, 101–110.

Levett-Jones, T., Sundin, D., Bagnall, M., et al., 2010. Learning to think like a nurse. Handover – Hunter N. Engl. Nurs. J. 3, 15–20.

Linn, A., Khaw, C., Kildea, H., et al., 2012. Clinical reasoning: a guide to improving teaching and practice. Austr. Fam. Phys. 41, 18–20.

Lundgrén-Laine, H., Salanterä, S., 2010. Think-Aloud technique and protocol analysis in clinical decision-making research. Qual. Health Res. 20, 565–575.

Mangena, A., Chabeli, M.M., 2005. Strategies to overcome obstacles in the facilitation of critical thinking in nursing education. Nurse Educ. Today 25, 291–298.

McGaghie, W., 2008. Research opportunities in simulation-based medical education using deliberate practice. Ann. Emerg. Med. 15, 995–1001.

Miller, G., 1956. The magical number seven, plus or minus two: some limits on our capacity to process information. Psychol. Rev. 63, 81–97.

Phillips, N., Duke, M., 2001. The questioning skills of clinical teachers and preceptors: a comparative study. J. Adv. Nurs. 33, 523–529.

Phillips, N.M., Duke, M.M., Weerasuriya, R., 2017. Questioning skills of clinical facilitators supporting undergraduate nursing students. J. Clin. Nurs. 26, 4344–4352.

Profetto-McGrath, J., Bulmer Smith, K., Day, R.A., et al., 2004. The questioning skills of tutors and students in a context based baccalaureate nursing program. Nurse Educ. Today 24, 363–372.

Rajkomar, A., Dhaliwal, G., 2011. Improving diagnostic reasoning to improve patient safety. Perm. J. 15, 68–73.

Rencic, J., 2011. Twelve tips for teaching expertise in clinical reasoning. Med. Teach. 33, 887–892.

Todhunter, F., 2015. Using concurrent think-aloud and protocol analysis to explore student nurses' social learning information communication technology knowledge and skill development. Nurse Educ. Today 35, 815–822.

34

SPEECH-LANGUAGE PATHOLOGY STUDENTS
Learning Clinical Reasoning

BELINDA KENNY ▪ RACHEL DAVENPORT ▪ ROBYN B. JOHNSON

CHAPTER AIMS

The aims of this chapter are to:

▪ provide a framework and tools that clinical educators may apply to facilitate speech-language pathology students' clinical reasoning and

▪ show how clinical educators may explicitly focus on different reasoning elements to support students who are struggling to develop competency and to extend students who are approaching entry-level competence.

KEY WORDS

International Classification of Functioning, Disability and Health (ICF)

Continuum of clinical reasoning

Speech-language pathology

ABBREVIATIONS/ ACRONYMS

E3BP Three components of evidence-based practice (research evidence, clinical data and informed client choice)

CBOS Competency-based occupational standards in speech pathology

CE Clinical educator

COMPASS® Competency-based assessment in speech pathology

ICF International Classification of Functioning, Disability and Health

PBL Problem-based learning

SLE Simulated learning environment

SLP/SLPs Speech-language pathology/speech language pathologists

WHO World Health Organization

INTRODUCTION

In the last edition of this book, our colleagues Lindy McAllister and Miranda Rose (2008) suggested there was confusion in terminology use between 'clinical decision making' and 'clinical reasoning'. They argued that the process of making clinical decisions, i.e., the reasoning, was not explicit and that it needed to be. They presented curriculum options that might develop clinical reasoning skills in SLP such as PBL and ideas that '… will serve as a catalyst for discussion of clinical reasoning in our profession' (p. 403).

The scope of SLP practice has continued to change, and we now have a standardized assessment tool, COMPASS® (McAllister et al., 2006), for assessing SLP students on clinical placements, which is used in Australia and overseas. One of the four core professional competency units of assessment in the tool is 'reasoning'. These core competencies support the development and maintenance of the seven occupational competencies (Speech Pathology Association of Australia, 2011). Clinical reasoning is now an explicit component of the education of student speech pathologists and is a common term in the professional vocabulary of students and CEs. COMPASS® requires students to demonstrate thinking skills and show how they integrate collaborative and holistic viewpoints into their reasoning, i.e., the client and caregivers' views, opinions and wishes, along with current best evidence, which might inform students' decision making. The E3BP and ICF frameworks can also assist students and clinicians to integrate information into the reasoning process.

Despite these shifts, making clinical reasoning more explicit, how good are we at actually describing and modelling to students how we do the 'reasoning'? How do we reason and make clinical decisions? Researchers in the UK found that speech pathology students struggled with developing clinical reasoning skills in similar ways to medical students and other healthcare professional students (Hoben et al., 2007). These researchers suggested that gathering information might be more difficult for novices because novices have a less accessible, and less structured, knowledge base. Therefore recognition and interpretation of salient cues are also difficult. Discriminating between the relevant and irrelevant is difficult for novices. Hoben et al. (2007) went on to suggest that virtual intelligent tutors could be used in simulations to employ explicit teaching strategies, such as formulating testable hypotheses. Another explicit teaching strategy is to foster reflective practice.

Hill et al. (2012) suggested that active reflection is a core skill needed to reason and make clinical decisions. They examined reflective journals of novice speech pathology students and found that students had some features of being 'reflectors', but few were able to critically reflect. They therefore suggested proactively teaching reflective practice to enhance students' clinical reasoning skills. Besides critical reflection, other clinical reasoning skills include integrating holistic viewpoints, being able to critically evaluate, interpret and synthesize information from a variety of sources, using metacognitive thinking skills to monitor strategies and reflecting on the reasoning process itself to identify gaps and any additional information that may be required. Because of work like this, we are now more aware of what struggles novice speech pathology students might have, and this chapter provides some suggestions of how we might go about addressing these needs. In particular, we propose and outline how the ICF model can be used to facilitate the clinical reasoning skills of all students, no matter what ability level they are.

ICF AS A FRAMEWORK FOR CLINICAL REASONING

The ICF (World Health Organization, 2001) provides SLPs with a framework for professional scope of practice, quality care and intervention (Speech Pathology Association of Australia, 2003). We believe that an ICF framework also provides an effective tool for facilitating students' clinical reasoning. A key consideration, underpinning SLP clinical reasoning, is the importance of communication and swallowing to an individual's health and well-being. The ICF framework makes these explicit. The framework is also useful in capturing the complexity of other healthcare needs in individuals and communities.

According to the ICF framework, health issues may be classified under two major parts, each comprising specific health components. Part 1 addresses the effects of Functioning and Disability on an individual's health. Health components underlying functioning and disability include Body Structures (an anatomical component) and Functions (a physiological component) and Activities (task execution) and Participation (involvement in life situations). Part 2 addresses Contextual Factors affecting health. The health context may include Environmental Factors (physical, social issues and community attitudes toward communication and swallowing impairment) and Personal Factors (internal factors) (World Health Organization, 2001). Each part and component contributes to effective clinical reasoning during SLP assessment and intervention. Indeed, the ICF framework has been used in diverse areas of speech pathology practice, including developmental speech and language impairment (McLeod, 2004) and acquired neurological motor speech, language and swallowing impairments (Ptyushkin et al., 2010). Wide professional application of the ICF framework may support students to use standardized approaches to clinical reasoning across caseloads and placements and develop professional competence.

Applying the ICF framework requires SLPs to adopt holistic management for clients with communication and swallowing impairments. Although health is classified under parts and components, the ICF framework presents a dynamic, interactional perspective on health. An underlying assumption is that disease, or disorder, alone does not determine an individual's health outcomes in a simplistic cause/effect relationship. Functional outcomes are influenced by the complex interaction of health components, including the nature of an individual's impairment and environment (Allen et al., 2006). This interactional aspect of health care represents a significant move from biomedical to biopsychosocial perspectives on health and resonates with more progressive, participatory models of SLP practice. For students, developing insights into inter-actional aspects of health can help them transition from clinician-focussed to more client-focussed practice as they consider their clients from a holistic perspective. Students may learn the importance of more meaningful goals and activities that meet clients' communication needs rather than simply dealing with impairments.

Examples of client-focussed practice are to use the ICF framework as a tool for joint goal setting with adults with aphasia (Worrall et al., 2011) and children with speech impairments (McLeod and Bleile, 2004). The ICF may also inform outcome measures by addressing the effects of communication and swallowing on everyday life (O'Halloran and Larkins, 2008) or identifying environmental factors that support clients' transfer of new skills and strategies in their community (Howe, 2008). When SLP clients are perceived as active healthcare decision makers with individual needs, clinicians must change from experts, with all the knowledge, to facilitators who recognize that clients have something important to contribute to their own assessment and management (Threats, 2008). For many clients, quality outcomes involve living successfully with a communication or swallowing disorder rather than curing it (Kagan, 2011), an important concept for students to grasp. Another benefit of the holistic ICF framework is that it offers a shared language for interprofessional care (Allen et al., 2006).

We believe that the ICF framework may be used to identify and support students who are struggling with clinical reasoning. As Fig. 34.1 (Johnson et al., 2016) shows, the ICF framework may be readily applied to students' knowledge, skills and professional attitudes as they develop along a continuum of competence. Novice SLP students may master the scientific basics yet struggle to acquire a client-focussed and holistic perspective during assessment and intervention. Intermediate SLP students may have insight into the importance of functional activities but have limited skills, experience and confidence in planning and delivering coordinated care. Even strong students benefit from focussing upon clinical reasoning. Adopting an ICF framework may encourage students to 'think like a speech pathologist' and consider interprofessional, educational and advocacy aspects of their professional roles.

REFLECTION POINT 1

Consider how CE questioning could focus students on specific components of the ICF:

What do you know about the trigeminal nerve, maxillary branch?

How safely will your client manage thin fluids at home?

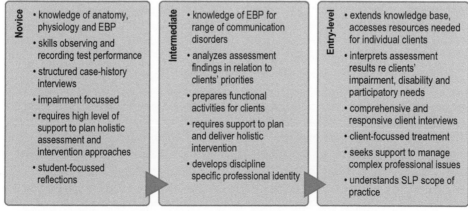

Novice
- knowledge of anatomy, physiology and EBP
- skills observing and recording test performance
- structured case-history interviews
- impairment focussed
- requires high level of support to plan holistic assessment and intervention approaches
- student-focussed reflections

Intermediate
- knowledge of EBP for range of communication disorders
- analyzes assessment findings in relation to clients' priorities
- prepares functional activities for clients
- requires support to plan and deliver holistic intervention
- develops discipline specific professional identity

Entry-level
- extends knowledge base, accesses resources needed for individual clients
- interprets assessment results re clients' impairment, disability and participatory needs
- comprehensive and responsive client interviews
- client-focussed treatment
- seeks support to manage complex professional issues
- understands SLP scope of practice

Fig. 34.1 ▪ Clinical reasoning in novice, intermediate and entry-level SLP student practice.

In the following sections, we suggest strategies to facilitate students' clinical reasoning during different stages of the competence continuum.

FACILITATING CLINICAL REASONING

There is presently no one theory, or approach, that fully describes the complex nature of clinical reasoning. Experienced clinicians use a combination of approaches, including, for example, 'both analytical (hypothetico-deductive reasoning) and nonanalytical (pattern recognition) processes' (Audétat et al., 2013, p. e394). McAllister and Rose (2008) discuss the intangible nature of clinical reasoning, noting that, to student speech pathologists, the clinical reasoning process can seem like a 'black box'. This is not unique to speech pathology (Delany et al., 2013). The first step towards effectively facilitating students' clinical reasoning is for CEs to reflect on and understand their own clinical reasoning skills and strategies.

CEs should provide student clinicians with a clear structure to develop the 'x-ray vision' to see into the black box and access the clinical reasoning process. Delany et al. (2013) aimed to expose the process of clinical reasoning for students by investigating the questions experienced allied health clinicians ask themselves during the process of clinical reasoning. They found that experienced clinicians use a combination of approaches, asking themselves questions about their role, specialist knowledge and experience (hypothetico-deductive) and their clients' individual needs and context (sociocultural).

Ginsberg et al. (2016) also sought to shed light on the thinking of experienced clinicians, specifically around diagnostic reasoning, to facilitate effective teaching of students. They describe a hierarchy of thinking used by experienced clinicians and suggest potential stepwise development for student clinicians through this hierarchy. Themes in the thinking of expert and student clinicians were 'seeking outside input, rationalizing, hypothesizing, differentiating, summarizing, deferring, comparing, specific planning, general planning and treatment planning' (p. 93). These reflect the range of reasoning models used effectively by experienced clinicians and less effectively and not as comprehensively by student clinicians. Clearly, CEs have an essential role in providing structured tasks (such as questions or a

hierarchy) and modelling and clearly articulating the process of clinical reasoning.

Audétat et al. (2013) aimed to identify common difficulties in clinical reasoning to help CEs support struggling medical trainees. They started from a series of assumptions (p. e985) that hold as true for SLPs as for doctors. They emphasized the similarity between clinical reasoning and educational reasoning, helping CEs to understand that the process of supporting a struggling student was not outside their scope of expertise. The five areas of difficulty they identified (in Table 1 on p. e987) are equally applicable to SLP students:

1. Difficulties in developing hypotheses, noting cues and collecting data
2. Ceases problem solving/reasoning too early
3. Difficulties identifying salient information
4. Difficulties in seeing the big picture of the clinical situation
5. Difficulties developing an adequate management plan

Students with difficulties such as these have trouble taking account of all aspects of the ICF, resulting in a potential lack of holistic client care. Structured clinical reasoning questions or tasks could be implemented in any of these areas as required.

CLINICAL REASONING APPROACHES

Hypothetico-deductive reasoning is a way of making a diagnosis/decision, through forming hypotheses from clinical data, comparing it to other evidence (such as theory or experimental data) and refining or rejecting hypotheses until one remains. Novice clinicians almost always have to use this method of clinical reasoning, as they have not had the opportunity to build a bank of knowledge and experience required for pattern recognition or forward reasoning as experts do. In contrast, expert clinicians are more likely to tap into their wide experience of cases and clinical clues to come to an accurate hypothesis, often using backward reasoning to check their final hypothesis against the case and its details.

In pattern recognition, clinicians use their specialist knowledge and experience, of many case narratives, to compare a new client to previous clients with similar difficulties and apply a similar solution, if possible. As experience increases, knowledge and reasoning become integrated. It is then possible to see how multiple client behaviours can fit into a range of case narratives. This makes pattern recognition more efficient (in the same way that experienced readers do not sound out every word from the letters but recognize words as whole, meaningful units).

Other forms of reasoning can be integrated into clinical reasoning. Taking a wider worldview and understanding how the client and the clinician fit into their society involve sociocultural reasoning. Putting the clients and their stories at the centre of the clinician's thinking involves narrative reasoning. Exploring the values that inform a patient's worldview might involve feminist thinking. All these can provide some holistic depth to clinicians' decision making.

Fig. 34.2 (Johnson et al., 2016) describes the way these clinical reasoning approaches fit within the ICF.

REFLECTION POINT 2

Encourage students to talk about the process of clinical reasoning, not just the outcome. Discuss your own thinking and clinical reasoning process, or use the questions and themes discussed earlier in the chapter (Delany et al., 2013; Ginsberg et al., 2016). Show students that hypothetico-deductive reasoning

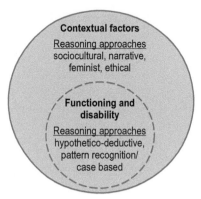

Fig. 34.2 ■ Clinical reasoning approaches and the ICF.

is only a beginning and that to be a fully holistic clinician other approaches must be tried.

The first case study (Case Study 34.1) is a synthesis of student and CE experiences of student struggles in the clinical setting, taken from recent doctoral research in the area of student struggle and failure. The research outcomes suggest that many struggling students have difficulties in more than one domain, i.e., academic, clinical and/or other (personal, health related) (Shapiro et al., 2002). Therefore, when working to problem-solve a student's issues, a holistic approach should be adopted.

CASE STUDY 34.1

Supporting a Student

Sam is a final-year speech pathology student, on her final placement. Common themes have arisen in the feedback from CEs in all Sam's placements to date. She has just managed to reach the pass criteria in previous placements. Issues include lots of support needed for decision making during sessions; gaps in the connections between observations and the clinical presentation of the client; and problems sorting relevant from irrelevant information (including observations) – often hones in on the irrelevant. When prompted by her CE, she can describe her observations at a physical, impairment level but cannot relate these to the patient as a person and how they may affect the patient's life. She struggles to incorporate the

client's and caregivers' wishes, opinions and needs into her planning. When asked to research specific information, she gets sidetracked and returns with lots of extraneous, irrelevant information. She does not often initiate discussion with her CE, Chris, and her post-session reflections are very concrete and self-focussed. When asked what she is finding difficult, Sam struggles to answer. She says, 'I just don't know where to start. I get lost in a sea of information. I don't know what's relevant or irrelevant'.

Although Chris finds COMPASS® useful to pinpoint Sam's reasoning as an area of concern, she would like more support to structure Sam's learning and develop her clinical reasoning skills.

ICF AND CLINICAL REASONING IN PRACTICE (CASE STUDY 34.1 ANALYSIS)

Consider Fig. 34.1 in the ICF section earlier in the chapter. Can we pinpoint where Sam is getting stuck? Thinking about clinical reasoning in developmental terms can assist here; most of Sam's skills currently sit in the first box (novice). Her thinking is at the impairment (structures and functions) level, and she is not yet considering the client's priorities and needs (contextual factors). She needs assistance from Chris to link her observations to research evidence, client function, participation and the contextual factors. Initially Chris needs to ensure that Sam's theoretical knowledge base is sound. Use the model later in the chapter for more suggestions of how these early skills can be facilitated.

How can Chris break down the information Sam needs to 'sort' through to be able to reason clinically and plan for her clients, using the suggestions mentioned earlier regarding integrating ICF and E3BP frameworks? Chris could start by verbalizing her own reasoning skills (make the implicit explicit). Experienced clinicians frequently operate with automaticity, not overtly thinking about how they make their clinical decisions. They are able to link multiple pieces of information from different sources and sort the relevant from the irrelevant quickly. Chris and Sam could work through some simple cases together with Chris modelling her thinking and reasoning. Chris could explicitly model different types of clinical reasoning to demonstrate how these are relevant to being a competent SLP.

REFLECTION POINT 3

How might a structured reflection tool be useful for CEs and students to help facilitate the development of student reasoning skills?

Developing a student's reflection skills can assist in developing his or her reasoning skills. As Sam's skills appear to be at a novice level, structuring her reflection of observations in clinical sessions would be useful in facilitating the breakdown of what she is seeing and doing into smaller elements. Chris will need to model this for her initially. When students are struggling during the latter stages of their course, it is natural to assume they should have some of the skills they are not

demonstrating. It is important that Chris goes back to an earlier developmental level and provides Sam with modelling and explicit verbalizing of what she expects Sam to do. Chris could also be working with Sam to check for other reasons why Sam might find it difficult to demonstrate her reasoning skills. Clinical placements are a complex melting pot of personal and environmental factors; students may be more stressed about their own health or other issues and are less likely to perform to their potential (Gan and Snell, 2014).

In the second case study, Alex is expected to reach professional entry-level competence by the end of this placement. Consider Alex's clinical reasoning skills in Case Study 34.2.

STRONG CLINICAL REASONING INCLUDES CONSIDERATION OF ALL AREAS OF ICF (CASE STUDY 34.2 ANALYSIS)

This supervisory interaction suggests that Alex is developing competent skills for an entry-level student. Key indicators include:

- Alex's reasoning incorporates an ICF framework. Alex considers potential effects of Jim's physical and cognitive impairments (Body Functions). Treatment goals are linked to Jim's functional communication needs (Activities) and facilitation of his social/leisure activities (Participation). Alex includes Jim's wife in treatment, identifies her need for communication partner education (Environment) and acknowledges family concerns regarding Jim's safety (Environment/Body functions). Alex has attended to Jim's frustration with word finding difficulties and responded by adopting a multimodal intervention approach (Personal/Activities).
- In keeping with an ICF framework, Alex's concept of professional role includes discipline-specific intervention, education and interdisciplinary teamwork.

STRATEGIES FOR CES: USING THE ICF TO EXTEND STUDENTS' CLINICAL REASONING SKILLS

We propose the model in Fig. 34.3 (Johnson et al., 2016) as a framework that will help CEs facilitate clinical

---

CASE STUDY 34.2

Extending a Student

Lee (CE): OK Alex, how do you think your sessions went today?

Alex (Student): Overall, well. I really focussed on time management and prioritized key goals today. So Jim still achieved his important goals even though his taxi was late. And I'm learning more about my clients so I can plan goals and activities that are relevant for them.

Lee: Yes, your time management has improved, and Jim responded to your football activity—much more interaction, well done!

Alex: Jim was initiating conversation with me about football. I've got my data here—he was 70% successful with nouns and verbs today. Having the sports section from the newspaper helped. We worked longer on that activity because Jim was so engaged and communicating his messages with speech and gestures. Jim's wife mentioned

how much he enjoyed going to the football game. It was good to include her in the activity and demonstrate strategies for helping Jim to communicate. She was still 'testing' Jim sometimes. Next time I'll respond more quickly and re-explain our intervention approach when Jim shows frustration.

Lee: Good idea. What else will you focus on next week?

Alex: Word retrieval related to Jim's interests in football and fishing. He's not doing those activities yet because his family is worried about his right-sided weakness and memory issues. I need to contact Jim's OT and Physio for an update on his other rehabilitation goals. Can I review my information and questions with you before I call them?

---

reasoning with students at different skill levels. This indicates the importance of supplementing clinical learning experiences with structured tasks, interprofessional tasks and ethical practice to enhance clinical reasoning skills.

Structured Tasks

- If possible, develop simulated/standardized patients and compile research for complex cases (Sabei and Lasater, 2016). Working in interprofessional teams would further extend students. Miles et al. (2016) found that the students' clinical reasoning skills, among other measures, significantly improved after undergoing interprofessional simulation-based dysphagia training. Some believe that the use of simulated learning environments (SLEs) has much potential for improved clinical reasoning. For example, MacBean et al. (2013) found that the current use of SLEs in speech pathology education was limited, but there were many possible benefits in the future use of SLEs.
- Explain to students how deep critical reflection on the process of clinical reasoning can open the 'black box'. Sabei and Lasater (2016) found that

using structured debriefing in SLEs, including critical reflection, allowed students to comment on the level of 'their cognitive, affective, and psychomotor performance' (p. 46) in the context of their developing clinical reasoning skills.

- Use structured questions or hierarchies (Delany et al., 2013; Ginsberg et al., 2016).

Interprofessional Tasks

- Set up opportunities for students to share theoretical knowledge – with students or staff from SLP or the wider team.
- Encourage students to explore the range of roles within the interdisciplinary team and reflect on the way the whole team delivers holistic care.
- Set up interprofessional student team tasks, as good teamwork skills predict good clinical outcomes (Shrader et al., 2013).

Ethical Practice

- Discuss ethical reasoning skills (Kenny et al., 2010) to ensure students understand that effective clinical reasoning is underpinned by sound application of professional codes of ethics. Students' insights

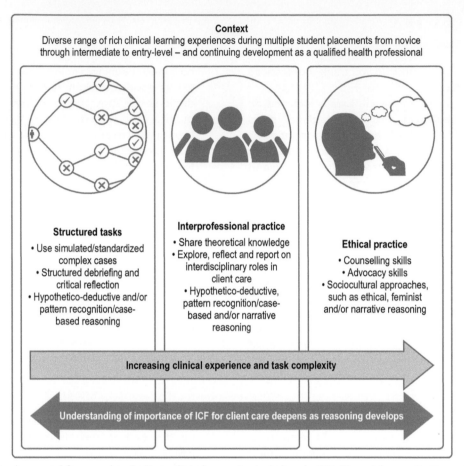

Fig. 34.3 ■ Developmental framework to facilitate clinical reasoning including the ICF. (From Johnson, R., Kenny, B., Davenport, R., 2016. Using the ICF to facilitate development of clinical reasoning. figshare.com, with permission.)

into perceived benefits, potential harms, client autonomy and access to quality services may be facilitated by discussing ethical implications of different intervention options.

- Ensure that students consider using the counselling skills they have learnt. These skills are essential in encouraging clients and carers to comfortably disclose their requirements, both in functional and contextual terms, and thus make fullest use of available services.
- Discuss the importance of developing advocacy skills, as many clients require support to make their requirements known in a range of contexts.

CHAPTER SUMMARY

In this chapter, we discussed:

- that as a profession, we have progressed our understanding of how students develop their clinical reasoning skills,
- how clinical reasoning is now a core competency in becoming a graduate speech-language pathologist,
- how using the ICF and E3BP models can assist students and CEs in identifying where a student's clinical reasoning skills are at developmentally and

■ suggestions for how to further develop these skills at various levels (see Fig. 34.3).

We presented practical suggestions to use in everyday clinical situations to support struggling students and extend students' clinical reasoning including:

■ structured debriefing,
■ using student reflection journals,
■ overtly modelling own reasoning skills,
■ learning in interprofessional teams,
■ working through cases and
■ simulation.

This information may help CEs decide where to start with a student. We hope that this will provide CEs with a framework and suggestions for facilitating students' clinical reasoning to the next level, regardless of the level of their existing clinical competence.

REFLECTION POINT 4

The challenge for every CE is to customize the use of the ICF and E3BP models to support every student in further developing clinical reasoning skills required for work readiness.

Acknowledgement

The authors wish to acknowledge Professor Lindy McAllister, Associate Dean, Work Integrated Learning, Faculty of Health Sciences, The University of Sydney, for her support and advice during the planning and preparation of this chapter.

REFERENCES

Allen, C.M., Campbell, W.N., Guptill, C.A., et al., 2006. A conceptual model for interprofessional education: the International Classification of Functioning, Disability and Health (ICF). J. Interprof. Care 20, 235–245.

Audétat, M.C., Laurin, S., Sanche, G., et al., 2013. Clinical reasoning difficulties: a taxonomy for clinical teachers. Med. Teach. 35, e984–e989.

Delany, C., Golding, C., Bialocerkowski, A., 2013. Teaching for thinking in clinical education: making explicit the thinking involved in allied health clinical reasoning. Focus Health Prof. Educ. 14, 44.

Gan, R., Snell, L., 2014. When the learning environment is suboptimal: exploring medical students' perceptions of 'mistreatment'. Acad. Med. 89, 608–617.

Ginsberg, S.M., Friberg, J.C., Visconti, C.F., 2016. Diagnostic reasoning by experienced speech-language pathologists and student clinicians. Contemp. Issues Commun. Sci. Disord. 43, 87.

Hill, A.E., Davidson, B.J., Theodoros, D.G., 2012. Reflections on clinical learning in novice speech–language therapy students. Int. J. Lang. Commun. Disord. 47, 413–426.

Hoben, K., Varley, R., Cox, R., 2007. Clinical reasoning skills of speech and language therapy students. Int. J. Lang. Commun. Disord. 42, 123–135.

Howe, T.J., 2008. The ICF contextual factors related to speech-language pathology. Int. J. Speech Lang. Pathol. 10, 27–37.

Johnson, R., Kenny, B., Davenport, R., 2016. Using the ICF to facilitate development of clinical reasoning. Viewed 24 March 2017. Available from: https://figshare.com/articles/Using_the_ICF_to_facilitate_development_of_clinical_reasoning/4235942/1.

Kagan, A., 2011. A-FROM in action at the Aphasia Institute. Semin. Speech Lang. 32, 216–228.

Kenny, B., Lincoln, M., Balandin, S., 2010. Experienced speech-language pathologists' responses to ethical dilemmas: an integrated approach to ethical reasoning. Am. J. Speech Lang. Pathol. 19, 121–134.

MacBean, N., Theodoros, D., Davidson, B., et al., 2013. Simulated learning environments in speech-language pathology: an Australian response. Int. J. Speech Lang. Pathol. 15, 345–357.

McAllister, L., Rose, M., 2008. Speech-language pathology students: learning clinical reasoning. In: Higgs, J., Jones, M.A., Loftus, S., et al. (Eds.), Clinical Reasoning in the Health Professions, third ed. Elsevier, Edinburgh, pp. 397–404.

McAllister, S., Lincoln, M., Ferguson, A., et al., 2006. COMPASS: Competency Assessment in Speech Pathology. Speech Pathology Association of Australia, Melbourne, VIC.

McLeod, S., 2004. Speech pathologists' application of the ICF to children with speech impairment. Adv. Speech Lang. Pathol. 6, 75–81.

McLeod, S., Bleile, K., 2004. The ICF: a framework for setting goals for children with speech impairment. Child Lang. Teach. Ther. 20, 199–219.

Miles, A., Friary, P., Jackson, B., et al., 2016. Simulation-based dysphagia training: teaching interprofessional clinical reasoning in a hospital environment. Dysphagia 31, 407–415.

O'Halloran, R., Larkins, B., 2008. The ICF activities and participation related to speech-language pathology. Int. J. Speech Lang. Pathol. 10, 18–26.

Ptyushkin, P., Vidmar, G., Burger, H., et al., 2010. Use of the International Classification of Functioning, Disability and Health (ICF) in patients with traumatic brain injury. Brain Inj. 24, 1519–1527.

Sabei, S.D.A., Lasater, K., 2016. Simulation debriefing for clinical judgment development: a concept analysis. Nurse Educ. Today 45, 42–47.

Shapiro, D.A., Ogletree, B.T., Dale Brotherton, W., 2002. Graduate students with marginal abilities in communication sciences and disorders: prevalence, profiles, and solutions. J. Commun. Disord. 35, 421–451.

Shrader, S., Kern, D., Zoller, J., et al., 2013. Interprofessional teamwork skills as predictors of clinical outcomes in a simulated healthcare setting. J. Allied Health 42, 1E–6E.

Speech Pathology Association of Australia, 2003. Scope of Practice in Speech Pathology. Speech Pathology Association of Australia, Melbourne, VIC.

Speech Pathology Association of Australia, 2011. Competency Based Occupational Standards for Speech Pathologists: Entry Level, revised ed. Speech Pathology Association of Australia, Melbourne, VIC.

Threats, T., 2008. Use of the ICF for clinical practice in speech-language pathology. Int. J. Speech Lang. Pathol. 10, 50–60.

World Health Organization, 2001. International Classification of Functioning, Disability and Health (ICF). World Health Organization, Geneva, Switzerland.

Worrall, L., Sherratt, S., Rogers, P., et al., 2011. What people with aphasia want: their goals according to the ICF. Aphasiology 25, 309–322.

35

CLINICAL REASONING AND BIOMEDICAL KNOWLEDGE
Implications for Teaching

DAVID R. KAUFMAN ■ NICOLE A. YOSKOWITZ ■ VIMLA L. PATEL

CHAPTER AIMS

The aims of this chapter are to:

■ discuss the relationship between basic science knowledge and clinical reasoning,

■ identify the nature of biomedical knowledge and challenges integrating it in clinical contexts,

■ review assumptions underlying different curricular models and

■ present findings from cognitive research that address these matters.

KEY WORDS

Clinical reasoning

Biomedical knowledge/basic science knowledge

Conventional curricula

Problem-based learning

Knowledge encapsulation

Two-world hypothesis

ABBREVIATIONS/ ACRONYMS

AAMC Association of American Medical Colleges

BSK Basic science knowledge

CC Conventional curricula

PBL Problem-based learning

INTRODUCTION

Health care is undergoing profound changes that are likely to shape clinical practice for decades to come. There are competing views concerning the role of biomedical knowledge and its proper place in a health science curriculum. In this chapter, we consider some of these arguments in the context of empirical evidence from cognitive studies in medicine. Biomedical knowledge has undergone a dramatic transformation over the past 30 years, presenting formidable challenges to medical education (Martin et al. 2004). There remains uncertainty concerning the relationship between basic science conceptual knowledge and the clinical practice of physicians (Kulasegaram et al., 2015). In the past, medical schools have typically responded by adding new biomedical science content to existing courses, increasing the number of lectures and textbook readings (D'Eon and Crawford, 2005). This has changed as clinical courses have become more routine in the first 2 years of medical school (Martin et al., 2004) as has the format of teaching, which places a premium on active learning in clinically relevant contexts (Stott et al., 2016). In addition, basic science courses are increasingly competing with new curricular demands and objectives – for example, to improve professionalism and patient-centred care (Association of American Medical Colleges [AAMC], 2006, 2011).

In the past 25 years, information technology has had a profound effect on the practice of medicine, providing access to a wealth of information and decision support tools that have the potential to improve patient care substantially (Shortliffe and Blois, 2014; Hersh et al., 2014). Concerns have been raised about whether future health practitioners will continue to require the kinds of scientific training that their predecessors received. Although discoveries in science will continue to provide physicians with increasingly powerful investigative tools, it seems likely that the best clinical judgement will require a broader understanding of both biology and medicine than ever before (Prokop, 1992). For example, it is likely that advances in bioinformatics will continue to affect clinical medicine and necessitate changes to medical curricula to meet these advances. Clinicians who have a deeper understanding of basic science knowledge (BSK) will be better prepared to address more complex clinical situations and novel therapeutic strategies (Finnerty, 2012).

CURRICULAR AND EPISTEMOLOGICAL ISSUES

Clinical knowledge includes knowledge of disease entities and associated findings, and BSK incorporates subject matter such as biochemistry, anatomy and physiology. It had been widely believed that biomedical and clinical knowledge can be seamlessly integrated into a coherent knowledge structure that supports clinical reasoning (Feinstein, 1973). Medical educators and researchers have argued over how to best promote clinical skill and foster robust conceptual change in students (Boshuizen and Schmidt, 1992; Clough et al., 2004; Patel and Groen, 1986).

Traditionally, the curricula of most medical schools during the first and second years involves preclinical courses that predominantly teach the basic sciences and clinical sciences in subsequent years. This began to change with problem-based learning (PBL), with instruction involving clinically meaningful problems being introduced at the beginning of the curriculum. This practice is guided by the assumption that scientific knowledge taught abstractly does not help students to integrate it in clinical practice (Norman and Schmidt, 2000). Many medical schools have embraced the idea of emphasizing a more clinically relevant basic science curriculum. The Association of American Medical Colleges (AAMC) (e.g., 2004, 2006, 2011) advocates reforming medical education to promote a more

patient-centred approach and a more rigorous approach for ensuring that students and residents are acquiring the knowledge, skills, attitudes, values and teamwork orientation deemed necessary to provide high-quality patient care. The renewed focus on clinical skills and competencies introduces additional demands on an already crowded undergraduate curriculum. Similarly, the volume of information in the basic science disciplines is so vast that it is unreasonable to expect that medical students can fully integrate the range of relevant biomedical concepts with knowledge of associated disease entities and findings in a short time span.

As expertise develops, the disease knowledge of a clinician becomes more dependent on clinical experience, and clinical problem solving is increasingly guided by the use of exemplars, becoming less dependent on a functional understanding of the system in question (Patel and Kaufman, 2014). Biomedical knowledge, by comparison, is of a qualitatively different nature, embodying elements of causal mechanisms and characterizing patterns of perturbation in function and structure. Fig. 35.1 presents the knowledge organization reflected in the basic science disciplines with a deeper dive into cardiovascular physiology. Although it is a very basic organizing scheme, it is helpful to think how certain concepts may inform clinical reasoning in adjacent areas.

REFLECTION POINT 1

Reflect on how knowledge in medicine has changed and continues to change. How can the issues addressed in this section inform curricular change?

RESEARCH IN CLINICAL REASONING

In this section, we review some of the pertinent research in medical reasoning, particularly research that addresses the role of BSK in clinical medicine.

Clinical Reasoning Strategies and Expertise

Lesgold et al. (1988) investigated the abilities of radiologists, at different levels of training and expertise, to interpret chest x-ray pictures. Experts were able to initially detect a general pattern of disease with a gross anatomical localization, serving to constrain the possible interpretations. Novices had greater difficulty focussing on the important structures, being more likely to

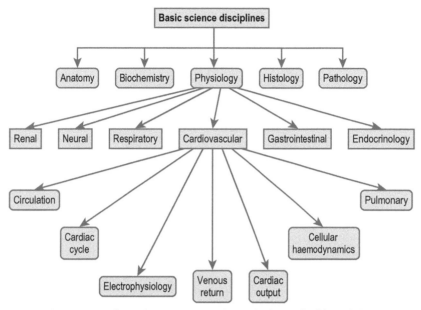

Fig. 35.1 ■ Classical organization scheme for biomedical knowledge.

maintain inappropriate interpretations despite discrepant findings in the patient history. The authors concluded that the knowledge that underlies expertise in radiology includes the mental representation of anatomy, a theory of anatomical perturbation and the constructive capacity to transform the visual image into a three-dimensional representation. The less expert subjects had greater difficulty in building and maintaining a rich anatomical representation of the patient. Crowley et al. (2003) documented differences among subjects at varying levels of expertise in breast pathology corresponding to accuracy of diagnosis and aspects of task performance including feature detection, feature identification and data interpretation.

Norman et al. (1989) compared dermatologists' performance at various levels of expertise in tasks that required them to diagnose and sort dermatological slides according to the type of skin lesion. Expert dermatologists were more accurate in their diagnoses and took significantly less time to respond than novices. Experts grouped the slides into superordinate categories such as viral infections, which reflected the underlying pathophysiological structure. Novices tended to classify lesions according to surface features such as scaly lesions. The implication is that expert knowledge is organized around domain principles, which facilitate the rapid recognition of significant problem features. Experts employ a qualitatively different kind of knowledge to solve problems based on a deeper understanding of domain principles.

The picture that emerges from research on expertise across domains is that experts use a quite different pattern of reasoning from that used by novices or intermediates and organize their knowledge differently. Three important aspects are that experts a) have a greater ability to organize information into semantically meaningful, interrelated chunks, b) selectively focus on relevant information and c) in routine situations, tend to use highly specific knowledge-based problem-solving strategies (Ericsson and Smith, 1991).

The use of knowledge-based strategies has given rise to an important distinction between a data-driven strategy (forward reasoning) in which hypotheses are generated from data and a hypothesis-driven strategy (backward reasoning) in which one reasons backward from a hypothesis and attempts to find data that elucidate it. Forward reasoning is based on domain knowledge and is thus highly error-prone in the absence of adequate domain knowledge. Backward reasoning is slower and may make heavy demands on working memory and is most likely to be used when domain knowledge is inadequate. Backward reasoning is characteristic of nonexperts and experts solving nonroutine problems (Patel et al., 1989). In Fig. 35.2, forward reasoning is illustrated in a case of acute bacterial endocarditis. Clinical findings (e.g., fever and chills) coupled with clusters of other findings are suggestive of intermediate diagnostic constructs (often called 'facets') such as endocarditis. The cluster of facets led to the forward inference of acute bacterial endocarditis with aortic insufficiency. Notice that there are no bidirectional or backward inferences.

In experiments with expert physicians in cardiology, endocrinology and respiratory medicine, clinicians showed little tendency to use basic science in explaining cases, whereas medical researchers showed preference for detailed, basic scientific explanations, without developing clinical descriptions (Patel et al., 1989). The pathophysiological explanation task requires subjects to explain the causal pattern underlying a set of clinical symptoms (Feltovich and Barrows, 1984). In one study (Patel and Groen, 1986), expert practitioners (cardiologists) were asked to solve problems within their domain of expertise. Their explanations of the underlying pathophysiology of the cases, whether correctly or incorrectly diagnosed, made virtually no use of BSK.

In a similar study (Patel et al., 1990), cardiologists and endocrinologists solved problems both within and outside their domains of expertise. The clinicians did not appeal to principles from basic biomedical science, even when they were working outside their own domain of expertise; rather, they relied on clinical associations and classifications to formulate solutions. The results suggest that basic science does not contribute directly to reasoning in clinical problem solving for experienced clinicians. However, biomedical information was used by practitioners when the task was difficult or when

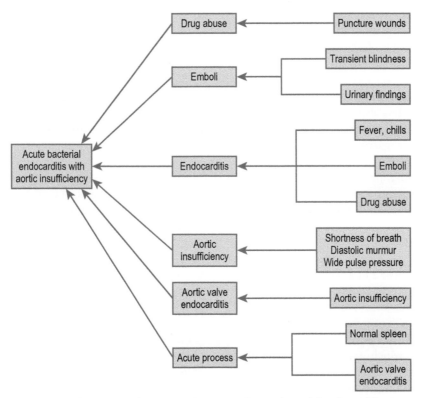

Fig. 35.2 ■ Forward reasoning in a case of acute bacterial endocarditis.

they were uncertain about their diagnosis. In these cases, biomedical information was used in a backward-directed manner, providing coherence to the explanation of clinical cues that could not be easily accounted for by their primary diagnostic hypothesis.

There have been many other studies highlighting the difficulty of integrating basic and clinical knowledge (e.g., Boshuizen and Schmidt, 1992; Patel et al., 1993; Kulasegaram et al., 2015; Woods, 2007). Pathophysiological information is used by physicians and senior medical students either when the problem-solving process breaks down or to explain findings that cannot be accounted for by the diagnostic hypotheses. In general, there is evidence to suggest that unprompted use of biomedical concepts in clinical reasoning decreases as a function of expertise. In addition, students have difficulty in applying basic science concepts in contexts that differ from the initial conditions of learning (Patel et al., 1990). On the other hand, the visual diagnosis studies suggest a more immediate role for BSK than does the work on expertise in the domains of cardiology and endocrinology. Certain domains necessitate a greater use of core biomedical concepts in understanding even basic problems.

We investigated subjects' mental models of cardiac output (Kaufman et al., 1996). The study characterized the development of understanding of the system as a function of expertise. The research also documented various conceptual flaws in the subjects' models and how these flaws affected subjects' predictions and explanations of physiological manifestations. Clinicians and medical students have variably robust representations of the structure and function of the system. We observed a progression of mental models as a function of expertise, as evidenced in predictive accuracy that increased with expertise and in the quality of explanations (Kaufman and Patel, 1998; Kaufman et al., 2008). Progression was also noted in the quality of explanations in response to individual questions and problems and in terms of the overall coherence of subjects' representations of the cardiovascular and circulatory system (Patel et al., 2000).

The study documented a wide range of conceptual errors in subjects at different levels of expertise. There were particular misconceptions that, according to our analyses, were more likely to be a product of formal learning.

REFLECTION POINT 2

Why do you think students have such difficulty assimilating basic science knowledge into clinical reasoning? What is different about visual diagnostic tasks?

Basic Science in Students' Explanations of Clinical Cases

A series of experiments were conducted to elucidate the role of basic science in clinical reasoning (Patel et al., 1990). In one study, medical students (who were either first-year students, second-year students who had completed all basic medical sciences but had not begun any clinical work or final-year students) were presented with three basic science tests (e.g., microcirculation) immediately before a clinical case of acute bacterial endocarditis (Patel et al., 1989). Subjects read basic science texts, recalled them in writing and then explained the clinical problem drawing on these texts. Subjects' recall of the basic science texts was poor, indicating a lack of well-developed knowledge structures in which to organize this information. Recall of the clinical text appeared to be a function of clinical experience, but there was no similar correlation between basic science and experience. In the explanation of the problem, second-year students made extensive use of BSK. Fourth-year students gave explanations that resembled those of expert physicians outside their domain of specialization, except that they more liberally used basic science information. The results indicate that BSK was used differently by the three groups of subjects.

In a second experiment (Patel et al., 1989), students recalled and explained cases when basic science information was provided after the clinical problem. Fourth-year students were able to use the basic science information in a highly effective manner. Second-year students were also able to use this information effectively, but diagnostic reasoning was not facilitated. First-year students were not able to use basic science information any more effectively when it was given after the clinical problem than when it was given before the clinical problem. These results suggest that reasoning towards a diagnosis from the facts of a case was frustrated by attempting to use BSK unless the student had already developed a strong diagnostic hypothesis. The addition of BSK seemed to improve the accuracy of diagnoses offered by final-year medical students but did not improve the accuracy of diagnoses by first- and second-year students. It is likely that final-year students, who had had some clinical experience, relied on clinically relevant features in a case to (broadly) classify the diagnosis and make selective predictions of features that could be explained by basic science concepts. This tendency of clinical solutions to subordinate basic scientific ones, and for basic science not to support the clinical organization of facts in a case, was evident among expert physicians, as discussed earlier. These results were also consistent with other findings, suggesting that unprompted use of biomedical concepts in clinical reasoning decreases as a function of expertise (Boshuizen and Schmidt, 1992).

Research evaluating the performance of PBL and conventional curricula (CC) programs has found negligible differences in terms of clinical skills (Jolly, 2006). Nevertheless, the different curricula are predicated on different assumptions about how best to foster conceptual change. PBL programs are based on the necessity of connecting scientific concepts to the conditions of application, whereas CC programs emphasize the importance of fostering a foundation of general scientific knowledge that is broadly applicable. The CC runs the risk for imparting inert knowledge, much of which is not retained beyond medical school and is not readily applicable to clinical contexts. On the other hand, PBL curricula may promote knowledge that is so tightly coupled to specific contexts as to have minimum generality beyond the immediate problem set.

Patel et al. (1993) attempted to replicate the studies mentioned earlier in an established PBL medical school. Results showed that when basic science information was provided before the clinical problem, there was once again a lack of integration of basic science into the clinical context. This resulted in a lack of global coherence in knowledge structures, errors of scientific fact and disruption of the diagnostic reasoning process. When basic science was given after the clinical problem, there was integration of basic science into the clinical context. It was concluded that clinical problems cannot be easily embedded into a basic science context, but basic science can be more naturally embedded within a clinical context. It is our belief that when one is attempting to learn two unknown domains, it is better to learn one well so that it can be used as an 'anchor'

for the new domain. BSK may serve as a better anchor than clinical knowledge. It may be useful to introduce some core basic science at the beginning of the curriculum, followed by an early introduction of clinical problems that are thematically connected to the specific scientific concepts.

The findings of these studies suggest that in conventional curricula, a) basic science and clinical knowledge are generally separate, b) clinical reasoning may not require BSK, c) basic science is spontaneously used only when students have difficulty diagnosing the patient problem and d) basic science serves to generate globally coherent explanations of the patient problem with connections among various components of the clinical problem. It is proposed that in a conventional curriculum, the clinical aspect of the problem is viewed as separate from the biomedical science aspect, the two having different functions. In the PBL curriculum, basic science and clinical knowledge are spontaneously integrated. However, this integration results in students' inability to decontextualize the problem and draw on basic science concepts in other contexts. There are multiple competencies involved in the practice of medicine, some of which are best fostered in the context of real-world practice and others best acquired through a process of formal learning (Patel and Kaufman, 2014).

REFLECTION POINT 3

Consider this discussion of curricula. How did you experience these learning sequences in your own course? If you are a teacher, does the curriculum of your students differ from your own? Do you see a link between knowledge and clinical reasoning capacity development?

KNOWLEDGE ENCAPSULATION OR TWO WORLDS

We consider two theoretical hypotheses that differ on the role of biomedical knowledge in clinical reasoning. Patel and Groen (1991) proposed that clinical and BSK bases constitute 'two worlds' connected at discrete points. Schmidt and Boshuizen offered a more integrative theoretical perspective, built around a learning mechanism, *knowledge encapsulation*, which explains how biomedical knowledge becomes subsumed under clinical knowledge in the development of expertise (Schmidt and Boshuizen, 1993). The process of knowledge encapsulation involves the subsumption of biomedical propositions and associative relations under a small number of higher-level clinical propositions with the same explanatory power. These authors argued that through repeated application of knowledge in medical training and practice, networks of causal biomedical knowledge become incorporated into a comprehensive clinical concept (Van De Wiel et al., 2000).

The crux of the two-worlds hypothesis is that these two bodies of knowledge differ in important respects, including the nature of constituent knowledge elements and the kinds of reasoning they support. Clinical reasoning involves the coordination of diagnostic hypotheses with clinical evidence. Biomedical reasoning involves the use of causal models at varying levels of abstraction (e.g., organ and cellular levels). The evidence suggests that routine diagnostic reasoning is largely a classification process in which groups of findings become associated with hypotheses. BSK is not typically evident in expert think-aloud protocols in these circumstances.

Under conditions of uncertainty, physicians resort to scientific explanations that provide coherence, even when inaccurate. The role of basic science, aside from providing the concepts required to formulate clinical problems, is to create a basis for establishing coherence in the explanation of biomedical phenomena. Basic science does not provide the abstractions required to support clinical problem solving. Rather, it provides the principles that make it possible to organize observations that defy ready clinical classification and analysis. Biomedical knowledge also provides a means for explaining, justifying and communicating medical decisions. In the absence of basic science, the relationships between symptoms and diagnoses seem arbitrary.

The two-worlds hypothesis is consistent with a model of conceptual change in which clinical knowledge and BSK undergo both a joint and separate processes of reorganization. This is partly a function of the kinds of learning experience that students undergo. The premedical years are focussed primarily on the acquisition of biomedical knowledge. As students become increasingly involved in clinical activities, the prioritization of knowledge also shifts to concepts that support the process of clinical reasoning. Schmidt and Boshuizen (1993) proposed a developmental process in which

students early in their training acquire 'rich elaborated causal networks explaining the causes and consequences of disease' in terms of biomedical knowledge (p. 207). Through repeated exposure to patient problems, the BSK becomes encapsulated into high-level simplified causal models explaining signs and symptoms. The knowledge structures remain available when clinical knowledge is not adequate to explain a clinical problem.

Intermediates require additional processing time to accomplish a task compared with experts and, at times, even novices. For example, in pathophysiology explanations, intermediates generate lengthy lines of reasoning that employ numerous biomedical concepts. On the other hand, experts use shortcuts in their line of reasoning, skipping intervening steps. A common finding is that intermediates recall more information from a clinical case than either novices or experts. Novices lack the knowledge to integrate the information, whereas experts selectively recall relevant information. Similarly, in pathophysiological explanation tasks, intermediates tend to use more biomedical knowledge and more elaborations than either novices or experts. The extra processing is caused by the fact that these subjects have accumulated a great deal of conceptual knowledge but have not fully tuned it to the performance of clinical tasks.

REFLECTION POINT 4

Reflect on the two proposed theories, namely, knowledge encapsulation and the two-worlds hypothesis. Can you think of different learning experiences that may be better explained by one theory or the other? The differences may be having an experience in which your knowledge appears to be seamless. On the other hand, sometimes you may have to do extra cognitive work to use basic science knowledge in addressing a clinical problem.

Schmidt et al. (Van De Wiel et al., 2000; Schmidt and Boshuizen 1993) conducted several studies in which they varied the amount of time that an individual was exposed to stimulus materials. They demonstrated that intermediates were negatively affected by having less time to process the stimulus material, whereas experts were largely unaffected by a reduction in time. The argument is that the immediate activation of a small number of highly relevant encapsulating concepts enables experts to rapidly formulate an adequate representation of a patient problem. On the other hand, students have yet to develop knowledge in an encapsulated form, relying more on biomedical knowledge and requiring more time to construct a coherent case representation. In other studies, Schmidt and Boshuizen (1993) demonstrated that expert clinicians could unfold their abbreviated lines of reasoning into longer chains of inferences that evoked more elaborate causal models when the situation warranted it.

The knowledge encapsulation theory may on the one hand overstate the capabilities of experts to rapidly activate elaborated biomedical models. On the other hand, by its focus on lines of reasoning, the theory may undermine the generative nature of expert knowledge. Lines of reasoning would suggest that experts have access to limited patterns of inference resulting from repeated exposure to similar cases. It is apparent that people learn to circumvent long chains of reasoning and chunk knowledge across intermediate states of inference as circumstances warrant this (Van De Wiel et al., 2000). This results in shorter, more direct inferences that are stored in long-term memory and are directly available to be retrieved in the appropriate contexts. We agree that repeated exposure to recurrent patterns of symptoms is likely to result in the chunking of causal inferences that will subsequently be available for reuse (Kaufman and Patel, 1998).

However, experts are also capable of solving novel and complex problems that necessitate the generation of new causal models based on a deep understanding of the system. This enables them to work out the consequences of a pathophysiological process that was never previously encountered (Kaufman and Patel, 1998). Mastery of biomedical knowledge may be characterized as a progression of mental models that reflect increasingly sophisticated and robust understandings of pathophysiological processes. Given the vast quantities of knowledge that need to be assimilated in 4-year medical curricula, it is not likely that one can develop robust understanding of the pathophysiology of disease. Clinical practice offers selective exposure to certain kinds of clinical cases. Even experts' mental models can be somewhat brittle when stretched to the limits of their understanding (Kaufman and Patel, 1998). Knowledge encapsulation may partially account for the process of conceptual change in biomedicine.

Learning Mechanisms

Clearly, the diversity of biomedical knowledge and clinical reasoning tasks requires multiple mechanisms of learning. BSK plays a different role in different clinical domains (such as dermatology and radiology) this requires a relatively robust model of anatomical structures, which is the primary source of knowledge for diagnostic classification (Norman, 2000). In other domains, such as cardiology and endocrinology, BSK has a more distant relationship with clinical knowledge. Furthermore, the misconceptions evident in physicians' biomedical explanations would argue against well-developed encapsulated knowledge structures, where BSK can easily be retrieved and applied when necessary. Our contention is that neither conventional nor problem-based curricula can foster the kind of learning suggested by the encapsulation process. The challenge for medical schools is to strike the right balance between presenting information in applied contexts and allowing students to derive the appropriate abstractions and generalizations to further develop their models of conceptual understanding. The two-worlds hypothesis implies that each body of knowledge be given special status in the medical curriculum and that the correspondences between the two worlds need to be developed.

The design and reform of educational curricula in complex advanced knowledge domains, such as biomedicine, depend on the identification of those concepts and knowledge that are considered necessary to become an effective and skilled scientist-practitioner (Patel et al., 2009). Successful knowledge integration is predicated on presenting basic science information in a manner that creates explicit relationships between basic and clinical science (Kulasegaram et al., 2015). Diemers et al. (2015) similarly concluded the need to provide students with varied patient experiences with the same underlying pathophysiological mechanism and encourage students to link biomedical and clinical knowledge.

CHAPTER SUMMARY

There has been a long-standing concern that the amount of time devoted to basic science in medical curricula is decreasing. The concern is made more acute by the fact that new knowledge in the biological sciences is increasing rapidly and by the emergence of comparatively new scientific domains bioinformatics and personalized medicine 'that promise paradigm shifts in clinical thinking'. Although medical cognition research continues to flourish, less attention has been paid to the problem of integrating basic science knowledge into clinical reasoning. Given the enormous advances in basic medical science and the changing character of clinical practice, the time may be ripe to revisit old debates, invigorate new research efforts and determine how to best inform the biomedical curriculum for the forthcoming decades.

REFLECTION POINT 5

In what ways (if any) has your view of the place of BSK in clinical reasoning and the education of healthcare professionals changed as a result of reading this chapter?

REFERENCES

Association of American Medical Colleges (AAMC), 2004. Educating doctors to provide high quality medical care: a vision for medical education in the United States. Report of the Ad Hoc Committee of Deans. AAMC, Washington, DC.

Association of American Medical Colleges (AAMC), 2006. Implementing the vision: group on educational affairs responds to the IIME Dean's Committee report. AAMC, Washington, DC.

Association of American Medical Colleges (AAMC), 2011. Core competencies for interprofessional collaborative practice. Report on an expert panel. AAMC, Washington, DC.

Boshuizen, H., Schmidt, H.G., 1992. On the role of biomedical knowledge in clinical reasoning by experts, intermediates and novices. Cogn. Sci. 16, 153–184.

Clough, R.W., Shea, S.L., Hamilton, W.R., et al., 2004. Weaving basic and social sciences into a case-based, clinically oriented medical curriculum: one school's approach. Acad. Med. 79, 1073–1083.

Crowley, R.S., Naus, G.J., Stewart, J., 3rd, et al., 2003. Development of visual diagnostic expertise in pathology: an information-processing study. J. Am. Med. Informat. Assoc 10, 39–51.

D'Eon, M., Crawford, R., 2005. The elusive content of the medical-school curriculum: a method to the madness. Med. Teach. 27, 699–703.

Diemers, A.D., Wiel, M.W., Scherpbier, A.J., et al., 2015. Diagnostic reasoning and underlying knowledge of students with preclinical patient contacts in PBL. Med. Educ. 49, 1229–1238.

Ericsson, K., Smith, J., 1991. Toward a General Theory of Expertise. Cambridge University Press, New York, NY.

Feinstein, A.R., 1973. An analysis of diagnostic reasoning I: the domains and disorders of clinical macrobiology. Yale J. Biol. Med. 46, 212–232.

Feltovich, P.J., Barrows, H.S., 1984. Issues of generality in medical problem solving. In: Schmidt, H.G., De Volder, M.L. (Eds.), Tutorials in Problem-Based Learning: New Directions in Training for the Health Professions. Van Gorcum, Assen/Maastricht, The Netherlands, pp. 128–142.

Finnerty, E.P., 2012. The role and value of the basic sciences in medical education: an examination of Flexner's legacy, Medical Science Educator, 20.

Hersh, W.R., Gorman, P.N., Biagioli, F.E., et al., 2014. Beyond information retrieval and electronic health record use: competencies in clinical informatics for medical education. Adv. Med. Educ. Pract. 5, 205–212.

Jolly, B., 2006. Problem-based learning. Med. Educ. 40, 494–495.

Kaufman, D.R., Keselman, A., Patel, V.L., 2008. Changing conceptions in medicine and health. In: Vosniadou, S. (Ed.), International Handbook of Research on Conceptual Change. Routledge, New York, NY, pp. 295–327.

Kaufman, D.R., Patel, V.L., 1998. Progressions of mental models in understanding circulatory physiology. In: Singh, I., Parasuraman, R. (Eds.), Human Cognition: a Multidisciplinary Perspective. Sage, New Delhi, India, pp. 300–326.

Kaufman, D.R., Patel, V.L., Magder, S.A., 1996. The explanatory role of spontaneously generated analogies in reasoning about physiological concepts. Int. J. Sci. Educ. 18, 369–386.

Kulasegaram, K., Manzone, J.C., Ku, C., et al., 2015. Cause and effect: testing a mechanism and method for the cognitive integration of basic science. Acad. Med. 90 (Suppl. 11), S63–S69.

Lesgold, A., Rubinson, H., Feltovich, P., et al., 1988. Expertise in a complex skill: diagnosing x-ray pictures. In: Chi, M.T.H., Glaser, R., Farr, M.J. (Eds.), The Nature of Expertise. Lawrence Erlbaum, Hillsdale, NJ, pp. 311–342.

Martin, J., Alpern, R., Betz, A., et al., 2004. Educating Doctors to Provide High Quality Medical Care: A Vision for Medical Education in the United States. Association of American Medical Colleges, Washington, DC.

Norman, G., 2000. The essential role of basic science in medical education: the perspective from psychology. Clin. Invest. Med. 23, 47–51.

Norman, G.R., Rosenthal, D., Brooks, L.R., et al., 1989. The development of expertise in dermatology. Arch. Dermatol. 125, 1063–1068.

Norman, G.R., Schmidt, H.G., 2000. Effectiveness of problem-based learning curricula: theory, practice and paper darts. Med. Educ. 34, 721–728.

Patel, V.L., Evans, D.A., Groen, G.J., 1989. Reconciling basic science and clinical reasoning. Teach. Learn. Med. 1, 116–121.

Patel, V.L., Evans, D., Kaufman, D., 1990. Reasoning strategies and the use of biomedical knowledge by medical students. Med. Educ. 24, 129–136.

Patel, V.L., Groen, G.J., 1986. Knowledge based solution strategies in medical reasoning. Cogn. Sci. 10, 91–116.

Patel, V.L., Groen, G.J., 1991. The general and specific nature of medical expertise: a critical look. In: Ericsson, K.A., Smith, J. (Eds.), Toward a General Theory of Expertise: Prospects and Limits. Cambridge University Press, New York, NY, pp. 93–125.

Patel, V.L., Groen, G.J., Norman, G.R., 1993. Reasoning and instruction in medical curricula. Cogn. Instruc 10, 335–378.

Patel, V.L., Kaufman, D.R., 2014. Cognitive science and biomedical informatics. In: Shortliffe, E.H., Cimino, J.J. (Eds.), Biomedical Informatics: Computer Applications in Health Care and Biomedicine, fourth ed. Springer-Verlag, New York, NY, pp. 133–185.

Patel, V., Kaufman, D., Arocha, J., 2000. Conceptual change in the biomedical and health sciences domain. In: Glaser, R. (Ed.), Advances in Instructional Psychology: Educational Design and Cognitive Science. Lawrence Erlbaum Associates, Mahwah, NJ, pp. 329–392.

Patel, V.L., Yoskowitz, N.A., Arocha, J.F., et al., 2009. Methodological review: cognitive and learning sciences in biomedical and health instructional design: a review with lessons for biomedical informatics education. J Biomed. Informat. 42, 176–197.

Prokop, D.J., 1992. Basic science and clinical practice: How much will a physician need to know? In: Marston, R.Q., Jones, R.M. (Eds.), Medical Education in Transition. Robert Wood Johnson Foundation, Princeton, NJ, pp. 51–57.

Schmidt, H.G., Boshiozen, H.P., 1993. On acquiring expertise in medicine. Educ. Psychol. Rev. 5, 205–221.

Shortliffe, E.H., Blois, M.S., 2014. Biomedical informatics: the science and the pragmatics. In: Shortliffe, E.H., Cimino, J.J. (Eds.), Biomedical Informatics: Computer Applications in Health Care and Biomedicine, fourth ed. Springer-Verlag, New York, NY, pp. 3–37.

Stott, M.C., Gooseman, M.R., Briffa, N.P., 2016. Improving medical students' application of knowledge and clinical decision-making through a porcine-based integrated cardiac basic science program. J. Surg. Educ. 73, 675–681.

Van De Wiel, M.W., Boshuizen, H.P., Schmidt, H.G., 2000. Knowledge restructuring in expertise development: Evidence from pathophysiological representations of clinical cases by students and physicians. Eur. J. Cogn. Psychol. 12, 323–356.

Woods, N.N., 2007. Science is fundamental: the role of biomedical knowledge in clinical reasoning. Med. Educ. 41, 1173–1177.

36

CULTIVATING A THINKING SURGEON, USING A CLINICAL THINKING PATHWAY AS A LEARNING AND ASSESSMENT PROCESS
Ten Years on

DELLA FISH ■ LINDA DE COSSART

CHAPTER AIMS

The aims of this chapter are to:

- review the basic components of our Clinical Thinking Pathway (CTP) as presented in a previous edition,

- share for critique the extension of our educational understandings and practice in respect of the need to broaden the basis of the our teaching into more moral and ontological areas and to develop further resources focussed on the development of character and the virtues in postgraduate medical practice to aid both teaching and assessment and

- present our newer developments and understandings of the clinical uses of our CTP.

KEY WORDS

Clinical Thinking Pathway
Clinical reasoning
Deliberation
Phrónêsis
Praxis
Personal professional judgement
Product professional judgement
Teaching in the moral mode of practice

ABBREVIATIONS/ACRONYMS

CBD Case-based discussion
CPD Continuing professional development
CTP Clinical Thinking Pathway
GMC General Medical Council (UK)
PGME Postgraduate medical education
RSCE Royal College of Surgeons of England

INTRODUCTION

We wrote *Cultivating a Thinking Surgeon* in 2005 and presented our CTP in the 2008 edition of this present book. One of us had already published qualitative research on professional judgement in health care (Fish and Coles, 1998). In 2005, we had found no evidence of the recognition in postgraduate medical education (PGME) of the relevance of Aristotle's Ethics (Aristotle, 2004) to the education of practicing medical professionals. Now, in the light of increasing understanding of phrónêsis and its illumination of professional judgement in medical practice (Conroy, 2016) and its more widely discussed relevance to professional education in general (Schwartz and Sharpe, 2010) and with the publications of Birmingham University's Jubilee Centre[i] from 2012 onwards, it is timely to consider the continued evolution and development of our ideas since 2005.

Between us, we have decades of working in surgical practice and surgical education. Linda was a vascular and general surgeon, an associate postgraduate dean, and in 2008–2009, vice president of the Royal College of Surgeons of England. Della worked in schools, teacher education and, for the past 18 years, in PGME with an interest in teaching and learning in the practice setting. We have worked together since 2002. Both of us have also published extensively. The past decade has crystallized for us a number of insights about clinical wisdom and practical knowledge and about the crisis in professional medical practice and in PGME and has revealed the slide towards overregulation and control of this whole field in both the UK and around the world. This in turn has driven us to extend our thinking and attempt to refocus education for all doctors beyond the technical to the moral mode of practice (Fish, 2012).

We offer first a brief resumé of the key components of the Clinical Thinking Pathway (CTP) as a basis for discussing our newer, revised thinking.

THE CLINICAL THINKING PATHWAY: THE BASIC COMPONENTS

The CTP highlights two main and highly contrasting forms of reasoning within clinical thinking (Fig. 36.1). These are clinical reasoning (the top end of the CTP) and deliberation (the bottom end). Running longitudinally throughout the pathway is what we have characterized as personal professional judgement, and the pathway ends in a final product professional judgement, leading to wise action (de Cossart and Fish, 2005). Our way of conceiving the role of professional judgement as running throughout the pathway and generating the end product was the really new insight. Aristotle described having the capacity for professional judgement (phrónêsis) as having the intellectual ability and emotional capacity to recognize the need for such judgement, together with the motivation, willingness and ability to exercise such judgement in practice and ultimately to engage in wise action (praxis). Aristotle's

ideal was that the practitioner should love 'getting this right for its own sake' and not for other reward.

Clinical reasoning (de Cossart and Fish, 2005), as used at the top end of the pathway, operates through a formula to solve a clinical problem and come to a conclusion (clinical solution) by using mainly a straightforward set of rules, with the assumption that what counts as evidence would be agreed by everyone. In its simplest and purest form, this construes the complex clinical problem as a technical one. From this viewpoint, clinical reasoning can be seen as a biomedical process that distinguishes the disease from the patient and regards the problem as to do with malfunctioning parts of the patient. It is a technical problem, requiring technical competence from the practitioner. It is based on rigorous logic and order, collects predictable categories of evidence and uses a formulaic approach to reach a clinical decision (the right thing to do generally). It claims a scientific basis and stems from a worldview that sees facts as objective, precise and absolute and 'truth' as 'out there', waiting to be discovered. It assumes that scientific theory can be directly translated into practice. This process is first taught at medical school and in various forms is used by many other healthcare professionals. This part of the pathway allows only a limited scope for the practitioner's own professional judgement, but it does require some (e.g., how many tests to send for).

Deliberation (de Cossart and Fish, 2005) is found at the bottom end of the pathway and, by contrast, demands that the practitioner starts from the clinical solution and tailors this, in the best possible interests of the individual, by taking account of the context of the patient as a whole person, the treating doctor(s) as people and professionals and the institution. It is the process through which the right general decision becomes the best possible action (or nonaction) for the individual patient here and now. It turns a working diagnosis into a treatment plan for a particular patient, which has been both understood and agreed by that patient and others involved. It requires the considerable exercise of professional judgement at all points, in taking account of a full range of human factors and recognizing the complexity at the core of clinical thinking. This process sees clinical problems as humane dilemmas and is grounded in the professional's humanity and concerned with the patient's social being in the world.

---

[i]<www.jubileecentre.ac.uk>

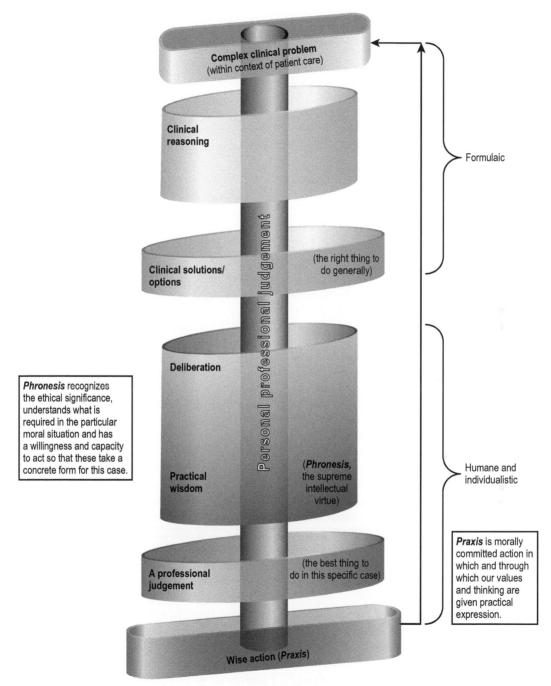

Phronesis recognizes the ethical significance, understands what is required in the particular moral situation and has a willingness and capacity to act so that these take a concrete form for this case.

Complex clinical problem
(within context of patient care)

Clinical reasoning

Clinical solutions/options   (the right thing to do generally)

Deliberation

Practical wisdom   (*Phronesis*, the supreme intellectual virtue)

Personal professional judgement

A professional judgement   (the best thing to do in this specific case)

Wise action (*Praxis*)

Formulaic

Humane and individualistic

Praxis is morally committed action in which and through which our values and thinking are given practical expression.

Fig. 36.1 ▪ The Clinical Thinking Pathway.

Here, the possible moral, humane and clinical priorities within a patient case compete for choice and are considered in an order that must arise from the particularities of the individual patient's problem(s). It thus eschews formulae for thinking, using instead an investigative approach to unearthing all the pertinent elements and a reflective and critical approach to prioritizing and weighing them up. This process is based on a view of the world as complex, ambiguous and uncertain and works from practice to theory. Typically, it involves clinicians in appreciating patients' experiences and ways of understanding their illness, the effect of this on their lives, their expectations about what should be done and their sense of control or powerlessness in relation to their situation (Higgs et al., 2004). Practitioners thus focus on and are sensitive to the moral and ethical dimensions involved and come to the 'product' judgement that is the final point of the entire thinking process. Aristotle refers to the subsequent wise action as 'praxis'. Inexperienced surgeons are often shocked to discover the central importance of deliberation and consideration of all elements (the entire bottom half of the pathway), expecting instead to follow protocols!

Deliberation, then, calls upon imagination and compassion in practitioners and involves the artistry of practice. It draws on knowledge of science and life, sensitivity to language, understanding of social interaction and recognition of and imagination about what is involved at a human level in being a patient. Further, it admits the existence of emotional elements in the patient's story and the practitioner's response. It sees disease as a breakdown of the patient's social world and crucially acknowledges that in human interaction, one person's way of making meaning out of a situation can never precisely match another's, thus recognizing both the social construction of knowledge and multiple versions of reality.

We wish to make very clear, however, that this model (like all diagrams) simplifies and reduces real-life complexities. For example, we do not see these processes as solitary activities leading to decisions by lone professionals. Nor do we see them as necessarily short and simple in a linear time scale. We also recognize with White and Stancombe (2003, p. 14) that, 'case formulations often remain unarticulated in encounters with patients ... and may not exist as single events produced spontaneously on discrete occasions ... [but] emerge gradually over time and through conversation with colleagues'. Further, narrative and interactive reasoning often occur in the clinical setting where multiprofessional teams are involved so that decision making itself is often a collective organizational activity.

The CTP and its components have, almost without exception, been acknowledged by all those we have worked with over the past 10 years as resonating with how they (subconsciously) think in their own clinical practice and as needing to be made explicit. However, over the years, we have gained a number of insights that have caused us to extend our understanding and develop further resources. The following two sections firstly offer these insights and secondly share some important literature and new resources.

KEY INSIGHTS FROM 10 YEARS OF WORK

These key insights lie in both the clinical and the educational realms. They have arisen through careful reflection by us on the teaching processes we have used, the comments by our teacher-learners and through them the young learning surgeons they supervise and also draw on four formal evaluations by outside researchers (Brown et al., 2016; Bullock et al., 2012; Thomé 2012, 2013).

Clinical Insights

The CTP, with its unpacking of phrónêsis (professional judgement) and praxis (wise action) was, in 2005, a revolutionary way of helping surgical teachers to attend to what we see as the heart of a surgeon's practice in respect of specific individual real cases in their practice. We have never denied the importance of surgeons' technical expertise, but we see this as driven by six key invisible elements that had always been left tacit in clinical practice and therefore had not easily been developed in a guided way. These are considering the importance of the context of that case; the person the surgeon personally brings to that case; the kind of professional he or she is within that case; his or her knowledge as brought to the case; the specifics of the surgeon's decision making within the case; and his or her professional judgements made during the case. All these 'invisibles', we contend, are implicit drivers of the final wise action (praxis) to be taken at that point in the patient's journey.

In teaching the teachers of those young surgeons, we now have evidence of how powerful the CTP and the invisible drivers that underpin it are, in both transforming the understanding of teachers about surgical expertise and facilitating young surgeons' ways of recognizing and developing their thinking. In short, we have learned the following about the CTP:

1. The CTP can act as a focus and guide for oral and written reflection for learning from specific clinical cases about the quality of the professional judgements being made in practice and what invests into them: (see Paper 2: A Case of Reflective Writing: A Rainbow Draft [Ed4MedPrac Ltd, no date]).
2. The CTP can be used as an assessment process across several cases during an attachment that shows the deepening insight of the trainee (or lack of it): see later for our enriched version of the case-based discussion (CBD), which is a required assessment tool at all stages in the postgraduate surgical curriculum.
3. It can be used as a guide for reflection on cases for continuing professional development (CPD) (at consultant level, where there is no longer a curriculum) and for appraisal (to show the heart of the professional's expertise and the judgement of individuals) (Fish and de Cossart, 2013).

We have also gained the following insights about the implementation process and present and future challenges:

1. Although there has been some rapid adoption of these ideas, the profession as a whole is slow to change its educational and assessment habits and still does not generally include in their teaching ways of exploring their thinking, decision making and professional judgements. This is probably because they are still not ready to see that words are better than numbers when it comes to placing on record the invisible qualities of their practice.
2. The prevailing public climate currently is in favour of the technical and rule-governed approach to life (Schwartz and Sharpe, 2010; Walker and Ivanhoe, 2007), but there are emerging signs of progress in how curriculum design in surgery is

moving: Version 10 of the Intercollegiate Surgical Curriculum Programme (ISCP) (Joint Committee for Higher Surgical Training, 2016).

3. There is much more consideration needed by learning surgeons in respect of the person they bring to their work. We had previously included this as one of the invisibles but had not recognized it in full until 2012 (Fish, 2012). The character and virtues of the professional (their personhood and 'being') are the core qualities that drive the surgeon's practice. This led us to see that the gap in the CTP was ontological. That is, there was not enough about the person the surgeon is and his or her professional identity. Further, it caused us to challenge the way that professionalism is currently developed in postgraduate practice. In returning to Aristotle, we have more recently developed a unit on character development and the virtues as part of a new way of teaching professionalism (Fish, 2015).
4. The moral and ethical dimensions of clinical practice were not being fully attended to in the CTP, and this also linked with not only the processes and foci of deliberation within a case but also was grounded in the virtuous aspiration of the practitioner.
5. We need to teach more ontological aspects of practice and to develop resources that enable surgeons to explore the character and virtues they bring to a case and that a case demands (Fish et al., 2015a, 2015b, 2015c). The subsection later in the chapter called 'Exploring the Character and Virtues' also provides background on the ontological aspects of practice found in key cases in medical practice.

Educational Insights

Educationally, we have refined our thinking and practice in respect of teaching the teachers of young surgeons in practice. Some of this is, inevitably, about teaching itself. Here we both model and also teach more directly a number of educational principles that have not, by their own frequent admission, been understood before by most surgeon teachers. This is because they were prepared for this obligatory part of their clinical contract by very short courses, which have inevitably left them with a highly technical and narrow view of teaching as the transmission of knowledge and the development of technical skills.

The following three key issues have been paramount:

1. We need to help surgical teachers to see that both medicine and education are practices in their own rights and that they are both moral practices, which in turn have serious implications for how learners are seen and treated and how teachers prepare for educating them.
2. We need to explicate what is involved in offering worthwhile education and in working as a teacher who is grounded in the moral mode of practice.
3. We need to be constantly alert to the ever-changing context in which doctors are working and the strangle-hold of the curriculum, which makes it harder and harder to maintain the teacher's own agency and to help learners manage the uncertainty of practice.

With these in mind, we have now developed and extended our work in two main ways as the following section demonstrates.

CRYSTALLIZING THE DISCOURSE AND OFFERING FURTHER EDUCATIONAL RESOURCES

During the past 10 years, we have learned to refine our ways of explaining, working on and modelling for surgeon teachers two key underpinning educational ideas: 1) what we mean by 'worthwhile education' and 2) by 'working in the moral mode of practice'. We have also developed a number of further resources for teaching. A critical component for implementation of these educational ideas is securing the full support for education from the executive board of hospitals where we work.

'Worthwhile Education' and 'Teaching in the Moral Mode of Practice'

The term 'worthwhile education' is, of course, tautological (worthwhile being an intrinsic characteristic of true education). We use it, however, to help us emphasize that education is a virtuous activity, leading to good ends for the public, so that no practice can be claimed as educational unless it is underpinned by an under-

standing of what it is 'to act educationally.' We believe this term establishes for surgical and medical teachers in clinical practice a stable and clear set of educational concepts and provides a principled underpinning to their practice, which can also be clearly articulated to their learners.

Educators cultivate learners' *understanding*, which involves coming to a view about a matter or matters as they seek to open up the learner's mind and contribute to their growth as a person (Pring, 2000). We would argue (and it is broadly agreed by educators, e.g., Oakeshott, 1967; Carr, D., 2004; Carr, W., 1995; Dewey, 1938; Freire, 1970) that to act educationally is to open minds, liberate thinking, encourage critique, explore the foundations of good practice, develop creativity and nurture and involve the learner in intrinsic motivation, to conduce to their flourishing as a person and a professional. Thus where learners are enabled to think in broader rather than narrower terms, have their confidence well grounded and fuelled rather than drained and have their engagement with the world deepened, then their teachers may, irrespective of their educational 'know-how' or skills, claim to offer worthwhile education (Carr, W., 1995, p. 160). By contrast, where learners are not so developed, no amount of technically well-performed teaching skills and clever strategies will compensate, and no technical know-how will make the experience educational for learners. Thus asking learners to ignore their personal perspectives including their own values, attitudes and feelings, suspend their thinking, shut down their critical faculties, abandon their moral awareness and merely parrot a performance (as seen in some training activities) would be neither ethical nor educational.

When we use the term 'the moral mode of practice' (following such writers as Carr, D., 2004; Carr, W., 1995; Dunne and Hogan, 2004; Pring, 2000), we are claiming the following. Firstly, education, like all professional practice, is a moral enterprise. This is well articulated in the most recent policy publication from the Jubilee Centre at Birmingham University in the UK: 'Statement on Character, Virtue and Practical Wisdom in Professional Practice' (2016). The policy statement expects that teachers should first determine what they care about (in terms of the qualities of practicing doctors) and then shape their educational aims and craft a conception of teaching that facilitates that end (Hansen 2001,

p. 4). Working in the moral mode of educational practice requires teachers to give their planning and their practice moral substance. It expects that teachers will give sustained intellectual and humane attention to their learners and help them to grow as persons, by focussing on what learners know, can do, feel and think. To *grow as a person* means to become more rather than less thoughtful about ideas and more rather than less sensitive to others' views and concerns. Teachers need to be mindful that every learner is unique, with a distinctive set of dispositions, capabilities, understandings and outlooks.

Thus the concept 'person' is central to the practice of teaching (and of course, of learning). The person you are as a teacher has a great bearing on how you interact with learners. For this reason, we take the word 'conduct' to say that what we do is driven by what we believe in and what we are, rather than by diktats or rules imposed from outside that do not resonate with our beliefs. We talk about the 'moral sensibility' of the teacher to indicate the overall attitude and sensitivities a teacher brings to bear in teaching and the intellectual and moral presence a teacher develops. We argue that learners learn as much from a teacher's conduct as from the subject he or she teaches. We suggest that teachers conduct themselves like this not as a means to an end but because that is what they see as 'being a teacher' (see also the works of Parker, 1998, and Hansen, 2001). All of these thoughts, ideas and theories have enriched and deepened the language we now use with learners and influenced how we develop surgical teachers.

Two of Our Newer Educational Resources

Each of the following subsections offers a resource that we have more recently developed. The first is an enriched version of one of the profession's assessment tools. The second is about our new approach to developing character and the virtues in professional practitioners.

Case-Based Discussion Plus

Case-based discussion (CBD) is now an assessment requirement endemic to PGME in the UK. It often fails to reach its full teaching potential in understanding professional judgement as a form of reasoning. To extend its educational value, we have created both a table of Aristotle's three forms of reasoning (Table 36.1) and

TABLE 36.1			
An Aristotelian Classification of Forms of Reasoning			
	Theoretical Reasoning	**Technical Reasoning**	**Practical Reasoning**
Disposition	*Epistêmê* The disposition to seek knowledge for its own sake	*Téchnê* The disposition to act in a rule-governed way to make a preplanned artefact	*Phrónêsis* The disposition to act wisely or prudently in a specific situation
Aim *(telos)*	To seek truth for its own sake … Seeking to achieve eternal and pure truth	To produce some object or artefact (e.g., a chair or a house or something a craftsperson has made *to a pre-conceived design*) This would produce craft, but not art	To do what is ethically right and proper in a *particular,* practical situation The basis of art that includes craft
Form of action	*Theoria* Contemplative action	*Poesis* Instrumental action that requires mastery of the knowledge, methods and skills that together constitute technical expertise	*Praxis* Morally committed action in which, and through which, our values are given practical expression
Form of knowing	Philosophy or abstract reasoning	Applied knowing or technical reasoning (Greek craftsmen and artisans applied their knowledge – the principles, procedures and operational methods – to achieve their predetermined aims)	Knowledge-in-use or practical reasoning (e.g., clinical reasoning/ professional judgement/going beyond protocols) – in relation to a specific case

See Fish 2012, p. 41.
(Figure owned by the authors, no copyright required. See Fish 2012, published by Aneumi Publications, a branch of Ed4MedPrac Ltd.)

TABLE 36.2		
The Qualities of Professional Judgement		
Kind of Professional Judgement	**Response to Patient Case**	**Motivation**
Wise Judgement (enlightenment and growing evidence of confidence fluency of thought and action)	Sees each case as needing to be enquired into beyond the obvious, defines what is needed for the best for the patient, can do/obtain what is needed (as a learner checks with senior as appropriate) and then does it. Can make rational sense out of intuitive judgement and use CTP Treats all judgements as potentially provisional and requiring revisiting Able to confidently and with evidence defend the judgement made	Willing and able to put patient's interests first at all times in decision making, even if this risks own interests and position in some way
Maturing Judgement (developing insight)	Open-minded to the complexity of each case; builds on experience. Has a proper respect for conservative management but beginning to balance safety of patient with carefully judged risks	Beginning to put patient first in decision making but still lacks experience and confidence to step outside own needs in favour of patient's interests Beginning to see that you can play it too safe
Self-Defensive Judgement (need for considerable developmental work)	Selects tactics known to please; and are safe; close-minded about choices Chooses what fits limited experience rather than seeing the wider context	Choice of decisions and resultant behaviour designed to enhance own performance and achievements in eyes of seniors
Hasty/Habitual Judgement (unsatisfactory)	Knee jerk reaction/going through the motions unthinkingly	Has not even considered that choices are available

CTP, Clinical Thinking Pathway.
(Authors own the copyright. Modified from Fish., de Cossart 2007, pp. 152–153)

also what we have called CBD Plus (See Paper 4[ii]). This case approach makes more demands of the learner, who along with his or her teacher will need to be familiar with the invisibles as described earlier and our medical reflective writing process, which uses different colours to indicate the different invisible drivers intrinsic to the decision-making processes being charted in the discussion of the case (Fish and de Cossart, 2013).

The rewards, however, as found by those we have taught to do this, are that it encourages the learner to demonstrate self-criticism, criticality and scepticism and be alert to the subtle help that his or her supervisor may be offering. It also leads to a deeper and wider professional conversation between teacher and learner more akin to two professionals having a dialogue than just a 'test.' The writing deepens the thinking of the learner and, when used for three or four cases over a

period of time (e.g., 6 months), puts on record hard evidence of the quality of his or her growing ability to make professional judgements. In Table 36.2, we distinguish a range of different levels of quality of professional judgement.

Exploring the Character and Virtues Called on in Key Cases in Medical Practice

We now seek to help consultant surgeons who are teachers in the clinical setting to start our courses with a detailed exploration of the person they bring to their medical and educational practice and also consider their professional identity (Trede and McEwen, 2012). In addition, we use stories, literature, poetry and the arts in considering the development of the learner's character (Gregory, 2009). We also seek to establish a clearer understanding of the role of the virtues in professional practice. As part of this, we ask learners to explore some of the literature and the concepts associated with the

[ii]<www.Ed4MedPrac.co.uk>

virtues (Annas, 2011; Aristotle, 2004; Arthur et al., 2015; Carr D., 2004; Dunne and Hogan, 2004; Pellegrino, 2006; Pellegrino and Thomasma, 1993, 1996). We ask them to think about these questions: What as a person do they bring to their supervision of doctors? What is required of them by their professional body as clinical supervisors in the literature of their professional body, the General Medical Council (GMC) (2011, 2012)? How do they see virtues, values, character education and professionalism? How do they construe the nature of clinical practice, and why does that matter? How do they view the nature and status of medical knowledge? How do they see patients and the relative priorities of patient care and supervision (Fish, 2015)?

CHAPTER SUMMARY

In this chapter, we have outlined that:

- the relevance of the CTP and the invisibles remains potent for teaching, learning and assessment in PGME and that the principles mentioned earlier resonate with the understanding and thinking of all of the doctors we have taught;
- we have come to believe that our resources, especially the CTP and teaching in the moral mode of practice and our processes for reflecting on cases, are highly relevant to developing quality clinical practice in the interest of safe patient care and for the flourishing of medical/surgical practitioners;
- more and more, we are finding the importance of ontology and doctors learning more deeply about themselves and therefore becoming more self-confident;
- the considerable significance of both medicine and education being moral practices demands the development of professionals' character and virtue in the practice setting;
- what is required in PGME is one-to-one teaching by a capable teacher/supervisor in well-prepared for and rigorous short teaching sessions that draw their learners to explore in detail for individual cases their decision making and the quality of their practical wisdom;
- although the context for clinical practice and the development of practitioners will change as the century progresses, the principles of teaching and

the importance of developing and recording sound clinical thinking in learners will remain powerful and

- engaging the executive boards of specific medical institutions to support the time available for the growth of surgeons and physicians in teaching and learning these critical concepts is crucial to the development of professionals whose wise decisions and actions are at the heart of safe patient care.

REFLECTION POINT 1

Reflection questions for consideration:

1. Explore the important teaching implications for engaging in the moral mode of educational practice by taking a case from your own practice and using the educational resources offered in the chapter to identify the character and virtues that that case demanded of you as a practitioner.
2. What kind of learning experiences help teachers learn more deeply about themselves through critical self-reflection and build their self-confidence?
3. Identify teaching and learning strategies that can be implemented in the practice setting to facilitate the development of the professionals' character and virtue.
4. What could executive boards of medical institutions do to support teachers and learners in implementing learning experiences that lead to a moral mode of practice?

REFERENCES

Annas, J., 2011. Intelligent Virtue. Oxford University Press, Oxford, UK.

Aristotle, 1955, revised ed, 2004. The Ethics of Aristotle: The Nicomachean Ethics, trans. JAK Thomson. Penguin Books, London, UK.

Arthur, J., Kristjanssen, K., Thomas, H., et al., 2015. Virtuous Medical Practice: Research Report. Jubilee Centre, Birmingham University, Birmingham, UK.

Brown, J., Leadbetter, P., Clabburn, O., 2016. Evaluation at East Lancashire Hospitals Trust (ELHT) of the Impact of the Project: 'Supervision Matters: Clinical Supervision for Quality Medical Care'. Edge Hill University, Lancashire, UK.

Bullock, A., Handyman, J., Phillips, S., 2012. Quality Teaching and Learning in Clinical Practice for F2 Teachers and Learners: An Executive Summary. Cardiff University, Cardiff, UK.

Carr, D., 2004. Rival conceptions of practice in education and teaching. In: Dunne, J., Hogan, P. (Eds.), Education and Practice: Upholding the Integrity of Teaching and Learning. Blackwell Publishing, Oxford, UK, pp. 102–115.

Carr, W., 1995. What is an educational practice? In: Carr, W. (Ed.), For Education: Towards Critical Educational Enquiry. Open University Press, Buckingham, UK, pp. 60–73.

Conroy, M., 2016. Pronesis and the medical community. Viewed 21 November 2016. Available from: www.researchgate.net/project/Phronesis-and-the-Medical-Community.

de Cossart, L., Fish, D., 2005. Cultivating a Thinking Surgeon: New Perspectives on Clinical Teaching, Learning and Assessment. TfN Publications, Shrewsbury, UK.

Dewey, J., 1938. Experience and Education. Colliers, New York, NY.

Dunne, J., Hogan, P. (Eds.), 2004. Education and Practice: Upholding the Integrity of Teaching and Learning. Blackwell Publishers, Oxford, UK.

Ed4MedPrac Ltd, n.d. Viewed 23 March 2015. Available from: http://www.ed4medprac.co.uk/.

Fish, D., 2012. Refocusing Postgraduate Medical Education: From the Technical to the Moral Mode of Practice. Aneumi Publications, Gloucester, UK.

Fish, D., 2015. Starting With Myself as Doctor and a Supervisor. Booklet 1 of Medical Supervision Matters. Aneumi Publications, Gloucester, UK.

Fish, D., Coles, C. (Eds.), 1998. Developing Professional Judgement in Health Care: Learning Through the Critical Appreciation of Practice. Butterworth Heinemann, Oxford, UK.

Fish, D., de Cossart, L., 2007. Developing the Wise Doctor. Royal Society of Medicine Press, London.

Fish, D., de Cossart, L., 2013. Reflection for Medical Appraisal. Aneumi Publications, Cranham, Gloucester, UK.

Fish, D., de Cossart, L., Wright, T., 2015a. Practical Dilemmas About Assessment and Evaluation. Booklet 4 of Medical Supervision Matters. Aneumi Publications, Gloucester, UK.

Fish, D., de Cossart, L., Wright, T., 2015b. Practical Dilemmas About Supervision and Teaching. Booklet 2 of Medical Supervision Matters. Aneumi Publications, Gloucester, UK.

Fish, D., de Cossart, L., Wright, T., 2015c. Practical Dilemmas About the Learner and Learning. Booklet 3 of Medical Supervision Matters. Aneumi Publications, Gloucester, UK.

Freire, P., 1970. Pedagogy of the Oppressed. Penguin, Harmondsworth, UK.

General Medical Council (GMC), 2011. The Trainee Doctor. GMC, London, UK. Viewed 30 November 2015. Available from: http://www.gmc-uk.org/Trainee_Doctor.pdf_39274940.pdf.

General Medical Council (GMC), 2012. Recognising and Approving Trainers: The Implementation Plan. GMC, London, UK. Viewed 24 August 2016. Available from: http://www.gmc-uk.org/education/10264.asp.

Gregory, M., 2009. Shaped by Stories: The Ethical Power of Narratives. University of Notre Dame, South Bend, IN.

Hansen, D., 2001. Exploring the Moral Heart of Teaching: Towards a Teacher's Creed. Teachers College Press, London, UK.

Higgs, J., Jones, M., Edwards, I., et al., 2004. Clinical reasoning and practice knowledge. In: Higgs, J., Richardson, B., Abrandt, B., et al. (Eds.), Developing Practice Knowledge for Health Professionals. Butterworth-Heinemann, Edinburgh, UK, pp. 181–199.

Joint Committee for Higher Surgical Training, 2016. Intercollegiate Curriculum Programme (ISCP), Version 10 2016. Viewed 22 November 2016. Available from: https://www.iscp.ac.uk/.

Jubilee Centre, Birmingham University, 2016. Statement on Character, Virtue and Practical Wisdom in Professional Practice. Birmingham University, Birmingham, UK. Viewed 9 November 2016. Available from: http://www.jubileecentre.ac.uk/userfiles/jubileecentre/pdf/Statement_Character_Virtue_Practical_Wisdom_Professional_Practice.pdf.

Oakeshott, K., 1967. Learning and teaching. In: Peters, R.S. (Ed.), The Concept of Education. Routledge and Kegan Paul, London, UK, pp. 156–176.

Parker, P.J., 1998. The Courage to Teach: Exploring the Inner Landscape of a Teacher's Life. Jossey-Bass, San Francisco, CA.

Pellegrino, E., 2006. Character formation and the making of good physicians. In: Kenny, N., Shelton, W. (Eds.), Lost Virtue: Professional Character Development in Medical Education, vol. 10. Advances in Bioethics. Elsevier JAI, Amsterdam, pp. 1–15.

Pellegrino, E., Thomasma, D.C., 1993. The Virtues in Medical Practice. Oxford University Press, Oxford, UK.

Pellegrino, E., Thomasma, D.C., 1996. The Christian Virtues in Medical Practice. Georgetown University Press, Washington, DC.

Pring, R., 2000. Philosophy of Educational Research. Continuum Books, London, UK.

Schwartz, B., Sharpe, K.E., 2010. Practical Wisdom: the Right Way to Do the Right Thing. Riverhead Books, New York, NY.

Thomé, R., 2012. Educational Practice Development: An Evaluation: An Exploration of the Impact on Participants and Their Shared Organisation of a Postgraduate Certificate in Education for Postgraduate Medical Practice 2010–2011. Aneumi Publications, Gloucester, UK.

Thomé, R., 2013. Educational Practice Development: An Evaluation of the Second Year 2011–12: An Exploration of the Impact on Participants and Their Shared Organization of Year Two of the Postgraduate Masters in Education for Postgraduate Medical Practice. Aneumi Publications, Gloucester, UK.

Trede, F., McEwen, C., 2012. Developing critical professional identity. In: Higgs, J., Barnett, R., Billet, S., et al. (Eds.), Practice Based Education: Perspectives and Strategies. Sense Publications, The Netherlands, pp. 27–40.

Walker, R.L., Ivanhoe, P.J. (Eds.), 2007. Working Virtue: Virtue Ethics and Contemporary Moral Problems. Clarendon Press, Oxford, UK.

White, S., Stancombe, J., 2003. Clinical Judgement in Health and Welfare Professions: Extending the Evidence Base. Open University Press, Berkshire, UK.

37

INTERPROFESSIONAL PROGRAMS TO DEVELOP CLINICAL REASONING

ROLA AJJAWI ■ ROSEMARY BRANDER ■ JILL E. THISTLETHWAITE

CHAPTER AIMS

The aims of this chapter are to:

- clarify key concepts in relation to interprofessional education (IPE) and collaborative practice and clinical reasoning,
- integrate research and practice knowledge in relation to IPE and clinical reasoning and
- have a greater understanding of how to teach interprofessional clinical reasoning.

KEY WORDS

Interprofessional learning
Interprofessional education
Collaborative practice
Clinical reasoning

ABBREVIATIONS

CAIPE Centre for the Advancement of Interprofessional Education
CIHC Canadian Interprofessional Health Collaborative
HCTC Health Care Team Challenge
IPE Interprofessional education
IPL Interprofessional learning
IPTWs Interprofessional training wards
WHO World Health Organization

INTRODUCTION

Clinical reasoning is a key capability for every health-care professional. There is a great deal of overlap between the way clinical reasoning is conceptualized and taught across the professions, with differences arising from variations in professionals' roles, responsibilities and scope of practice. However, healthcare professional learners throughout the continuum of training tend to be segregated from each other on uniprofessional programs or through profession-specific continuing professional development. This has frequently resulted in poor communication between practitioners, leading to compromised patient safety and less than optimal client outcomes. For example, the Garling report published in New South Wales, Australia, after a number of patient safety problems occurred in the state's hospitals, recommended that 'clinical education and training should be undertaken in a multiprofessional environment which emphasizes interprofessional team based patient centred care' as a means of improving patient care (Garling 2008, p. 11).

Interprofessional education (IPE) has been recommended as a method of 'learning together to work together' (WHO, 2010). In this chapter, we focus on the rationale for IPE and its feasibility as a means of helping students develop clinical reasoning in preparation for working collaboratively and in teams. Key terms are defined in Box 37.1.

BACKGROUND

The history of IPE is one of waxing and waning of popularity and institutional commitment. The early advocates realized the illogicality of each health profession being educated in a silo with little interaction with other professions (e.g., Barr, 1996). They argued that uniprofessionally trained practitioners typically move into a healthcare system in which clients interact with a diverse range of providers, yet the newly fledged professional, straight out of a higher education system, may have had little experience of this way of working. Modern health care is delivered by many different people – some in bounded, colocated and well-established teams; others coming together for certain tasks; and some meeting collaboratively through referrals and consultations. Clients with complex needs and long-standing chronic conditions frequently require a team-based or collaborative approach to diagnosis and management, as one profession may not be equipped with the capability to do everything necessary. The rationale for interprofessional learning (IPL) is therefore to facilitate such interactions through giving students a grounding in teamwork and

its theory. IPL affords opportunities to learn together, with commonly defined learning outcomes and time for discussion of the values that each profession brings to client care. For the development of clinical reasoning, students require time to observe and discuss their own profession's approach to decision making, the process when more than one profession is involved and the interprofessional negotiation that may be required, together with the client's input, to agree with a plan of care.

The push to incorporate IPE into university-based prequalification healthcare professional education programs has gained momentum because accreditation bodies in many countries have included IPL outcomes or competencies into their standards. A problem, however, is that these outcomes are frequently expressed in different words without consensus across all professions. This can hinder planning educational activities as each profession tries to meet its own requirements. Language may also be a major barrier to successful implementation of IPE; even agreeing on terminology, such as patient, client or service-user, may be difficult. We are at a time of change when, as some are trying to maintain traditional professional boundaries, healthcare systems are developing new roles and delineations, which is a major challenge for healthcare professional education and IPL (Thistlethwaite, 2012). However, when delivered effectively, IPE can foster an understanding of the broad range of healthcare professions, the ways in which they interact with clients and how they complement each other.

LEARNING OUTCOMES

A number of frameworks defining IPL outcomes or the competencies required for interprofessional practice have been published (Thistlethwaite et al., 2014). There is some commonality across these in terms of broad outcomes (Box 37.2), and they may be used as the basis for developing IPL activities focussing on clinical reasoning. It is important for learners to be aware of what they are expected to achieve, not only in terms of subject content (e.g., diagnostic reasoning categories) but also 'with, from and about' their peers from the professions involved. The rationale for IPE needs to be discussed with learners and its importance for clinical practice.

INTERPROFESSIONAL LEARNING ACTIVITIES FOR CLINICAL REASONING

At the prequalification level, clinical reasoning is frequently taught within a specific profession. However, once qualified, the practitioner is immediately thrust into a complex network that demands clinical reasoning not only within a profession but also across professions and sectors. In addition, not only does the practitioner need to develop the skills to engage in collaborative decision making, but also he or she must be able to discern which professions, specialists and community partners are required for successful diagnosis and care. It follows that developing an understanding of clinical reasoning with respect to collaborative competencies across professions and sectors at an early stage of career development would be an asset.

LEARNING THROUGH STRUCTURED OPPORTUNITIES IN THE CLASSROOM

Activities that promote discussion and shared thinking, about a real or hypothetical client case, are ideal IPL opportunities for promoting clinical reasoning. Many such examples exist in the literature based on problem-based learning (e.g., Ajjawi et al., 2010), case-based learning (e.g., Lindqvist et al., 2005) and team-based learning (e.g., Fatmi et al., 2013). In these collaborative inquiry-based approaches, students exchange their ideas, identify their knowledge deficits, agree on solutions and develop a care plan. In so doing, they learn with each other about particular client presentations, the roles of other healthcare professionals in exploring clients' stories and caring for clients and how to improve their understanding of other healthcare professional roles and contributions.

The design of cases and scenarios can be quite sophisticated. For example, Jorm et al. (2016) utilized complexity theory to deliver IPL activities for 1220 healthcare students through developing complicated client cases that required more than simple application of each student's profession-specific knowledge. These cases were designed to ensure that students engaged with IPL because of their perceived relevance, which provided a context for meaningful interaction. The issue of scenario realism, the degree to which a scenario is likely to be similar to participants' experiences in real life, has been found to be crucial for student engagement (van Soeren et al., 2011). Realistic clinical scenarios allowed participants to practice their profession-specific knowledge in an interprofessional context. Client scenarios can be extended beyond the classroom into the simulated setting, where aspects of realism and fidelity may be more closely maintained.

LEARNING THROUGH SIMULATION

Simulations of collaborative reasoning and decision making can provide prequalification learners' opportunities to develop competence in the skills required for successful collaboration, and simulations have been developed for many IPL activities. Indeed, learning through simulation has the potential to enable students and clinicians to critically analyze their own actions, reflect on their skills and critique the clinical decisions of others (van Soeren et al., 2011). One such learning activity is the Health Care Team Challenge (HCTC)™. In this learning activity, students form interprofessional teams to participate in a friendly competition. Students are provided with a case that has information about a

CASE STUDY 37.1

Preparing for Team Work

Your IPL group, which consists of students from medicine, nursing, nutrition, pharmacy and physiotherapy, is asked to consult with Rosie, a 77-year-old patient attending the community clinic to which you are attached. Rosie's GP letter advises that she has been referred to the clinic to help with pain and poor mobility caused by osteoarthritis in both knees. Her body mass index is 31, and she is taking medication for type 2 diabetes, hypertension and pain. This is the first time you have worked together in this group. Before you interact with Rosie, how do you prepare to work as a team? What do you hope to learn from this encounter, and what is the value of collaborating with students from other health professions? If you were the educator facilitating the interprofessional management plan, how might you help students to understand different professional groups' perspectives on diagnosis and care?

---

client and the client's family and community and are tasked to develop a client-centred collaborative plan of care, reinforced with evidence and best practice, which they present to a panel of judges. The educational process centres on group learning with authentic teamwork over time and culminates in a formal presentation to an audience (Newton et al., 2013).

The HCTC™ process is rigorous and follows stipulated competition rules. Students develop knowledge of their own and each other's roles and abilities tailored within the team and for the unique simulated case. They can develop high-level teamwork skills, for example, in conflict resolution and collaborative leadership, as they work together through the client's case and negotiate a best plan of care. Students become more knowledgeable about common healthcare regulatory issues and anticipate safety issues for service users and for healthcare workers. Together they build trust, dispel professional stereotypes and strengthen their competence for collaborative practice. The HCTC™ also holds other competitions at regional, national and international levels, in turn providing new, unique and varied team learning experiences across diverse provinces/states and countries.

LEARNING THROUGH COMMUNITY ENGAGEMENT, PARTNERSHIPS AND SERVICE

Prequalification learners frequently tell us that application of interprofessional principles in the workplace is difficult. Higgs et al. (2008) describe the development of clinical reasoning ability as beginning with theoretical knowledge that is used to make sense of clinical findings.

This ability can then be used to start developing practice wisdom that incorporates the understanding of complex social interactions, ethical subtleties and individual situations and context. It takes considerable time and exposure to clinical realities to develop practice wisdom. To provide this exposure, many IPE centres have sought to engage community and practice healthcare teams in educating prequalification learners. These opportunities provide new learning spaces.

Learning spaces, which bridge workplace learning and classroom learning, have been extended in many different and creative ways. Student-centred approaches in which educators partner with community healthcare teams and can share their stories of success and challenges with students are commonly used. Hearing about the experiences from authentic interprofessional teams provides a 'reality check' and enables students to extend their imaginations into, and further their understandings of, clinical practice. Through critical discussion with each other, plus guided faculty and clinician facilitation, students can sort through such domains as individual and team roles, communications and actions taken and propose questions and alternative solutions for the scenarios presented.

A mutually beneficial approach, centred on both student and community needs, has also demonstrated successful learning outcomes. Students are introduced to interprofessional clinical reasoning opportunities in structured curricular activities to learn together in the workplace and/or in service learning opportunities (Brander et al., 2015a). For example, in a recent project sponsored by the Associated Medical Services and Queen's University, both in Ontario, Canada, healthcare students who were scheduled for placements in primary care clinics were organized to spend time together to review and discuss educational modules purposefully created for IPL about compassion in primary care. This opportunity encouraged students to develop clinical reasoning skills related to collaborative practice and compassion in the primary care context, which they could extrapolate to other healthcare contexts (Donnelly et al., 2016).

Other initiatives have focussed on the development of interprofessional student-led outpatient and hospital clinics, student-run community clinics and interprofessional training wards (IPTWs). Linköping University (Sweden) has led the way with IPTWs, which have now been replicated in Australia, Canada, the United States and the UK in various ways. Typically, these are well received by students as offering meaningful learning activities. These settings have been found to increase students' understanding of their future professional roles and the roles of the other professions and highlight the value of teamwork for client care (Falk et al., 2013). The proximity among students, sharing of responsibility and authentic tasks were found to enable collaborative practice and development of professional knowledge, e.g., through round-table discussions of client care, negotiations and decision making about specific clients. Students on the IPTW can work with the task of clarifying how their respective professional roles and practical understandings of care contribute to the team and ultimately to the welfare of the client. This produces valuable opportunities to learn from and about other professions and enriches the learning relating to specific client cases. Interestingly, the IPTW raised awareness of some unexpected issues where students experienced dissonance between the reality of collaborative practice and expectations of their own professional role (Falk et al., 2013). Being able to discuss and manage all students' expectations is important for optimizing their engagement and learning within the IPTW.

Community engagement and community partnerships are inextricably linked for the creation of useful and accountable learning opportunities. Relationships with community partners that are genuinely productive for the local population are the foundation for fruitful project development, implementation and outcomes. Partnerships can include many different healthcare teams across a wide variety of contexts. A variety of IPL experiences with real healthcare teams will assist students to develop clinical reasoning skills in preparation for demanding healthcare careers, where interprofessional acumen and success are required for the delivery of safe and quality care. In addition, interprofessional faculty and clinicians working together to deliver successful educational initiatives are provided with robust prospects to role-model the realization of collaboration, reveal some of the hidden curriculum and lead learners to professional behaviour growth. Fig. 37.1 shows the different models of interaction of IPE.

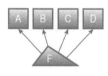

Multiprofessional: facilitator talking to students – minimal interaction between students

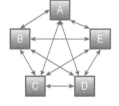

Interprofessional: interactive; students learning with, from and about

Students interviewing a patient together

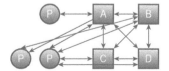

IP training ward or clinic: students interacting with patients and each other

Fig. 37.1 ■ Examples of multiprofessional and interprofessional activities. A, B, C, D, E, students from different health professions; F, facilitator; P, patient.

LEARNING ABOUT COLLABORATIVE LEADERSHIP

There is evidence that shared responsibility for clinical reasoning and decisions augments safety, provides quality outcomes and improves client and staff experiences within the workplace (WHO, 2010). However, a recent scoping review revealed that little has been established about frames of reference, definitions, or theory about leadership in health care and especially in regards to interprofessional practice (Brewer et al., 2016). More concerning are findings from a recent narrative study of leadership-followership indicating that static and hierarchical leadership relationships remain the norm, despite the espoused rhetoric of distributed leadership relationships within the health-care literature (Gordon et al., 2015). This points to a strong need for critical discussion and robust research regarding leadership frameworks within the health sector.

Collaborative leadership is a newer and more complex form of leadership that has emerged to better fit with collaborative client-centred care and the realities of current-day regulations and practice. Collaborative leaders 'engage one another in such a way that leaders and followers raise one another's levels of motivation and morality and nurture interdependencies among multiple parities' (VanVactor, 2012, p. 555) for the achievement of collective goals and successful outcomes.

Four key leadership competencies of collaborative teams include being authentic, empowering, facilitating and sustaining (Brander et al., 2015b). These competencies emerged after extensive literature and scoping reviews, an environmental scan of health leadership programs and key informant interviews of Canadian health leaders, practitioners and students. The goal was to guide the development of a health leaders' collaborative leadership pilot curriculum. Orchard and Rykhoff (2015) proposed a complementary framework of leadership that depicts reciprocity between vertical/hierarchical and collaborative leadership theory and that builds relationships among interprofessional team members. They surmised that today's interprofessional leadership was developed from an evolution of leadership styles to best fit the delivery of collaborative client-centred care. These studies begin to describe emergent competencies and theories related to collaborative

leadership. However, much more work is needed to develop these findings before we can implement them.

Dow et al. (2013) suggested a framework to assist with curriculum planning for collaborative practice for healthcare workers, which includes the development of knowledge, attitudes and behaviours across four concepts. Two of these four concepts focus on leadership. The first concept, 'leadership and followership', is described as being coproduced by the healthcare workers and requires the ability to move between leading and following roles. The second concept, 'locus and formality of leadership', is demonstrated by the ability to modify leadership behaviours based on a leader's relationship to the team and the formality of leadership required for any unique situation (Dow et al., 2013, p. 954). Dow et al. claim that learners, at all levels, who develop the clinical reasoning and skills related to these concepts will be better team members and leaders. They also review a continuum of learning experiences, from the classroom, to simulation, to the clinic, as important to develop the needed team competencies for successful outcomes in healthcare professional learners.

Students indicate that there often is a disconnect between their education about principles for effective collaborative practice, teamwork and leadership and their experiences in clinical settings. One way that faculty have attempted to bridge this gap at Queen's University, Kingston, Canada, is in conducting an educational event to practice all six teamwork competencies (CIHC, 2010) and in particular with a focus on the development of the competencies of collaborative leadership and conflict resolution within their student interprofessional teams.

In this simulation activity, students meet in inter-professional teams with a 'community mentor', who shares his or her healthcare story. Interprofessional student teams are then asked to develop interprofessional care plans reflective of the mentor's priorities and concerns using evidence-based and best-practice–based research. The teams present their rationale and teamwork skills to a panel of faculty, clinician and community judges and are questioned about their strategies for success and challenges with any of the teamwork competencies. This task requires the students to exchange knowledge and clinical reasoning frames, which in turn gives them active instruction in learning to work as a team towards a considered and comprehensive care plan focussed on the community mentor.

CHALLENGES OF IPE

Introducing and sustaining IPL activities is a challenging task for many reasons. Descriptions of IPE frequently cite the main problems as being logistical including large numbers of learners in undergraduate programs across multiple departments and schools; timetabling as each healthcare professional course has its own system and clinical placements; curriculum space; and varying requirements for supervision. With committed educators and careful planning, the logistics may be overcome, and there are many examples of innovative ways of doing this. In our experience the major barriers are rather professional hierarchies, lack of understanding of what IPE is and may achieve and concerns about professional identity and scope of practice. It is very important that everyone involved in the development of IPE agrees on the learning outcomes and/or competencies to be achieved, the activities that are necessary for that achievement, the type and timing of assessment and what faculty development is required.

Different health professions have different foci for clinical reasoning, which lead to different content, different data collection and different clinical action for the same client (Sheehan et al., 2005). Healthcare professional educators may need to discuss how clinical reasoning is conceived by the different professions and what implications this has for interprofessional teaching and learning. Professionals typically approach client problems based on profession-specific ways of knowing and being because of the socialization of professionals into particular ways of thinking, talking and being (Ajjawi and Higgs, 2008). Students working interprofessionally may need to move from their usual professional responsibilities to negotiate and make decisions collectively for the care of the client (Falk et al., 2013). These 'boundary zones' can be sites of struggle, where educator support and debrief are essential.

REFLECTION POINT 1

How might you identify that a student is struggling with collaborative practice and decision making? How could you tackle this?

FACULTY DEVELOPMENT

Highly skilled and experienced teachers, facilitators and supervisors working within the dominant uniprofessional education model may have initial difficulties with IPE. A robust program of faculty development for IPE is necessary to enable staff to acquire the attributes required for effective interprofessional facilitation (see Reflection Point 2). Such development should be devised and delivered by an interprofessional group. As IPL activities for clinical reasoning may take place within a diverse range of locations such as the classroom, clinical environment, community and hospital, faculty development is a complex process. An interprofessional educator should be attuned to the dynamics of IPL and skilled in optimizing learning opportunities while valuing each participating profession's experience and expertise (Barr, 1996).

A study into educators facilitating IPE programs found that not all brought positive attitudes towards interprofessional collaborators. Time, reflection and caution were needed for educators to explore implications of past interprofessional experiences on educators' current approaches to IPL and their development of shared purpose for working with other educators (Croker et al., 2016). Interprofessional facilitators need to develop awareness of how students are interacting and are able to involve students in feedback dialogue about team processes and their roles, responsibilities and language. The facilitator may need to challenge stereotyping, encourage students to challenge this themselves and compare group work as students do teamwork in clinical settings. Focussing students on the needs of the clients, rather than specific professional roles, can be valuable for educators to break down boundaries through shared negotiation and decision making.

REFLECTION POINT 2

Reflect on the attributes listed below that are necessary for effective interprofessional facilitation: how do these match your own experiences and capacity? How might you tackle these in a faculty development program?
• Knowledge of the rationale and evidence for IPE
• Motivation for and commitment to IPE

- Thorough knowledge of the roles, responsibilities and scope of practice of a wide range of healthcare professionals
- Understanding of teamwork theory and team building
- Experience of working in an interprofessional healthcare team
- Understanding of collaborative practice and what it looks like in the workplace
- Understanding of the process of professional identity formation and socialization and how these might affect interprofessional practice
- Skills in negotiation and conflict resolution

CHAPTER SUMMARY

- There are similarities in the way clinical reasoning is conceptualized and taught across the professions, with differences arising from variations in professionals' knowledge, roles, responsibilities and scope of practice.
- The development of clinical reasoning requires students to observe and discuss their own profession's approach to decision making, the process when more than one profession is involved and the negotiation that may be required interprofessionally, and with the client, to agree on a management plan and carry it out.
- Learning to reason interprofessionally can be taught through the formal (e.g., case-based learning, simulation) and the informal (e.g., community placements and IPTWs) curriculum.
- Making the reasoning focus explicit allows for discussion and exploration of how others think in practice.
- The role of the educator is complex and nuanced, with specific faculty development required.

REFLECTION POINT 3

For further reading and reflection:
Reeves, S., Fletcher, S., Barr, H., Birch, I., Boet, S., Davies, N, et al., 2016. A BEME systematic review of the effects of interprofessional education: BEME Guide No. 39. Med. Teach. 38 (7), 656–668.

REFERENCES

Ajjawi, R., Higgs, J., 2008. Learning to reason: a journey of professional socialisation. Adv. Health Sci. Educ. Theory Pract. 13, 133–150.

Ajjawi, R., Thistlethwaite, J.E., Williams, K.A., et al., 2010. Breaking down professional barriers: medicine and pharmacy students learning together. Focus Health Prof. Educ. 12, 1–10.

Barr, H., 1996. Ends and means in interprofessional education: towards a typology. Educ. Health 9, 341–352.

Brander, R., Bainbridge, L., Van Dijk, J., et al., 2015a. Transformative continuing interprofessional education and professional development to meet patient care needs: a synthesis of best practices. In: Orchard, C., Bainbridge, L. (Eds.), Interprofessional Client-Centred Collaborative Practice: What Does It Look Like? How Can It Be Achieved? Nova, Hauppauge, NY, pp. 113–130.

Brander, R., MacPhee, M., Careau, E., et al., 2015b. Collaborative leadership for the transformation of health systems. In: Forman, D., Jones, M., Thistlethwaite, J. (Eds.), Leadership and Collaboration: Further Developments for Interprofessional Education. Palgrave MacMillan, London, UK, pp. 153–166.

Brewer, M.L., Flavell, H.L., Trede, F., et al., 2016. A scoping review to understand 'leadership' in interprofessional education and practice. J. Interprof. Care 30, 408–415.

Centre for the Advancement of Interprofessional Education (CAIPE), 2002. Viewed 1 March 2017. Available from: http://caipe.org.uk/resources/defining-ipe/.

Canadian Interprofessional Health Collaborative (CIHC), 2010. A national interprofessional competency framework. Viewed 1 March 2017. Available from: http://www.cihc.ca/files/CIHC_IPCompetencies_Feb1210.pdf.

Croker, A., Wakely, L., Leys, J., 2016. Educators working together for interprofessional education: from 'fragmented beginnings' to being 'intentionally interprofessional'. J. Interprof. Care 30, 671–674.

Donnelly, C., Brander, R., Watson, S., et al., 2016. Teaching compassionate care in primary care using enhanced online delivery methods, paper presented at the Canadian Conference for Medical Educators, 18 April. Montreal, Canada, Abstract #OF 1–3, p. 103.

Dow, A.W., DiazGranados, D., Mazmanian, P.E., et al., 2013. Applying organizational science to health care: a framework for collaborative practice. Acad. Med. 88, 952–957.

Falk, A.L., Hult, H., Hammar, M., et al., 2013. One site fits all? A student ward as a learning practice for interprofessional development. J. Interprof. Care 27, 476–481.

Fatmi, M., Hartling, L., Hillier, T., et al., 2013. The effectiveness of team-based learning on learning outcomes in health professions education: BEME Guide No. 30. Med. Teach. 35, e1608–e1624.

Freeth, D., Hammick, M., Reeves, S., et al., 2005. Effective Interprofessional Education: Development, Delivery and Evaluation. Blackwell Publishing, Oxford, UK.

Garling, P., 2008. Final report of the Special Commission of Inquiry: Acute Care Services in NSW Public Hospitals. State of NSW through the Special Commission of Inquiry, NSW.

Gordon, L.J., Rees, C.E., Ker, J.S., et al., 2015. Leadership and followership in the healthcare workplace: exploring medical trainees' experiences through narrative inquiry. BMJ Open 5, e008898.

Higgs, J., Jones, M.A., Titchen, A., 2008. Knowledge, reasoning and evidence for practice. In: Higgs, J., Jones, M.A., Loftus, S., et al.

(Eds.), Clinical Reasoning in the Health Professions, third ed. Elsevier Health Sciences, Philadelphia, PA, pp. 151–161.

Jorm, C., Nisbet, G., Roberts, C., et al., 2016. Using complexity theory to develop a student-directed interprofessional learning activity for 1220 healthcare students. BMC Med. Educ. 16, 199.

Lindqvist, S., Duncan, A., Shepstone, L., et al., 2005. Case-based learning in cross-professional groups: the development of a pre-registration interprofessional learning programme. J. Interprof. Care 19, 509–520.

Newton, C., Bainbridge, L., Ball, V.A., et al., 2013. Health care team challenges: an international review and research agenda. J. Interprof. Care 27, 529–531.

Orchard, C., Rykhoff, M., 2015. Collaborative leadership within interprofessional practice. In: Forman, D., Jones, M., Thistlethwaite, J. (Eds.), Leadership and Collaboration: Further Developments for Interprofessional Education. Palgrave MacMillan, London, UK, pp. 71–94.

Sheehan, D., Robertson, L., Ormond, T., 2005. An exploration of the impact of professional experience and background on clinical reasoning. Focus Health Prof. Educ. 7, 99–113.

Thistlethwaite, J., 2012. Interprofessional education: a review of context, learning and the research agenda. Med. Educ. 46, 58–70.

Thistlethwaite, J., Forman, D., Matthews, L.R., et al., 2014. Competencies and frameworks in interprofessional education: a comparative analysis. Acad. Med. 89, 869–874.

van Soeren, M., Devlin-Cop, S., MacMillan, K., et al., 2011. Simulated interprofessional education: an analysis of teaching and learning processes. J. Interprof. Care 25, 434–440.

VanVactor, J.D., 2012. Collaborative leadership model in the management of health care. J. Bus. Res. 65, 555–561.

World Health Organization, 2010. Framework for action on interprofessional education and collaborative practice. WHO, Geneva.

38 ASSESSING CLINICAL REASONING

LAMBERT W.T. SCHUWIRTH ▪ STEVEN J. DURNING ▪
GEOFFREY R. NORMAN ▪ CEES P.M. VAN DER VLEUTEN

CHAPTER AIMS

The aims of this chapter are to:

- describe the developments in assessment of clinical reasoning and
- explain the possibilities and limitations in further developments.

KEY WORDS

Clinical reasoning

Clinical decision making

Assessment methods

Domain specificity and sampling

ABBREVIATIONS/ ACRONYMS

EMQ Extended matching question

KFP Key Feature Problem

MCQ Multiple-choice question

OSCE Objective Structured Clinical Examination

PMP Patient Management Problem

SCT Script Concordance Test

INTRODUCTION

Central to being a clinician is arriving at diagnoses and management by gathering data from history-taking, physical examination and laboratory tests. The process is described by a variety of terms, such as 'clinical reasoning' and 'decision making'. Many distinctions can be made, but perhaps the most important one is that reasoning focusses on the thought processes, with studies of clinicians and learners typically using psychological and observational methods. Decision making examines the optimal outcome of the process with studies using epidemiological data and methods such as decision analysis.

There has been increased interest in both domains over the past decade, stimulated by two important documents from the Institute of Medicine in the United States: 'To Err Is Human', a review of management errors (Kohn et al., 2000), and 'Improving Diagnosis in Health Care' (Balogh et al., 2015), which focussed specifically on diagnostic errors. This increased interest has led to many studies and papers describing theories of clinical reasoning and subsequent educational strategies to reduce error (Croskerry, 2003; Norman, 2005).

Early Research on Clinical Reasoning

In the 1970s and 1980s several studies showed that although expert clinicians systematically outperformed less experienced doctors on a variety of simulations of clinical diagnosis, there was little difference in the nature of problem-solving processes they used. This led to a new direction in fundamental research, guided by cognitive psychology (Eva, 2004; Norman, 2005; Regehr and Norman, 1996; Schmidt et al., 1990), which led to a further understanding that problem-solving ability is not a separate teachable skill and that it cannot be measured independently of relevant content knowledge. More important than the amount of knowledge are the ways in which it is structured, stored, accessed and retrieved (de Bruin et al., 2005). An essential facet in this storage and retrieval of knowledge is the understanding of the so-called deep structure – the fundamental ideas that shape our understanding of the problem (Chi et al., 1982). From this perspective, expertise is a function of how well the problem at hand is understood as a specific instance of the deep structure, which then allows us to understand differences and similarities between seemingly different problems. For example, there are the similarities and differences between an aspirin overdose and hyperventilation; both may have different symptoms and aetiologies, but both are a disturbance of the acid-base balance.

An alternative developmental theory of knowledge organization (Schmidt et al., 1990) proposes three different kinds of knowledge relevant to solving clinical problems. The most elementary is knowledge of disease processes and causal relationships, the basic science of medicine, followed by the acquisition of so-called 'illness scripts', which are quite literal, listlike structures relating signs and symptoms to disease prototypes. At the highest level of functioning, the expert uses a sophisticated form of pattern recognition, called 'nonanalytic' or 'exemplar-based' reasoning, characterized by speed and efficient use of information (Schmidt et al., 1990). It appears that pattern recognition is, in fact, recognition at a holistic level of the similarity between the present patient and previous patients (Hatala and Norman, 1999). More recent theories (Croskerry, 2003; Norman, 2005) collapse the distinction between process and knowledge and instead propose a 'dual-process' model in which problems can be solved by either unconscious application of experiential knowledge (System 1) or conscious application of analytical knowledge (System 2).

The more experience a person has had with a given type of clinical problem, the more likely he or she is to employ a faster and less effortful System 1 problem-solving process. However, if the solution is not recognized as a pattern, more effortful and analytical problem-solving processes must be brought into play. Any individual will demonstrate a range of approaches, both within and across problems, depending on previous experience and exposure to similar problems. Problem-solving ability is therefore not a characteristic of the clinician but an interaction between the nature (including complexity) of the problem and the clinician's knowledge and problem-specific expertise. These insights help to explain the findings of idiosyncrasy and domain specificity of patient management problems. Experts employ more nonanalytical reasoning and pattern recognition and are therefore able to solve a problem more efficiently requiring less information than clinicians of more intermediate ability.

RESEARCH ON DECISION MAKING

Since the 1970s, research on decision making has taken a very different direction, driven by searches for optimal approaches to decision making. This research typically takes the form of investigations of the extent to which human decision makers (doctors) are suboptimal in their decisions and the causes of these suboptimal decisions, typically framed as heuristics and biases (cf. Plous, 1993); hence, there is some overlap with the clinical reasoning literature.

Implications for Assessment of Clinical Reasoning

Although the two domains of clinical reasoning and clinical decision making appear very different, in assessment the distinction blurs. For that reason, we will treat clinical decision making as part of clinical reasoning, and we will describe the developments in assessment of decision making and reasoning, limiting our discussion primarily to methods designed to elucidate the cognitive thinking processes involved in reasoning. We acknowledge that clinical reasoning can also be assessed with performance-based measures such as the OSCE (Objective Structured Clinical Examination) or in real-life clinical practice, but it is first and foremost an activity of the mind.

Assessment methods typically begin with the presentation of a clinical problem, either in sequential fashion (e.g., history, physical) or as a whole case description. The associated questions focus either on the decisions or the reasoning behind them. Variations may range from simple to complex and can be linked with different question and response formats. We will describe some of the more common approaches.

REFLECTION POINT 1

No single assessment method will be able to capture the whole process of clinical reasoning and decision making. A combination of instruments will have to be used in an assessment program.

AN HISTORICAL PERSPECTIVE ON ASSESSMENT

In the 1960s and 1970s, the focus was on the development of methods that assessed 'clinical problem-solving skills'. The main thrust was to mimic authentic clinical situations optimally in a paper-based format. One popular variant, the Patient Management Problem (PMP), attempted to simulate the process by which a doctor obtained information from history and physical examination. A typical PMP began with an initial complaint and brief demographic details of the patient. The candidate was then requested to collect further data, sequentially in a branched fashion, e.g., with a 'rub out' pen that exposed the answer (or later on with computers). Then, the candidate could select investigations and/or make diagnostic and management decisions. A criterion panel of physicians would decide a priori on the weight assigned to each option, typically from +2 to −2. The candidate would then receive a variety of scores (Proficiency, Efficiency, Competence, Errors of Omission) based on various approaches to aggregating the weights over all components of the problem.

A number of psychometric problems with the PMP (Swanson et al., 1987) emerged. First, different experts used different pathways to solve the same problem, so it was difficult to get consensus on the scoring of each individual decision in the problem-solving process. Second, because the various scoring methods ultimately rewarded thoroughness, and expert physicians took shortcuts, junior doctors often received higher scores than experts. A third problem was that studies that directly compared PMP performance to performance on the same problem with a live simulated (standardized) patient showed that people selected about twice as many data options in the PMP as they did with the live patient, which was a fundamental threat to the validity of the method. Finally, the most striking and counterintuitive finding was that performance on one PMP was a poor predictor of performance on any other

PMP. Correlation across problems was typically around 0.1 to 0.3 (Norman et al., 1985), which seriously undermined the hypotheses that problem solving was a generic ability or skill, independently assessable of the underlying knowledge structure. The explanation of this phenomenon is referred to as content or case specificity (Elstein et al., 1978). Because candidates took too long to work through a single case of a PMP, typically 30 to 45 minutes, large numbers of cases and considerable testing time were needed to produce acceptably reliable results. This finding of case or domain specificity is not unique to PMPs but is also seen in other methods that assess clinical competence and performance.

A final consequence of these early studies was a renewed focus on knowledge as a prerequisite for clinical decision making and reasoning. Efficient measures of knowledge such as multiple-choice questions (MCQs) remain a mainstay of testing agencies because we now recognize, as we did not in the 1960s, that knowledge is central to expertise. Some studies, for example, have shown that written knowledge tests, oriented to the kind of clinical knowledge central to clinical practice, are better predictors of competence in medical practice 5 to 20 years later than more 'authentic' performance tests (Tamblyn et al., 2007; Wenghofer et al., 2009). The centrality of knowledge is not limited to medicine; research in the development of expertise in many domains comes to the same conclusions (Ericsson, 2007).

Also, these studies suggest that highly authentic (and expensive) test situations do not automatically lead to useful assessment information. LaRochelle has shown that students can learn clinical reasoning using written cases just as effectively as they can with more realistic formats (La Rochelle et al., 2012). Norman et al. (2012) showed that low-fidelity simulations are as effective in learning transferrable skills as much more expensive high-fidelity simulations.

NEWER ASSESSMENT DEVELOPMENTS

The evidence thus far leads to a number of conclusions. First, assessment must be anchored in case-based material presented in a way that will induce and sample clinical reasoning activities (Schuwirth et al., 2001). Second, laboriously taking a student through the full data gathering and investigational phase of a real or simulated clinical case is an inefficient approach when the purpose is to evaluate clinical reasoning, because of content specificity. For example, up to 8 hours of testing time would be required to achieve reliable assessments with PMPs (Norcini et al., 1985), demonstrating that testing methods require more time-efficient sampling.

A useful distinction is between stimulus formats and response formats (Norman et al., 1996). The stimulus format refers to the task presented to the candidate. This may range from very simple short questions to very complex and time-consuming questions. The stimulus format typically ends with one or more questions asking the candidate to connect the information in the stimulus with the required response. Typical lead-ins are 'What is the most likely diagnosis?' or 'What are the most indicated next steps in the management?'

The response format refers to the way the response of the candidate is captured. It can consist of a short menu of options (MCQs), long extensive (computerized) menus, a short write-in format, a long write-in format (essay-type questions), an oral response or an observed behaviour either in a simulated environment (e.g., OSCE) or in a real-life context.

Two recent developments, the key feature approach (Page et al., 1990) and extended matching items, exemplify the divergence of response approaches.

Key Feature Problem Approach

The basic idea behind Key Feature Problems (KFPs) is to focus only on essential aspects of clinical cases, allowing more cases to be asked per hour and providing more efficient sampling. Also, by asking essential decisions only, quick pattern recognition and expert efficiency are not 'penalized' as with PMPs. Key features are the decisions pivotal to the successful outcome of the case, e.g., a particular diagnosis, a critical test or the next management steps. More detailed item construction tips are provided elsewhere (Farmer & Gordon Page, 2005; Page and Bordage, 1995; Schuwirth et al., 1999). Questions relating to the key features can use a variety of response formats (e.g., short-answer, MCQs or selection from longer menus of options), but they should be such that the candidate must read the whole case and synthesize the necessary information. The KFP allows 40 to 50 cases to be administered in the same time as needed for 12 to 15 PMPs. Studies so far have indicated substantially better reliability than with PMPs

but, still, 2 to 5 hours of testing time is required. Medical Council of Canada data showed a reliability of 0.80 with approximately 40 cases in 4 hours of testing time (Page and Bordage, 1995). A recent study showed that two to three items (questions) per case are optimal for maximum reliability (Norman et al., 2006); reading time will compromise reliability when fewer items are used, and information redundancy will compromise reliability when more items are used.

Validity studies investigating correlations with other measures typically show moderate correlations. More compelling are studies using think-aloud strategies when comparing stimulus formats, showing that case-based stimulus formats elicit other cognitive processes than fact-oriented stimulus formats (Schuwirth et al., 2001). Although the more factual questions elicited more or less simple black-and-white or 'yes/no' thinking steps, the case-based questions elicited probabilistic reasoning weighing different bits of information from the case against each other. Response formats that use menus instead of write-ins may cue the candidate to both correct and incorrect answers with slightly higher scores as a net effect, naturally depending on the number of alternatives in the menu (Schuwirth et al., 1996). Score correlations across these response formats, however, are invariably high.

A modern variation of the key feature format is the use of computers for test administration, allowing more flexible use of pictorial and audio information. Many variants of computer-based 'virtual patients' now exist. A recent systematic review (Cook et al., 2010) examined 50 studies of the use of virtual patients for learning reasoning and concluded that they have no systematic advantage over simpler formats.

Multiple-Choice Questions and Extended-Matching Items

In their simplest format, simulations take the form of vignette-based MCQs. Short cases are presented that require a judgement or decision about data gathering, case management or any other phase of the clinical problem. These questions are, with some initial training, relatively easy to write, particularly because they come close to what clinicians do in actual clinical practice. The response format is a menu. The length of the menu does not need to be fixed but is usually as long as there are meaningful alternatives.

Virtual Patients in Student Assessment

Dr. Dawson is a busy clinician with a huge interest in medical education and clinical reasoning. He is contacted by a friend, who has recently developed a new virtual reality engine and now suggests that Dr. Dawson develop some authentic virtual patients. The friend suggests that they can use them to assess the clinical reasoning ability of medical students for their final examinations.

This thought is very appealing to Dr. Dawson, given his interest in clinical reasoning, but he decides to ask for advice from medical education experts first. The medical education experts explain that the research into clinical reasoning and decision making has shown that fidelity/authenticity is not the same as validity and that the history of high-fidelity simulations for the assessment of clinical reasoning and decision making has been sobering. They explain that various concerns with this approach have been identified, with the most important being the so-called 'domain specificity'. So, regardless of how well designed the virtual reality engine and how authentic the simulation is, it does not alter the fact that to get a reliable and valid assessment of a student's clinical decision-making and reasoning ability, many cases need to be processed by the student. They further tell him that, up until now, the most promising developments have been with short cases and a limited number of questions per case and that low-fidelity simulations seem to be as valid as high-fidelity simulations for the assessment of clinical decision making and reasoning. Dr. Dawson decides to read this literature himself and comes to the same conclusion. He is glad he has consulted the medical education experts and has thus avoided wasting considerable time and resources on an approach that has been demonstrated to be unsuccessful.

The lesson from this case is that much of the research outcome in the field of assessment of clinical decision making and clinical reasoning is counterintuitive, and consulting with people who have a good knowledge of this literature is helpful in preventing busy people from spending their precious time on unsuccessful approaches.

Another MCQ type – proposed by the US National Board of Medical Examiners (NBME) – is the Extended Matching Questions (EMQs) (Case and Swanson, 1993). Students are presented with a series of brief case scenarios based on a single chief complaint (e.g., shortness of breath) and must select the most appropriate diagnosis or action from a menu of options. EMQs are relatively easy to construct. They represent clinical reasoning assessments in their simplest form, with an authentic stimulus in combination with a closed response. Reliability is similar to that of normal MCQs. Stimulus formats with richer (and longer) vignettes contain more 'measurement information' and contribute more to reliability than other vignettes. Longer menu response formats may appear to be better, but evidence suggests no advantage over simple five-option MCQs. More complex response formats (e.g., using multiple best answers or allowing logical operators between different elements) and more complex scoring systems (like penalties and partial credit) are not recommended.

Simple single best-answer formats and simple scoring systems are advised. Excellent manuals for writing these MCQs are available through the NBME[i] or from the Australian Office for Learning and Teaching (OLT)[ii].

BUT WHAT ABOUT CLINICAL REASONING?

The assessment methods described earlier may have good psychometric properties, but many people feel that they do not fully capture the clinical reasoning process (e.g., Charlin et al., 2000). To fill this gap, Charlin et al. proposed a new type of assessment using cognitive expertise theory and the Script Concordance Test (SCT)

[i] US National Board of Medical Examiners (NBME): www.nbme.org
[ii] Australian Office for Learning and Teaching (OLT): https://www.acer.edu.au/files/quality-determination-of-assessment-items-amac-resource.pdf

(Charlin et al., 2000). The assumption is that most clinical problems are ill defined, and experts are not expected to always collect exactly the same information. They challenged the MCQ formats because these always required agreed-upon solutions to well-defined problems (Charlin et al., 2000). SCT questions focus on essential decisions in a case like the KFP but allow for variability between experts. For this, Charlin suggested using ill-defined problems with a previously published aggregate scoring method. A clinical scenario is presented that provides a challenge to the candidate because not all data are provided for solution of the problem. However, the question format is constrained to questions whose answers can be scales on a +2 to –2 scale. An example is presented in Box 38.1.

The scoring reflects the variability experts demonstrate in the clinical reasoning process. Credits on each item are derived from the answers given by a reference panel, with each score being proportional to the number of reference panel members who have provided that answer. Studies into the validity of the SCT have been conducted, and reliability studies show that 0.80 can be reached with approximately 1 hour of testing using about 80 items.

REFLECTION POINT 2

For each case, there may not be a single best way of clinical reasoning. Assessment should focus on distinguishing between good or acceptable reasoning processes and bad or unacceptable reasoning processes.

CURRENT DEVELOPMENTS

Current theories acknowledge that analytical and nonanalytical processes work in conjunction and interact with each other continually (Norman, 2005), and any separation of these processes leads to oversimplification. Instead of trying to focus on single points in the process, modern assessment seeks to develop rigorous ways of assessing clinical reasoning heeding the complexity of the whole process. This means that they do not attempt to assess the single-best reasoning process but acknowledge that there are multiple equally acceptable reasoning processes for any given case (Durning et al., 2013) but that there are also unacceptable 'solutions'. Answer keys – descriptions of the correct answers – are not based on a single best solution but on defining boundaries between admissible and inadmissible solutions. Such boundaries are not clearly definable, and much research is aimed at understanding the complexity associated with such reasoning (Checkland, 1985). Another consequence is a reappraisal of human judgement in assessment and the incorporation of qualitative approaches in assessment (Driessen et al., 2005). In a nutshell, clinical reasoning expertise is now seen as the ability to avoid overstepping boundaries of the 'problem space', the possession of a repertoire of strategies to manage the case (instead of a one-size-fits-all) and the agility to switch strategies or solutions.

It is clear that human judgement will play a role in the assessment of clinical reasoning, and there is a reappraisal in the literature of understanding the quality of human judgement and how it can be supported in valid assessment. Gingerich et al. (2011), for example, explored the different perceptions of different examiners, not from the viewpoint that differences equate to error but that different perspectives produce a more complete picture. Ginsburg et al. (2015) explored the 'narratives' that examiners use when providing judgement. Their work shares the foundation that human judgement in assessment does not have to be as fallible as some of the biases and heuristics literature (cf. Plous, 1993) lead us to believe, as long as it is based on the judgement of an examiner with assessment expertise or assessment literacy. Unfortunately, in assessment of clinical reasoning, there is still some ground to be covered in terms of examiner development (Berendonk et al., 2013).

GAPS AND REMEDIES

Although assessment methods do mirror the various components of competence elucidated by fundamental research, this appears to occur haphazardly rather than by design. Basic research supports the dual-process model but by extension serves to underline that the two processes are very different, derive from different kinds of learning (formal rules and mechanisms for System 2, experience and exemplars for System 1) and warrant different assessment methods. As an example of the dilemma, the SCT, described earlier, purports to derive from research on clinical reasoning. However, its focus is entirely on the candidate's ability to 'correctly' (consistent with a panel of experts) enter the relation between features and diagnoses on a +2 to −2 scale. Leaving aside the validity of reducing complex judgement processes to a simple arithmetic sum of weights, the focus is entirely on the interpretation of diagnostic cues. No attention is paid to data gathering, to the generation of hypotheses or to management decisions. As such, a test, whatever its psychometric properties, lacks face validity as a single measure of reasoning.

We earlier commented on the dearth of basic research around actual management decision making. To some degree, assessment may be in better shape. Measures like the key feature test, or even MCQs, are easily adapted to examine management decision making. Although they may not explore the thinking processes underlying these decisions, they remain a credible approach to assessing the appropriateness of management decisions.

IMPLICATIONS AND ADVICE FOR THE TEACHER

The question remains as to what lessons can be drawn from these historical and ongoing developments. What should we educators do in day-to-day practice? Are there guidelines that could be developed from the findings allowing us to proceed with some forms of assessment of clinical reasoning? Unfortunately there are no fixed answers, and answers are quite different for tests with different main purposes. There are several key points though.

First, it is difficult to imagine a credible assessment of clinical competence that does not attempt to evaluate clinical reasoning. An assessment using less-than-perfect instruments is preferable to no assessment of this component at all. This validity issue must apply to the whole assessment procedure. Second, perhaps one of the most ubiquitous findings from the literature is 'context specificity'. General clinical reasoning skills or abilities simply do not exist. Nothing has emerged more recently that disproves this universal, and so any credible assessment must be based on a substantial number of cases. A third compelling argument against discarding our imperfect instruments is the powerful relationship between assessment and student learning. Students will try to identify and study what they believe will be in their examinations, and they will learn purely from taking the assessment. This is inevitable, if not desirable, and requires a good match between the assessment and the expected outcomes of the course. This education effect may be as important as the psychometric properties.

Finally, because there are many ways to assess clinical reasoning, and no single measure is the best measure, the choice is really yours. Which method appeals to you or your institution? How much effort do you wish to invest in writing simple or more complex stimulus formats? How many resources would you like to spend on the response format? What sort of reliability is required in your setting? What kind of effect do you strive for? What affinity or convention exists in your situation in relation to clinical reasoning assessment? Answers to these questions may vary across different education contexts. A deliberate and motivated choice among the many possibilities that the literature now has to offer is on your agenda. The simpler your selected approach, the more you can rely on existing technologies and procedures and the less you will need to invest in unique solutions.

CHAPTER SUMMARY

In this chapter, we have:

- described the developments in assessment of clinical reasoning and
- explained the possibilities and limitations in further developments.

REFLECTION POINT 3

Assessment of clinical reasoning is never an objective activity; it is a combination of information about a learner's clinical reasoning and an interpretation of this information. Interpretation is a process of expert-human judgement.

REFERENCES

Balogh, E.P., Miller, B.T., Ball, J.R. (Eds.), 2015. Improving Diagnosis in Health Care. National Academies Press, Washington, DC.

Berendonk, C., Stalmeijer, R.E., Schuwirth, L.W.T., 2013. Expertise in performance assessment: assessors' perspectives. Adv. Health Sci. Educ. 18, 559–571.

Case, S.M., Swanson, D.B., 1993. Extended-matching items: a practical alternative to free response questions. Teach. Learn. Med. 5, 107–115.

Charlin, B., Roy, L., Brailovsky, C., et al., 2000. The script concordance test: a tool to assess the reflective clinician. Teach. Learn. Med. 12, 185–191.

Checkland, P., 1985. From optimizing to learning: a development of systems thinking for the 1990s. J. Oper. Res. Soc. 36, 757–767.

Chi, M.T.H., Glaser, R., Rees, E., 1982. Expertise in problem solving. In: Sternberg, R.J. (Ed.), Advances in the Psychology of Human Intelligence 1. Lawrence Erlbaum Associates, Hillsdale, NJ, pp. 7–75.

Cook, D.A., Erwin, P.J., Triola, M.M., 2010. Computerized virtual patients in health professions education: a systematic review and meta-analysis. Acad. Med. 85, 1589–1602.

Croskerry, P., 2003. The importance of cognitive errors in diagnosis and strategies to minimize them. Acad. Med. 78, 775–780.

de Bruin, A.B., Schmidt, H.G., Rikers, R.M., 2005. The role of basic science knowledge and clinical knowledge in diagnostic reasoning: a structural equation modelling approach. Acad. Med. 80, 765–773.

Driessen, E., van der Vleuten, C.P.M., Schuwirth, L.W.T., et al., 2005. The use of qualitative research criteria for portfolio assessment as an alternative to reliability evaluation: a case study. Med. Educ. 39, 214–220.

Durning, S.J., Artino, A.R., Schuwirth, L., et al., 2013. Clarifying assumptions to enhance our understanding and assessment of clinical reasoning. Acad. Med. 88, 442–448.

Elstein, A.S., Schulmann, L.S., Sprafka, S.A., 1978. Medical Problem-Solving: An Analysis of Clinical Reasoning. Harvard University Press, Cambridge, MA.

Ericsson, K.A., 2007. An expert-performance perspective of research on medical expertise: the study of clinical performance. Med. Educ. 41, 1124–1130.

Eva, K.W., 2004. What every teacher needs to know about clinical reasoning. Med. Educ. 39, 98–106.

Farmer, E.A., Gordon Page, G., 2005. A practical guide to assessing clinical decision-making skills using the key features approach. Med. Educ. 39, 1188–1194.

Gingerich, A., Regehr, G., Eva, K., 2011. Rater-based assessments as social judgments: rethinking the etiology of rater errors. Acad. Med. 86, S1–S7.

Ginsburg, S., Regehr, G., Lingard, L., et al., 2015. Reading between the lines: faculty interpretations of narrative evaluation comments. Med. Educ. 49, 296–306.

Hatala, R., Norman, G.R., 1999. Influence of a single example upon subsequent electrocardiogram interpretation. Teach. Learn. Med. 11, 110–117.

Kohn, L.T., Corrigan, J.M., Donaldson, M.S. (Eds.), 2000. To Err Is Human: Building a Safer Health System. National Academies Press, Washington, DC.

La Rochelle, J.S., Durning, S.J., Pangaro, L.N., et al., 2012. Impact of increased authenticity in instructional format on Preclerkship students' performance: a two-year, prospective, randomized study. Acad. Med. 87, 1341–1347.

Norcini, J.J., Swanson, D.B., Grosso, L.J., et al., 1985. Reliability, validity and efficiency of multiple choice question and patient management problem item formats in assessment of clinical competence. Med. Educ. 19, 238–247.

Norman, G.R., 2005. Research in clinical reasoning: past history and current trends. Med. Educ. 39, 418–427.

Norman, G., Bordage, G., Page, G., et al., 2006. How specific is case specificity? Med. Educ. 40, 618–623.

Norman, G., Dore, K., Grierson, L., 2012. The minimal relationship between simulation fidelity and transfer of learning. Med. Educ. 46, 636–647.

Norman, G., Swanson, D., Case, S., 1996. Conceptual and methodology issues in studies comparing assessment formats, issues in comparing item formats. Teach. Learn. Med. 8, 208–216.

Norman, G.R., Tugwell, P., Feightner, J.W., et al., 1985. Knowledge and clinical problem-solving. Med. Educ. 19, 344–356.

Page, G., Bordage, G., 1995. The Medical Council of Canada's key features project: a more valid written examination of clinical decision-making skills. Acad. Med. 70, 104–110.

Page, G., Bordage, G., Harasym, P., et al., 1990. A new approach to assessing clinical problem-solving skills by written examination: conceptual basis and initial pilot test results. In: Bender, W., Hiemstra, R.J., Scherpbier, A., et al. (Eds.), Teaching and Assessing Clinical Competence: Proceedings of the Fourth Ottawa Conference. Boekwerk Publications, Groningen, The Netherlands.

Plous, S., 1993. The Psychology of Judgment and Decision Making. McGraw-Hill, New York, NY.

Regehr, G., Norman, G.R., 1996. Issues in cognitive psychology: implications for professional education. Acad. Med. 71, 988–1001.

Schmidt, H.G., Norman, G.R., Boshuizen, H.P.A., 1990. A cognitive perspective on medical expertise: theory and implications. Acad. Med. 65, 611–622.

Schuwirth, L.W.T., Blackmore, D.E., Mom, E., et al., 1999. How to write short cases for assessing problem-solving skills. Med. Teach. 21, 144–150.

Schuwirth, L.W., van der Vleuten, C.P., Stoffers, H.E., et al., 1996. Computerized long-menu questions as an alternative to open-ended questions in computerized assessment. Med. Educ. 30, 50–55.

Schuwirth, L.W., Verheggen, M.M., van der Vleuten, C.P., et al., 2001. Do short cases elicit different thinking processes than factual knowledge questions do? Med. Educ. 35, 348–356.

Swanson, D.B., Norcini, J.J., Grosso, L.J., 1987. Assessment of clinical competence: written and computer-based simulations. Assess. Eval. Higher Educ. 12, 220–246.

Tamblyn, R., Abrahamowicz, M., Dauphinee, D., et al., 2007. Physician scores on a national clinical skills examination as predictors of complaints to medical regulatory authorities. JAMA 298, 993–1001.

Wenghofer, E., Klass, D., Abrahamowicz, M., et al., 2009. Physician scores on national qualifying examinations predict quality of care in future practice. Med. Educ. 43, 1166–1173.

Section 6 LEARNING CLINICAL REASONING

39 LEARNING TO COMMUNICATE CLINICAL REASONING

ROLA AJJAWI ■ JOY HIGGS

CHAPTER AIMS

The aims of this chapter are to:

- reflect on core processes of communicating clinical reasoning,
- consider strategies for learning to communicate clinical reasoning and
- reflect on learning to communicate clinical reasoning.

KEY WORDS

Communication of clinical reasoning

Learning

Reflection

ABBREVIATIONS/ ACRONYMS

BTE Bedside teaching encounters

INTRODUCTION

Clear and effective communication of clinical reasoning is essential for all healthcare professional practice, especially in the current healthcare climate. Increasing litigation leading to legal requirements for comprehensive information exchange between healthcare professionals and clients (including their carers) and the drive for active consumer involvement are just two factors that emphasize the importance of clear communication

and collaborative decision making. Poor communication skills affect patient safety and quality of care (Levett-Jones et al., 2010), and good communication is an important factor in patient satisfaction (Hills and Kitchen, 2007).

REFLECTION POINT 1

Often students in health science courses focus on learning knowledge and skills. Do you? Does your course help you learn about doing clinical reasoning and communicating it? How well are you able to communicate your reasoning? What are the challenges you experience in communicating your reasoning?

Healthcare professionals are accountable for their decisions and service provision to various stakeholders, including clients, health sector managers, policy-makers and colleagues. An important aspect of this accountability is the ability to clearly articulate and justify management decisions. Beyond this, communication of clinical reasoning is necessary for novice healthcare professionals to develop their clinical reasoning and the ability to communicate this reasoning appropriately to the various people they deal with and are responsible to in their clinical practice encounters.

In this chapter, we present the core processes of communicating clinical reasoning along with ways learning in these areas can be enhanced through classroom and workplace learning. This is supported by a synthesis of research investigating how healthcare professionals develop the ability to unpack and communicate their clinical reasoning and a discussion of ideas for teachers regarding supporting students' learning and faculty development initiatives.

COMMUNICATION OF CLINICAL REASONING

Because of its rapid, complex and often subconscious nature, practitioners and students cannot easily recall and explain the fine details and nuances of their own reasoning. Also, clinical reasoning is not a single process; it varies with expertise, discipline and individual practice models. However, it is possible to 'slow down' and systematically examine some of the processes involved in reasoning to reflect on them more clearly, thereby facilitating articulation of clinical reasoning. For instance, novices frequently use and are taught a more 'studied' form of reasoning such as hypothetico-deductive reasoning (see Chapter 3) and are encouraged to 'think aloud' about the various alternative possibilities (of differential diagnosis, investigation options, treatment alternatives, prognosis pathways and client choices). These approaches are useful to build sound reasoning practices that avoid errors such as quickly choosing the most obvious answer/solution or failing to carefully consider the pros and cons of different treatment decisions in relation to the client's particular context. Talking aloud or explaining our reasoning also helps check our knowledge and understanding of what is going on – both in relation to the clinical situation and the client's life and well-being.

REFLECTION POINT 2

In Section 4, the chapters consider how reasoning is conducted and interpreted in different professions. Have a look at the chapters most relevant to your situation, and reflect on how your disciplinary perspective influences your reasoning and how you communicate it. How do other disciplinary perspectives influence the reasoning of practitioners in these disciplines?

Effective communication of clinical reasoning involves a depth of knowledge and understanding of clinical reasoning and all the factors involved in and influencing the decision-making process. Practitioners, both novice and experienced, must draw on multiple forms of knowledge (formal, professional/experiential and personal) to inform the content and process of communicating reasoning. In addition, communication of clinical reasoning in practice is multifactorial, requiring cognitive and metacognitive processing of many factors about the co-communicator(s), the message to be communicated and the environmental context in which the communication takes place. We also use metalanguage to think about and evaluate our language choices and effect during communication. In all of this, we need to remember that communication cannot be thought of as a discrete skill that can be learned separate of the underlying thinking and content (Ajjawi and Higgs, 2012).

REFLECTION POINT 3

Metacognition is 'thinking about what you are thinking about'. This is an invaluable skill and process to bring into your reasoning and communicating. For instance, when you are talking with a child, parent or colleague, how do you change your language? And even in the process of speaking, you can ask yourself: Have I got my thinking right about what they can understand and what is important to them? Am I using metalanguage as well metacognition? How well do you understand, monitor and adapt the language you use in different circumstances?

Articulating reasoning does not completely reflect actual reasoning processes but represents a (re)construction and (typically) a simplification of the more complex, rapid and multilayered processes that operate in practice. These communications are constructed in ways that are perceived as being most relevant to the audience, context and purpose of the communication. With experience, communicating reasoning becomes almost 'second nature' and so requires effort to bring these circumstances and processes of reasoning to consciousness, often after the event as a posthoc rationalization or justification and reporting of the decisions reached.

LEARNING TO COMMUNICATE CLINICAL REASONING: WHAT'S INVOLVED?

There has been limited research in the health sciences into how healthcare professionals learn to communicate clinical reasoning in practice. Learning of such a complex skill begins at university and continues after graduation in practitioners' chosen career paths. In this chapter we are taking a broad view of learning as *becoming* (e.g., becoming a nurse and learning to think and practice like a nurse), where individuals and their social cultures are enmeshed, with each influencing and changing the other (Hager et al., 2012). This reframing of the nature of learning combines construction and a sense of belonging, where individuals construct and reconstruct their understanding, knowledge, skills and practices entailing shifts in 'habitus' and identity. Similarly, the contexts in which learning takes place are constructed and reconstructed (Hager and Hodkinson, 2009).

Learning is neither simply the acquisition of knowledge and skills nor a straightforward process of participation and joining a community of practice. Students and novice practitioners need to learn how to learn differently in classroom, online and workplace learning situations and to consider what this means for their developing professional identity. For instance, in practical classes they can 'try out' their reasoning and get feedback without any consequences for clients, and it is safer to say 'I don't know'. In real workplaces when working, reasoning and communicating with real clients, it is a challenging task to simultaneously deal with unfamiliar situations (and possibly make mistakes and have to change their decisions) and maintain the trust of clients and ensure client safety, see Box 39.1.

BOX 39.1
A MESSAGE TO EDUCATORS

Educating students, in particular, prompts practitioners to break down more automated reasoning to first principles to reduce the complexity of reasoning for students and to provide a structure upon which the students could start to develop their own illness scripts. This dual mode of performance (what practitioners think/do – and how they explain it more simply to students) is a necessity because of the nature of expert-novice differences in clinical reasoning and the dynamic nature of communication (Ajjawi and Higgs, 2012). Further, from the perspective of the rhetoric and language of clinical reasoning, this reconstruction can be seen as a tool for persuading others (clients, students, peers) and oneself of the cogency of the underlying reasoning and the actual decisions made (Nugus et al., 2009).

Researching Reasoning and Communication

In our own research into clinical reasoning (Ajjawi and Higgs, 2008, 2012), we looked at aspects of learning how to reason and how to communicate reasoning. In particular, Rola's doctoral research (Ajjawi, 2009) examined how experienced physiotherapists learn to communicate clinical reasoning. This research highlighted the interplay between individuals and their learning culture. Practitioners in her research talked about the opportunities they had in their everyday work to use their prior knowledge to practice communication of clinical reasoning with a wide variety of people, which aided in the development of their communication ability. These opportunities were often unplanned and revolved around 'authentic contribution' in work practices, communicating with clients about their conditions and management plans, helping students develop their own reasoning and communicating in team meetings and continuing education lectures.

The participants spoke about their learning journeys as being supported and developed through communities of practice. A community of practice is defined as a 'set of relations among persons, activity and world, over time and in relation with other tangential and overlapping communities of practice' (Lave and Wenger, 1991, p. 98). Learning in communities of practice takes place through engagement in actions and interactions that are embedded in the culture and history forming the community of practice. Such learning and the emphasis on the cultural learning process can be seen as essential parts of the broader concept and process of professional socialization (Abrandt et al., 2004), which is based on learning the particular profession's socially constructed norms, values and beliefs through interaction within workplace and cultural situations.

Experience-based learning strategies such as the combination of explicit guidance, observation, modelling, discussion and feedback in workplace learning were reported as being effective for the development of skills required to communicate reasoning. Participants found that learning to perform (and communicate) in the way their profession demanded of them involved active participation based on their personal community.

Implications for University Curricula

Communication skills training is a central component of health professions curricula, sanctioned by regulatory bodies (Kurtz et al., 2005). Communication of clinical reasoning with different stakeholders (clients, colleagues, supervisors) should be an explicit goal of health professions curricula, and its place in formal curricula needs to be clearly defined. Experiential learning strategies are typically recommended for communication skills training, such as simulation, role-modelling and case discussion (Rider and Keefer, 2006) plus inbuilt opportunities for peer, teacher and self-reflexive feedback. Other creative endeavours include narrative journaling and storytelling about clients' journeys (Charon, 2001). Blogging in fieldwork education has also been used as a means of promoting reflection and self-regulation of clinical reasoning in final-year physiotherapy students (Tan et al., 2010). Findings from experimental research with medical students highlight how self-explanation can be used to improve diagnostic accuracy and performance, with best results documented for the group who also listened to a near-peer's self-explanation of the same case (Chamberland et al., 2015). Common to these strategies is the opportunity for active processing and articulation of clinical reasoning.

One study examined a subject developed to teach second-year medical students the important link between communication and clinical reasoning (Windish et al., 2005). The subject ran for 6 weeks and used mainly experiential learning methods such as role-play, videotaped encounters and feedback through self-reflection, peers and faculty. Compared with a control group, the experimental group scored higher in establishing rapport as rated by the standardized patients and elicited more psychosocial history items in communication. Evaluation feedback on the course indicated that 95% of the participants considered integrated learning of communication and clinical reasoning was beneficial. Windish et al. (2005) claimed that this integration allowed students to understand the important relationship between the biomedical and psychosocial aspects of patient care. The value of this research lies in recognition of the need to teach both processes in parallel and to make explicit the important link between reasoning and communication.

Recognition by faculty of the importance of learning and teaching of these two phenomena (reasoning and communicating reasoning) for future professionals, and their core place in curricula, is one key strategy to minimize the negative effects on student learning of

typical 'hidden curriculum' emphasis on prioritizing knowledge retention and technical skills. Hidden curriculum messages play a forceful role in the socialization of students, as they absorb values, beliefs and attitudes (that may be projected intentionally or unintentionally) of educators and healthcare professionals; these messages may well be inconsistent with the intended and explicit curriculum objectives (Hafferty, 1998). It is important to explicitly define the skills of clinical reasoning and its communication and to draw them to the learners' attention by making them readily identifiable within their courses. The place of communication and clinical reasoning in university curricula needs to be clearly defined, with close integration between classroom activities and fieldwork placements. Curriculum developers should also aim to foster skills in collaboration, critical self-evaluation and feedback seeking. Reflective learning could be built into the curriculum and could be modelled for students by academics and healthcare professionals via articulation of thought processes. Students could be encouraged to evaluate their practice and that of others against rubrics, which explicate standards. Seeking feedback is important to help calibrate judgements and improve the quality of clinical reasoning, see Box 39.2.

Implications for Workplace Learning

Workplaces lend themselves to helping students learn to communicate clinical reasoning particularly because they are places where real people engage in authentic practices and experience the consequences of practice interventions that can be sound or unsound, beneficial or harmful and relevant to the client or not. Strategies for learning about reasoning and communication are many and varied, including observation and feedback, role modelling, bedside teaching encounters (BTEs), self-reflection, peer learning and case discussion. Individuals need to seek out opportunities to observe senior practitioners and educators and to seek feedback

---

BOX 39.2
A MESSAGE TO EDUCATORS

What is your role in learning or fostering learning about reasoning and communication of reasoning within the formal and informal curriculum? How might you give or seek feedback on these capabilities?

from various people, including their clients and peers. Discussions about learners' perceptions of their learning compared with observations of and by teachers at university or seniors in the workplace may aid the development of learners' critical self-assessment skills (Paschal et al., 2002).

Research highlights the valuable role of mentors and role models in the development of communication abilities, particularly in the professional development of novice practitioners (Ajjawi and Higgs, 2008, 2012). This development may be spurred by generating regular opportunities for new graduates to discuss their reasoning about their clients and to ask questions of the senior practitioners. Incorporating self-explanation and prompt questions between learners at different levels is another strategy (Chamberland et al., 2015) amenable to workplace learning situations where students from different year levels work with new graduates and more experienced colleagues. Seniors, educators and facilitators need to be aware of their professional responsibilities in guiding and mentoring novice practitioners. These professional responsibilities extend beyond the possession of formal knowledge and technical skills to include attitudes, values and beliefs of senior colleagues or role models, which strongly influence the development of students' professional identities. This role transcends what is articulated explicitly; it encompasses the behaviour and values that embody a profession; these may be implicit or tacit and remain highly influential in learning and professional development.

Research into BTEs as an essential mode of workplace learning provides important insight into the communication of clinical reasoning. Bedside teaching brings together distinct but overlapping activity systems of patient care and student education (Ajjawi et al., 2015). In this way, BTEs offer important opportunities for students to learn how to communicate clinical reasoning through observation, modelling, practice, feedback and assessment. However, practitioners in trying to educate students while caring for their clients may inadvertently exclude their clients through the use of jargon, bodily positioning and referring to them, for instance, in the third person or as an object or disease (Ajjawi et al., 2015). Similarly, students often report feeling confused when communicating clinical reasoning, as to whether they should be performing within the client care system and/or performing for the clinical educator, who is often

also their assessor. When students adopt this latter genre of communication of clinical reasoning, they also tend to adopt jargon, refer to clients in the third person and shift their gaze away from their clients, therefore excluding them from the clinical communication, as they talk *about* rather than *with* clients (Elsey et al., 2016). Being clear about expectations within BTEs, being careful with language and engaging both students and clients within the communication, i.e., privileging the student-client relationship, can be effective ways of including all as actors in the interaction. The time after the consultation can then be utilized by clinical educators/practitioners and students to discuss particular decisions made with the patient and the underlying reasoning in more depth.

REFLECTION POINT 4

What is your experience when you are working in student-client-educator situations? How do you deal with the competing priorities of learning and client care? Do your reasoning, communication and actions change because there is a clinical educator observing and/or assessing you?

Implications for Faculty Development

Although clinical educators broadly see communication skills as essential for student-client communication, there is less recognition of the need for learning about communication of the students' developing reasoning. Clinical educators have been found to focus on procedural aspects of gathering information and communicating a management plan as necessary for student-client communication (Woodward-Kron et al., 2012) and excluding the communication of reasoning. This is disappointing, as encouraging students to make their thinking explicit would be an effective strategy to help them improve their clinical reasoning and their communication of it (Ajjawi and Higgs, 2008). And, perhaps going unnoticed is the clinical educators' role in modelling this communication to the students and the importance of seeing clinical workplaces as ideal for opportunistic learning. We can never predict all the possibilities and unexpected occurrences in the workplace that provide opportunities for learning.

Understanding the powerful influence of the workplace culture on learning enables practitioners to adopt a critical and reflective stance with regard to the activities of their workplaces. This understanding also encourages them to be strategic in their learning and professional development and to be active agents in choosing both what is learned and the process of learning within the community. Therefore healthcare professionals (novice and experienced alike) need to combine giving deliberate attention to their work activities with self-monitoring, rather than relying on unreflective and unchallenged routine and habit. A core goal in learning to communicate clinical reasoning is developing abilities and habits of reflexivity. Reflexivity goes beyond reflection, by attending also to learning and improving practice as a result of reflection and critical self-assessment.

According to de Cossart and Fish (2005), three main processes that develop good reflective practice are a) following a rigorous process for reflection (that is particular to each individual), b) engaging in dialogue with teachers and peers (including talking and writing as key means of developing reflection) and c) recognizing proper ethical and moral obligations to clients and colleagues (e.g., maintaining confidentiality). These could be key processes used within faculty development initiatives, for instance, around client cases and/or for mentoring relationships. In their faculty development program, Delany and Golding (2014) explored how to make thinking visible by identifying and then 'repackaging' the thinking steps used by experts when they engage in clinical reasoning in 'thinking routines'. These thinking routines consisted of short, repeatable actions that unpack lines of thinking and provide heuristics or 'tools' for enabling and promoting this thinking. Clinical educators are encouraged to first identify the types of knowledge they are privileging, the cognitive processes they are using and the connections they are making in their mind. They then refine this thinking to concrete steps or thinking routines that capture the specific clinical context. These steps help to make the structure of clinical educators' thinking visible, a necessary precondition to teaching clinical reasoning (Delany and Golding, 2014).

CHAPTER SUMMARY

In this chapter we have:

■ argued that communication cannot be thought of as a discrete skill that can be learned separate

of the underlying thinking (reasoning and decision making) and content of practice: It is multifactorial and context-specific;

■ discussed strategies that promote this learning, including practice, reflection, modelling, role-play, self-appraisal and feedback from others and

■ encouraged readers to engage in reflexivity and explicit learning about how to communicate clinical reasoning and remember that developing these abilities is the responsibility of individuals, universities and the workplace.

REFLECTION POINT 5

Having read this chapter, now consider: What have you learned that you can use to help develop your reasoning (or your students'), and how can this be communicated?

REFERENCES

Abrandt Dahlgren, M., Richardson, B., Sjöström, B., 2004. Professions as communities of practice. In: Higgs, J., Richardson, B., Abrandt Dahlgren, M. (Eds.), Developing Practice Knowledge for Health Professionals. Butterworth-Heinemann, Edinburgh, pp. 71–88.

Ajjawi, R., 2009. Learning Clinical Reasoning and Its Communication. VDM Verlag Dr. Müller, Saarbrücken, Germany.

Ajjawi, R., Higgs, J., 2008. Learning to reason: a journey of professional socialisation. Adv. Health Sci. Educ. Theory Pract. 13, 133–150.

Ajjawi, R., Higgs, J., 2012. Core components of communication of clinical reasoning: a qualitative study with experienced Australian physiotherapists. Adv. Health Sci. Educ. Theory Pract. 17, 107–119.

Ajjawi, R., Rees, C., Monrouxe, L.V., 2015. Learning clinical skills during bedside teaching encounters in general practice: a video-observational study with insights from activity theory. J. Workplace Learn 27, 298–314.

Chamberland, M., Mamede, S., St-Onge, C., et al., 2015. Self-explanation in learning clinical reasoning: the added value of examples and prompts. Med. Educ. 49, 193–202.

Charon, R., 2001. Narrative medicine: a model for empathy, reflection, profession, and trust. JAMA 286, 1897–1902.

de Cossart, L., Fish, D., 2005. Cultivating a Thinking Surgeon: New Perspectives on Clinical Teaching, Learning and Assessment. tfm Publishing, London, UK.

Delany, C., Golding, C., 2014. Teaching clinical reasoning by making thinking visible: an action research project with allied health clinical educators. BMC Med. Educ. 14, 1–10.

Elsey, C., Challinor, A., Monrouxe, L.V., 2016. Patients embodied and as-a-body within bedside teaching encounters: a video ethnographic study. Adv. Health Sci. Educ. Theory Pract. 1–24.

Hafferty, F.W., 1998. Beyond curriculum reform: confronting medicine's hidden curriculum. Acad. Med. 73, 403–407.

Hager, P., Hodkinson, P., 2009. Moving beyond the metaphor of transfer of learning. Br. Educ. Res. J. 35, 619–638.

Hager, P., Lee, A., Reich, A., 2012. Problematising practice, reconceptualising learning and imagining change. In: Hager, P., Lee, A., Reich, A. (Eds.), Practice, Learning and Change: Practice-Theory Perspectives on Professional Learning. Springer, New York, NY, pp. 1–14.

Hills, R., Kitchen, S., 2007. Satisfaction with outpatient physiotherapy: focus groups to explore the views of patients with acute and chronic musculoskeletal conditions. Physiother. Theory Pract. 23, 1–20.

Kurtz, S., Silverman, J., Draper, J., 2005. Teaching and Learning Communication Skills In Medicine. Radcliffe Publishing, Oxford, UK.

Lave, J., Wenger, E., 1991. Situated Learning: Legitimate Peripheral Participation. Cambridge University Press, Cambridge, UK.

Levett-Jones, T., Hoffman, K., Dempsey, J., et al., 2010. The 'five rights' of clinical reasoning: an educational model to enhance nursing students' ability to identify and manage clinically 'at risk' patients. Nurse Educ. Today 30, 515–520.

Nugus, P., Bridges, J., Braithwaite, J., 2009. Selling patients. BMJ 339, b5201.

Paschal, K.A., Jensen, G.M., Mostrom, E., 2002. Building portfolios: a means for developing habits of reflective practice in physical therapy education. J. Phys. Ther. Educ 16, 38–51.

Rider, E.A., Keefer, C.H., 2006. Communication skills competencies: definitions and a teaching toolbox. Med. Educ. 40, 624–629.

Tan, S.M., Ladyshewsky, R.K., Gardner, P., 2010. Using blogging to promote clinical reasoning and metacognition in undergraduate physiotherapy fieldwork programs. AJET 26, 355–368.

Windish, D.M., Price, E.G., Clever, S.L., et al., 2005. Teaching medical students the important connection between communication and clinical reasoning. J. Gen. Intern. Med. 20, 1108–1113.

Woodward-Kron, R., van Die, D., Webb, G., et al., 2012. Perspectives from physiotherapy supervisors on student-patient communication. Int. J. Med. Educ. 3, 166–174.

40 DEVELOPING CLINICAL REASONING CAPABILITY

NICOLE CHRISTENSEN ■ GAIL M. JENSEN

CHAPTER AIMS

The aims of this chapter are to:

■ explore the concept of capability as an adaptive learning outcome,

■ discuss a proposed model of clinical reasoning capability,

■ explore the relationship of clinical reasoning capability and development of adaptive expertise and

■ discuss future implications for educators of tomorrow's healthcare professionals.

KEY WORDS

Adaptive expertise

Adaptive learner

Capability

Clinical reasoning

INTRODUCTION

The work of the health professions is inherently complex and, more often than not, situated in what Schön (1987) famously described as a 'swampy' and uncertain practice environment. Many, if not most, health professions educational institutions claim critical thinking (seen as analytical thinking) rather than clinical reasoning as a central learning outcome for their students. Yet when critical thinking is taught as the primary cognitive skill set applied in clinical decision making, we can lose the ability to develop healthcare professionals capable of clinical reasoning in the 'swampy' and uncertain environments mentioned by Schön. Under conditions of uncertainty, true experts in the practice of health care have the capability to engage in collaborative clinical reasoning leading to wise judgements. These are also people whose knowledge base is continually evolving. Why is that? This chapter addresses important concepts about the development of thinking and learning skills that underlie clinical reasoning and the development of clinical reasoning capability, essential to the preparation of practitioners for the constantly changing and uncertain practice of health care.

CAPABILITY AS A LEARNING OUTCOME

The concept of 'capability', described in the higher education literature originally by Stephenson (1998), comprises a particular set of attributes and abilities. Capability is a key outcome for graduates of higher education, enabling them to more effectively and substantively contribute to the work of their professions and to the broader society. Capability is a demonstrable and justifiable confidence and ability to interact effectively with other people and to undertake tasks in known and unknown contexts, both now and in the future (Stephenson, 1998). Capability is demonstrated through:

■ confident, effective decision making and associated actions in practice,

427

- confidence in the development of a rationale for decisions made,
- confidence in working effectively with others and
- confidence in the ability to navigate unfamiliar circumstances and learn from the experience.

In addition to development of justifiable confidence in one's own effectiveness as a collaborator and a decision maker, in both known and unknown contexts, capability is also characterized by a motivation to intentionally and continuously develop one's own knowledge through reflective learning in clinical practice (Doncaster and Lester, 2002). This aspect of capability as an educational outcome aligns well with another concept with roots in the education and expertise literature: the adaptive learner.

Adaptive Learners

Adaptive learners are described as able to thrive in changing environments by learning in, and for, practice and adapting as necessary (Cutrer et al., 2017). Characteristic of these individuals is their engagement in continuous learning and self-improvement. Adaptive learners achieve this through active self-monitoring and critical reflection, integrated with actively sought external feedback. They are motivated, and skilled, in learning from their experiences to change and grow. When needed, they can innovate, enabling themselves to continue to perform well when encountering complex, uncertain and novel situations (Cutrer et al., 2017; Schumacher et al., 2013). The justifiable confidence, or self-efficacy, of a capable individual in his or her ability to make well-reasoned decisions collaboratively, in both known and unknown circumstances, is the result of adaptive learning. This, in turn, is related to transformative learning theory.

Transformative learning theory (Cranton, 2006; Mezirow, 2009) is a branch of constructivist learning theory that can provide a foundation for educational strategies that facilitate clinical reasoning capability in learners. In healthcare education, these strategies are often based on clinical reasoning experiences. Transformative learning takes place when a learner uses a prior understanding to construct a new or revised interpretation to guide future action, thereby transforming him or herself through the emergence of new knowledge and understanding (Mezirow, 2009). This view meshes well

with the way adaptive learners are thought to generate new knowledge to make wise decisions.

REFLECTION POINT 1

As a student, do you recognize attributes in yourself that fit with descriptions of capable, adaptive learners? What are those attributes? What aspects of the description of a capable, adaptive learner do you feel you need to develop further?

As an educator, do you intentionally design learning activities to develop capability? How can you change or add to what you currently do to facilitate capability?

CLINICAL REASONING CAPABILITY

Building on the model of capability as a desirable outcome for higher education, Christensen et al. (Christensen, 2009; Christensen et al., 2008b; Christensen & Nordstrom, 2013) described clinical reasoning capability as confidence in the ability to effectively integrate key thinking and learning skills to make sense of and learn collaboratively from clinical experiences, in both known and unknown clinical contexts (Fig. 40.1). The model of clinical reasoning capability is informed by an understanding of the key characteristics of the clinical reasoning of physiotherapist experts and identified gaps between these experts and the clinical reasoning of novices (Christensen et al., 2008a, 2009; Edwards et al., 2004). The model proposed four key areas of thinking and experiential learning skills, directly related to descriptions of skills inherent in the clinical reasoning of expert physiotherapists across all practice settings. These skills sets, linked to the development of excellence as both a clinical reasoner and an experiential learner, are reflective thinking, critical thinking, complexity thinking and dialectical thinking (Christensen, 2009; Christensen et al., 2008a, 2008b).

These proposed clinical reasoning capability skills are consistent with the literature on capability, especially the emphasis on coping with new and previously unknown contexts (Doncaster and Lester, 2002; Stephenson, 1998). However, these skills are not intended to represent a definitive or exhaustive list of all aspects of thinking and learning important to developing excellence in clinical reasoning. For example, although

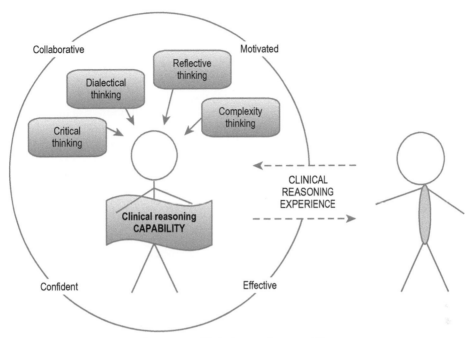

Fig. 40.1 ■ Clinical reasoning capability.

not the focus of this chapter, other more affective qualities of experienced clinical reasoning such as emotional intelligence have become a focus of research more recently (e.g., Chaffey et al., 2012; Marcum, 2013).

Essential Thinking and Experiential Learning Skills for Clinical Reasoning Capability

Descriptions of each of the thinking and experiential learning skill sets proposed to be essential to the development of clinical reasoning capability follow.

Reflective Thinking

Reflective thinking is thinking about a situation to make sense of it. In clinical reasoning, this involves evaluating the influence of all relevant aspects of the situation and individuals involved (e.g., clinician, patient, clinical setting, resources available, time constraints). Reflection allows for interpretation of experience. The thinker also attempts to know the 'why' of a situation by subjectively and objectively reconsidering the context to bring to light the underlying assumptions used to justify beliefs (Mezirow, 2000). When reflective thinking calls into question the adequacy of the clinician's knowledge, then the clinician is prompted to learn something new and/

or revise prior knowledge. Schön (1987) describes various moments in time when reflection is integral to making sense of and eventually improving practice: reflection-on-action, reflection-for-action and reflection-in-action. As applied to a clinical reasoning encounter, reflection-on-action occurs after the clinical action is completed and involves cognitive organization of experiences to make sense of what happened. Reflection-for-action involves planning for future encounters by thinking back on past experiences. This includes reflecting on the adequacy of the knowledge available to the clinical reasoner during those past encounters, identifying and actively seeking to fill any gaps in existing knowledge and making links between past experiences and anticipated future events.

Reflection-in-action occurs in the midst of an experience and allows for modification of clinical reasoning by 'thinking on your feet' to best adapt to an emerging understanding of a situation. To successfully employ reflection-in-action to modify decision making in the moment, a clinician must be able to readily access contextually relevant knowledge from memory. This is closely related to the idea of metacognition (Higgs et al., 2008; Marcum, 2012; Schön, 1987), which is self-awareness and monitoring of one's own thinking while in action. Wainwright et al. (2010) describe how reflection at different times in relation to a clinical encounter was used by both novice and experienced clinicians. Their research findings include the observation that novices less commonly used reflection-in-action, and when it was used it focussed mainly on the patient's performance. More experienced clinicians reflected in action more often and were focussed not only on the patient's performance but were also focussed on self-monitoring of their own reasoning in action. These findings highlight the importance of facilitation of reflection and evaluation of one's reasoning as essential to developing expertise in clinical reasoning.

Critical Thinking

Critical thinking is intimately linked to reflective thinking and involves the disciplined process of actively conceptualizing, synthesizing, analyzing and evaluating information; this information can be gathered or generated from observation, experience, interaction, reasoning and reflection and serves as a guide toward action (Paul and Elder, 2006). In this context, critical thinking is conceived as a way of thinking about thinking, with an emphasis on questioning and clarifying erroneous assumptions. It is a skill that promotes learning from and about thinking. In this way, similar to reflective thinking, critical thinking is also linked to metacognition.

In the context of clinical reasoning capability, critical thinking applies to both the examination and management of a particular patient's clinical presentation and to the critical evaluation of one's own thinking or reasoning used to engage in, interpret and synthesize that patient's clinical information (Christensen, 2009, 2008b). Critical thinking also attempts to bring to light blind spots or gaps in knowledge that may be adversely affecting a clinician's clinical reasoning in a given context. Critical thinking has an important role in exploring the potential for biases, incorrect assumptions and inadequate knowledge and detecting unconscious errors of interpretation in clinical reasoning.

Complexity Thinking

Complexity thinking acknowledges the dynamic interdependencies at work between the many elements and players influencing a given situation (Plsek and Greenhalgh, 2001). Therefore complexity thinking is linked to the recognition and consideration of the

relative weighting of all relevant internal (within the person) and external (the context in which the person is functioning) factors influencing a given clinical presentation (Christensen et al., 2008b; Christensen and Nordstrom, 2013). Skilled clinical reasoning has been shown to be, in part, characterized by this ability to see and appropriately address all influences (both biological and psychosocial) at play in a particular clinical presentation, leading to a plan of care that clinician and patient can mutually accept (Edwards et al., 2004). The ability to see a situation from multiple frames of reference is a key aspect of complexity thinking in clinical reasoning. Both students and practitioners must be able to use analytical and interpretative skills in managing uncertain situations.

Capability in clinical reasoning is also characterized by motivation and skill in learning from clinical experiences (Christensen, 2009; Christensen et al., 2008b). Consistent with a complexity science perspective on learning, clinical experience alone is not enough to bring about learning; rather, experience is viewed as a trigger, or an opportunity, for learning to emerge from interactions with other individuals (Davis and Sumara, 2006). Complexity thinking, therefore, is also a key element that enables a capable clinician to consider and appreciate the importance and implications of establishing a collaborative relationship with the patient. Collaboration is an essential component of clinical reasoning because of the complex interactive social systems through which decisions emerge. This collaborative interaction between participants in clinical reasoning is an important hallmark of clinical reasoning capability (Christensen, 2009; Christensen et al., 2008b).

Complexity thinking allows us to integrate an understanding of both the physical and biological aspects of a patient's presentation together with the psychosocial and behavioural aspects in a comprehensive biopsychosocial approach. Interestingly, Alhadeff-Jones (2012) proposed that a trigger for transformative learning is a recognition of some of the challenges raised by the complexity inherent in particular contexts such as collaborative clinical reasoning. Alhadeff-Jones also proposed that complexity thinking can be 'a method of learning involving human error and uncertainty … taking into consideration both the individual and collective experiences grounding any activity' (p. 190). In this way, complexity thinking is again closely linked to collaborative clinical reasoning and the learning that can emerge for all involved. Complexity thinking is also consistent with the dialectical reasoning approach observed in the reasoning of experts (Edwards and Jones, 2007).

Dialectical Thinking

The clinical reasoning of experts, as described by Edwards and Jones (2007), is characterized by a fluidity of reasoning between deductive thinking and inductive thinking within each of the clinical reasoning strategies (Edwards et al., 2004). Dialectical thinking is seen when expert physiotherapists move in their reasoning between contrasting biological and psychosocial poles in a fluid and seemingly effortless manner. This dialectical thinking ability is necessary for a holistic understanding that considers the clinical presentation of a patient's problem(s) in the context of the patient as a person and is consistent with a biopsychosocial approach to clinical reasoning (Edwards and Jones, 2007). Development of dialectical thinking allows for clinicians to achieve a more complex and contextual understanding of situations both affecting, and affected by, a patient's presentation. Dialectical thinking and complexity thinking can be seen as interdependent and promote capability in clinical reasoning. This is because capability includes effectiveness in working with others to achieve collaborative and productive working relationships (Doncaster and Lester, 2002; Stephenson, 1998). An advanced reasoning ability is the perception of what is important information and being able to interpret its implications for all aspects of the biopsychosocial approach. This ability needs to be developed through practice and assistance.

REFLECTION POINT 2

As a student, are you aware of using all four of the thinking and experiential learning skill sets that capable clinical reasoners use in your own clinical reasoning? Do you have any ideas about how you can strengthen your skills and integrate them into your clinical reasoning?

As an educator, are there any thinking and experiential learning skill sets that you focus on developing more than others, when facilitating clinical reasoning development? Can you think of ways to strengthen the skills you have not focussed on in the past?

FACILITATING CLINICAL REASONING CAPABILITY AND ADAPTIVE EXPERTISE

The interdependence between clinical reasoning ability and the development of clinical knowledge is a well-known dimension of expertise. Experts are those who both know a lot and are skilled at learning from their clinical experiences. Expertise is not a static concept or a goal that one reaches passively through accumulation of years of experience or achievement of credentials. The foundations are the continual learning and innovative problem solving that are crucial to wise decision making in conditions of uncertainty. This type of expertise has been termed 'adaptive expertise' and can only be achieved through adaptive learning.

Adaptive expertise is described as a 'context appropriate, balanced cluster of learning oriented, self-regulatory and metacognitive processes that moderate and mediate the application of abilities and previously acquired knowledge to problem solution, future knowledge acquisition and ultimately effective leadership' (Birney et al., 2012, p. 563). Adaptive expertise demands flexibility in knowledge structures and performance, to effectively respond in novel situations, and is highly metacognitive (Hatano et al., 1986). Therefore, there are clear connections to the aspects of capability described previously. These are the thinking and experiential learning skills essential to clinical reasoning capability and the notion of adaptive expertise development in the context of learning in, and from, clinical reasoning experiences.

FUTURE IMPLICATIONS

Our challenge then is to foster the development of the adaptive learner. Recently calls for explicit curricular focus on the promotion and development of adaptive learners have been well argued in the current literature (Jensen et al., 2017a; Mylopoulos et al., 2016). Capability in learning how to learn from clinical reasoning experiences continues to be a critical missing link between our desired, and our actual, educational outcomes in the context of professional education of today's healthcare professionals.

Jensen et al. (2017a, 2017b) recently published findings of a national study of physiotherapy education in the United States, characterizing excellence in professional and postprofessional education. Their findings described ways in which creative teachers provided learning contexts for their students that promoted the developmental skills, attributes and dispositions that characterize an adaptive learner. These included:

- placing students early on in their curriculum in situations where they could safely struggle and experiment in complex and uncertain practice situations;
- providing practice-based learning environments with multiple teachers and learners at multiple levels of development and professional education, all engaged in frequent feedback exchanges, reciprocal teaching and learning processes and mutual inquiry around complex, uncertain clinical problems and situations and
- fostering a culture of excellence, continuous feedback and improvement and transparency in the goals and intended outcomes for all learning activities.

Although Jensen et al.'s study was focussed on excellence in education, as a whole, their findings are clearly relevant to creating optimal contexts within which learners can be encouraged to develop clinical reasoning capability. Indeed, one of the recommendations these authors put forward, to promote intentional educational excellence across education programs, is that the profession develop a longitudinal view and strategy for development of clinical reasoning that spans from professional-entry through to postgraduate education and is continued on throughout a learner's career (Jensen et al., 2017a). Adaptive learners are nurtured in authentic, complex, practice-based learning environments across the developmental continuum from novice to expert; it is precisely these environments that can promote the development of justifiable (i.e., can be tested and proven) confidence in their abilities to reason their way through any situation they encounter. Although novices cannot be directly taught to be expert clinical reasoners, they can be taught to rely on their thinking and experiential learning skills to guide them while in action. Critical reflection on their reasoning experiences can reveal areas ripe for new knowledge development.

Essential to the development of capability in clinical reasoning is facilitation of, and provision of, formative feedback about a learner's critical self-reflection abilities,

when evaluating their own clinical reasoning performance. Self-directed learning, an essential value and behaviour exhibited by both capable and adaptive learners, builds on the ability to critically self-assess one's own performance; this is a precursor to development of flexible expertise (Birney et al., 2012).

Ultimately, as healthcare educators and students, we should be working toward the establishment of explicit educational outcome goals for development of adaptive learners, capable in clinical reasoning. This would, eventually, be very likely to increase the number of practitioners who would go on to develop adaptive expertise. As Bransford et al. (2009) explain, isolated pockets of expertise hold less potential to bring about transformational change than distributed adaptive expertise across individuals, organizations, communities and professions. If we can shift our focus in professional education to the development of excellent adaptive learners who are capable in clinical reasoning, then we can transform the variable experiences of care our patients are living through today for the better.

CHAPTER SUMMARY

In this chapter, we have outlined:

- qualities and attributes that characterize capable, adaptive learners who are motivated and justifiably confident in their abilities to make sound, collaborative decisions and to learn and adapt in known and unknown situations;
- the thinking and experiential learning skill sets that must be integrated into reasoning to optimize clinical reasoning capability; these comprised reflective thinking, critical thinking, complexity thinking and dialectical thinking and
- the role of clinical reasoning capability in the development of adaptive expertise and the implications for educators of healthcare professionals.

REFLECTION POINT 3

As a student, are you provided with feedback about how well you are able to critically self-reflect on your clinical reasoning? Can you think of ways to improve on your capability in this area?

As an educator, do the learning activities you provide for learners intentionally include opportunities to clinically reason in brand new (to them), complex situations? In the practice setting, how do you facilitate the development of learners' skills in critical self-reflection and self-directed learning?

REFERENCES

Alhadeff-Jones, M., 2012. Transformative learning and the challenges of complexity. In: Taylor, E.W., Cranton, P., Associates, (Eds.), The Handbook of Transformative Learning: Theory, Research, and Practice. Jossey-Bass Wiley, San Francisco, CA, pp. 178–194.

Birney, D.P., Beckmann, J.F., Wood, R.E., 2012. Precursors to the development of flexible expertise: metacognitive self-evaluations as antecedents and consequences in adult learning. Learn. Indiv. Diff 22, 563–574.

Bransford, J., Mosborg, S., Copland, M.A., et al., 2009. Adaptive people and adaptive systems: issues of learning and design. In: Hargreaves, A., Lieberman, A., Fullan, M., et al. (Eds.), Second International Handbook of Educational Change, Part 1. Springer, Dordrecht, The Netherlands, pp. 825–856.

Chaffey, L., Unsworth, C.A., Fossey, E., 2012. Relationship between intuition and emotional intelligence in occupational therapists in mental health practice. Am. J. Occup. Ther. 66, 88–96.

Christensen, N., 2009. Development of clinical reasoning capability in student physical therapists, PhD thesis. University of South Australia, Adelaide, SA. Viewed. 1 July 2017. Available from: http://trove.nla.gov.au/work/36257790.

Christensen, N., Jones, M., Edwards, I., et al., 2008a. Helping physiotherapy students develop clinical reasoning capability. In: Higgs, J., Jones, M.A., Loftus, S., et al. (Eds.), Clinical Reasoning in the Health Professions, third ed. Elsevier, Edinburgh, pp. 389–396.

Christensen, N., Jones, M., Higgs, J., et al., 2008b. Dimensions of clinical reasoning capability. In: Higgs, J., Jones, M.A., Loftus, S., et al. (Eds.), Clinical Reasoning in the Health Professions, third ed. Elsevier, Edinburgh, pp. 101–110.

Christensen, N., Nordstrom, T., 2013. Facilitating the teaching and learning of clinical reasoning. In: Jensen, G.M., Mostrom, E. (Eds.), Handbook of Teaching and Learning for Physical Therapists, third ed. Butterworth-Heinemann Elsevier, St. Louis, MO, pp. 183–199.

Cranton, P., 2006. Understanding and Promoting Transformative Learning: A Guide for Educators of Adults, second ed. Jossey-Bass Wiley, San Francisco, CA.

Cutrer, W.B., Miller, B., Pusic, M., et al., 2017. Fostering the development of master adaptive learners: a conceptual model to guide skill acquisition in medical education. Acad. Med. 92, 70–75.

Davis, B., Sumara, D., 2006. Complexity and Education: Inquiries into Learning, Teaching, and Research. Lawrence Erlbaum Associates, Mahwah, NJ.

Doncaster, K., Lester, S., 2002. Capability and its development: experiences from a work-based doctorate. Stud. Higher Educ. 27, 101.

Edwards, I., Jones, M., 2007. Clinical reasoning and expert practice. In: Jensen, G., Gwyer, J., Hack, L., et al. (Eds.), Expertise in Physical Therapy Practice, second ed. Saunders Elsevier, St. Louis, MO, pp. 192–213.

Edwards, I., Jones, M., Carr, J., et al., 2004. Clinical reasoning strategies in physical therapy. Phys. Ther. 84, 312–330.

Hatano, G., Inagaki, K., 1986. Two courses of expertise. In: Stevenson, H., Azuma, H., Hakuta, K. (Eds.), Child development and education in Japan. WH Freeman and Company, New York, NY, pp. 262–272.

Higgs, J., Fish, D., Rothwell, R., 2008. Knowledge generation and clinical reasoning in practice. In: Higgs, J., Jones, M.A., Loftus, S., et al. (Eds.), Clinical Reasoning in the Health Professions, third ed. Elsevier, Edinburgh, pp. 163–172.

Jensen, G.M., Hack, L., Nordstrom, T., et al., 2017a. National study of excellence and innovation in physical therapist education: part 2 – a call to reform. Phys. Ther. 97, 875–888.

Jensen, G.M., Nordstrom, T., Mostrom, E.M., et al., 2017b. National study of excellence and innovation in physical therapist education: part 1—design, method, and results. Phys. Ther. 97, 857–874.

Marcum, J.A., 2012. An integrated model of clinical reasoning: dual-processing theory of cognition and metacognition. J. Eval. Clin. Pract. 18, 954–961.

Marcum, J.A., 2013. The role of emotions in clinical reasoning and decision making. J. Med. Philos. 38, 501–519.

Mezirow, J., 2000. Learning to think like an adult: core concepts of transformation theory. In: Mezirow, J. (Ed.), Learning As Transformation: Critical Perspectives on a Theory in Progress. Jossey-Bass, San Francisco, CA, pp. 3–33.

Mezirow, J., 2009. Transformative learning theory. In: Mezirow, J., Taylor, E.W., Associates, (Eds.), Transformative Learning in Practice: Insights from Community, Workplace, and Higher Education. Jossey-Bass Wiley, San Francisco, CA, pp. 18–31.

Mylopoulos, M., Brydges, R., Woods, N.N., et al., 2016. Preparation for future learning: a missing competency in health professions education? Med. Educ. 50, 115–123.

Paul, R., Elder, L., 2006. The Miniature Guide to Critical Thinking: Concepts and Tools, fourth ed. The Foundation for Critical Thinking, Santa Rosa, CA.

Plsek, P.E., Greenhalgh, T., 2001. Complexity science: the challenge of complexity in health care. Br. Med. J. 323, 625–628.

Schön, D., 1987. Educating the Reflective Practitioner. Jossey-Bass, San Francisco, CA.

Schumacher, D., Englander, R., Carraccio, C., 2013. Developing the master learner: applying learning theory to the learner, the teacher, and the learning environment. Acad. Med. 88, 1635–1645.

Stephenson, J., 1998. The concept of capability and its importance in higher education. In: Stephenson, J., Yorke, M. (Eds.), Capability and Quality in Higher Education. Kogan Page, London, UK, pp. 1–13.

Wainwright, S.F., Shepard, K.F., Harman, L.B., et al., 2010. Novice and experienced physical therapist clinicians: a comparison of reflection is used to inform the clinical decision-making process. Phys. Ther. 90, 75–88.

41

REMEDIATING LEARNING AND PERFORMANCE OF REASONING

JEANNETTE GUERRASIO ■ JUAN N. LESSING

CHAPTER AIMS

The aims of this chapter are to:

■ understand students who struggle with clinical reasoning,

■ describe a methodical approach for teaching and learning clinical reasoning and

■ encourage students to engage self-guided learning to improve clinical reasoning.

KEY WORDS

Remediation

Remedial teaching

Framework

ABBREVIATIONS/ ACRONYMS

CEX Clinical examination

OSCE Observed structured clinical encounter

H&P History and physical

SNAPPS Summarize the case, narrow the differential, analyze the differential, probe the preceptor, plan management, select an issue for self-directed learning

RIME Reporter, interpreter, manager, educator (developmental framework)

HPI History of present illness

NSAIDS Nonsteroidal anti-inflammatory drugs

PT Physical therapy/physiotherapy

CAN CLINICAL REASONING BE LEARNED?

Throughout health professions education, students are exposed to new information in the form of facts and concepts, with the expectation that they will be able to learn, expand and apply their medical knowledge. The ability to learn new information is assessed through a series of mostly written examinations. As students pass examinations, they are deemed to possess sufficient knowledge to progress through the next stages of education and eventually independent practice. Medical knowledge serves as a required foundation for the development of clinical reasoning skills. However, merely having knowledge and passing examinations do not confer the ability to access or appropriately apply that knowledge to specific clinical problems and individual patients.

A student may score at the top of his or her class on written examinations yet struggle to decide which questions to ask while interviewing a patient, which physical examination manoeuvres or laboratory tests are most pertinent, how to select and rank differential diagnoses, or how to choose an appropriate and prioritized patient-specific diagnostic and treatment plan. For years, there has been debate as to whether clinical reasoning, like problem solving, can be learned or if clinical reasoning is an innate skill or trait, like being left-hand dominant or having blue eyes (Schuwirth, 2002). In large part, this debate continued because clinical educators did not have a structured or systematic approach for remediation and therefore expressed scepticism about the effect remediation can have on clinical reasoning skills. Teaching and learning methods continue to be developed to help settle this debate. In this chapter, one specific method for learning and teaching clinical reasoning skills is described. This is a method that can benefit both underperforming and passing learners who wish to improve their clinical skills through a systematic approach to clinical reasoning.

REFLECTION POINT 1

Struggling with clinical reasoning is NOT uncommon, and it can be taught. The key is to address deficits in knowledge before focussing on clinical reasoning.

IDENTIFICATION OF STUDENTS WHO STRUGGLE WITH CLINICAL REASONING

For the majority of learners, exposure to the standard curriculum and education provided by their professional schooling is sufficient to develop the necessary knowledge, skills and attitudes to achieve an acceptable level of competence. This is not, however, true for all learners (Olmesdahl, 1999; Paul et al., 2009). When medical students were studied (Guerrasio et al., 2014; Olmesdahl, 1999; Paul et al., 2009), approximately 15% of all students required some form of remediation or additional teaching and learning strategies beyond that provided by the general curriculum to achieve competence. Of these 15% of medical students, one-third were found to struggle with elements related to clinical reasoning.

Students who struggle with clinical reasoning can be identified by direct observation of patient encounters, during patient presentations and by chart review. In studies of the struggling medical learner (Guerrasio, 2013; Guerrasio and Aagaard, 2014), those who struggle with clinical reasoning typically:

1. In patient encounters
   ■ collect too much extraneous information and
   ■ perform a generic, nontargeted physical examination
2. Patient presentations and chart review

■ recite what they have learned from the patient, in the words of the patient, rather than synthesize the story,
■ include irrelevant information,
■ provide unreasonable differential diagnosis or none at all,
■ struggle to prioritize diagnoses,
■ have difficulty analyzing their differential diagnoses,
■ order excessive and often unhelpful tests and
■ rely heavily on diagnostic tools and algorithms, without the ability to adapt to the individual patient or situation.

As an example, a student struggling with clinical reasoning may have difficulty recognizing that the more urgent priority in the care of a patient with active life-threatening bleeding and a non–life-threatening blood clot is to the more immediately dangerous condition. This concern may then be communicated back to the learner via direct feedback, rotation evaluations, clinical examinations (CEX) or mini clinical examinations (mini-CEX) and/or observed structured clinical encounters (OSCEs).

If a student is identified as having both medical knowledge and clinical reasoning deficits, we contend that medical knowledge must be remediated first. When core knowledge is insufficient, students cannot aptly demonstrate clinical reasoning, and their ability to showcase clinical reason remains untested until their medical knowledge improves. Students can clinically reason with whatever knowledge they possess, but in the absence of critical knowledge, reasoning will be deficient.

REFLECTION POINT 2

There are discrete signs, such as collecting too much information or not synthesizing the patient's story, that help identify the learner struggling with clinical reasoning.

UNDERSTANDING STRUGGLING LEARNERS

To gain expertise in any skill area (i.e., diving, playing the oboe or clinical skills), one must engage in deliberate practice. Deliberate practice consists of an ongoing repetitive circle of practicing a specific, and ideally, well-defined skill, receiving meaningful performance feedback, reflecting on that feedback to improve practice and practising that same skill again (Fig. 41.1).

In our experience, most learners engage in this cycle of practice, feedback and reflection unconsciously and also consider how new information fits within their larger understanding of a topic. Struggling learners do not intuitively learn this way. Struggling learners will practice a skill over and over and over and over … and yet never achieve mastery. Why? Struggling learners have trouble recognizing and therefore also applying feedback, as they do not learn from the hidden curriculum. The hidden curriculum describes the transmission of norms and values and practices that are not explicitly taught. Struggling learners must be told directly and concretely what to do next. Once feedback is identified for them (rather than by them), they struggle to actualize that feedback and need assistance to put feedback into action. Additionally, struggling learners often have knowledge memorized and stored in isolated

blocks that lack a connection or scaffold to other information that they have learned.

If these areas of weakness are not realized, a large mismatch exists between how teachers are teaching and what learners are learning. Teachers tend to teach to the course objectives rather than start at the learner's level of competence and need. Teachers assume that learners have a scaffold onto which to add new information, but struggling students often lack that framework that gives knowledge meaning and structure. Teachers expect learners to absorb hidden, unconscious curriculum messages that often are fairly abstract, but these struggling learners need concrete instruction. In these instances, teachers provide feedback and directions that are not received.

Struggling learners may not learn the same as most learners, but they are teachable. They are most often motivated and hard-working. They have foundational knowledge and skills to build upon. In many instances, having progressed this far in their education, struggling learners are often great memorizers and then can learn from the concrete rather than the abstract.

REFLECTION POINT 3

Struggling learners need something other than the typical curriculum. The struggling learner does not intuit the way most nonstruggling learners do. Struggling learners need a different approach. Feedback and next steps must be identified for them, as opposed to by them, and described concretely rather than fluidly. Struggling learners may not learn the same as most learners do, but they are teachable.

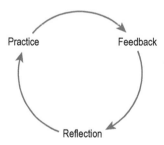

Fig. 41.1 ▪ Cyclic model of deliberate practice. This model of learning, established by Ericsson (2004), describes how to learn new skills and eventually develop expertise.

CASE STUDY 41.1

Learning Clinical Reasoning

Jay sees a patient with a new cough. After asking history questions of the patient, the attending physician tells Jay that there are two additional questions that he should have asked. Jay then reflects on why those questions were important and how the patient's responses to those questions can be used to distinguish between cough related to asthma and cough related to gastroesophageal reflux disease. Later the same

week, when Jay interviews a patient with a new cough, he includes these two questions. The attending physician then suggests a new question, because this latest patient grew up in Nepal. Jay discusses with his attending how living in Nepal would affect the working differential diagnosis and data collected during the history of present illness (HPI). Jay decides that he will incorporate this into his future practice.

UNIQUE CHALLENGES TO LEARNING CLINICAL REASONING

One main challenge of teaching and learning clinical reasoning is that the phenomenon of clinical reasoning is inherently abstract, making concepts difficult to understand for concrete struggling learners. The skill set to improve clinical reasoning, however, need not be abstract. Secondly, there are multiple methods for approaching clinical reasoning (e.g., hypothetico-deductive reasoning, pattern recognition, schema group diagnostics of either pathophysiology/causality or algorithms). Because each individual clinical case can be approached from different or even multiple perspectives or strategies, teachers have a harder time interpreting a learner's thought process and more difficulty providing meaningful feedback. Thirdly, in naming the multiple approaches to clinical reasoning, it becomes evident that this topic alone has its own unique and extensive language. Although there are several great texts (Higgs et al., 2008; Kassirer et al., 2010; Trowbridge et al., 2015) on improving clinical reasoning skills and on advanced clinical problem solving, these resources are too complex and advanced for the struggling student or beginner. These texts assume that one can embark on the clinical reasoning continuum rather than teach it from the ground up.

We describe a method for learning and teaching clinical reasoning that aims to combat many of the aforementioned challenges. This method starts from the earliest steps of the clinical reasoning process. It provides concrete steps to follow. It limits or at least addresses subject-related jargon. It standardizes the approach to allow for more specific feedback. It provides opportunity to use the feedback to improve practice. It helps students compare and contrast information and build scaffolds for organizing and applying their knowledge. At the same time, this method incorporates the concepts of deliberate practice, with the cycle of practice, feedback and reflection imbedded.

AN APPROACH TO THE REMEDIATION OF CLINICAL REASONING

In this section we describe a structured, systematic approach to evaluation and remediation of clinical reasoning skill, which is one effective method to improving clinical reasoning skills. This approach to remediation of clinical reasoning is adapted from Guerrasio and Aagaard (2014) and Guerrasio (2013). This step-by-step approach is written such that a student can initiate and engage in the improvement process him or herself. To complete the steps, the student will need someone to engage in the feedback and reflection portions of the approach. This person can be a faculty member, resident or mentor. For consistency, this individual will be referred to as a mentor. Ideally, this process will be most effective if there is a mentor who is familiar with this framework, or at least has access to this chapter, and who is available for the entire process. Given the short length of most clinical rotations, this degree of consistency may not be feasible. If this is the

---

CASE STUDY 41.2 (PART A)

Being a Novice Reporter

Michael has completed the preclinical courses for medical school and has passed all of his examinations with above-average scores. Six months into his first clinical year, he became frustrated by his clinical grades. He was no longer honouring courses but just passing all of his rotations. He sat down to review all of the feedback and evaluations that he had received, trying to determine how to improve his grades. A common theme emerged: 1) His presentations were too long, yet he missed key questions; 2) His physical examinations were always the same; and 3) He needed to work hard on creating differentials. In sum, he had the necessary medical knowledge but could not apply it to individual patients and could not synthesize patient cases succinctly. Per the RIME developmental model (reporter, interpreter, manager, educator), Michael was a novice reporter but struggled to interpret information.

case, the student will need to seek multiple mentors for feedback and reflection along this journey.

REFLECTION POINT 4

Consider the applicability of this approach to your teaching situations.

A Step-by-Step Approach to the Remediation of Clinical Reasoning

1. Review three frameworks for creating a differential diagnosis, and discuss them with a mentor. Here are three commonly used frameworks:
   a. Anatomical framework
      1) For example, what anatomical structures are in or refer to the abdominal left lower quadrant that could cause pain experienced there?
   b. Systems framework
      1) Acronym VINDICATE AIDS
         V – Vascular
         I – Infectious
         N – Neoplastic
         D – Degenerative
         I – Inflammatory
         C – Congenital
         A – Autoimmune
         T – Traumatic
         E – Endocrine and Metabolic
         A – Allergic
         I – Iatrogenic
         D – Drugs
         S – Social
   c. Pathophysiological framework
      1) For example, in the workup of anaemia, your differential diagnosis can be subdivided into conditions that cause macrocytic, normocytic or microcytic anaemia.
2. Practice creating differentials based on age, gender, race/ethnicity and chief complaint.
   a. Choose cases based on the most common presentations for your upcoming or current rotation (i.e., 20-year-old Caucasian woman with shortness of breath). For each common presentation, create three lists: List A is a comprehensive list of diagnoses, list B consists of the most likely four to five diagnoses based on prevalence and list C is the top two to three diagnoses that are most important to not miss. For feedback, compare your lists with a differential diagnoses reference, and discuss the lists with a mentor. Is your differential diagnosis appropriate? What diagnoses did you miss? Which diagnoses are too rare to reasonably include in list B?

3. Write history questions that you would ask your patient to rule-in or rule-out each of the diagnoses on lists B and C. Build a grid similar to Table 41.1, filling in the first column with the diseases identified in lists B and C and the second column with your history questions. Be as concise as possible. These grids should fit onto a large index card. Seek feedback on your list of history questions from a mentor. Reflect on key questions missed and extraneous questions.
   a. What questions did you ask appropriately?
   b. What questions did you forget to ask?
   c. Did you ask too many extraneous questions?
4. Write the physical examination manoeuvres on the grid that you would perform and the signs you would look for to rule-in or rule-out each of the diagnoses in lists B and C. Obtain feedback at each step of the process as you did earlier, and update the list of physical examination manoeuvres and signs based on feedback. Reflection on any discrepancies is preferred over memorization.
   a. What physical examination elements did you remember to perform?
   b. What physical examination elements did you forget to perform?
   c. Are you performing too many extraneous examination elements?
5. Repeat Steps 2 to 4 with multiple case scenarios until you or a mentor determines that this skill is mastered on all of the most common presentations for that rotation. This usually takes 10 to 20 cycles. Make photocopies of these tables upon which you can highlight and take notes for individual future patients.
6. While seeing patients, complete history and physical written notes (H&P). Based on your leading diagnosis, highlight the information on

TABLE 41.1

Clinical Reasoning Grid[1]

Learners were asked to create grids based on the most common patient presentation for their clinical rotation or specialty to help compare and contrast information between diagnoses with the same chief complaint.

Example Chief Complaint: 43-Year-Old Caucasian Woman With Chest Pain

Differential Diagnosis	Symptoms and Historical Information	Signs	Diagnostic Workup	Treatment
Gastroesophageal reflux disease	Subacute, epigastric, burning, supine, relief with antacids	Tenderness to palpation of epigastrium	History alone, trial of H_2 blocker or PPI, abnormal EGD	Raise head of bed, change diet, avoid tobacco and alcohol, weight loss, H_2 blocker or PPI, follow up in 12 weeks
Muscular strain	Pain in muscle, worse with use of muscle, acute injury or repetitive use	Tenderness to palpation of muscle, +/− mild swelling	History and physical alone	Rest, ice, NSAIDs, follow up in 4–8 weeks for PT referral for strengthening and mechanics
Costochondritis	Female, sharp, worse with deep inspiration	Tenderness to palpation of costochondral junction	+/− erosions on x-ray if chronic	Rest, ice, NSAIDs, follow up if doesn't resolve in 8 weeks

[1]Additional columns may also be added for pathophysiology, especially for medical students who rely more heavily on basic science principles or complications for procedure-based specialties.

Adapted from Guerrasio & Aagaard, 2014

your table that supports that diagnosis in green and the information that refutes the diagnosis in red, and cross out distracting, unhelpful or irrelevant information. Repeat this with multiple cases, and for each case obtain feedback from a mentor.

a. Would the mentor have highlighted the H&P differently?

b. Did the mentor agree with your choice for most likely diagnosis?

   1) If not, repeat this exercise with the diagnosis that a mentor thinks is most likely, again highlighting the grid, and then *compare* and *contrast*. This will provide a concrete visual representation of the most likely diagnosis – the sheet with the most green and least red highlighter, proportionally, represents the most likely to be a correct diagnosis.

   2) Note the information that was crossed out and deemed extraneous. You probably can skip this information next time (unless needed to create an adequate treatment plan).

7. Using the same case as in step 6, create a table of symptoms and signs, rating their relevance for the top three diagnoses on your differential (Table 41.2). In this table, the top three differential diagnoses are listed down the first column, and pertinent (positive and negative) signs and symptoms are listed across the top row. This top row represents the problem list. This chart is used to help you understand gradations of supporting and refuting data with arrows either up for supporting or down for refuting information, with the number of arrows indicating the degree of influence on the diagnostic decision. An equal sign may be used to represent data that neither increase nor decrease the probability of the disease. *Compare* and *contrast*. Once again, seek feedback, and engage in reflection with a mentor.

8. Steps 6 and 7 are also repeated with multiple case scenarios until you or a mentor feels that the skill has been mastered.

9. Use summarizing words called 'semantic qualifiers' (examples listed below) to summarize each case.

TABLE 41.2

Weighing Data in the Clinical Reasoning Process

Differential Diagnosis	Female	Left Sided	Pleuritic Pain	Shortness of Breath	Pregnancy	Hypotension	Elevated JVP
Gastroesophageal reflux disease	=	↓	↓↓	↓↓	↑↑	↓↓	↓↓↓
Muscular strain	=	↑	↑	↑	=	↓↓	↓↓↓
Myocardial infarction	↓	↑	↓	↑↑	=	↑↑	↑↑

JVP – Jugular Venous Pressure.
Adapted from Guerrasio & Aagaard, 2014

 a. Patient characteristics – young, middle-aged, elderly, race, gender

 b. Onset – slow, sudden, acute, subacute, chronic

 c. Site – bilateral, unilateral, central, peripheral

 d. Course – constant, intermittent, episodic, progressive

 e. Severity – mild, moderate, severe

 f. Context – rest, activity, lying, seated

 Ask a mentor to provide feedback on your current ability to represent the patient's problem(s) using semantic qualifiers. After feedback, practice resummarizing the case based on this feedback.

10. Return to the original grids created in steps 3 and 4. Create a diagnostic workup for each of the diagnoses, considering the following categories: monitor the patient, order laboratory(s), order test(s) and/or prescribe a therapeutic trial of medication. Write down the diagnostic workup necessary for each common presentation. To assist with prioritization, circle the workup that is required immediately. Check references, including practice guidelines and algorithms for feedback, and discuss with a mentor.

 a. Confirm the appropriate workup.

 b. Which diagnostic elements did you correctly choose?

 c. Which diagnostic elements did you incorrectly choose and why?

 d. What are you missing and why?

 e. Did you circle the appropriate urgent elements of the workup?

11. Stop to reflect. When seeing the patient, have the grids available. Ask yourself, 'Have I read about a similar case before? How is this case similar, and how is it different?' *Compare* and *contrast*. Consider how this patient may be the same or different from the typical patients described in the grids. This process teaches you how to better discuss your clinical judgement and decisions and how to frame specific and productive questions for faculty and other more senior peers. Feedback and reflection are a key component to all steps.

12. Finally, create a treatment plan for each of the diagnoses created in the grids from steps 3, 4 and 10. Consider the following categories: monitor the patient, order prescription and nonprescription treatment, provide education, place referrals and review follow-up needs. Prioritize the treatment plan, circling the treatment that is required most urgently. Complete the final column of the grid, and seek feedback and reflection with a mentor.

 a. Review treatment options.

 b. Discuss with a mentor the potential consequences of treatment choices, including benefits and complications.

 c. For patient cases, state your final treatment recommendation. Learning how to commit to one's beliefs is a crucial step in improving clinical reasoning skills.

USING THE TOOLS AND GRIDS IN THE CLINICAL ENVIRONMENT

When a student is in the clinical environment, he or she may need to be reminded to use these tools and grids for reference. For example, the student can identify key questions and physical examination manoeuvers based on the reported chief complaint before going to see a patient. Inpatient follow-up visits are excellent for this. For instance, if your patient was admitted 2 days ago with pneumonia, what information would be most helpful for a student to assess to adjust the treatment plan? Have the learner start with open-ended questions with the patient, but be sure to include and adapt the prepared questions. Even before students review a patient's medical record, they should ask themselves what information they are specifically looking for, given the demographic information and chief complaint. We often refer to reviewing the old record as a 'chart biopsy'. A biopsy doesn't examine an entire organ; it looks at areas likely to give the highest yield.

To continue to obtain this high-level feedback in the clinical setting, students should be encouraged to explain their reasoning on all active problems or at least all major clinical decisions. Consider providing a structured means for communicating their clinical reasoning, such as using the SNAPPS model (Wolpaw et al., 2003) (Box 41.1). This will allow for errors in reasoning to be identified and corrected immediately and for a mentor to model a different thought process. If you find this very challenging and are unable to come up with a plan, a learner can ask faculty to resist giving 'the answer', but rather to teach him or her where to go to find the answer.

CHAPTER SUMMARY

In this chapter, we have outlined:

■ how to identify students who struggle with clinical reasoning,
■ unique challenges of learners who struggle with clinical reasoning,
■ how to adapt the teaching and learning of clinical reasoning so that it is congruent with the strengths of underperforming students and

---

BOX 41.1
THE SNAPPS MODEL

S—Summarize history and findings
N—Narrow the differential to two to three most likely diagnoses
A—Analyze the differential by comparing and contrasting
P—Plan treatment and further workup
P—Probe the preceptor about uncertainties and alternatives
S—Select an issue related to the care for self-directed learning

Adapted from Wolpaw, Wolpaw and Papp, 2003.

CASE STUDY 41.2 (PART B)

Improving Reasoning

Once Michael decided to work to improve his clinical reasoning, he realized that he did not have a strategy to do so. Determined to improve his grades, be better prepared for residency and be the best possible physician, Michael decided to try out the step-by-step approach for improving clinical reasoning. He found a mentor, Dr. Jones, who was willing to review the approach and provide feedback and opportunities for reflection. He then set up meetings with Dr. Jones twice a week for 2 months to create a time and space to review his progress and to get feedback.

Methodically, Michael worked through the steps one by one. During the first meeting, he and Dr. Jones reviewed the strategies for creating a differential diagnosis, and he asked Dr. Jones to help him identify the most common chief complaints and presentations for his upcoming rotation – Neurology. There were six common presentations, and Michael worked to build grids for each. He also collected cases from his rotation for steps 6, 7, 9 and 11.

The process of going through all of the steps was time-consuming, but Michael noticed an improvement in his performance on rounds. He emphasized his clinical reasoning on rounds using the SNAPPS method of presentation and listened to the feedback that he was given. He became more interested in the work he was doing and more engaged with patient care. Michael then noticed a change in his evaluations, and his course grades and performance on OSCEs began to improve.

■ a step-by-step approach for learning and teaching clinical reasoning.

REFLECTION POINT 5

This resource/time-intensive strategy is an effective method to raise most strugglers to the level of passing/competence. For teachers and learners outside of medicine – consider how this approach could be modified for your discipline.

REFERENCES

Ericsson, K.A., 2004. Deliberate practice and the acquisition and maintenance of expert performance in medicine and related domains. Acad. Med. 79, S70–S81.

Guerrasio, J., 2013. Remediation of the struggling medical learner. Association for Hospital Medical Education, Irwin, PA.

Guerrasio, J., Aagaard, E.M., 2014. Methods and outcomes for the remediation of poor clinical reasoning. J. Gen. Intern. Med. 29, 1607–1614.

Guerrasio, J., Garrity, M.J., Aagaard, E.M., 2014. Learner deficits and academic outcomes of medical students, residents, fellows and physicians referred to a remediation program: 2006–2012. Acad. Med. 89, 352–358.

Higgs, J., Jones, M., Loftus, S., et al. (Eds.), 2008. Clinical Reasoning in the Health Professions, third ed. Elsevier, Edinburgh.

Kassirer, J.P., Wong, J., Kopelman, R., 2010. Learning Clinical Reasoning, second ed. Lippincott Williams & Wilkins, Philadelphia, PA, pp. 1–307.

Olmesdahl, P.J., 1999. The establishment of student needs: an important internal factor affecting course outcome. Med. Teach. 21, 174–179.

Paul, G., Hinman, G., Dottl, S., et al., 2009. Academic development: a survey of academic difficulties experienced by medical students and support services provided. Teach. Learn. Med. 21, 254–260.

Schuwirth, L., 2002. Can clinical reasoning be taught or can it only be learned? Med. Educ. 36, 695–696.

Trowbridge, R.L., Rencic, J.J., Durning, S.J. (Eds.), 2015. Teaching Clinical Reasoning. American College of Physicians, Philadelphia, PA.

Wolpaw, T.M., Wolpaw, D.R., Papp, K.K., 2003. SNAPPS: a learner-centered model for outpatient education. Acad. Med. 78, 893–898.

LEARNING ABOUT FACTORS INFLUENCING CLINICAL DECISION MAKING

MEGAN SMITH ■ JOY HIGGS

CHAPTER AIMS

The aims of this chapter are to:

■ present a contemporary understanding of how clinical decision making can be influenced by contextual factors,

■ reflect on the interaction between decision makers' frame of reference and their decision making,

■ assist beginning healthcare professionals to learn to account for these factors in their clinical decision making and

■ assist educators to consider learning opportunities to develop clinical decision-making capability.

KEY WORDS

Context
Situatedness
Frame of reference
Influences

INTRODUCTION

Clinical decision making is both an outcome and a component of clinical reasoning. A contemporary understanding of decision making is that it is bound to the context in which it occurs (Durning et al., 2011). Quality health care occurs when practitioners are able to understand when factors influencing decision making contribute to errors, mistakes and potential adverse outcomes for healthcare participants and recipients and when factors influencing decision making can be manipulated to enhance healthcare experiences or outcomes. Learning to make sound clinical decisions, therefore, requires the ability to learn to identify and understand how contextual factors influence decision making.

CLINICAL DECISION MAKING

Decision making refers to the process of making a choice between options as to categories (e.g., diagnoses, areas of responsibility), courses of action (e.g., clinical testing, communication, treatments) and judgements (e.g., evaluation of treatment outcomes). Clinical decision making by healthcare professionals is a complex process, requiring more of individuals than making defined choices between limited options. Healthcare professionals make decisions with multiple foci, in dynamic contexts, using a diverse knowledge base (including an increasing body of evidence-based literature), with multiple variables and individuals involved. In addition, clinical decisions are characterized by situations of uncertainty in which not all the information needed to make them is, or can be, known. Clinical decision making may involve individual healthcare practitioners making decisions on behalf of patients, or there may be a collaborative process, involving shared and parallel decision making with patients and teams of healthcare professionals. The collaborative nature of decision making means that we must consider factors that can influence individual practitioners and the teams they work in (see Chapters 15 and 17 for further discussion of shared decision making).

Learning to make clinical decisions involves an understanding of the nature of decision making in dynamic contexts (e.g., healthcare, industry and educational settings). These contexts include characteristics such as those described by Orasanu and Connolly (1993):

- problems that are ill-structured and made ambiguous by the presence of incomplete dynamic information and multiple interacting goals,
- decision-making environments that are uncertain and may change while decisions are being made,
- goals that may shift, compete or be ill-defined,
- decision making that occurs in the form of action–feedback loops, where actions result in effects and generate further information that decision makers have to react to and use to make further decisions,
- decision situations that contain elements of time pressure, personal stress and highly significant outcomes for participants,
- multiple players who act together with different roles and
- organizational goals and norms that influence decision making.

REFLECTION POINT 1

Think about clinical decision making as a process of making choices. Sometimes the choices we make in our personal and professional lives are small with limited consequences. Sometimes they are major with potentially very significant consequences to the quality and even continuity of our lives and the lives of others. The importance of considering carefully a range of factors that can influence such choices is generally much greater in the latter case.

Factors Influencing Decision Making

In this chapter, we describe factors influencing decisions in terms of four key areas including:

- clinical task complexity,
- internal context and capabilities of the decision maker,
- decision-making environment and
- level of shared decision making with clients.

These areas interact to shape the nature and outcomes of decision making (Table 42.1). We have included in this table reference to the shared nature of decision making, especially as it relates to decision making with clients. As this topic is explicitly discussed in depth elsewhere in this book (see Chapters 15 to 20), we have not explored it in any further detail here.

A Model of Factors Influencing Clinical Decision Making

Doctoral research by Megan Smith (Smith, 2006; Smith et al., 2007, 2008a, 2008b, 2010) explored clinical decision making by physiotherapists practicing in acute care settings (hospitals). This research revealed decision making about individual patient care to be a complex and contextually dependent process. Although the research focus was on physiotherapy and the acute care setting, in this chapter we provide alignment of the outcomes with more recently published literature. This alignment will illuminate the potential implications of the research for learning to make decisions more broadly.

This research generated a model of clinical decision making (Fig. 42.1) in which:

- decision making is a process (where decisions are made about patients' healthcare problems, appropriate therapeutic interventions, optimal modes of interaction and methods of evaluation) that is dependent on attributes of the task such as difficulty, complexity and uncertainty;
- decision making involves a dynamic, reciprocal process of engaging with and managing environmental factors in the immediate context to identify and use these factors in making decisions and carrying out an optimal course of action;
- practitioner factors, such as their frames of reference, individual capabilities and experience of physiotherapy decision making in the relevant work contexts, influence the decisions practitioners make;
- decision making is situated within a broader contextual ethos, with dimensions particular to the practice in the specific workplace and

TABLE 42.1			
Interpretation of Factors Influencing Decision Making			
Practitioner's Personal and Professional Frame of Reference	***Capabilities***	***Decision-Making Difficulty***	
	Practitioner's level of decision-making expertise and knowledge	LOW ◄─────────────────────────► HIGH	
		Task complexity	
		Shared decision making	
		Environmental challenges to decision making	
Range of individual practice models, personal frames of reference including values, beliefs and attitudes and personal dispositions particularly around interpersonal interactions	***Novice***	***Interaction With Context***	
	Focus on:	■ textbook approaches satisfy demands of low-difficulty and low-complexity tasks	■ insufficient knowledge, experience and reasoning capacity to deal with task and environment complexity
	■ process of reasoning		
	■ biomedical knowledge		■ limited ability to deal with the human complexities of shared decision making
	■ hypothetico-deductive reasoning		
	■ practitioner-led reasoning		
	■ limited experience in reasoning and judgement		
	Intermediate		
	Focus on:	■ ability and experience-based confidence to explore more advanced reasoning approaches (e.g., pattern recognition, shared decision making) in simpler cases and contexts	■ limited ability to deal with highly complex cases and very challenging situations
	■ growing clinical knowledge and judgement		■ reversion to hypothetico-deductive reasoning in unfamiliar and context situations
	■ expanding clinical knowledge base		
	■ growing set of illness scripts based on clinical experience building on textbook learning		
	■ expanding interpersonal communication and collaboration skills		
	Expert		
	Focus on:	■ typically use advanced reasoning approaches built on clinical knowledge	■ considerable experience in working with a range of clients and situations makes experts highly capable of dealing with most complex cases and settings and working with a wide range of patients and patients' preferences for shared decision making
	■ rich, extensive clinical knowledge base		
	■ many illness and instantiated scripts	■ much expertise and capacity to engage in shared decision making (if this is the chosen collaboration strategy)	
	■ well-developed clinical practice model		
	■ rich experience with involving patients in decision making		

Informed by the work of Boshuizen and Schmidt, 2008, and Smith, Higgs and Ellis, 2008a, 2008b

■ traversing all of these factors, to manage and make sense of them, requires four key capabilities: cognitive, emotional, social and reflexive.

Learning to Identify and Integrate Strategies for Dealing With Clinical Task Complexity Into Decision Making

The task of decision making is to make action-related choices (including, if necessary, deciding not to act). Decisions can be defined in terms of attributes such as stability, certainty, familiarity, urgency, congruence, risk, relevance and a number of additional variables (Fig. 42.2). Megan's research found that these attributes shape clinical task complexity. These tasks can have poles of complexity (e.g., stable vs. unstable, familiar vs. unfamiliar), with further difficulty and complexity arising from the summation and interplay between attributes (Smith et al., 2008a). The research found that attributes that made a decision relatively simple were familiarity, certainty, limited variables, stability, congruence and low risk. Decisions became more difficult if there were uncertainty, conflict, unfamiliarity, changing conditions,

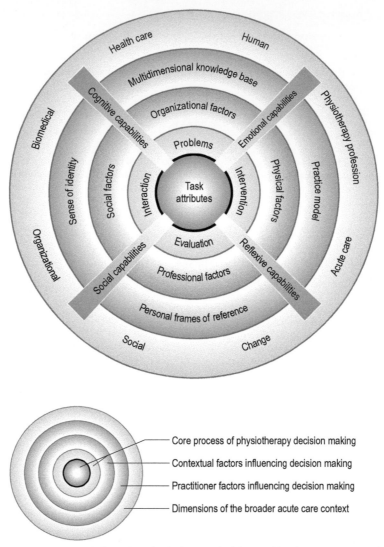

Fig. 42.1 ■ Factors influencing physiotherapy decision making in acute care settings.

multiple relevant variables and high risk. In the research, difficult decisions also had an ethical and emotional dimension that the participants found challenging.

Task complexity has an important relationship with the experiences of the decision maker that contributes to the perceived difficulty of decision making and learning to make decisions (McLellan et al., 2015; Parkes, 2017). Megan's research found that, when making decisions in acute care settings, participants responded to simple decisions by choosing a usual mode of practice, selecting an intervention that they found usually worked and modifying their choice to fit the unique situation by adopting more creative and novel approaches to intervention. In contrast, when decisions were difficult, participants were more likely to experiment, draw upon the knowledge of other people, weigh up the competing aspects of the decision, follow protocols or rules and seek less opportunity for creativity (Smith et al., 2007).

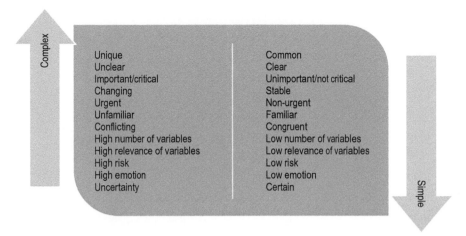

Fig. 42.2 ■ Levels of clinical task complexity.

As we have illustrated in Table 42.1, the practitioner's level of expertise and clinical experience is recognized to have an influence on these matters also.

Learning to make decisions can be aided by the novice learning to break down the clinical task to understand its complexity and context. Conceptualizing the complexity of decision tasks can provide opportunities for educators and facilitators to consider how to structure and scaffold learning for new practitioners. For example, an educator working with new paramedic students might choose an initial learning scenario with relatively low risk and that has stable variables with limited changes. As decision-making speed and accuracy improve with experience, the educator could vary the scenario to introduce additional, inconsistent and changing variables.

Learning About Your Capabilities and Experience as a Decision Maker

Megan's research (Smith et al., 2007) identified that practitioners' decision making was influenced by their capabilities, confidence, self-efficacy, emotions, frames of reference and degree of expertise. She found that physiotherapists, in acute care settings, had a number of personal qualities and decision-making capabilities that enabled them to make effective decisions in relation to the nature of the task and the context of practice. The capabilities of the physiotherapists in the study are illustrated in Fig. 42.3; these were categorized as cognitive, reflexive, social and emotional.

Megan's research revealed that in clinical decision making by acute care physiotherapists, self-efficacy and confidence in decision making were important determinants of the decisions that were made. Physiotherapists' feelings and levels of self-efficacy resulted from a) evaluating their level of knowledge, particularly in comparison to the knowledge levels of other healthcare professionals with whom they were working; b) having experienced success and failure; and c) knowing the likely responses to interventions and the likelihood of adverse events occurring. When self-efficacy was higher, there was a greater willingness to take risks and greater confidence in decision making, as opposed to relying on others or deferring decision making. As an example of understanding emotional capability, she found decision makers' emotions and feelings of confidence and controllability influenced participants' decision making as they sought to control negative outcomes and emotions, particularly under conditions of risk and uncertainty.

An important attribute that influences decision making is the decision maker's level of expertise. Experts are considered to be superior decision makers, making decisions that are faster and more accurate and using their experience of similar situations to address more effectively the perceived difficulty of decision-making tasks. A distinction is typically made between the extremes of novice and expert; however, individual practitioners are more appropriately viewed as being

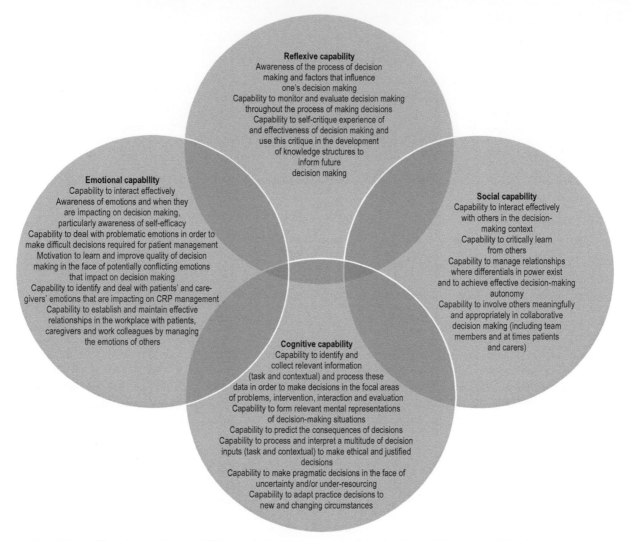

Fig. 42.3 ■ Clinical reasoning capabilities to deal with the nature of the decision-making task and the decision context.

in varying degrees of transition between more and less experienced and expert. As such, they will demonstrate characteristics consistent with their own variable pathways towards expertise, dependent on their unique experiences and the current clinical situation and task. In learning decision making, helping learners to understand how experience shapes decision making could be used to guide expectations of their decision making and the reflective learning activities that are used to learn from decision making.

The more experienced physiotherapists in Megan's study (Smith et al., 2010) adopted an approach to decision making that was more specific, creative and refined towards the individual needs of patients and the unique contextual dimensions. Compared with less experienced physiotherapists, they used more interpretation and critique in their decision making, being comparatively more confident and self-reliant. They handled uncertainty in decision making more effectively by adopting a higher level of practical certainty. This means they were better able to engage in wise risk-taking and possessed a greater knowledge base that decreased the relative uncertainty of decision making. Their knowledge base was broader and deeper than that of the novices and contained a greater level of experience-based knowledge. Their knowledge base was personalized and multidimensional; it included a better awareness of the limits of their knowledge and what could be known. More experienced physiotherapists also had more advanced cognitive capabilities for decision making, being more flexible, adaptive and capable of predicting outcomes, as well having higher levels of emotional capability. They were able to separate emotion from task and knew how to use their own personality in their decision making. They also had a higher awareness of patients' experiences of illness.

The frames of reference of more experienced practitioners are different from those of novices. Expert decision makers critically apply norms and criteria of decision making. Where novices choose simply to follow rules and value the safety of working within rules, experts understand the bases for the rules and thus apply them more variably and wisely. The more experienced physiotherapists in this study had more developed personal theories of practice consisting of their own set of criteria for practice. These were more important than using rules and guidelines for practice derived from their university education or work-based protocols. The contrast was that less experienced practitioners framed decision making as needing to make the right decision, whereas more experienced practitioners sought optimal decisions given the circumstances.

More experienced practitioners were also more capable of managing the context, being more aware of the influences and better able to pragmatically interact with and manipulate contextual factors to achieve optimal decision outcomes. The knowledge base of experts has been found to extend beyond direct patient care to include knowledge of their work context in terms of the physical environment and organizational structures (Ebright et al., 2004), see Box 42.1.

REFLECTION POINT 2

Consider your own clinical work. What are the key contextual factors you generally want to take into consideration for your patients? What effect do such factors make in relation to your clinical decision making, the patient's key concerns and treatment outcomes?

BOX 42.1
EMOTIONAL CAPABILITIES

In guiding learning to make decisions, educators could explore the notion of emotional capabilities and how managing emotions can be integral to decision-making outcomes. A learning situation could be constructed that challenges novice decision makers to notice the role their emotions play in making a clinical decision. Examples include if they try to avoid negative emotions by postponing a decision, letting others make the decision, maintaining the status quo, choosing an option that is easy to justify to others and avoiding specific aspects of the decision that they find distressing. Further examples of implementing educational strategies to develop capabilities can be found in Ajjawi and Smith (2010).

Learning About the External Context and Decision-Making Environments

A key focus of Megan's research was to explore the influence of the external context of practice on decision making. The research showed that the physiotherapists' decision making could not be separated from the context in which it occurred. They changed or modified decisions in response to contextual factors. They also learned the value of developing strategies to manage and control the context of their practice. In this way, the interaction between context and decision making was seen to be reciprocal, complex and dynamic. The influence of specific contextual factors upon decision making was dependent on the unique features of the decision being undertaken at the time. Context was not a fixed entity but was found to be dynamic and variable. A key finding of this research was that contextual factors influencing practitioners' decision making could not be consistently ranked according to their prevalence or importance. Rather, different contextual factors assumed different importance according to the unique circumstances at a given time. We see through these findings that practitioners need to make decisions about their decision making (i.e., use metacognition) in addition to making the decisions themselves (i.e., using cognition).

The broader context of clinical decision making can be seen to consist of different types of factors that become relevant to particular decisions; these include social, organizational and physical dimensions. In the following case study, these research findings have been applied to the implementation of a simulated learning activity that could be used to develop skills in clinical decision making.

CHAPTER SUMMARY

Quality decision making is an essential component of good clinical practice. If we are to understand, critique and improve clinical decision making, it is imperative that, in addition to understanding the elements of the immediate clinical problem, we make explicit the contextual factors that we need to take into account when making decisions. When seeking to improve decision making, a broad perspective needs to be adopted that considers factors such as the individual's decision-making attributes and the influence of the external context on decision making. As teachers, we need to explore our own, and our students', ability to use metacognition to critically appraise these factors in decision making in particular cases. We also need to consider how our decision-making practices need to evolve in response to patient, practitioner and environmental factors that affect decisions and decision making.

Evidence-based practice is consistently advocated as a means for improving the quality of clinical practice. A broader perspective on factors influencing decision making illustrates how evidence-based practice needs to be integrated with the many other influences on practice.

CASE STUDY 42.1

Using Simulated Learning Experiences to Assist Students to Learn Clinical Decision Making Under Different Environmental Conditions

Environmental Dimension	Example of Use During Simulation	Debrief – Positive Implications	Debrief – Negative Implications
Social	Learning decision making can be assisted by deliberately constructing social situations in scenarios involving varying perceived difficult decision making ■ allowing conferring with others to check their decision making ■ using others to generate novel perspectives ■ anchoring their decision making to decisions others made in the past	Debrief with learners about the positive role social interaction had on their decision making such as ■ using other individuals to check for errors, ■ using positive synergies arising from the combination of team members' knowledge and ■ recognizing that there is an increased likelihood of generating novel solutions and diverse perspectives when more people are consulted in decision making.	Debrief with learners about the negative role social interaction had on their decision making such as how they might ■ choose to do what others do to avoid social rejection, ■ take advantage of others' decision making rather than being responsible for their own decision making, ■ perpetuate dominant workplace norms (people can be inhibited from offering or adopting different perspectives) and ■ not developing individual expertise.

Using Simulated Learning Experiences to Assist Students to Learn Clinical Decision Making Under Different Environmental Conditions (Continued)

Environmental Dimension	Example of Use During Simulation	Debrief – Positive Implications	Debrief – Negative Implications
Organizational systems	Introduce organizational variables into scenarios such as ■ variable workloads, ■ interruptions and ■ decision-making aids and guidelines.	Debrief on the effect of systems in place to guide decision making, such as clinical pathways, policies, protocols and system definitions and how these were relied upon in the decision making.	■ Where workload resulted in limited time availability, were any compromises made in the decisions that could be made? ■ What were the effects of systems on prioritization? ■ What were the effects of time pressures, such as less thinking time, less effective interventions, streamlining assessment, choosing less creative options for treatment, less time for offering patients choice in decision making and choosing interventions that would be adequate rather than optimal? ■ How did time pressures influence decision making by affecting the capacity of decision makers to develop rapport with patients? Did the learner feel he or she had the capacity to get to know patients and their condition? ■ How did interruptions add to the complexity of the decision-making process and affect the cognitive capacity to recall information and make decisions?

Continued on following page

CASE STUDY 42.1

Using Simulated Learning Experiences to Assist Students to Learn Clinical Decision Making Under Different Environmental Conditions (Continued)

Environmental Dimension	Example of Use During Simulation	Debrief – Positive Implications	Debrief – Negative Implications
Physical	Adjusting scenarios to vary the physical environment ■ resources available such as the location and supply of equipment ■ room layout	What was the effect of familiarity on the efficiency of their decision making?	■ How effective was their response to limited resources?

Consideration of personal, social and organizational dimensions of context is critical in optimizing the quality of clinical decision making. If we are to help learners develop effective decision making, we need to understand how we can best teach decision making that considers and manages the multiplicity of factors that influence it rather than focusing only on the immediate clinical decision-making tasks of diagnosis and intervention.

REFLECTION POINT 3

Think about your role as educator or learner. What key messages about factors influencing decision making from this chapter will change the way you teach or learn in the future?

Acknowledgement

Elizabeth Ellis contributed to a previous version of this chapter.

REFERENCES

Ajjawi, R., Smith, M., 2010. Clinical reasoning capability: current understanding and implications for physiotherapy educators. Focus Health Prof. Educ 12, 60–73.

Boshuizen, H., Schmidt, H., 2008. The development of clinical reasoning expertise. In: Higgs, J., Jones, M., Loftus, S., et al. (Eds.), Clinical Reasoning in the Health Professions, third ed. Elsevier, Edinburgh, pp. 113–121.

Durning, S., Artino, A.R., Jr., Pangaro, L., et al., 2011. Context and clinical reasoning: understanding the perspective of the expert's voice. Med. Educ. 45, 927–938.

Ebright, P.R., Urden, L., Patterson, E.S., et al., 2004. Themes surrounding novice nurse near-miss and adverse-event situations. J. Nurs. Admin. 34, 531–538.

McLellan, L., Yardley, S., Norris, B., et al., 2015. Preparing to prescribe: how do clerkship students learn in the midst of complexity? Adv. Health Sci. Educ. 20, 1339–1354.

Orasanu, J., Connolly, T., 1993. The reinvention of decision making. In: Klein, G.A., Orasanu, J., Calderwood, R., et al. (Eds.), Decision Making in Action: Models and Methods. Ablex, Norwood, NJ, pp. 3–20.

Parkes, A., 2017. The effect of individual and task characteristics on decision aid reliance. Behav. Inf. Technol. 36, 165–177.

Smith, M., 2006. Clinical decision making in acute care cardiopulmonary physiotherapy. PhD thesis. The University of Sydney, Sydney, Australia.

Smith, M., Higgs, J., Ellis, E., 2007. Physiotherapy decision making in acute cardiorespiratory care is influenced by factors related to the physiotherapist and the nature and context of the decision: a qualitative study. Aust. J. Physiother. 53, 261–267.

Smith, M., Higgs, J., Ellis, E., 2008a. Characteristics and processes of physiotherapy clinical decision making: a study of acute care cardiorespiratory physiotherapy. Physiother. Res. Int. 13, 209–222.

Smith, M., Higgs, J., Ellis, E., 2008b. Factors influencing clinical decision making. In: Higgs, J., Jones, M., Loftus, S., et al. (Eds.), Clinical Reasoning in the Health Professions, third ed. Elsevier, Edinburgh, pp. 89–100.

Smith, M., Higgs, J., Ellis, E., 2010. Effect of experience on clinical decision making by cardiorespiratory physiotherapists in acute care settings. Physiother. Theory Pract. 26, 89–99.

43

LEARNING REASONING USING SIMULATION

NICOLE CHRISTENSEN ■ CELESTE VILLANUEVA ■ SUSAN GRIEVE

CHAPTER AIMS

The aims of this chapter are to:

- introduce simulation-based learning (SBL) in the education of healthcare professionals as a bridge between academic and workplace learning contexts,
- discuss ways that simulation can be used to facilitate the learning of clinical reasoning and
- describe how principles of cognitive load theory can guide the design of simulation-based learning activities for learners along the developmental continuum.

KEY WORDS

Clinical reasoning
Cognitive load
Debriefing
Simulation-based learning

ABBREVIATIONS/ACRONYMS

CBS Computer-based simulation
CLT Cognitive load theory
MBS Manikin-based simulation
SBL Simulation-based learning
SP Standardized patient
WM Working memory

INTRODUCTION

Educators of health professions students, in the academic setting, are challenged to adequately prepare students to enter into the workplace-situated phases of their curricula. In the workplace, students must be capable of applying the knowledge they have acquired during their didactic education and prepared to learn from their clinical education experiences. The lack of connection between academic and clinical learning environments has been identified by multiple disciplines as a priority in revising health professions education today (e.g., Cooke et al., 2010; Benner et al., 2009). Within the academic environment, therefore, the integration of activities that facilitate application of knowledge in realistic clinical reasoning experiences is essential to connect the gap. To achieve optimal graduate outcomes, the focus in both learning contexts must be the development of professionals who are able to efficiently and effectively apply the knowledge gained through their academic education to clinical reasoning in the workplace.

Facilitation of learning from experience has long been accepted in the social-constructivist educational literature as requiring reflection, interaction with others and critical evaluation of one's own thinking and past learning in light of new clinical experiences (Dewey, 1933; Schön, 1987). Education within constructivist traditions aims to provide learners with experiences that can help them develop new perspectives. It has been argued that the existence of multiple, individual, differently constructed perspectives on reality help when it comes to problem solving and decision making in a real healthcare context (Yardley et al., 2012).

The learning required for students to cope in clinical settings should also include a focus on how to benefit from one's own clinical reasoning experiences. Situated, immersive learning through simulation is a rapidly developing mode of education in the academic environment that is perfectly positioned to prepare learners to cross the bridge from academic to workplace learning contexts. Learning clinical reasoning within a relevant practice context is an effective way to engage in thinking for, in, and on practice actions, while in a safe and controlled environment. There are many benefits. For example, pauses in action to intentionally facilitate reasoning, decision making and critical reflection on those decisions are possible in simulated practice experiences in ways not feasible in authentic practice settings. Simulation also allows for planned curriculum to be executed in a sequence and according to a timeline in ways that cannot be guaranteed in authentic practice settings. A strong argument can be made that highly realistic patient simulation is, in fact, a type of authentic clinical experience (Yardley et al., 2012). Simulation, therefore, can be an ideal teaching and learning strategy that prepares students in the health professions to thrive in their workplace learning experiences.

WHAT IS SIMULATION-BASED LEARNING?

At its core, SBL is an instructional methodology used to provide learners with highly contextualized practice experiences to promote experiential learning. SBL in health care encompasses many different techniques, using different types and levels of technology. Irrespective of the technique used, effective SBL should be constructed such that two requirements are met: (1) the learning activity is experiential, and (2) there is a facilitated reflective learning follow-up activity. This activity is referred to as 'debriefing', which we will discuss after first reviewing the various categories of simulation and simulator technologies associated with each one.

Types of Simulation

The healthcare simulation community is international, interprofessional and multicultural. Given the fact that simulation is also heavily influenced by rapidly changing trends in technology and healthcare delivery, the language used to describe healthcare simulation is often inconsistent, and this can be a problem. We have chosen the Healthcare Simulation Dictionary, published by the Society for Simulation in Healthcare (SSH), for simulation definitions (Lopreiato et al., 2016).

Manikin-Based Simulation

Manikin-based simulation (MBS) utilizes manikins to represent patients using heart and lung sounds, palpable pulses, voice interaction, movement (e.g., seizures, eye blinking), bleeding and other human capabilities that may be controlled by a trained facilitator using computers and software. Fundamentally, a *human patient simulator* comprises three components: 1) a human-like manikin controlled by 2) software contained in a desktop/laptop computer or any number of handheld computers and 3) the simulated physical and psychosocial environment in which a simulation exercise would be set. Manikin-based simulation is often used for immersive teaching scenarios in which the simulated patient is required to exhibit physiological signs and symptoms requiring clinical interventions that cannot be authentically and safely replicated on a human being (e.g., a patient with chest pain who deteriorates to a cardiac arrest or a patient in an intensive care unit who is on mechanical ventilation and requires routine daily care). Typically, an MBS scenario will include the presence of a simulated family member, a healthcare professional or other characters deemed necessary to meet the objectives of the learning activity, which significantly enhances the realism of the situation. The key to optimally using MBS is to match the level of fidelity (i.e., the degree of realism presented to the learner via the manikin and/or the situated learning environment) most appropriate to the desired learning outcomes. This type of simulation is frequently used to present clinically complex situations replete with confounding data sets, which foster the development of clinical reasoning.

Standardized Patient Simulation

The best preparation for the interpersonal, empathic aspects of health care is practice with real people. Therefore educators often engage a simulated/standardized patient (SP) as a 'human simulator' for SBL activities. An SP is a person who has been carefully coached to simulate an actual patient so accurately that the simulation cannot be detected by a skilled clinician (this usually excludes physical examination). In addition to the physical symptoms of a specific medical diagnosis, an SP is prepared to tell stories, express emotions, show stress and exhibit the full range of attitudes towards the healthcare professionals as required to meet the learning objectives of the simulation activity. Their purpose is threefold:

- SPs create a safe environment for practice. By interacting with SPs, learners gain firsthand experience in making clinical decisions without jeopardizing the health, welfare and privacy of real patients.
- SPs allow for immediate feedback and reflection. In the debriefing session that follows the simulation, students receive feedback from faculty facilitators, fellow learners, the SPs themselves and often from a video playback of their own performance and critical reflection on their own performance and the performance of others.
- SPs provide an authentic, direct measure for evaluation. Because SPs are trained to reproduce predetermined behaviours and attributes with each performance, faculty may compare students' performances with expected outcomes.

Hybrid Simulation

This technique involves the union of two or more modalities of simulation with the aim of providing a more realistic experience. In healthcare simulation, hybrid simulation is most commonly applied to the situation where a part task trainer (e.g., a urinary catheter model or an intramuscular injection model) is realistically affixed to an SP, allowing for teaching and assessing technical and communication skills in an integrated fashion.

Mixed-Methods Simulation

Commonly, different simulation techniques are used within one simulation session. The use of a variety of different simulation modalities (e.g., screen-based + manikin-based + procedural) is differentiated from hybrid simulation in that it is not characterized by the combination of one type of simulation to enhance another (as described earlier). The use of different simulation modes here aims to accomplish different learning objectives or may be a logistical solution to limited faculty resources when teaching large learner groups. Examples include a scenario in which a manikin simulator is the patient and an SP is a family member. This scenario may be one station in a session composed of several stations. Students rotate through the various stations in timed intervals, each station involving a different type of simulation.

Procedural Simulation

This type of simulation entails the use of a simulator modality (e.g., a task trainer, a manikin or a computer) to assist in the process of learning to complete a technical skill(s) or procedure. A task trainer is a device designed for deliberate practice to achieve technical mastery in the key elements of the procedure or skill being learned. Examples include lumbar puncture, chest tube insertion, central line insertion or medication injections into joints.

Computer-Based Simulation (Also Referred to As Screen-Based Simulation)

This type of simulation comprises the modelling of real-life processes with input and output exclusively confined to a computer and is usually associated with a computer monitor and a keyboard or other simple assistive device. Subsets of computer-based simulation (CBS) include virtual patients, virtual reality task trainers (usually a haptic device integrated with software and graphics displayed on a computer screen) and immersive virtual reality simulation.

Manikins and SPs are likely to continue as mainstays of SBL for the foreseeable future. A robust body of evidence now exists to support these and other simulation techniques as effective for learning (e.g., Issenberg et al., 2005; McGaghie et al., 2010) and improved patient/client outcomes (e.g., Griswold et al., 2012). CBS techniques are gaining traction in health professions education, in large part because of the expectation that SBL will need to be far more accessible, affordable and scalable than it currently is. Well-designed CBS is based on the theoretical foundations of MBS and SPS; the differentiating factor in CBS is the technology used to implement instructional design. A review of the full range of CBS techniques is beyond the scope of this chapter, so we will limit the discussion to the CBS subcategories that lend themselves to the development of clinical reasoning: virtual reality and virtual worlds.

Virtual Reality and Virtual World Simulation

Virtual reality is a computer-generated, interactive, three-dimensional environment in which objects have a sense of spatial presence. The artificially generated environment creates an immersion effect. Virtual reality simulation is defined as simulation that uses any of the variety of immersive, highly visual, three-dimensional characteristics to replicate real-life situations and/or healthcare procedures (Lopreiato et al., 2016). Virtual reality and virtual world are often used synonymously. However, distinguishing between virtual *reality* (VR) and virtual *world* (VW) is helpful when comparing the simulation techniques associated with each type of environment (De Gagne et al., 2013). In VR, individuals typically experience simulation by wearing headsets, which are head-mounted displays with screens placed in the user's visual field. Alternatively, headsets are worn in a simulation theatre with up to six wall-mounted screens in a room-sized cube; high-resolution images are projected on the screens to produce the immersive experience. The VW, in contrast, is a completely portable experience because it is generated wholly on a computer in a web-based software platform. Virtual worlds essentially combine the characteristics of the virtual community (best exemplified by Facebook®) with the synchronous, graphically intense environment of online video games (De Gagne et al., 2013). Both VR and VW simulations are designed so that participants can inhabit the environment and interact with avatars, graphical representations of living beings. In the VW, each participant normally has his or her own avatar that represents him or her.

The sophistication of today's video games fosters learning, socialization and collaboration in addition to relaxation. The serious game (a game designed for a primary purpose other than pure entertainment) is a core concept underlying healthcare simulations using both VR and VW environments. Games or simulations, both products of game-based learning, aim to facilitate development of skills and abilities in learners that results in safe, effective care in the complex and changing healthcare environment.

To date, healthcare simulation using the VW is more prevalently used and studied than is VR, although both techniques are in nascent stages of development (De Gagne et al., 2013; Ghanbarzadeh et al., 2014). Of the VWs, Second Life[i] is the platform most commonly employed, although VW platforms specific to healthcare simulation are rapidly emerging: Virtual Heroes;[ii] BreakAway Games;[iii] CliniSpace;[iv] and SimTabs.[v]

Manikin-based based simulation, although a proven learning strategy, is very labour- and equipment-intensive. It requires the presence of skilled facilitators and can be prohibitively costly, especially for institutions with limited fiscal resources and/or high volumes of learners. Maintaining an active SP program can also drain fiscal and personnel resources. Simulations using VR or VW technology can also be expensive to build. However, they are relatively inexpensive to maintain and are far more scalable, distributable, personalized and adaptable. Duff et al. (2016) reviewed simulation studies implemented in virtual environments and assessed them for their potential to foster diagnostic reasoning skills and found that, although the literature is sparse in this particular area, initial evidence indicates a positive trend in the use of these types of simulations for the development of reasoning skills required for clinical practice. This finding aligns with De Gagne et al. (2013), who reported that clinical reasoning and student-centred learning were among the positive attributes of VW curricula, contributing to its feasibility and acceptability.

REFLECTION POINT 1

SBE is an emerging and expanding educational modality in the health professions. In thinking about the types of simulation commonly used in today's educational practice and those under development:

1. As an educator, which modes or types of simulation do you see as most promising in helping to bridge the gap between academic and clinical practice? Why? How might your students react to different modes of simulation? Why might they react this way?

---

[i]http://www.secondlife.com
[ii]http://www.virtualheroes.com
[iii]http://www.breakawaygames.com
[iv]http://virtualsimcenter.clinispace.com/home.html
[v]http://www.simtabs.com

2. As a student, which types or modes of simulation do you feel most comfortable engaging with currently? How close are these types of simulation to mimicking realistic clinical practice? Do you see a benefit to experiencing all types of simulation in your development as a healthcare professional? Why or why not?

FACILITATING CLINICAL REASONING DEVELOPMENT THROUGH SIMULATION-BASED LEARNING

Situated learning literature describes the nature of experiential learning as inherently social. The construction of unique experiential knowledge is achieved through interactions with others, situated in the context of the shared values and perspectives of a particular practice community or profession (Greeno, 1998; Lave and Wenger, 1991; Wenger, 1998). Integral to SBL is Dewey's (1933) original concept of reflection as engendering learning through an active, dialogical process. Reflection is viewed as 'a meaning-making process that moves a learner from one experience into the next with deeper understanding of its relationships with and connections to other experiences and ideas' (Rogers 2002, p. 845).

This philosophy of learning facilitation is enacted during the reflective debriefing activities that follow simulated clinical reasoning practice experiences. Debriefing in SBL is the recognized component that allows learners to relate doing and thinking in their individual minds (Fanning and Gaba, 2007). Dreifuerst (2009, p. 111) delineated defining attributes of simulation debriefing as follows:

- Reflection: the opportunity to reexamine the [simulated] experience
- Emotion: facilitation of emotional expressions from all participants in the learning activity
- Reception: openness to feedback by both the learner and the debriefing facilitator
- Integration: embedding elements of the simulated experience into a relevant conceptual framework scaffolding that the learner is familiar with and can access in future situations
- Assimilation: providing opportunities to articulate what one has learned and how that learning will be transferred to the next experience, whether in simulation or in actual clinical practice

There are multiple approaches to the debriefing process, each one based in different constructivist theoretical frameworks (e.g., Eppich and Cheng, 2015; Palaganas et al., 2016). No single approach to debriefing has been established as the gold standard or best practice; however, what all debriefing strategies have in common is the that the focus must always be related to the primary learning goal(s) of the simulation exercise. The skill of the individual assigned to facilitate any simulation debriefing is paramount to learning success (Waxman and Miller, 2014).

Optimal facilitation of clinical reasoning development requires a revisioning of the role of teacher to that of a learning facilitator, focussed on development of ways to meaningfully interpret experience. When considering how best to facilitate the learning of clinical reasoning through debriefing simulated practice encounters, it is essential that the discussion explicitly focus on various aspects or foci of clinical reasoning enacted by those directly participating in the simulation and those observing the encounter but not directly participating. Examples of such foci may include diagnostic or examination activities; procedural or technical skills performance; communication among healthcare team members, patient, family members or other carers; attempts at collaboration; and a vast array of contextual factors that must be perceived, interpreted and managed. Context can include psychosocial factors, environmental factors, work, family, personal circumstances and financial factors, beliefs and values of the patient, resources available, culture and values of the practice setting and health system factors.

The key to effective debriefing after simulation activities is facilitation of critical reflection on clinical reasoning experiences and involves dialogue and questioning in a collaborative environment. Questions can establish a dynamic whereby learners can 'figure things out' for themselves. The facilitator helps students think about, and make explicit, their own thinking to an external audience (Cranton, 2006). The intent is to help learners realize what they know, reasoned about and did well and also to facilitate self-identification of any gaps in knowledge or reasoning skills that can focus efforts for future learning and improved performance.

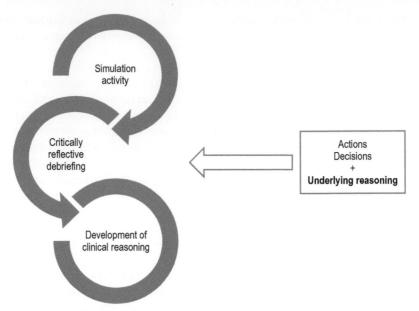

Fig. 43.1 ▪ Relationship of simulation-based learning event and development of clinical reasoning.

By engaging learners with strategic questions to stimulate constructive dialogue rather than by 'teaching' or 'telling' learners what educators believe they 'need to know', learners can construct new understandings and revise problematic knowledge they see as inadequate for their reasoning.

In this way, the debriefing discussion can explore not only the actions performed and the decisions made but also, and most importantly, the reasoning underlying those actions and decisions. This in turn facilitates exploring, evaluating and potentially refining, revising and/or constructing new practice knowledge through critical reflection about the clinical reasoning that the simulation experience engendered (Fig. 43.1).

REFLECTION POINT 2

The framework presented based on CLT can be very helpful for educators in creating new or critiquing existing simulation experiences and learning activities and for students in understanding their frustrations with a simulation experience or learning activity.

1. As an educator, reflecting on a recently created learning activity (simulation or otherwise) can you now alter that activity based on your understanding of cognitive load? How might you

alter task fidelity, complexity and support, and what effect on load would you expect?

2. As a student, reflect on your participation in a recent simulation experience or with a novel learning activity. How engaged were you in learning from the experience or activity? Can you link your answer to your understanding of cognitive load and provide suggestions that might improve the activity for your learning?

COGNITIVE LOAD CONSIDERATIONS FOR SIMULATION-BASED LEARNING

How people learn is an important consideration in the design of optimal SBL environments. Cognitive load theory (CLT) is one of many information processing theories that has found recent application to medical education curricular design. The theory provides a useful framework for understanding how people learn and is based on the foundations of human cognitive architecture, focussing specifically on the limits of working memory (WM) (Sweller et al., 1998). CLT posits that when learners are immersed in realistic environments without consideration for the potential cognitive overload of working memory (WM), any potential for learning becomes increasingly difficult or impossible.

SBL provides an optimal instructional methodology for intentional manipulation in order to optimize 'load' on WM (to promote learning) during simulated clinical reasoning experiences.

The basics of human cognitive architecture, illustrating the relationship between sensory, working and long-term memory, are described in the seminal three-stage memory model attributed to Atkinson and Shiffrin (1968). Limited in storage capacity, WM is often described as the bottleneck of the memory system, as both sensory and long-term memory have limitless capacity. WM can hold on to only five to seven 'chunks' or information elements at one time (Miller, 1956), and if rehearsal of an element does not occur within 15 to 20 seconds it disappears from WM storage (Cowan, 1988). Additionally, WM can only manipulate two to four elements at once, which defines the upper limits of human active processing capacity (Cowan, 2001). Overloading WM by exceeding these limits decreases the effectiveness of active processing and therefore adversely affects learning. This is precisely what CLT attempts to address: how to best optimize load on WM to promote learning. Doing so maximizes a learner's active processing potential, leading to the integration of new information with existing related knowledge organized and stored in long-term memory.

A tenet of CLT is that there are different types of load imposed on the limited WM resources. Resources devoted to dealing with the inherent complexity of the learning environment, task or problem are referred to as 'intrinsic cognitive load', whereas resources devoted to understanding the manner in which a learning environment, task or problem is presented are referred to as 'extraneous cognitive load'. Germane cognitive load or germane resources refers to WM resources needed in revising existing knowledge and or creating new knowledge (Kalyuga, 2011; Sweller, 2010; Sweller et al., 1998).

Intrinsic cognitive load cannot be altered by instructional design or method as it is inherent to the environment, task or problem presented. Intrinsic cognitive load for a given learning activity does, however, vary depending on the level of learner experience in a particular domain. Extraneous cognitive load, on the other hand, is entirely dependent on how the learning environment, task or problem is presented and therefore can be altered, ideally lowered, by intentional design strategies. Decreasing extraneous cognitive load frees WM resources for use as germane resources devoted to creating new knowledge or revising existing knowledge (Sweller, 2010).

Leppink and van den Heuvel (2015) recently developed a framework grounded in CLT that considers three dimensions in designing learning activities in medical education: task fidelity, task complexity and instructional support. Within the framework, each dimension is titrated in an attempt to promote an optimal load balance for the level of the learner. Use of the framework has been applied to designing layered competency modules in medical education (Leppink and Duvivier, 2016). Task fidelity applied to simulation design is determined by the types of simulation used in an encounter: Higher fidelity equates with higher realism. Task complexity considers the number of interacting elements designed into a simulation encounter. Lastly, instructional support involves the intentional use, or not, of different instructional methods to provide learner support during a simulation experience. High instructional support, low task fidelity and low task complexity are generally associated with decreasing extraneous cognitive load in learners.

We now provide examples of grading a simulation environment for a more effective cognitive load balance in novice, intermediate and experienced learners (Table 43.1). We use the dimensions of fidelity, complexity and support to grade the cognitive load in each context.

REFLECTION POINT 3

Skilled debriefing is paramount to development of learning for clinical reasoning in healthcare professional students.

1. As an educator, can you identify strategies you currently use to foster the learning of clinical reasoning? Have you applied these strategies to debriefing a simulation experience? If yes, do your strategies go beyond reflection on actions performed and decisions made? If no, how might you ensure that the debrief focusses on the reasoning underlying actions and decisions?

2. As a student, when you last participated in a debriefing session, did the facilitator guide the discussion beyond what you did, how you did it and what you would do differently next time? Did you explore your thinking and reasons underlying

TABLE 43.1

Grading a Simulated Environment for Appropriate Cognitive Load Balance According to Level of Learner

Learner → Dimensions↓	Novice	Intermediate	Experienced	Considerations	Cognitive Load Effect
Fidelity	▪ MBS; lines/tubes, eye blink, limited voice interaction ▪ Standard hospital patient room	▪ MBS similar to novice with increased voice interaction and physiological responses ▪ ICU or step-down unit	▪ SP ▪ Any practice setting	▪ MBS provides enhanced realism for learners unfamiliar with an environment and/or patient interaction. ▪ Manikin eye blink and increased voice interaction enhance realism. ▪ SPs provide the highest level of realism aside for actual patient interaction.	▪ Moving from simplistic to more realistic MBS increases both intrinsic and extraneous load. ▪ SPs can be used with novice learners, but care should be taken with titrating complexity and support so as not to overload WM novice learners.
Complexity	▪ Manikin eye blinks will only respond when spoken to. ▪ Monitor with continuous run arrhythmia, BP/HR ▪ Lines; ECG leads, IV hep lock, BP cuff	▪ Manikin initiates conversation with preplanned questions or spontaneous comments ▪ Monitor alternating between normal rhythm and arrhythmia, BP/HR, RR, SpO$_2$ ▪ Lines; ECG leads, IV hydration fluids, BP cuff, pulse-ox	▪ SP with levels of alertness, orientation and anxiety ▪ Monitor starts with normal rhythm and deteriorates to significant arrhythmia. BP/HR, RR, SaO$_2$. All changing in concert with rhythm ▪ Lines; ECG leads, IV medication, BP cuff, pulse-ox, catheters	▪ When adding elements, only add those that a learner is familiar with. ▪ When using a manikin or SP to add complexity, vocal prompts or responses are carefully planned. ▪ Monitor variables should start by being displayed in limited quantity and representing stable non–life-threatening values, progressing as appropriate.	▪ SBL provides a myriad of options from which to design complexity. ▪ Awareness that complexity can easily overload WM resources through both intrinsic load and extraneous load if not titrated appropriately is of paramount importance.
Support	▪ Presimulation review module and question-and-answer period before start ▪ Facilitator acting as a willing clinical instructor fielding learner-initiated questions during simulation	▪ Question-and-answer period only before start ▪ Facilitator present during simulation acting in capacity as interprofessional team member. May answer questions if asked	▪ No review module, limited question-and-answer period ▪ Actors play additional roles (family members, friends, other providers), may provide additional information to the learner if asked	▪ Presimulation review to hidden support through actors providing information through interaction during an SP illustrates several of many methods to titrate support. ▪ A variety of methods should be attempted.	▪ Higher levels of support tend to decrease extraneous load in novice learners and provide hints to enhance germane processing. ▪ Higher levels of support provided to experienced learners can increase extraneous load.

your actions and decisions? How might you contribute to deeper facilitation of your own learning if you find yourself debriefing with a less skilled facilitator?

FUTURE IMPLICATIONS

Though the logic and value of widespread application of a single framework for SBL are intuitively reasonable, the realization of a standard, universally adopted, theoretical framework has been challenging and will require significantly more educational research. The important message is that educators responsible for developing simulation-based curricular components should invest time investigating and developing an understanding of theoretical foundations of SBL as well as educational strategies and principles that support how people learn such as CLT.

Several recent systematic reviews of the efficacy of SBL demonstrate that we should no longer be asking whether or not learners are satisfied with their simulation experiences, or if they value simulation or if they gain confidence after undergoing simulation (e.g., Cook et al., 2011; Issenberg et al., 2011). The focus now must be on answering questions such as How does simulation work (as a learning strategy)? What techniques are best to use for particular learning outcomes? What aspects of an instructional design make it more effective than another? What is the rationale for using a particular instructional design? Educational research designed to answer these higher-level questions will require knowledge of the vast selection of theoretical frameworks upon which to build a meaningful line of inquiry.

CHAPTER SUMMARY

In this chapter, we have discussed:

- SBL as an emergent and expanding educational modality to assist learners in crossing the bridge from academic to workplace learning contexts in the health professions,
- using CLT as a framework for guiding the design and development of simulation experiences, so as to optimally load and avoid overloading a learner's working memory, potentially maximizing learning through SBL and

- the importance of skilled debriefing to the facilitation of learning of clinical reasoning in SBL. This facilitation is achieved though explicit discussions of not just the actions taken and decisions made during a simulated encounter but also the clinical reasoning underlying those decisions and actions.

REFLECTION POINT 4

Further reading:

- Nestel, D., Bearman, M., 2015. Theory and simulation-based education: definition, worldviews and applications. Clin Simul. Nurs. 11, 349–354.
- Young J.Q., van Merrienboer J., Durning S., Ten Cate O., 2014. Cognitive load theory: implications for medical education: AMEE Guide No. 86. Med. Teach. 36, 371–384.
- The International Nursing Association for Clinical Simulation and Learning (INACSL) has published 'Standards of best practice: simulation'. This resource has been widely adopted across the health professions with active simulation communities. These standards have been published in various peer-review journals. The Society for Simulation in Healthcare partners with the INACSL for many major educational initiatives. This information is valuable for anyone designing and facilitating SBL: https://www.inacsl.org/i4a/pages/index.cfm?pageid=3407

REFERENCES

Atkinson, R.C., Shiffrin, R.M., 1968. Human memory: a proposed system and its control process. In: Spence, K.W., Spence, J.T. (Eds.), The Psychology of Learning and Motivation. Academic Press, New York, NY.

Benner, P., Sutphen, M., Leonard, V., et al., 2009. Educating Nurses: A Call for Radical Transformation. Jossey-Bass, San Francisco, CA.

Cook, D.A., Hatala, R.A., Brydges, R., et al., 2011. Technology-enhanced simulation for health professions education: a systematic review and meta-analysis. JAMA 306, 978–988.

Cooke, M., Irby, D.M., O'Brien, B.C., 2010. Educating Physicians: A Call for Reform of Medical School and Residency. Jossey-Bass, San Francisco, CA.

Cowan, N., 1988. Evolving conceptions of memory storage, selective attention and their mutual constraints within the human information processing system. Psychol. Bull. 104, 163–191.

Cowan, N., 2001. The magical number 4 in short term memory: a reconsideration of mental storage capacity. Behav. Brain Sci. 24, 87–185.

Cranton, P., 2006. Understanding and Promoting Transformative Learning: A Guide for Educators of Adults, second ed. Jossey-Bass Wiley, San Francisco, CA.

De Gagne, J.C., Oh, J., Kang, J., et al., 2013. Virtual worlds in nursing education: a synthesis of the literature. J. Nurs. Educ. 52, 391–396.

Dewey, J., 1933. How We Think: A Restatement of the Relation of Reflective Thinking to the Educative Process. Heath and Company, Boston, MA.

Dreifuerst, K.T., 2009. The essentials of debriefing in simulation learning: a concept analysis. Nurs. Educ. Perspect. 30, 109–114.

Duff, E., Miller, L., Bruce, J., 2016. Online virtual simulation and diagnostic reasoning: a scoping review. Clin. Simul. Nurs. 12, 377–384.

Eppich, W., Cheng, A., 2015. Promoting excellence and reflective learning in simulation (PEARLS): development and rationale for a blended approach to health care simulation debriefing. Simul. Healthc. 10, 106–115.

Fanning, R.M., Gaba, D.M., 2007. The role of debriefing in simulation-based learning. Simul. Healthc. 2, 115–125.

Ghanbarzadeh, R., Chapanchi, A.H., Blumenstein, M., et al., 2014. A decade of research on the use of three-dimensional virtual worlds in health care: a systematic literature review. J. Med. Internet Res. 16, e47.

Greeno, J.G., 1998. The situativity of knowing, learning, and research. Am. Psychol. 53, 5–26.

Griswold, S., Ponnuru, S., Nishisaki, A., et al., 2012. The emerging role of simulation education to achieve patient safety: translating deliberate practice and debriefing to save lives. Pediatr. Clin. North Am. 59, 1329–1340.

Issenberg, S.B., McGaghie, W.C., Petrusa, E.R., et al., 2005. Features and uses of high-fidelity medical simulations that lead to effective learning: a BEME systematic review. Med. Teach. 27, 10–28.

Issenberg, S.B., Ringsted, C., Østergaard, D., et al., 2011. Setting a research agenda for simulation-based healthcare education: a synthesis of the outcome from an Utstein style meeting. Simul. Healthc. 6, 155–167.

Kalyuga, S., 2011. Cognitive load theory: how many types of load does it really need? Educ. Psychol. Rev. 23, 1–19.

Lave, J., Wenger, E., 1991. Situated Learning: Legitimate Peripheral Participation. Cambridge University Press, Cambridge, MA.

Leppink, J., Duvivier, R., 2016. Twelve tips for medical curriculum design from a cognitive load theory perspective. Med. Teach. 38, 669–674.

Leppink, J., van den Heuvel, A., 2015. The evolution of cognitive load theory and its application to medical education. Perspect. Med. Educ. 4, 119–127.

Lopreiato, J.O. (Ed.), Gammon, W., Lioce, L., Sittner, B., Slot, V., Spain, A.E. (associate Eds.), Terminology Concepts Working Group 2016. Healthcare Simulation Dictionary™. Viewed 10 June 2017. Available from: http://www.ssih.org/dictionary.

McGaghie, W.C., Issenberg, S.B., Petrusa, E.R., et al., 2010. A critical review of simulation-based medical education research: 2003–2009. Med. Educ. 44, 50–63.

Miller, G.A., 1956. The magical number seven, plus or minus two: some limits on our capacity for processing information. Psychol. Rev. 63, 81–97.

Palaganas, J.C., Fey, M., Simon, R., 2016. Structured debriefing in simulation-based education. AACN Adv. Crit. Care 27, 78–85.

Rogers, C., 2002. Defining reflection: another look at John Dewey and reflective thinking. Teach. Coll. Rec. 104, 842–866.

Schön, D., 1987. Educating the Reflective Practitioner. Jossey-Bass, San Francisco, CA.

Sweller, J., 2010. Element interactivity and intrinsic, extraneous, and germane cognitive load. Educ. Psychol. Rev. 22, 123–138.

Sweller, J., van Merrienboer, J., Paas, F., 1998. Cognitive architecture and instructional design. Educ. Psychol. Rev. 10, 251–295.

Waxman, K.T., Miller, M.A., 2014. Faculty development to implement simulations: strategies and possibilities. In: Jeffries, P.R. (Ed.), Clinical Simulations in Nursing Education: Advanced Concepts, Trends, and Opportunities. National League for Nursing, Baltimore, MD, pp. 9–21.

Wenger, E., 1998. Communities of Practice: Learning, Meaning, and Identity. Cambridge University Press, Cambridge, UK.

Yardley, S., Teunissen, P.W., Dornan, T., 2012. Experiential learning: AMEE Guide No. 63. Med. Teach. 34, e102–e115.

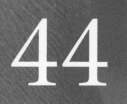

44

LEARNING TO USE EVIDENCE TO SUPPORT DECISION MAKING

JOY HIGGS ■ MERRILL TURPIN

■ ■

CHAPTER AIMS

The aims of this chapter are to:

■ examine different perspectives about the concept of 'evidence' in clinical decision making,

■ explain how clinical reasoning can be used to integrate information and knowledge from the different sources that are required for evidence-based practice,

■ understand what is meant by judgement and critical reflection and how these can support evidence-based practice and

■ connect evidence and good client care with the ability to justify and articulate clinical decisions.

KEY WORDS

Evidence

Decision making

Judgement

Critical reflection

ABBREVIATIONS/ ACRONYMS

CDM Clinical decision making

EBP Evidence-based practice

INTRODUCTION

Evidence-based practice aims to improve outcomes for healthcare clients. This goal appears uncontentious and would generally be accepted by a range of stakeholders in health: patients/clients, healthcare professionals, managers, funding bodies and policy-makers. Chapters in Section 1 of this book have presented various interpretations of clinical reasoning. Building on the idea of clinical reasoning as a client-centred approach to making decisions for and with the client to optimize their health, we focus in this chapter on understanding evidence and learning to use it wisely to make relevant, sound and defensible clinical decisions.

REFLECTION POINT 1

Before you read further: What are your opinions of evidence-based practice? How do you adopt this approach in your practice or teaching?

UNDERSTANDING EVIDENCE-BASED PRACTICE

Evidence-based practice (EBP) is a movement in health that aims to improve patient outcomes by supporting and expecting healthcare professionals to incorporate sound evidence into their practice. Sackett et al. (2000) provided a concise and useful definition of evidence-based medicine that emphasizes the complexity of the task that faces healthcare professionals in striving to create and sustain a practice that is evidence-based. The definition states that the process of evidence-based medicine requires 'the integration of best research evidence with clinical expertise and patient values' (p. 1). The practice context was added as a component in a fourth source (Rycroft-Malone et al., 2004). This perspective recognizes that research evidence alone is not sufficient for addressing the complex nature of professional practice and that the ability by health-care professionals to integrate information and that knowledge from different sources is required.

Health practitioners must engage in clinical decision making (CDM), a process of making professional judgements underpinned by a range of forms of evidence. Professional judgement lies at the core of professional practice, EBP and CDM. Healthcare professionals warrant the title of *professional* because of their ability to use judgement and reasoning combined with a credible knowledge base to enable them to make sound decisions. CDM is not, and EBP cannot be, a simplistic process of application of knowledge and practice rules designed by others and blindly following externally regulated demands or standards. Such actions would reduce the healthcare practitioner to the role of a technician. Similarly, regarding EBP as a process of treatment prescription based on absolute and unequivocal research-driven evidence fails in several respects. It fails to acknowledge the complexity of human responses to ill health; to comprehend the epistemological rules of knowledge creation (including the use of probability in empirico-analytical research to produce knowledge claims); and to recognize that medicine is an inexact science in which not everything can be known or predicted and where many decisions need to be made in the face of uncertainty.

In both EBP and CDM:

■ Health practitioners are using judgements and making decisions.
■ Critical reflection is a key element of practice.
■ Evidence of multiple forms is required to support these decisions.
■ Actions arising within and from CDM (including choices of investigations, treatments and evaluations) result from decisions at micro, macro and meta levels.
■ Practitioners need to be able to use a range of evidence (research and practice-based knowledge and clinical data) to make and justify their decisions.
■ The evidence used needs to be trustworthy because its use affects clients' quality of life and sometimes

life or death. Judgement is needed to assess the trustworthiness and relevance of evidence and in making decisions and taking actions based on the evidence.
■ Practitioners need to have access to the latest generalized, scientific, propositional knowledge (based on theory and research) to use in supporting decisions. This includes, for example, knowledge of the incidence and prevalence of diseases, knowledge of the likely prognosis of different diseases, knowledge of the effect of various disabilities on people's abilities and knowledge of the effect of various treatments on people's medical conditions.
■ With growing expertise, practitioners build rich knowledge bases where complex clinical, experience-based knowledge replaces learned discrete or clustered biomedical knowledge as the primary foundation for CDM and EBP (see Chapter 5).

REFLECTION POINT 2

In your practice and teaching, what information and knowledge do you use to evidence your decisions, and where do you source it from? How has your knowledge base grown and changed as your expertise has increased?

To practice in an evidence-based way, healthcare professionals need to integrate their clinical experience, research findings, information about the preferences and circumstances of their patients and an understanding of the demands and expectations of the practice context. The process by which healthcare professionals integrate this information is clinical reasoning.

WHAT CONSTITUTES EVIDENCE?

The Evidence-Based Practice Movement's Concept of Evidence

The assumption underpinning the perceived need for an evidence-based practice is that basing practice on rigorously produced information or evidence will lead to enhanced patient outcomes. Given the complex range of factors that can affect patient outcomes, how can we be sure that basing our practices on such evidence will improve them, and what kinds of information and knowledge constitute appropriate and sufficient evidence? In the definition of evidence-based practice by Sackett et al. (1996), the term 'current best evidence' was introduced as the criterion for satisfactory evidence. Predictably, clarifying the nature of 'best' evidence is a central concern of the evidence-based practice movement.

Knowledge Paradigms and Evidence

The empirico-analytical paradigm, also known as the scientific paradigm, is the dominant philosophy that underpins medicine. According to Higgs et al. (2008), this paradigm 'relies on observation and experiment in the empirical world, resulting in generalisations about the content and events of the world which can be used to predict the future' (p. 155). From the perspective of the empirico-analytical paradigm, the best form of evidence is that produced through rigorous scientific enquiry, particularly randomized controlled trials. It has been assumed that such rigour can be achieved best through the methods of research, especially quantitative research (Rycroft-Malone et al., 2004). Qualitative research methods across the interpretive research paradigm and the critical paradigm are being increasingly valued as approaches to providing research evidence for the utility of interventions and the experiences of particular groups of people or individuals (Pearson, 2004).

The position that scientific knowledge is the sole key to evidence has been questioned by a number of writers (Higgs et al., 2004; Jones et al., 2006a; Jones et al., 2006b) who have argued that research evidence alone is not sufficient for addressing the complexities of professional practice and that the ability to generate and integrate different types of evidence from different sources is also required. Critics of evidence-based practice argue that there are problems with the production, relevance and availability of research evidence. Furthermore, it has limited capacity to address the human and clinical problems of practice and enhance decision making in the context of complex practice and life situations (Small, 2003). Examples of criticisms include 1) the research that is undertaken is often dependent on funding, and, therefore, what is researched can be influenced by factors other than need and importance; 2) the research undertaken can

reflect what is easier to measure more than what is important to understand or most important to professional practice; and 3) often, research findings are not presented in forms that are easily accessible to healthcare professionals.

Although the evidence-based practice movement is centred on evidence derived from rigorously conducted research, it also recognizes that to practice in an evidence-based way, professionals need to integrate research findings with practice-based knowledge derived from rigorous reflection and testing of their clinical experience and with an understanding of the preferences and circumstances of their patients.

Types of Knowledge

Professional practice can be characterized as reasoned action, as it requires both knowing and doing. Different types of knowledge are required for healthcare professionals to undertake such reasoned action. Three types of knowledge (Higgs and Titchen, 1995) are required for practice (Table 44.1).

Types of Evidence

If we examine clinical reasoning deeply, a range of different types and levels of evidence becomes apparent (Higgs, 2018). For instance:

- evidence in the form of clinical data derived from observations and tests is needed to:
  a. assess the credibility of individual patient's history and
  b. help in establishing diagnoses in complex cases, cases with unusual presentations and multiple comorbidities;
- evidence in the form of experience-based illness scripts (Boshuizen and Schmidt, 1992, 2008) is invaluable for:
  a. understanding the nature of complex cases,
  b. appreciating the patient's perspective, responses (e.g., anxiety) and experiences,
  c. valuing the role the patient can play in clinical decision making,
  d. developing alternative narratives for treatment and prognosis and
  e. helping the patient understand his or her situation, treatment choices and potential health/illness progression;

	TABLE 44.1
	Types of Knowledge
Type	**Description**
Propositional knowledge	This is also known as theoretical and science-based knowledge. This is an explicit and formal type of knowledge that is generated through research and scholarship. This type of knowledge is often thought of as 'scientific knowledge' and has been emphasized in the main conceptualization of evidence-based practice to date.
Professional craft knowledge	This is grounded in practice experience and requires the rigour of review and reflection to justify the claim of being knowledge. It is often associated with the idea of an 'art' of practice and includes the particular perspectives that characterize each profession.
Personal knowledge	This refers to an individual healthcare professional's knowledge of his or her self in relation to others. This type of knowledge is important for professional practice because professional relationships are central to person-centred practice.
Professional craft knowledge and personal knowledge	Both are experience-based knowledge. They 'may be tacit and embedded either in practice itself or in who the person is' (Higgs et al., 2001, p. 5) and have been referred to collectively as 'nonpropositional' knowledge.

Derived from Higgs and Titchen, 1995

■ evidence in the form of research findings can assist, along with professional judgement, in:

   a. determining the best supported diagnosis and individual treatment options (taking a personalized medicine approach) and

   b. drawing up a list of treatment options (and potential risks/benefits) to discuss with patients;

■ evidence in the form of arguments constructed from first principles (e.g., using knowledge of biomedical science, psychology in support of clinical decisions in the absence of compelling clinical evidence) and

■ evidence in the form of theorization where the individual clinician has built his or her own body of practice knowledge grounded in and tested through practice. Such practice theories are part of the individual practitioner's knowledge base and practice model. Once presented to the practice community for peer review, they can become part of the profession's (collective) knowledge base.

This list presents evidence that is data, evidence that is knowledge and evidence that is argument. All three of these types of evidence fit the following definitions of evidence; evidence is 'grounds for belief' (*The Macquarie Concise Dictionary,* 1998), evidence is 'an outward sign' or 'something that furnishes proof' (*Merriam-Webster Dictionary,* n.d.).

REFLECTION POINT 3

Different ways of knowing and reasoning can provide evidence for reasoned action. Consider the types of evidence that provide a foundation for decisions and actions in your practice and teaching.

Considering Evidence From the Patient's Perspective

Bringing the patient's perspective into the evidence debate raises two key questions: 'What is going to make the biggest difference to my patient's life and health?' and 'What evidence is the patient in a better position to provide than the practitioner?' Answering the first question is addressed by understanding the part that situatedness and patient-centred care play in CDM. Basically, health care is for the benefit of individuals and groups and should be relevant to their interests, well-being, medical condition and preferences. Considerations of duty of care, ethics, patients' rights and choices are equally as important as generalized knowledge of best practice. Answering the second question requires the practitioner to share power in decision making, respect patients' knowledge of themselves and their health and value the role of the patient as a participant in decision making. Consider these arguments in case studies 44.1 and 44.2.

Patients seek professional services because they need something that they cannot obtain in other ways.

Understanding the Client's Situation

This case study draws upon the two processes of understanding and negotiating that are used when individualizing intervention (identified by Copley et al., 2008).

Val is a woman in her eighties who lives with her husband in a high-set house not far from a major regional centre. She has severe rheumatoid arthritis, particularly affecting her hands and hips. She has lived with her condition for many years but seeks assistance from healthcare professionals at times when the deterioration in her condition means that the routines and methods she has in place no longer support her participation. When working with her, the healthcare professional first tries to understand her particular situation, with a focus on what has worked for her in the past, her current concerns and circumstances and her goals for the future and

expectations of the healthcare professional. He listens closely for any cues that might indicate her attitudes to certain interventions or courses of action. He also pays attention to details about her circumstances, considering matters such as what she can afford and who is available to help her. While listening to Val, he is thinking about what is known about the issues being raised and other clients with whom he has worked previously and considers the relevance of all of this to Val's circumstances. As understanding of Val's situation and possible courses of action develop, the healthcare professional works towards a shared understanding with Val. In coming to this shared understanding, he has combined knowledge from a range of sources into the process of shared decision making.

Professional services often come at substantial financial costs (and other costs such as time and effort) to patients. Attending to patients' predicaments, rights and preferences requires a developed ability to understand people, both as individuals and as members of groups within the overall population. Examples of understanding preferences and rights include giving patients choices in relation to interventions (that is, considering their preferences) and understanding and advocating for the rights of people who are marginalized to participate in social roles such as work. Understanding 'predicaments' requires the ability to imagine patients within the context of their living situations and social roles (not just the service contexts in which they are seen). For example, a healthcare professional might have to consider the need for support from a patient's carer, the logistics of whether a patient is able to follow an intervention recommendation when the patient returns to daily life and his or her opportunities for social participation.

Although patients expect healthcare professionals to offer them services that will be effective, they also expect them to listen to their concerns and validate their experiences of health. Increasingly, patients also acquire healthcare knowledge and information from

sources such as the Internet. Consequently, they are likely to expect healthcare professionals to know about this information and help them to understand it and to appraise its relevance and appropriateness for them. In addition to the effectiveness of the interventions, patients might expect a greater role in shared decision making, 'evidence' of a healthcare professional's interpersonal skills (e.g., a professional's ability to listen to their concerns), 'value for money' and the accessibility (physical and temporal) of the services that are being offered. The importance of healthcare professionals being able to communicate effectively with their patients is vital.

EVIDENCE-BASED PRACTICE AND CLINICAL REASONING

Healthcare professionals deal with the complexity of professional practice using judgement (Coles, 2002) that relies on their clinical or professional expertise. The concept of professional expertise is central to the evidence-based practice process, which is made clear in discussions of evidence-based medicine by Sackett et al. (1996, 2000).

CASE STUDY 44.2

Using Different Knowledge Sources in Clinical Decision Making

This case study illustrates the process of prioritizing information about the client when using different sources of evidence as a basis for making clinical decisions, as outlined by Copley et al. (2010).

Luke is a young man in his late teens with an anxiety disorder. He has had substantial time away from school because of his anxiety and has taken longer than his peers to finish grade 12. He would like to go to university next year but is seeking help from healthcare professionals to plan for this. Prompted by this goal, the healthcare professional working with him accesses recent peer-reviewed journals and textbooks to ensure that her knowledge base includes up-to-date information and draws upon her clinical experience of other people whose life roles are disrupted by anxiety. This is done in preparation for seeing Luke and enables the healthcare professional to develop a generalized image. Forming generalized hypotheses can provide a point of comparison and shape the information she seeks from and about Luke.

In the first meeting with Luke and his mother, they talk about information they have gained from the Internet, and the healthcare professional is able to discuss this with them in light of her own knowledge of peer-reviewed literature. As she comes to know Luke and his circumstances more, the healthcare professional is able to reflect on the applicability of her knowledge base and retrieve knowledge that is most relevant. When making clinical decisions, the healthcare professional prioritizes information about Luke and his circumstances while using what is relevant from her body of knowledge. The healthcare professional engages in a process of reasoning-in-action, whereby CDM forms the basis for reasoned action, and the results of that action with Luke further inform clinical decisions and action. In this way, the healthcare professional is able to provide a service that is valuable to Luke and addresses his goals.

The practice of evidence based medicine means integrating individual clinical expertise with the best available external clinical evidence from systematic research. By individual clinical expertise we mean the proficiency and judgement that individual clinicians acquire through clinical experiences and clinical practice. Increased expertise is reflected in many ways, but especially in more effective and efficient diagnosis and in the more thoughtful identification and compassionate use of individual patients' predicaments, rights, and preferences in making clinical decisions about their care (Sackett et al., 1996, p. 71).

As this discussion makes clear, professional expertise includes thoughtfulness and compassion with effectiveness and efficiency.

Professional Expertise and Clinical Reasoning

Sociocultural theories of learning suggest that professional expertise develops through interaction with, and induction into, communities of practice (Lave and Wenger, 1991). These experiences enable healthcare professionals to learn the practices, activities and ways of thinking and knowing of their profession through participation in the community of practice. Expertise develops 'as an individual gains greater knowledge, understanding and mastery' (Walker 2001, p. 24) in his or her practice area.

Three models that interpret ways in which expertise is developed are as follows:

- The Stage Theory of the Development of Medical Expertise of Boshuizen and Schmidt (1992, 2008) (see Chapter 5) in which clinical reasoning development occurs alongside of, and reciprocally with, the acquisition and development of knowledge structures rather than being a separate skill that is acquired independently of medical knowledge and other diagnostic skills.
- The grounded theory of expert practice in physical therapy developed by Jensen et al. (Jensen et al., 2000, 2007) in which expertise in physical therapy

is understood as a combination of multidimensional knowledge, clinical reasoning skills, skilled movement and virtue (see Chapter 6).

■ The novice to expert model of Dreyfus and Dreyfus (1986) that illustrates how professional expertise develops with experience. These researchers characterized five stages through which professionals progress as they gain experience: novice, advanced beginner, competent, proficient and expert. Essentially, these stages reflect a movement from a practice that is based on context-free information and generalized rules to a sophisticated and 'embodied' understanding of the specific context in which the practice occurs. The earlier stages focus on the application of generalized knowledge. In the proficient and expert stages, healthcare professionals are able to recognize (often subtle) similarities between the current situation and previous ones and use their knowledge of previous outcomes to make judgements about what might be best in the current situation.

We see across these models three core elements: a strong link between knowledge and reasoning development, a transition in both of these dimensions commencing at the novice level and (for some) progressing to the level of expert (which itself involves ongoing development) and the importance of experience and experience-based knowledge and learned propositional knowledge.

REFLECTION POINT 4

Reflect on your own situation. What is your level of progression towards expertise? How is this reflected in your knowledge base, judgement and reasoning?

Making Decisions in Conditions Where Knowledge Is Uncertain

Healthcare professionals need to use their judgement to make decisions about the best course of action to take under conditions of uncertainty, within the given setting and client circumstances. Part of the complexity is dealing with different and often competing understandings from a variety of data and knowledge sources and considering the individual nature of patient circumstances, needs and preferences. Professional practice

is an ethical endeavour tailored to the individual patient and requires critical reflection, the credible use of theory and research, good judgement, metacognition and problem solving and the ability to implement protocols and procedures. Integrating information from research, clinical expertise, patient values and preferences and information from the practice context requires judgement and artistry with science and logic.

Combining Art and Science in Credible Evidence-Based Practice

Strategies for combining science and art in practice are embedded in the way that healthcare professionals think about their work. For example, in reference to occupational therapists, it has been stated that 'when occupational therapists refer to the paired concepts of art and science, they express their moral dissatisfaction with being constrained by either. In isolation, art somehow seems too soft and unquantifiable and science too hard and unyielding' (Turpin, 2007, p. 482). Although science is generally associated with rigour, reliability and predictability, artistry is associated with judgement and being able to deal with unpredictability. In Sackett et al.'s 1996 definition of evidence-based medicine, artistry is evident in the reference to 'thoughtful identification and compassionate use' of information that pertains to a particular patient. Although various health professions emphasize art and science to different degrees, they all appear to accept that a balance of these approaches is required for professional practice.

Making Practice Evidence-Based and Reasoning-Sound

Professional practice is a complex and fluid process that is characterized by high levels of uncertainty that arise from the context-dependent nature of the tasks that are undertaken. Professional practice is difficult to describe specifically, as it involves fulfilling particular professional roles with particular patients within particular contexts. Each of these factors contributes a unique aspect to the phenomenon, leading to a complex range of variations to what might be considered 'standard practice'.

There is no easy answer to the question 'How do I make my practice evidence-based?' However, a number of principles and tools can provide healthcare professionals with strategies for working towards improved

---

BOX 44.1
HOW DO I MAKE MY PRACTICE EVIDENCE-BASED?

Approaches include:

- **being systematic in the way information and knowledge** are collected and used to support the trustworthiness and relevance of these;
- **using sound and logical reasoning with compassion and understanding** when making decisions and being clear about the information and knowledge used as the basis of decision making;
- **having a good working knowledge of current discipline-based propositional knowledge**, being aware of the limits of my propositional knowledge and having a plan for expanding my knowledge base;
- **being aware of my current nonpropositional knowledge** (including professional craft knowledge and personal knowledge). Reflecting on this knowledge, asking myself, for instance: How have I systematically tested my practice experiences and derived knowledge from these experiences? Can I communicate this knowledge with credibility to my colleagues and patients and use it as sound evidence to support my practice? Is there personal knowledge derived from my life experiences (for example, working with people from different cultures) that I can use in my practice? What have I learned about communicating with people who speak different languages to me or who experience hardship, disability or illness/injury that I can use to enhance my practice?

Planning to systematically enhance or expand this type of knowledge is an excellent way of drawing on practice expertise and individualizing the services that I provide to patients;

- **engaging in empathic visioning and collaborative questioning with patients** about their experiences, knowledge and values. Listen to my patients' stories and experiences and try to understand their experience of and perspective on the situation. Ask them what they think would make the biggest difference in their life. Practice problem solving and mutual decision making with patients to expand my collaboration skills and improve my decision making;
- **being aware of the degree to which my actions are informed by the different sources of information** and knowledge: research evidence; your own clinical expertise; the patients' values, preferences and circumstances; and an understanding of the practice context and how it shapes my practice (e.g., what demands and expectations it places on me; in what ways it constrains what I can and cannot do);
- **using metacognition during reasoning** to bring evaluation and monitoring into my thinking during the act of thinking and
- **critically reflecting on and practicing articulating my reasoning** and professional practice model.

---

patient outcomes through a practice that is evidence-based (Box 44.1).

CHAPTER SUMMARY

In this chapter, we have explored a number of arguments:

- The notion of 'evidence' varies with different stakeholders and conceptual approaches.
- Integrating knowledge and data from different sources to create an evidence-based practice requires clinical reasoning and judgement.
- Integrating knowledge from research, clinical expertise, patient values and preferences and knowledge from practice requires judgement and artistry with science and reasoning.

REFLECTION POINT 5

Engage in critical reflection about the types of knowledge that you are using and how you are using

them, and ask yourself whether this constitutes appropriate evidence for the particular questions and problems about which you seek to be informed. Think about the cognitive and metacognitive processes that you are using to combine information from different sources within the context of your discipline and practice context.

REFERENCES

Boshuizen, H., Schmidt, H., 2008. The development of clinical reasoning expertise. In: Higgs, J., Jones, M., Loftus, S., et al. (Eds.), Clinical Reasoning in the Health Professions, third ed. Elsevier, Edinburgh, pp. 113–121.

Boshuizen, H.P.A., Schmidt, H.G., 1992. On the role of biomedical knowledge in clinical reasoning by experts, intermediates and novices. Cogn. Sci. 16, 153–184.

Coles, C., 2002. Developing professional judgement. J. Contin. Educ. Health Prof. 22, 3–10.

Copley, J., Turpin, M., Brosnan, J., et al., 2008. Understanding and negotiating: reasoning processes used by an occupational therapist to individualize intervention decisions for people with upper limb hypertonicity. Disabil. Rehabil. 30, 1486–1498.

Copley, J.A., Turpin, M.J., King, T.L., 2010. Information used by an expert paediatric occupational therapist when making clinical decisions. Can. J. Occup. Ther. 77, 249–256.

Dreyfus, H., Dreyfus, S., 1986. Mind over Machine. Free Press, New York, NY.

Evidence, 1998. The Macquarie Concise Dictionary, third ed. Macquarie Library, Sydney, NSW.

Evidence, n.d. Merriam-Webster Dictionary. Merriam-Webster, Springfield, MA. Viewed 28 February 2017. Available from: https://www.merriam-webster.com/dictionary/evidence.

Higgs, J., 2018. Judgment and reasoning in professional contexts. In: Lanzer, P. (Ed.), Catheter-Based Cardiovascular Interventions: Knowledge-Based Approach. SpringerNature, Berlin, Heidelberg, New York. In Press.

Higgs, J., Andresen, L., Fish, D., 2004. Practice knowledge: its nature, sources and contexts. In: Higgs, J., Richardson, B., Abrandt Dahlgren, M. (Eds.), Developing Practice Knowledge for Health Professionals. Butterworth-Heinemann, Oxford, pp. 51–69.

Higgs, J., Jones, M., Titchen, A., 2008. Knowledge, reasoning and evidence for practice. In: Higgs, J., Jones, M., Loftus, S., et al. (Eds.), Clinical Reasoning in the Health Professions, third ed. Elsevier, Edinburgh, pp. 151–161.

Higgs, J., Titchen, A., 1995. Propositional, professional and personal knowledge in clinical reasoning. In: Higgs, J., Jones, M. (Eds.), Clinical Reasoning in the Health Professions, second ed. Butterworth-Heinemann, Oxford, pp. 129–146.

Higgs, J., Titchen, A., Neville, V., 2001. Professional practice and knowledge. In: Higgs, J., Titchen, A. (Eds.), Practice Knowledge and Expertise in the Health Professions. Butterworth–Heinemann, Oxford, pp. 3–9.

Jensen, G.M., Gwyer, J., Hack, L.M., et al., 2007. Expertise in Physical Therapy Practice, second ed. Saunders-Elsevier, St. Louis, MO.

Jensen, G.M., Gwyer, J., Shepard, K.F., et al., 2000. Expert practice in physical therapy. Phys. Ther. 80, 28–43.

Jones, M., Grimmer, K., Edwards, I., et al., 2006a. Challenges in applying best evidence to physiotherapy. Internet J. Allied Health Sci. Pract. 4, 1–8.

Jones, M., Grimmer, K., Edwards, I., et al., 2006b. Challenges in applying best evidence to physiotherapy practice: part 2—reasoning and practice challenges. Internet J. Allied Health Sci. Pract. 4, 1–9.

Lave, J., Wenger, E., 1991. Situated Learning: Legitimate Peripheral Participation. Cambridge University Press, Cambridge.

Pearson, A., 2004. Balancing the evidence: incorporating the synthesis of qualitative data into systematic reviews. JBI Rep. 2, 45–64.

Rycroft-Malone, J., Seers, K., Titchen, A., et al., 2004. What counts as evidence in evidence-based practice? J. Adv. Nurs. 47, 81–90.

Sackett, D.L., Rosenberg, W.M.C., Muir Gray, J.A., et al., 1996. Evidence based medicine: what it is and what it isn't: it's about integrating individual clinical expertise and the best external evidence. BMJ 312, 71–72.

Sackett, D.L., Straus, S.E., Scott Richardson, W., et al., 2000. Evidence-Based Medicine: How to Practice and Teach EBM, second ed. Elsevier Churchill Livingstone, Edinburgh.

Small, N., 2003. Knowledge, not evidence, should determine primary care practice. Clin. Govern. 8, 191–199.

Turpin, M., 2007. The issue is … recovery of our phenomenological knowledge in occupational therapy. Am. J. Occup. Ther. 61, 481–485.

Walker, R., 2001. Social and cultural perspectives on professional knowledge and expertise. In: Higgs, J., Titchen, A. (Eds.), Practice Knowledge and Expertise in the Health Professions. Butterworth-Heinemann, Oxford, pp. 22–28.

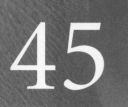

45

LEARNING TO RESEARCH CLINICAL REASONING

KATHRYN N. HUGGETT ■ NICOLE CHRISTENSEN ■
GAIL M. JENSEN ■ ANNA MAIO

CHAPTER AIMS

The aims of this chapter are to:

- discuss why educators should engage in research about clinical reasoning,
- summarize common purposes and types of educational studies in the health sciences,
- discuss considerations in selecting a conceptual framework to guide research,
- describe early steps in determining the research design and
- illustrate how an educator might propose to study a question from his or her teaching practice.

KEY WORDS

Research design
Research method
Conceptual framework
Clinical reasoning

ABBREVIATIONS/ ACRONYMS

AAMC Association of American Medical Colleges
AERA American Educational Research Association
AMEE Association for Medical Education in Europe
IAMSE International Association of Medical Science Educators
MERC Medical Education Research Certificate

RCT Randomized controlled trial
RESME Research Essential Skills in Medical Education

INTRODUCTION

Educational research may seem too far beyond the scope of customary activity for faculty who develop and implement clinical reasoning curricula. Some faculty feel unprepared to engage in educational research, citing lack of relevant social science research skills. There are at least three reasons, however, why educators should engage in research about clinical reasoning. First, as educators and scholars, it is critical that we share descriptions of our work with others. Descriptive studies offer ideas and guidance to other educators who may be seeking a similar innovation or application of a new method. Second, justification studies permit us to compare educational interventions to answer the questions 'Does it work?' and 'How well does it work?' (Cook et al., 2008). Finally, there is a rich history of scholarship describing theories of clinical reasoning, expertise and clinical decision-making methods. Clarification studies test predictions about these existing theories and models and answer questions such as 'How does it work?' and 'Why does it work?' (Cook et al., 2008). Building on this work through justification studies allows us to better understand which theories apply to a particular context or setting, under what conditions, and for whom.

Learning to research clinical reasoning can be the start of a new scholarly path. Traditionally, scientific inquiry pursued the creation of new knowledge. Ernest Boyer (1990, p. 24) challenged scholars to envision a wider understanding: 'What we urgently need today is a more inclusive view of what it means to be a scholar – a recognition that knowledge is acquired through research, through synthesis, through practice and through teaching'. This is particularly true for expanding knowledge and understanding of clinical reasoning. For example, the clinical learning environment is often interdisciplinary and interprofessional, providing opportunities for the discovery of new relationships, techniques and approaches. The insights and questions that emerge in clinical practice also contribute to knowledge development through synthesis, and these may advance knowledge in the form of policy papers and case reviews. New knowledge is also created through practical application, as questions emerge in practice and are explored when hypotheses are tested against clinical findings and pathophysiological principles. Likewise, the scholarship of practice can occur when technical skills are applied to develop quality indicators and innovations to improve healthcare systems and delivery. Finally, the scholarship of teaching and learning can enlarge knowledge of a clinical topic when educators create scholarly products to guide clinical practice such as textbooks, assessments and accreditation standards.

In this chapter, we offer ideas to help educators develop a research question supported by a conceptual framework. Next, we discuss early steps in determining the research design. Finally, we provide a case study to illustrate how an educator might propose to study a question from his or her teaching practice. If you are new to educational research, do not be intimidated. If you have participated in basic science or clinical research, you already possess some of the skills and habits of mind required for educational research. Above all, employ your skills of observation, and stay open to new questions that emerge during your clinical teaching. These often set the foundation for studies that answer our own local questions and initiate a wider conversation in our field.

DEVELOP A RESEARCH QUESTION

A question is the starting point, and refining that question is critical to developing a project. A literature search is always an early step to refine a question, to see what has been studied and what still needs to be explored. Starting broad with a goal and thinking of it in terms of what you want to measure, replicate, discover or

confirm begin the process. A working list of questions and ideas can be distilled by consulting and critiquing the literature. At a later date in the process, a method of inquiry is chosen. Keeping an open mind in this early phase is important.

A good question meets key criteria. Using a tool to assess questions is vital to development. One such tool is FINER (Hulley and Cummings, 1988). Using this acronym, F represents Feasible. Is the scope possible, and are there resources for the project (time and money)? I is Interesting. Why is it interesting to you, and who else is interested that can help with resources and promotion? N identifies Novel. Has this been done before, and how can this project be made unique? This is a signal to dive deeper into the literature. E is Ethical. Spend time thinking about your participants and any ethical issues that could arise. For example, a researcher may wish to conduct a think-aloud study to investigate how advanced nursing students solve complex cases and arrive at clinical decisions. The investigator is a faculty member who evaluates learners in a final capstone course and writes letters of recommendation. Thus students may feel compelled to participate in the study. To address these ethical considerations, the study protocol must offer voluntary participation and ensure protections such as confidential data collection and de-identification of data before review by this researcher-teacher. The researcher-teacher must not be able to find out who provided data and who did not. R stands for Relevant. Your proposed project should be useful in some way and relate to the current state of health sciences education. Even if your project is historical, understanding how things were done in the past can help us understand why the present situation has come about in the way that it has.

IDENTIFY A CONCEPTUAL FRAMEWORK

Conceptual frameworks are scaffolds that provide an important resource in helping the researcher explore the possible dimensions or components of your question or problem. In other words, the conceptual framework explains, either graphically or in some narrative form, the main things to be studied. The conceptual framework is a helpful structure for guiding you to think more deeply about the factors, constructs or variables and the relationships among them that you will be studying.

The framework is a dynamic structure that will continue to evolve as the research progresses. In other words, you can have multiple iterations of your framework throughout your research. Frameworks vary and can be descriptive and rudimentary, or they may be more theory-driven or have some combination of both (Bordage, 2009; Merriam, 1998; Miles et al., 2013).

For example, if you are using qualitative research methods to explore a phenomenon that is not well described or understood, such as how health professions students describe their reasoning processes in their first semester of study, you would first begin by interviewing and observing students. From this initial data collection, you could identify key concepts that might include how they describe their approach to reasoning and the processes they use to make decisions. To continue with this example, if you moved on to studying the development of clinical reasoning abilities of health professions students across all years of the educational program, you might use concepts from how learners organize knowledge (script theory) and dual-process theory (analytic and nonanalytic thinking), along with concepts you uncovered in your exploratory research from first-year students.

REFLECTION POINT 1

Reflection Questions for Students

Here are some questions to guide your research planning:

1. How could instruction for clinical reasoning be improved?
2. Where did the real learning occur?
3. What resources would have been useful to guide my learning?
4. What questions do I still have about clinical reasoning?

Step 1: Get a Central Focus

In clinical reasoning research, an initial question for developing the framework is: What is the central question or problem? Are you interested in:

1. learner development of clinical reasoning abilities?
2. the teaching of clinical reasoning?
3. the clinical reasoning process used in the context of practice?
4. understanding types or approaches to clinical reasoning used? (Khatami et al., 2012)

Step 2: Set Boundaries for the Framework

Once you have a central focus, then what actors will be studied or relationship explored? In other words, what are the boundaries of the study (what is included and what is excluded and why)? You cannot study everything, and setting boundaries for the framework or scaffold is a very important step in the process.

Step 3: Look to the Literature for Research *and* Theory

What do we already know about this problem in clinical reasoning from your profession and others? What are the recurring concepts, models and theories that you continue to see in the literature? Central to understanding the development of clinical reasoning abilities will be the learning sciences and educational theories. What current learning science theories may be helpful in your research?

Learning theories that are currently used in clinical reasoning include cognitive theories. Currently popular is dual-process theory, which can be described simply as fast thinking (nonanalytic thinking; also called pattern recognition or type 1 thinking) or slow thinking (analytic thinking; also called type 2 thinking). Another example is cognitive load theory, which has to do with information processing and how much a learner can handle. Clinical reasoning research can also use noncognitive theories, such as those from social cognitive work, and are focussed on the situativity of the situation and the interactions occurring in the learning environment and community of practice (Trowbridge et al., 2015).

Step 4: Make a Visual, One-Page Framework

Conceptual frameworks are sometimes best done as a graphic or visual. This helps you see the core concepts or constructs and the relationships among them. If you have more than one researcher, you may each want to develop an individual model and then come together to build a consensus model for the research.

REFLECTION POINT 2

Reflection Questions for Faculty

Here are some questions to guide your research planning:
1. Did the instructional method and assessment support the learning objectives?

2. Did learners achieve the learning objectives as expected?
3. Are there key concepts or processes that consistently challenge learners?
4. What contributed to or detracted from the learning experience?

SELECT THE RESEARCH DESIGNS AND METHODS

Once you have identified an area of interest and developed your conceptual framework, you are ready to consider which type of research design and associated methods will lead to answering your type of research question. Ringsted et al. (2011) describe a 'research compass' model of design approaches that is very helpful for guiding initial decisions about which direction to go with research design, depending on the purpose of the study (Table 45.1).

Perhaps an even simpler place to start in selecting an appropriate research design is to consider which research paradigm is most suited to answer the research question. Research paradigms are commonly separated into qualitative, quantitative or mixed-methods approaches to design. Qualitative approaches are well suited to answer open-ended exploratory research questions. Researchers working in the qualitative paradigm intentionally do not predetermine hypotheses related to what they expect or predict their possible outcomes to be. Rather, these designs have, as an outcome of the research, a description of 'what is there' in the phenomenon of interest or of what things mean to people. Quantitative approaches are well suited to answer closed-ended research questions; these are questions that test or measure 'what is there' as the outcome of research. The hypothesis being tested assumes that the entities being measured are there to begin with. Mixed-methods approaches to design are often used when, to develop a deeper or more contextualized understanding of a situation, the researcher chooses to explore both closed-ended and open-ended questions that are closely related. It is helpful to consider that the quantitative aspects of a mixed-methods design are intended to provide replicable evidence and therefore can contribute to the establishment of laws and principles, while the qualitative aspects, although not replicable, can provide essential context within which

to understand the quantitative findings (Leppink, 2017).

DEVELOP THE RESEARCH DESIGN

After you have selected the appropriate research design, you can proceed to develop the plan for your study. Remember that the research design will help you answer your research questions and guide the investigation in a purposeful and systematic way. Although an in-depth examination of research design elements is beyond the scope of this chapter, here are some considerations to guide your planning. For quantitative studies, randomized controlled trials (RCTs) should be considered for relatively standard interventions. RCTs require the random assignment of participants to treatments, and this randomization reduces bias. For this reason, RCTs are considered the gold standard in the clinical research paradigm. In educational settings, however, it is often difficult to randomize learners to different educational experiences. It is also challenging to standardize learning environments and experiences. Randomization will not control for sources of error such as variations in learner preparation and motivation, learning settings and intervention implementation. For these reasons, RCTs are recommended for situations in which the mechanism of learning is already understood, the outcome of the intervention is easily measured and accepted, the effect size of the intervention is small or the results from the trial may have a large effect. If any of these criteria are not met, then it can be difficult to justify the cost of an RCT (Norman, 2010).

There are many alternatives to the RCT, and it is not uncommon to use nonrandomized methods in education studies. In some educational settings, it is not appropriate to randomize learners. For example, if withholding the intervention or educational resource may disadvantage learners and jeopardize examination or course performance, it will be unfair to randomize learners. The complex design of health sciences education also makes it difficult to employ the RCT model. Learners are often assigned to different sites, rotations and preceptors at different times. This makes it logistically difficult to randomize learners and minimize confounding influences. In these cases, investigators must employ other research design strategies to overcome potential sources of bias. Some examples include comparison groups,

TABLE 45.1
Research Design Directions With Associated Approaches

Category of Study	Purpose	Research Approaches	Types of Research Questions Answered
Explorative	Modelling: identification and explanation of elements and establishing relationships between those elements in phenomena; aims to understand the whole of a phenomenon rather than reduce data through statistical analysis	Descriptive e.g., action research, case studies Qualitative e.g., ethnography, grounded theory, phenomenology Psychometric e.g., focussed on measurement and/ or development of a measurement instrument; establishment of validity (face, content, criterion, construct); establishment of reliability (reproducibility, internal consistency)	*What characterizes...?* *How do theories of learning inform the observation of...?* *What are students' perceptions of...?* *What is the nature of...?* *What is the validity and reliability of...?* *What are normative values for...?*
Experimental	Justification: Highly controlled experiments involving homogeneous group comparisons; seek evidence of the effects of an intervention	Randomized controlled trials (RCTs)	*Does this intervention work?* *Is this new intervention better/more efficient than the way things have been traditionally done?*
Observational	Prediction: Examination of naturally occurring or static groups (heterogeneous), to predict an outcome or relationship; causal studies	Cohort: inquiry starts with the predictor variable (an exposure to a particular educational event or characteristic that is different between cohorts) Case-control: inquiry starts with criterion variable (outcome that is different between groups) Associational: cross-sectional studies that provide a snapshot of certain variables in a variety of people, to investigate how they are associated; no use of groups for comparison	*Does attending a program that uses high-fidelity simulation activities predict future clinical competence?* *How do students who have educationally disadvantaged backgrounds perform in the first year of nursing school compared with students who do not have educationally disadvantaged backgrounds?* *What is the relationship between X (criterion variable) and Y (predictor variable)?*
Translational	Implementation: Knowledge and findings from research implemented in real-life complex settings with heterogeneous participants; may involve evaluation of process and outcome	Knowledge creation (reviews): Investigations of prior research (e.g., systematic reviews, critical, narrative reviews) Knowledge implementation: Systematic efforts to change existing educational practices by distributing knowledge of and/or facilitating the implementation of new evidence-inspired educational practices Efficiency studies: address questions of what works, how, and for whom in real-life settings	*What is the evidence base for this approach to curricular design?* *Does the provision of educational best-practice guidelines to the faculty of a professional education program change teaching or assessment practices?* *Does this educational strategy work for first-year students in their early clinical rotations?*

Based on Ringsted, Hodges and Scherpbier, 2011

pretest/posttest, blinding of participants or teachers to the research hypothesis and increasing the sample size by waiting for several implementations of the intervention (Sullivan, 2011). Comparison groups offer an opportunity to investigate the outcome of an intervention when it is not feasible to create a control group. Comparison group designs may draw upon participants from other sites or historical groups (e.g., previous cohort). Another approach is to use a cross-over design in which control and experimental groups are created, but the groups switch halfway, thus ensuring each group receives the intervention. The pretest/posttest design is perhaps the most widely used research design for nonrandomized studies. This design provides comparison data because data are collected from the same group before and after the intervention. For a deeper explanation of these designs, their limitations and other approaches, consult an expert at your institution or resources such as the AMEE Guides published by the Association for Medical Education in Europe.

For quantitative and mixed-methods studies, schedule early consultations with a statistician to ensure you plan for an appropriate sample size to ensure statistical power. The statistician can also provide guidance on your study design, data collection and management strategies and data analysis plan. For qualitative and mixed-methods studies, be sure to consult an expert to help you select among many approaches, e.g., case study, phenomenology, grounded theory, narrative, ethnography. Each approach has its own procedures and standards for participant selection, data collection, data analysis and quality control.

When you have finalized your research plan and have sufficient detail to describe the research design, instrumentation, data collection, sample and plan for data analysis, you are ready to submit a proposal for formal ethical approval. Nearly all educational research projects require formal ethical approval of some sort. The committees/organizations that provide ethical review can go by a variety of titles. For example, in North America they are generally called Institutional Review Boards.

While you await ethical approval for your project, continue to read the literature and prepare the infrastructure to support your project work. For example, consult with a librarian to expand your literature review and construct a bibliography, perhaps using an online bibliography and citation application. If you will be conducting interviews or observations, begin to identify time in your schedule and place a hold on these times. Similarly, consider reserving physical facilities such as clinical simulation centre space. This is also a good time to anticipate equipment needs (e.g., video cameras or software) and place orders, especially if the item may be limited or difficult to find. Finally, begin to create any necessary files, spreadsheets and databases to manage data collection.

The protocol for your project will guide you through implementation, but you may wish to consult with colleagues about strategies and tips to guide your work. Setting deadlines, scheduling periodic consultations with key study personnel and reserving time on your calendar for uninterrupted project work are simple but effective strategies. These strategies are also useful when you have completed data collection and analysis and proceed to the writing stage. Finally, be mindful of quality standards and journal guidelines when writing up your study findings. There are many helpful resources including the Association of American Medical Colleges' Review Criteria for Research Manuscripts (Durning and Carline, 2015) that includes both a checklist and in-depth explanation of the criteria. For example, in the category 'Data Analysis and Statistics', there are six criteria, including 'Data analysis procedures are described in sufficient detail' and 'Power issues are considered in studies that make statistical inferences'. Although this checklist was designed for manuscript reviewers, it is equally valuable for authors. Using a checklist will make the process less daunting and ensure you do not omit an essential element in your manuscript.

Remember that most health sciences educators do not have training and expertise in education research, so you are not alone in seeking additional information and professional development. A growing number of institutions offer consultation, typically located in academies of educators, offices of research, departments of medical education or centres for teaching, learning and research. Many professional societies and organizations also offer professional development to foster educational research, including the American Educational Research Association (AERA), the Research Essential Skills in Medical Education (RESME) program of the Association for Medical Education in Europe

Learning Clinical Reasoning

The director of an ambulatory clinic rotation has at least one teaching session devoted to the importance of antibiotic stewardship. The medical students have already learned that most upper respiratory infections, sinus infections and bronchitis are caused by viruses and rarely on presentation require antibiotics. Several of the clinic providers (including physicians, nurse practitioners, physician assistants) provide feedback that the students seem to understand the differential diagnosis but still often want to give antibiotics in these situations. The reasons seem unclear, and some of the clinic providers speculate that these students may be responding to patients' requests for antibiotics.

The course director initially surveys the students about their thought processes. The survey provides quantitative data indicating that most of the students recognize that most upper respiratory infections, sinus infections and bronchitis are caused by viruses and rarely on presentation require antibiotics. Responses to other survey questions indicate that diagnostic uncertainty, office procedures, healthcare provider practices and patient requests may also influence

students' treatment plans. The survey responses alone do not provide sufficient insight into the reasons for why the students decide to treat with antibiotics. To better understand the clinical reasoning underlying the students' decision making, the director designs a qualitative study to explore more deeply the various meanings underlying the factors identified in the survey. Examples of research questions that could be developed further include:

- What is the relationship between patients and students?
- How do patients pressurize students into prescribing antibiotics?
- How do students justify prescribing antibiotics in these settings?
- To what extent do students understand the notion of antibiotic stewardship?
- Do students encounter a hidden curriculum at their clinical placement sites, i.e., do providers demonstrate different prescribing practices?
- Do beliefs about prescribing antibiotics vary by profession?

(AMEE), the International Association of Medical Science Educators (IAMSE) Medical Educator Fellowship program, and the Association of American Medical Colleges' (AAMC) Medical Education Research Certificate (MERC) program.

Case Study 45.1 outlines the kind of problem that can be turned into a research project in clinical reasoning.

CONCLUSION

The phenomenon of clinical reasoning is diverse enough, and rich enough, to be researched in many different ways. There are many disciplines and many theories that can be used, or combined, to provide a theoretical foundation for a research project. The nature of the research question will determine which theories will be most useful. The research question will also determine whether quantitative, qualitative or mixed methods will be appropriate. The case study provides a simple example

that can generate a number of research questions that can be researched in a variety of ways.

CHAPTER SUMMARY

In this chapter we have presented the following:

- Research about clinical reasoning is essential to understanding processes and conditions for optimal learning and assessment.
- A conceptual framework is a helpful structure for helping you think more deeply about the factors, constructs or variables and the relationships among them that you will be studying.
- The research design will help you answer your research questions and guide the investigation in a purposeful and systematic way.
- There are many alternatives to the RCT, and it is not uncommon to use nonrandomized methods in education studies.

REFLECTION POINT 3

Research into clinical reasoning can bring many benefits. Research can generate new knowledge that helps us to gain a better understanding of clinical reasoning, a worthwhile goal in itself. The same research may also help us improve our teaching with benefits for students, teachers and ultimately patients.

REFERENCES

Bordage, G., 2009. Conceptual frameworks to illuminate and magnify. Med. Educ. 43, 312–319.

Boyer, E.L., 1990. Scholarship Reconsidered: Priorities of the Professoriate. Princeton University Press, Lawrenceville, NJ.

Cook, D.A., Bordage, G., Schmidt, H.G., 2008. Description, justification and clarification: a framework for classifying the purposes of research in medical education. Med. Educ. 42, 128–133.

Durning, S.J., Carline, J.D. (Eds.), 2015. Review Criteria for Research Manuscripts, second ed. Association of American Medical Colleges, Washington, DC.

Hulley, S.B., Cummings, S.R. (Eds.), 1988. Designing Clinical Research: An Epidemiologic Approach. Lippincott Williams & Wilkins, Philadelphia, PA.

Khatami, S., MacEntee, M.I., Pratt, D.D., et al., 2012. Clinical reasoning in dentistry: a conceptual framework for dental education. J. Dent. Educ. 76, 1116–1128.

Leppink, J., 2017. Revisiting the quantitative–qualitative-mixed methods labels: research questions, developments, and the need for replication. J. Taibah Univ. Med. Sci. 12, 97–101.

Merriam, S.B., 1998. Qualitative Research and Case Study Applications in Education: Revised and Expanded from Case Study Research in Education. Jossey-Bass, San Francisco, CA.

Miles, M.B., Huberman, A.M., Saldana, J., 2013. Qualitative Data Analysis, third ed. Sage Publications, London, UK.

Norman, G., 2010. Is experimental research passé? Adv. Health Sci. Educ. Theory Pract. 15, 297–301.

Ringsted, C., Hodges, B., Scherpbier, A., 2011. 'The research compass': an introduction to research in medical education: AMEE Guide No. 56. Med. Teach. 33, 695–709.

Sullivan, G.M., 2011. Getting off the 'gold standard': randomized controlled trials and education research. J. Grad. Med. Educ. 3, 285–289.

Trowbridge, R., Rencic, J., Durning, S. (Eds.), 2015. Teaching Clinical Reasoning. American College of Physicians, Philadelphia, PA.

46

LEARNING CLINICAL REASONING ACROSS CULTURAL CONTEXTS

MAREE DONNA SIMPSON ■ JENNIFER L. COX

CHAPTER AIMS

The aims of this chapter are to:

■ identify and discuss the domains of culture of both the individual and professional,

■ highlight issues of culture that affect patients' beliefs, behaviours and patient care,

■ explore cultural influences on clinical reasoning and

■ provide readers with case studies and resources to enhance cultural awareness.

KEY WORDS

Culture

Professional practice

Cultural competency

Cultural awareness

INTRODUCTION

Increasingly, patients and communities are seeking and expecting provision of health services that are mindful and respectful of their cultural beliefs and practices. This may reflect the health experiences of minority populations but also the expectations of healthcare professionals from minority backgrounds. Therefore healthcare practitioners, healthcare organizations and providers of healthcare professional education benefit from developing an understanding of culture and the effect of their own culture and that of their coworkers and of their patients. In the literature and in professional competency standards, there are many expectations for today's healthcare providers, including cultural sensitivity, cultural awareness, and several seeking cultural competency.

However, although 'culture' could seem to be just another capability to be gained or imparted, we argue that it is an especially beneficial skill quite distinct from a professional courtesy. For example, consider an older female patient from a cultural group that values restrained, pragmatic behaviour. This patient may downplay her experience of pain so much that her healthcare providers consider that it is not an issue, neglect to seek further details, and then may overlook a life-threatening condition. People from different backgrounds bring to any health interaction different beliefs, behaviours and expectations, which may also vary by age and gender. These beliefs need to be factored into our decision making, because failure to do so can result in unfortunate outcomes.

When we start to consider the effects of culture on clinical decision making, the focus is not on the straightforward evidence-based activity that many of us have been taught to expect and to practice. In this chapter, we focus on culture and potential cultural differences, between and within professions, between individual patients and between the patient and the patient care team, and how they influence clinical reasoning.

PROFESSIONAL CULTURE AND LANGUAGE

Each health profession has a philosophy or paradigm that articulates the role and function of the profession. Many characteristics are common across professions such as ethical conduct with patients; however, others may be specific to one or more professions (e.g., issues of appropriate touch). In addition, not only do professions vary by philosophy but also by use of argot or jargon, though many healthcare professionals' terminology may be common or comparable.

With an increasing focus on interprofessional or multidisciplinary management of patient issues, it is essential that we understand our profession's culture, focus, communication and decision-making style and equally crucial that we reflect on our own cultural background when making clinical decisions. This becomes important when we engage with patients as they, like us, belong to a culture, communicate with referral networks (often lay referral networks centred on family, friends and colleagues) and have a decision-making style.

CULTURE, CONTEXT AND PROFESSIONAL PRACTICE

One of the more recently identified influences on clinical decision making is the context or social environment and the professional culture of the healthcare practitioners. However, this too needs to be contextualized as most healthcare professionals belong to multiple cultural groups even within their profession. Let's consider a rural pharmacist: He or she does belong to the broad professional culture of pharmacy but also may belong to community or hospital pharmacy culture, to rural as opposed to metropolitan culture. This also may affect medical practitioners, paramedics, Chinese traditional medicine practitioners, physiotherapists, nurses, dietitians and the whole gamut of other healthcare professionals.

So what is professional culture? Professional culture has been described and defined by numerous authors across a range of professions within and outside the health environments. The literature addresses many professions such as nursing, pharmacy, medical and social work but also human resources, accountancy and probation officers (e.g., Boutin-Foster et al., 2008; Hoeve et al., 2014; Kluijtmans et al., 2017; Rosenthal et al., 2015; Yu et al., 2015).

Although there are many definitions and descriptions, it is possibly simplest to consider a professional culture as the professional customs, habits and ways of life within a group of individuals who share a common professional socialization, education and capacity to demonstrate professional competencies and perform professional tasks. Therefore, professional cultures may endorse quite different values depending on the profession and, arguably, the recency of the profession. For example, it would be anticipated that the culture of medicine might be better known and defined compared with a newer profession such as exercise physiology or one that may be viewed as less mainstream such as osteopathy (Grace et al., 2016). Professional cultures may have differing values or characteristics, such as innovation, competitiveness, team or individual focus, supportiveness, risk-taking, collaboration, quality and achievement orientation. These differences may hinder or enhance communication between professions or with patients and, in larger professions such as medicine or nursing, may even affect communication within subcultures – for example, communications between the general practitioner and the specialist physician within medicine or between the registered nurse and the nurse practitioner within nursing.

REFLECTION POINT 1

Students: As you learn/have learned to become a member of your profession, how have you engaged with patients of the same background as yourself? Has that differed from patients of a different background? What changes did you make in your interaction? Why?

Educators: How do you incorporate reflection on your professional experiences with cultural diversity within your teaching? Why or why not?

WHAT IS CULTURAL COMPETENCE?

Preregistration training in healthcare professions aims to provide students with clinical training and experience to facilitate/develop the required competencies of that particular profession. In Australia, from 1 July 2010 a system of National registration of registered healthcare practitioners was adopted to enhance patient care. This was overseen by the Australian Health Practitioner Regulation Agency (AHPRA)[i]. Within that framework, the term 'competency' 'covers the complex combination of knowledge and understanding, skills and attitudes needed by a health graduate to practice effectively and equitably' (Australian Dental Council, 2016, p. 5). The Australian Nursing and Midwifery Accreditation Council (ANMAC) National Competency Standards for Registered Nurses, for example, states that 'The registered nurse recognises that ethnicity, culture, gender, spiritual values, sexuality, age, disability and economic and social factors have an effect on an individual's responses to, and beliefs about, health and illness, and plans and modifies nursing care appropriately' (Australian Nursing and Midwifery Accreditation Council, 2012, p. 1).

Culture has a powerful influence on development of a person's personality, identity, response to environmental stimuli, health beliefs and responses to health care including recovery from illness (Seibert et al., 2002). Understanding culture in the context of how people choose, access and respond to health care is therefore an essential skill for healthcare professionals. Cultural competence can be defined as 'having the knowledge, abilities, and skills to deliver care congruent with the client's cultural beliefs and practices' (Purnell, 2008, p. 6).

Papadopoulos et al. (1998) proposed a model for development of cultural competence that consists of

four separate stages: cultural awareness, cultural knowledge, cultural sensitivity and cultural competence. We believe, however, that interaction among these stages is a key element and that each of these stages, in fact, amplifies the previous stage. Thus we would propose an adaptation to this model to include patient assessment and professional activity as an additional stage to reflect our belief that cultural competence is always evolving and being informed by your experiences as a healthcare professional. Reflection on clinical reasoning and decision making within those professional experiences then provides stimulus for the growth and development of cultural competence (Fig. 46.1).

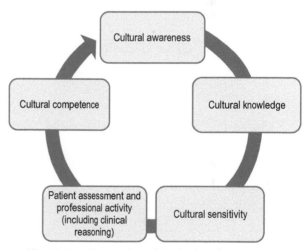

Fig. 46.1 ■ Proposed model of cultural competence development incorporating clinical reasoning.

[i]Australian Health Practitioner Regulation Agency (AHPRA): https://www.ahpra.gov.au/

CASE STUDY 46.1

Ethical Decision Making

Mr. Huang, a grey-haired older individual wearing glasses and of apparent Asian background, has been evaluated and taken to hospital after a heavy fall in a local Asian grocery store, a short distance from his home. Mr. Huang lives with his son and daughter-in-law but tells paramedics in halting English that he is keen to go to hospital rather than bother his family at work. When he arrives at the local hospital, the emergency department staff notice that he seems to have bruises on his back that the fall today would not usually cause. Elder abuse is raised as a possible explanatory factor. As the emergency doctor/nurse, what cultural factors could be taken into consideration in your clinical decision making and decision whether or not to report abuse?

Cultural Awareness

According to Norris and Allotey (2008), the first level of cultural competence is understanding and accepting that other people have different cultural positions/beliefs. That is, acknowledging that there are multiple truths. The ability to acknowledge multiple truths necessitates the healthcare practitioner to first understand and reflect on his or her own cultural awareness. The professional standard/competency statements of many healthcare professions reflect the importance of both the patient's and the healthcare practitioner's own cultural beliefs in providing health care and achieving the best possible health outcomes. Note, for example, how consideration and integration of culture are acknowledged in multiple sections within the Australian Competency Standards for Occupational Therapists in Mental Health (Occupational Therapy Australia, 1999) (Table 46.1).

The National Competency Standards for Dietitians in Australia (Dietitians Association of Australia, 2015) state that a practicing dietitian who demonstrates cultural competency:

- reflects on his or her own culture, values and beliefs and his or her influence on practice,
- seeks out culturally specific information to inform practice and
- works respectfully with individuals, groups and/or populations from different cultures.

The Australian Dental Council (2016) Professional Standards provide a more detailed statement regarding the requirements of cultural competency:

Culturally safe and culturally competent practice involves an awareness of the cultural needs and contexts of all patients to obtain good health outcomes. This includes: having knowledge of, respect for and sensitivity towards the cultural needs and background of the community practitioners serve, including those of Aboriginal and/or Torres Strait Islander Australians and those from culturally and linguistically diverse backgrounds; acknowledging the social, economic, cultural, historic and behavioural factors influencing health, both at individual and population levels; **understanding that a practitioner's own culture and beliefs influence his or her interactions with patients***; and adapting practice to improve engagement with patients and health care outcomes (p. 6).*

Thus to be deemed culturally competent in accordance with these professional standards, the healthcare professional must have an awareness of his or her own cultural values and beliefs. We may, however, not always be aware of our own cultural beliefs until we encounter someone from a different culture or a situation that confronts them.

TABLE 46.1		
Performance Criteria Involving Consideration or Incorporation of Culture		
Unit of Competency	**Element**	**Performance Criteria**
Facilitate Occupational Development with Individuals, Groups, Organizations and Communities	Engage consumers, carers and others in identifying occupational strengths, competence, needs, resources and opportunities.	Mental and physical health status, biopsychosocial functioning, language and **cultural factors** are explored and taken into account in the occupational analysis/assessment.
	Select and use suitable methods, tools and processes for information gathering, assessment and evaluation to facilitate occupational development.	Selection of tools, methods and implementation processes take account of mental and physical health status, biopsychosocial functioning, **culture** and rights of those involved.
Develop and Maintain Collaborative Partnerships with Consumers and Carers	Actively seek to understand the lived experience of consumers and carers.	Knowledge to develop and maintain effective and culturally sensitive partnerships is acquired.

Adapted from: Occupational Therapy Australia, 1999

Cultural Knowledge

In today's world, the population of many modern countries is made up of multiple ethnic communities. For example, within Australia alone, there are more than 200 ethnic communities. Therefore it is neither possible nor feasible for healthcare professionals to have intimate knowledge of every culture. An organizing framework such as the Purnell Model for Cultural Competence (Purnell, 2002) is one example of a clinical assessment tool that has been widely used by students in healthcare settings to assist in gaining cultural information about a particular patient and/or family (Table 46.2).

Although tools such as the Purnell Model for Cultural Competence can be used to gain information/ understanding of a patient's cultural beliefs/views/ context, it may not always be possible or practical (from a time economy perspective) to use such an extensive tool/gather every patient's full details, particularly when taking care of multiple patients and/or in contexts characterized by heavy workloads.

Cultural Sensitivity

Cultural knowledge does not necessarily create cultural sensitivity. However, sensitivity is a key factor required for competence (i.e., to provide culturally sensitive health care). For example, we may come from a cultural background with no expectations of dietary fasting and so may not factor fasting into our decision making when recommending a medication, diet or a food supplement to a patient. However for a patient from a Middle-Eastern background or an Asian background, fasting can be an important expectation that may place significant restrictions on the time during the day when food can be consumed (Kalra et al., 2015; Latt et al., 2014).

More importantly, health care is only considered culturally sensitive if it is viewed as such by the patient and/or family. So what is sensitivity, and how can it be enhanced? Seibert et al. (2002) developed a practical checklist to facilitate cultural sensitivity and awareness in practitioners (Table 46.3).

Cultural Competence

Just like any other continuous professional development and refinement of capacity to deliver health care, cultural competence should be considered as a process, not simply an outcome, always evolving and being informed by your experiences. It requires the synthesis and application of cultural awareness, knowledge and

---

TABLE 46.2

Cultural Domains and Example Concepts Underpinning the Purnell Model of Cultural Competence

Domain	Concept (Example)
Overview/heritage	Country of origin, politics, economics, educational status
Communication	Native/dominant languages; nonverbal communications such as facial expressions, use of hands
Family roles and organization	Gender roles; head of the household; social views towards sexual orientation; single parenting; divorce
Workforce issues	Gender roles; autonomy; assimilation
Biocultural ecology	Variations in skin colour; physical differences in body stature, genetic and hereditary diseases
High-risk behaviours	Use of tobacco, alcohol; nonuse of safety measures such as helmets
Nutrition	Food choices, rituals, taboos; use of food during illness
Pregnancy and childbearing practices	Birth control methods; views towards pregnancy; taboo practices
Death rituals	How the individual and culture view death; rituals and burial practices; bereavement behaviours
Spirituality	Religious practices, use of prayer
Healthcare practices	Traditional, magicoreligious and biomedical beliefs; self-medicating practices; views towards mental illness; response to pain
Healthcare providers	Status, use and perceptions of healthcare providers (e.g., traditional versus magicoreligious) and gender of healthcare provider

Adapted from Purnell, 2002

TABLE 46.3
Cultural Sensitivity and Awareness Checklist

Focus		Instructions
Communication	Effective communication is an important launching pad for effective health care. Miscommunication and language barriers can have adverse effects on patient decision making and health outcomes.	Identify the patient's preferred method of communication. Identify potential language barriers (both verbal and nonverbal). Involve the services of a translator if necessary.
Cultural identification	It is important to be aware of and sensitive to the patient's cultural customs and religious/spiritual beliefs as these can have a powerful effect on the patient's response to health care and recovery.	Identify the patient's culture and religious/spiritual beliefs. Make appropriate support contacts and, where possible, identify someone who is able to educate the caregivers about the target culture, its customs and possible associated needs that may play a role in recovery.
Comprehension	It is important that information is conveyed and received as intended.	Double-check that the patient and/or family comprehend the situation at hand. Continue checking for how and what the patient has heard and understood.
Trust	Lack of trust can impede health outcomes. If the patient and/or family do not trust the healthcare professional, they may withhold important health-related information and/or fail to follow crucial instructions.	Look for verbal and nonverbal cues to indicate whether the patient trusts the caregiver.
Recovery	Misconceptions or unrealistic expectations can impede a patient's decision-making process and subsequently his or her recovery from illness.	Double-check if the patient and/or family have misconceptions/unrealistic views about the treatment and/or recovery process. Ensure that the patient and/or family have had sufficient time to process the information given and gain familiarity with the situation. Provide an opportunity, later on, for those involved to ask any questions.
Diet	Appropriate nutrition is important for illness recovery.	Identify and address any culture-specific dietary regulations.
Assessments	Cultural differences in emotional expression and verbalizations of private information can have a significant influence on health assessments.	Conduct assessments with cultural sensitivity in mind. It may be necessary to use culturally specific questions.

Adapted from Seibert, Stridh-Igo and Zimmerman, 2002

sensitivity on a case-by-case basis. It is important to remember that cultures are dynamic and ever-changing, so although it is easy to consider one has 'achieved' cultural competence, we would argue that the evidence provided by previous stages, in fact, demonstrates a *level* of competence. See Box 46.1.

CONCLUSION

In our discussion of culture, we have discussed the importance of our own, our professions', our practice setting's and our patients' cultures in our professional quest for good health outcomes and effective patient engagement. In adding patient assessment and professional activity to the model that has been proposed (see Fig. 46.1), we assert that knowledge of culture and even certain patient engagement skills will continue to be shaped by ongoing experiences in our professional journey through life. Reflection on reasoning and decision making within those experiences as a healthcare professional provides stimulus for growth and development of cultural competence.

DISCUSSION OF CASE STUDY 46.1

Considerations in Ethical Decision Making

Mr. Huang may have been born overseas and may have immigrated to Australia as an adult and so may prefer to have a translator or a visit from the culturally specific patient support team, if available. Further, he may usually choose to use Asian treatment modalities and remedies and may prefer to discuss available treatment options that consider or include these. It is possible that he may seek treatments such as moxabustion and cupping, which can leave marks that may resemble bruises.[ii]

Further, many Asian societies have traditionally been founded on principles such as filial piety and respect for the elderly, and this may have been Mr. Huang's expectation. However, children raised within a Western society may not adopt the same values and may find it challenging to care and show respect for older family members who expect care as their due. Elder abuse is a possibility and may take many different patterns including verbal abuse or minor neglect, which can be challenging for frail, relatively isolated older individuals who may believe they have nowhere to go and no one to ask for help. So addressing Mr. Huang's injuries and exploring the 'bruises' on his back will need care and consideration.

[ii]https://www.cuppingresource.com/cupping-bruises-and-markings/

BOX 46.1
CULTURAL DECISION MAKING

Here are more case studies that you may like to consider:

1. Mary Harissa is a regular patient referred to your dietetic practice for dietary advice. Mary is of a Middle-Eastern appearance and dresses very modestly. She has been referred because she has been diagnosed with type 2 diabetes mellitus but finds that she is unable to follow the diet recommended, as her family prefers the food they usually eat and that Mary cooks so well. Her husband accompanies her and agrees that Mary needs to cook food that is acceptable to the family. Are there cultural issues that need to be addressed in your clinical decision making?

2. John Brown is a 70-year-old former painter who has been referred to your acupuncture clinic by his GP, Dr. Tatsoi, for lower back pain. You are a 34-year-old female of a Caucasian background qualified in acupuncture. Dr. Tatsoi is keen for John to try acupuncture, but John would prefer to take analgesics and is reluctantly attending your clinic. Are there cultural issues to consider as you decide how to approach John?

3. Keiko Nakamura is an older female of Japanese background whom you have identified as having osteoporosis. You have recommended that Keiko consume three servings of dairy products every day and have referred her to an exercise physiologist for development of a weight-bearing exercise program.

CHAPTER SUMMARY

In this chapter, we have:

- highlighted the effect and relevance of cultural factors on clinical decision making and health outcomes,
- framed cultural competence as an ongoing, lifelong process informed by professional experiences, not just an outcome of training,
- discussed the four stages of development of cultural competence and
- outlined the need for every healthcare professional/student to acknowledge and 'step outside' his or her own health beliefs to be able to ascertain and assess culturally relevant information from/about the patient.

REFLECTION POINT 2

What do you consider to be culturally appropriate care?

The following document could be a useful tool for reflecting on this question: https://www.jointcommission.org/assets/1/6/ARoadmapfor Hospitalsfinalversion727.pdf

REFERENCES

Australian Dental Council, 2016. Professional attributes and competencies of the newly qualified dentist. Viewed 2 December 2016.

Available from: http://www.adc.org.au/documents/Professional CompetenciesoftheNewlyQualifiedDentist-February2016.pdf.

Australian Nursing and Midwifery Accreditation Council, 2012. Registered Nurse Accreditation Standards 2012. Viewed 17 May 2017. Available from: http://www.anmac.org.au/sites/default/files/documents/ANMAC_RN_Accreditation_Standards_2012.pdf.

Boutin-Foster, C., Foster, J.C., Konopasek, L., 2008. Viewpoint: physician, know thyself: the professional culture of medicine as a framework for teaching cultural competence. Acad. Med. 83, 106–111.

Dietitians Association of Australia, 2015. National Competency Standards for Dietitians in Australia. Viewed 12 May 2017. Available from: https://daa.asn.au/maintaining-professional-standards/ncs/.

Grace, S., Orrock, P., Vaughan, B., et al., 2016. Understanding clinical reasoning in osteopathy: a qualitative research approach. Chiropr. Man. Therap 24, 1–10.

Hoeve, Y.T., Jansen, G., Roodbol, P., 2014. The nursing profession: public image, self-concept and professional identity: a discussion paper. J. Adv. Nurs. 70, 295–309.

Kalra, S., Bajaj, S., Gupta, Y., et al., 2015. Fasts, feasts and festivals in diabetes-1: glycemic management during Hindu fasts. Indian J. Endocrinol. Metab. 19, 198–203.

Kluijtmans, M., Haan, E., Akkerman, S., et al., 2017. Professional identity in clinician-scientists: brokers between care and science. Med. Educ. 51, 645–655.

Latt, T.S., Kalra, S., Sahay, R., 2014. Extensive clinical experience: rational use of oral antidiabetic drugs during War Dwin, the Buddhist Lent, Sri Lanka. J. Diabetes Endocrinol. Metab 3, 108–111.

Norris, M., Allotey, P., 2008. Culture and physiotherapy. Divers. Health Soc. Care 5, 151–159.

Occupational Therapy (OT) Australia, 1999. Australian Competency Standards for Occupational Therapists in Mental Health. OT Australia, Fitzroy, VIC.

Papadopoulos, I., Tilki, M., Taylor, G., 1998. Transcultural Care: A Guide for Health Care Professionals. Quay Books, Dinton, Wiltshire, UK.

Purnell, L., 2002. The Purnell Model for Cultural Competence. J. Transcult. Nurs. 13, 193–196.

Purnell, L., 2008. Transcultural diversity and health care. In: Purnell, L., Paulanka, B. (Eds.), Transcultural Health Care: A Culturally Competent Approach. FA Davis, Philadelphia, PA, pp. 1–18.

Rosenthal, M., Hall, K.W., Bussières, J.F., et al., 2015. Professional culture and personality traits of hospital pharmacists across Canada: a fundamental first step in developing effective knowledge translation strategies. Can. J. Hosp. Pharm. 68, 127–135.

Seibert, P.S., Stridh-Igo, P., Zimmerman, C.G., 2002. A checklist to facilitate cultural awareness and sensitivity. J. Med. Ethics 28, 143–146.

Yu, K.H., Kim, S., Restubog, S., 2015. Transnational contexts for professional identity development in accounting. Organ. Stud 36, 1577–1597.

47

PEER LEARNING TO DEVELOP CLINICAL REASONING ABILITIES

NICOLE CHRISTENSEN ▪ STEPHEN LOFTUS ▪ TERESA GWIN

CHAPTER AIMS

The aims of this chapter are to:

- introduce peer learning as an educational strategy to enhance professional education,
- discuss ways that peer learning can be used to facilitate the development of clinical reasoning and
- provide examples of peer learning activities that develop clinical reasoning in professional education.

KEY WORDS

Clinical reasoning

Peer assessment

Peer learning

ABBREVIATIONS/ ACRONYMS

PBL Problem-based learning

TBL Team-based learning

INTRODUCTION

Modern educational conceptions of peer learning describe it as a deliberate, learner-centred, educational strategy that aims to facilitate acquisition of knowledge and skills through active help and support among peers. With its roots in social constructivism, many trace the origins of peer learning to Vygotsky (1978). Based on his ideas, peer learning is a good way for learners to construct new conceptual understandings by experimenting with new concepts and discussing them with others to help link them to existing knowledge. Peer learning today is viewed as a collaborative, reciprocal, social interaction that involves learners who are not professional teachers, learning with and from each other (Boud, 2013a, 2013b; Topping, 2005).

PEER LEARNING FOR KNOWLEDGE AND METASKILLS DEVELOPMENT

Peer learning activities are planned and designed to use the social interactions that naturally arise within a group of peers to facilitate participants' learning while also contributing to the learning of others. This is effective when a group of peers succeeds in developing a trusting, nonhierarchical relationship with each other, making it more likely that individuals will willingly self-disclose instances of misinterpretation or gaps in knowledge in the course of working through problems together, thereby facilitating student-directed knowledge building and refinement (Topping, 2005). Therefore a primary focus of attention is what students are doing to facilitate their own learning, in activities that have been designed by faculty to leverage the social interactions peer learning requires.

An ideal peer learning context mitigates power dynamics and also provides learners with emotional support and empathy. The interactions among peers, while focussing on specific academic content, can also allow the emergence of a collaborative group learning dynamic that fosters the practice and development of important adult learning metaskill sets (Boud, 2013b; Ladyshewsky, 2010). These include:

■ critical thinking and questioning of assumptions,
■ articulation of knowledge and
■ dialogue and debate.

These metaskills contribute to the development of graduates able to think and learn through clinical reasoning experiences and of independent practitioners who are prepared to engage with colleagues constructively, collaboratively and productively. The development involved in becoming effective peer learners, as individuals and as members of a team, is just as important an area of intended learning outcomes as is understanding the discipline-specific knowledge and skills the learners are focussed on during peer learning activities (Boud, 2013b; Ladyshewsky, 2006).

PEER LEARNING ACTIVITY DESIGN CONSIDERATIONS

The most optimal peer learning contexts involve matched or near peers, so as to minimize differences between participants' levels of knowledge and confidence or practice experience. Greater cognitive differences may promote a group dynamic where less knowledgeable or experienced participants simply accept the contributions of others without questioning or discussion, or they may simply disengage from the process (Topping, 2005). Peer learning can promote development of good communication skills and confidence in being able to challenge and respond appropriately to cognitive challenges from others. Therefore effective peer learning experiences can also provide growth in conflict management abilities and the practice of negotiation skills.

With this in mind, peer learning activities should be designed so as to encourage participants to actively promote debate and questioning of assumptions. For example, participants might be prompted to play 'devil's advocate' with each other in order to gain confidence in their own and their peers' application of knowledge and reasoning as related to identifying solutions or answers throughout the learning activity. This activity design strategy is particularly helpful in peer groups where homogeneity of thinking is prevalent and questioning of each other may not arise spontaneously without facilitation.

Participants may never have been aware of the level to which they have understood various concepts until they are challenged by having to explain them in their own words, defend their interpretations, answer questions and/or support their hypotheses to others (Topping, 2005). Consequently, they also get practice in rethinking their positions publicly and acknowledging the contributions of others in the development of their own points of view.

Peer learning also promotes intrinsic motivation for learning and effective team interactions. This is achieved through role modelling among peers and near-peers, and the development of leadership skills and health educator skills (Boud, 2013a; ten Cate and Durning, 2007b). There is also the inherent requirement in all peer learning activities of having to collaboratively manage their own learning by exploring how best to learn together as a team.

ten Cate and Durning (2007a) discuss the importance of developing teaching skills as part of learning in medical education. Because peer learning provides the opportunity for students to learn from teaching their peers, these authors point out the importance, not only of teaching medical students to be reflective practitioners but also to be 'reflective educators and learn from teaching' (ten Cate and Durning, 2007a, p. 551). This call for an explicit focus on the value of developing the teaching and educational skills of medical students is echoed by Nelson et al. (2013), further highlighting the advantages inherent in students consolidating their learning while also becoming competent in a variety of transferable skills to be drawn upon as future educators of patients as well as students of the future.

REFLECTION POINT 1

For students: How much have you learned and do you learn from discussing ideas with other students?

For teachers: What opportunities and support do we provide to encourage students to learn from each other?

Peer Assessment

There is a need to monitor and assess the predetermined learning outcomes that provide the foundation of peer learning (Boud, 2013b). Peer assessment can play a part in this. Research reported by Tai et al. (2014) addressed commonly raised concerns that involving learners in assessment of their peers might foster competitiveness or inhibit self-disclosure and collaboration within peer learning activities. They found that although peer assessment did not foster competition or create social discord in medical student peers during clinical placements, students were reticent to provide feedback due to a lack of confidence in their own assessment capabilities and a lack of clarity about expected performance standards. These authors' findings highlighted the importance of the development of the metaskills involved in peer teaching and learning discussed previously. They concluded that to be optimally effective, peer learning requires explicit attention to development of these metaskills and practice in provision of performance feedback to others.

Maas et al. (2014) researched peer assessment in the context of undergraduate physical therapy education and found that peer assessment was most effective when provided formatively rather than summatively. In addition, peer assessment was not an adequate replacement for assessment by nonpeer skilled practitioners. Topping (2005) likewise argued for avoidance of summative assessment by peers. The rationale for this focus on formative peer assessment is grounded in the social aspects of provision of feedback among peers; peers tend to be uncomfortable with giving grades to each other, and this can promote provision of more superficial, less honest and less helpful feedback as a result. We support Topping's additional argument in support of the value of peers providing formative feedback to each other, acknowledging that it is more cognitively demanding for a peer assessor to develop detailed, qualitatively oriented formative feedback than to simply provide a quantitative score via a summative rubric, thereby facilitating learning on the part of the peer assessor and the assessed peer learners. In addition, it is likely to be more socially comfortable for all involved. Formative peer assessment can also enhance development of accurate self-assessment skills, contributing further to valuable metacognitive skills development (Topping, 2005).

REFLECTION POINT 2

For students: What kind of feedback from other students would be helpful and supportive for you?

For teachers: What support do we provide for students to learn how to give useful feedback to their peers?

FACILITATING CLINICAL REASONING DEVELOPMENT WITH PEER LEARNING

The learning of clinical reasoning is well suited for peer learning activities, in both academic and clinical contexts. Peer learning activities focussed on clinical reasoning development provide opportunities for learners to practice all of the metaskills required to capably navigate clinical reasoning and decision making with a real or simulated clinical scenario providing the context for the peer activity. These metaskills include:

- critical thinking, reflective thinking and dialectical (deductive and inductive) reasoning,
- engagement with complexity and exploring interdependencies of all aspects and individuals involved (Christensen et al., 2008) and
- communication, collaboration and teamwork.

In addition, through formative peer assessment, these activities have the potential to provide practice opportunities for giving and receiving immediate formative feedback on how well aspects of clinical reasoning are put into language and communicated to peers, both important aspects of learning clinical reasoning in a community of practice or profession (Ajjawi and Higgs, 2007; Loftus, 2009). Topping (2005) posits that peer learning facilitates engagement in fully conscious and explicit metacognition, which in turn promotes more effective learning and confidence in learning abilities and outcomes. Metacognition is a key metaskill associated with excellence in clinical reasoning, and confidence in one's reasoning abilities is a hallmark of clinical reasoning capability (Christensen et al., 2008).

When considering how best to facilitate the learning of clinical reasoning through peer learning activities, it is essential that the facilitation and guidance provided to the learners lead them to explicitly focus on various aspects or foci of clinical reasoning relevant to the activity. Examples of such foci may include:

- application of foundational knowledge to a clinical situation,
- diagnostic or examination activities,
- procedural or technical skills performance,
- communication among healthcare team members, the patient, family members or other carers,
- attempts at collaboration and

■ a vast array of contextual factors that must be perceived, interpreted and managed (e.g., psychosocial factors, environmental factors, work, family, personal circumstances and financial factors, beliefs and values of the patient, resources available, culture and values of the practice setting, health system factors).

Provision of sufficient structure for the peer learning activity is essential. The structure facilitates critical reflection on one's own or a peer's clinical reasoning and promotes group dialogue and reciprocal questioning in a supportive, safe environment. The intent is to facilitate learners to help their peers to recognize what they do understand and areas where they are unclear or have made errors and also to facilitate self-identification of any gaps in knowledge or reasoning skills.

Examples of Peer Learning Activities for Clinical Reasoning Development

There are several ways in which to provide peer learning opportunities for students. Some are well known such as problem-based learning (PBL) and team-based learning (TBL). There is a well-established literature on these approaches in particular. A common theme is that PBL and TBL need to be carefully managed so that peer learning is allowed to occur in a safe and supportive environment that takes advantage of the students' natural curiosity.

Peer learning can also happen in large lecture settings. For example, Mazur (1997) described how he used audience response systems to get students to teach each other. We recommend teachers be creative in thinking through ways to provide peer learning opportunities. We next provide examples of learning activities we have developed for students of health professions. These have a focus on facilitating clinical reasoning development.

Peer Learning With Simulation

Students of healthcare professions often begin a clinical or practice immersion during the first one or two semesters of their program. Therefore they are able develop a portfolio of case examples that can be used as the context for examples of their own developing clinical reasoning throughout their educational program. A peer learning activity using a simulation project was developed with this type of patient portfolio in mind;

students develop a simulation scenario using a real patient case example from their portfolio as the basis of the simulation (Gwin et al., 2017; McLaughlin et al., 2014).

For this activity, students are divided into peer learning groups, with up to 6 to 8 students per group. Each student proposes a clinical example from his or her patient case portfolio and describes it to their peers. The group critically examines each example and chooses one example they deem most likely to contribute to the learning of their classmates (peers in other small peer learning groups). A faculty instructor with simulation development expertise then guides the students in the creation of their simulation activity for the rest of the class and facilitates their identification of particular learning outcomes for the simulation experience that is relevant to the focus of the overall course. Working together in this manner fosters a collaborative approach to learning in that students are encouraged to accept others' clinical experiences and resultant knowledge as sufficiently valid to warrant translation into the simulation learning experience for the rest of their classmates. In having to create teachable simulation to peers, students learn how to distil from their case the essential elements for their peers to experience and reflect on within the simulation context, in order to achieve their identified learning outcomes. Because acute care patients in today's health systems have multiple complex issues, these simulation activities require students to develop their clinical reasoning in many aspects of the scenario, in particular related to the interdependent effects any clinical decisions can have on multiple body systems.

In addition to developing the simulation activity, the peer learning group is also responsible for assisting in the critically reflective debriefing session that follows. Debriefing sessions following simulation activities are considered the part of the simulation experience that facilitates maximal learning for students. Conducting a debriefing session requires development of skills in starting a conversation with open-ended questions and by active listening to foster reflective discussion. The student participants are thereby encouraged to practice and build their skills in providing constructive, formative feedback to their peers. This exercise is brought to a close with each student being asked to share his or her reflection on what he or she experienced and learned during his or her peers' simulation activity

Peer Learning in PBL

Margot took her seat in the tutorial room. As the other participants of the PBL session wandered in, she pulled out the notes she had gathered over the last few days. The facilitator soon arrived and began by asking the students to summarize the learning issues and the gaps in their knowledge that had emerged as a result of their work at the previous meeting. The patient case they had been working through was complex and focussed on having the group work through a systematic process of differential diagnosis. During their last session, the group had generated a long list of hypotheses about potential alternative diagnoses, and they had agreed to split up the research among them to give them a head start in working through the list in today's session. Each participant then shared back with the group what he or she had found out.

When Margot's turn came, she shared a copy of a review paper she had found on sarcoidosis, one of the group's hypotheses, and gave the group the citation details. While they located the paper online, she then summarized the key points of the paper. The others took up these points and used them to discuss whether or not sarcoidosis was still an item on their differential diagnosis. Now that they had more knowledge, the facilitator encouraged the group to discuss in more depth how or why sarcoidosis came to be on the differential diagnosis list in the first place and what they now thought about their reasoning in the last session that led to that as one of their hypotheses. In the end, the group decided that although they now considered sarcoidosis much less likely to be the definitive diagnosis, they were not yet ready to rule it out entirely just yet. The group then moved on to the next student, who shared what he had found out about tuberculosis, another one of their hypotheses. The group continued moving through each member's information until they had sorted through their differential diagnosis list and come up with their hypothesis for the most likely definitive diagnosis for the patient case.

At the end of their session, the facilitator asked participants to summarize what they had learned in terms of their medical knowledge and any insights they had today about additional gaps in their knowledge that they wanted to prioritize to address at the next session. The conversation was then guided to focus on the group's assessment of their own clinical reasoning through the differential diagnosis, as well as their self-evaluation of their group processing and teamwork that day. The facilitator guided them in comparing their performance today with a typical session at the start of the term, leading the participants to acknowledge that although they still had a lot to learn, they could see they were making progress in all areas. Finally, the group made agreements about what each participant would take responsibility for researching ahead of the next session so that they could move on to the next portion of the patient case they would tackle the following week.

---

and debriefing discussion. Those who participated in the development of the simulation and facilitated the debriefing discussion share their learning gained through the process of creating the experience. This final aspect of the exercise emphasizes the collaborative, critically reflective, social learning experience that has taken place among peers. Additionally, it promotes teaching and learning activity development skills in these learners, who will likely assume the role of educator for younger clinicians in their future careers.

Peer Learning in Interprofessional Clinical Settings

Students of all healthcare professions are required to spend certain numbers of hours in supervised clinical practice. When students are undertaking their clinical learning experiences in interdisciplinary care contexts such as community health settings, there are opportunities for educators to facilitate rich peer learning in and from interprofessional clinical reasoning experiences. These settings challenge the student to apply his or her knowledge to reasoning in the context of collaborative professional practice. Community health clinical placements facilitate students in learning with and from their peers about how to define and enact both the unique aspects of their discipline-specific professional role and also their collaborative contributions to the work of the collective team. Frequently, community health sites bring several disciplines together to work with one patient; these may include social workers, physiotherapists, nurses, pharmacists and others.

It is in the community health setting, working and learning with their peers from other disciplines, that students experience and are able to develop a deeper understanding of the value that each discipline potentially contributes to the care of patients and their families. The longer-term focus than would be found in an acute care setting is an additional dimension to the learning available. Critically reflective debriefing discussions help students to discuss, evaluate and critique their common clinical reasoning experiences. The debriefing sessions need to be systematic and placed at strategic points in the learning experience. In this way, peers can develop an understanding of how their own discipline's specific focus of care is a part of the whole of a larger comprehensive care approach to promoting the health of communities of individuals. This can expand their perspectives on the clinical reasoning of the interprofessional team and how their individual part of that reasoning process fits into the bigger picture. By articulating and discussing their own clinical reasoning, brought into focus through their specific professional lens, and by also engaging in discussion of the clinical reasoning of their peers who have different professional lenses, they are helped to expand their understanding of clinical reasoning from many perspectives. This kind of learning experience serves to further develop their abilities to collaborate with other healthcare professionals in the future. Therefore students' abilities to conceptualize multiple complementary approaches to person-focussed care also serve to expand their knowledge of clinical reasoning in practice.

CONCLUSION

The skilful and strategic implementation of peer learning strategies in the development of clinical reasoning capabilities is a critically important step in continuing efforts to reshape health professions' educational culture. The move away from passive knowledge transmission modes in all stages of learning and development is important for continued professional development among peers and eventually among professional colleagues and future students. Resultant elevation of practitioners' patient education skills is also critically important and enhanced by promotion of the teaching and learning metaskills developed through peer learning in the workplace (Nelson et al., 2013).

CHAPTER SUMMARY

In this chapter, we have discussed:

- peer learning as an effective educational strategy to enhance the education of health professions students for discipline-specific knowledge and teaching and learning metaskills development,
- ways that peer learning can be used to facilitate the development of clinical reasoning in the context of knowledge development and application and social interaction and collaborative practice and
- examples of peer learning activities that develop clinical reasoning in professional education.

REFLECTION POINT 3

For students: How have you made use of informal study groups that meet regularly to help and support each other? If so, would you describe them as true peer learning experiences, based on what our chapter has described about peer learning activities?

For teachers: What peer learning techniques or strategies do you know about or have you tried before? What skills do you need to facilitate these effectively?

REFERENCES

Ajjawi, R., Higgs, J., 2007. Using hermeneutic phenomenology to investigate how experienced practitioners learn to communicate clinical reasoning. Qual. Rep. 12, 612–638.
Boud, D., 2013a. Conclusion: challenges and new directions. In: Boud, D., Cohen, R., Sampson, J. (Eds.), Peer Learning in Higher Education: Learning From and With Each Other. Routledge, New York, NY.
Boud, D., 2013b. Introduction: making the move to peer learning. In: Boud, D., Cohen, R., Sampson, J. (Eds.), Peer Learning in Higher

Education: Learning From and With Each Other. Routledge, New York, NY.

Christensen, N., Jones, M., Edwards, I., et al., 2008. Helping physiotherapy students develop clinical reasoning capability. In: Higgs, J., Jones, M.A., Loftus, S., et al. (Eds.), Clinical Reasoning in the Health Professions, third ed. Elsevier, Edinburgh, pp. 101–110.

Gwin, T., Villanueva, C., Wong, J., 2017. Student developed and led simulation scenarios. Nurs. Educ. Perspect. 38, 49–50.

Ladyshewsky, R.K., 2006. Building cooperation in peer coaching relationships: understanding the relationships between reward structure, learner preparedness, coaching skill and learner engagement. Physiotherapy 92, 4–10.

Ladyshewsky, R.K., 2010. Building competency in the novice allied health professional through peer coaching. J. Allied Health 39, e77–e82.

Loftus, S., 2009. Language in clinical reasoning: towards a new understanding. VDM Verlag Dr Müller, Saarbrücken, Germany.

Maas, M.J., Sluijsmans, D.M., van der Wees, P.J., et al., 2014. Why peer assessment helps to improve clinical performance in undergraduate physical therapy education: a mixed methods design. BMC Med. Educ. 14, 117.

Mazur, E., 1997. Peer Instruction: A User's Manual. Prentice-Hall, Upper Saddle River, NJ.

McLaughlin, J.E., Roth, M.T., Glaff, D.M., et al., 2014. The flipped classroom: a course redesign to foster learning and engagement in a health professional school. Acad. Med. 89, 236–243.

Nelson, A.J., Nelson, S.V., Linn, A.M.J., et al., 2013. Tomorrow's educators…today? Implementing near-peer teaching for medical students. Med. Teach. 32, 156–159.

Tai, J.H.M., Haines, T.P., Canny, B.J., et al., 2014. A study of medical students' peer learning on clinical placements: what have they taught themselves to do. J. Peer Learn 7, article 6.

ten Cate, O., Durning, S., 2007a. Dimensions and psychology of peer teaching in medical education. Med. Teach. 29, 546–552.

ten Cate, O., Durning, S., 2007b. Peer teaching in medical education: twelve reasons to move from theory to practice. Med. Teach. 29, 591–599.

Topping, K.J., 2005. Trends in peer learning. Educ. Psychol. 25, 631–645.

Vygotsky, L., 1978. Mind in Society: The Development of Higher Psychological Processes. Harvard University Press, Cambridge, MA.

INDEX

Page numbers followed by "*f*" indicate figures, "*t*" indicate tables, and "*b*" indicate boxes.